Current Vascular Surgery

40th Anniversary of the Northwestern Vascular Symposium

Mark K. Eskandari, MD
James S.T. Yao, MD, PhD, Professor of Education in Vascular Surgery
Professor of Radiology and Cardiology
Chief, Division of Vascular Surgery
Department of Surgery
Northwestern University
Feinberg School of Medicine
Chicago, Illinois

William H. Pearce, MD
Violet R. and Charles A. Baldwin Professor of Vascular Surgery
Division of Vascular Surgery
Department of Surgery
Northwestern University
Feinberg School of Medicine
Chicago, Illinois

James S.T. Yao, MD, PhD
Professor Emeritus
Division of Vascular Surgery
Department of Surgery
Northwestern University
Feinberg School of Medicine
Chicago, Illinois

2016
PEOPLE'S MEDICAL PUBLISHING HOUSE—USA
SHELTON, CONNECTICUT

People's Medical Publishing House-USA
2 Enterprise Drive, Suite 509
Shelton, CT 06484
Tel: 203-402-0646
Fax: 203-402-0854
E-mail: info@pmph-usa.com

PMPH-USA

16 17 18 19 20/KING/9 8 7 6 5 4 3 2 1

ISBN-13 978-1-60795-195-7
ISBN-10 1-60795-195-9
eISBN-13 978-1-60795-941-0

Printed in the United States of America by King Printing Co., Inc.
Editor: Linda H. Mehta; Copyeditor/Typesetter: diacriTech; Cover designer: Mary McKeon

Library of Congress Cataloging-in-Publication Data

Text on file.

Sales and Distribution

Canada
Login Canada
300 Saulteaux Cr.
Winnipeg, MB R3J 3T2
Phone: 1.800.665.1148
Fax: 1.800.665.0103
www.lb.ca

Foreign Rights
John Scott & Company
International Publisher's Agency
P.O. Box 878
Kimberton, PA 19442, USA
Tel: 610-827-1640
Fax: 610-827-1671
rights@johnscottco.us

United Kingdom, Europe, Middle East, Africa
Eurospan Limited
3, Henrietta Street, Covent Garden
London WC2E 8LU, UK
Tel: Within the UK: 0800 526830
Outside the UK: +44 (0)20 7845 0868
http://www.eurospanbookstore.com

Singapore, Thailand, Philippines, Indonesia, Vietnam, Pacific Rim, Korea
McGraw-Hill Education (Asia)
1 International Business Park
#01-15A, The Synergy
Singapore 609917
Tel: (65) 6863-1580
Fax: (65) 6862-3354
(65) 6863-1580
mghasia.sg@mheducation.com

Australia, New Zealand, Papua New Guinea, Fiji, Tonga, Solomon Islands, Cook Islands
Woodslane Pty Limited
10 Apollo Street
Warriewood NSW 2102
Australia
Tel: 612-8445-2300
Fax: 612-9997-5850
www.woodslane.com.au

India, Bangladesh, Pakistan, Sri Lanka, Malaysia
Jaypee Brothers Medical Publishers Pvt. Ltd.
4838, 24 Ansari Road, Darya Ganj
New Delhi-110002, India
Phone: +91 11 23272143
Fax: +91 11 23276490
www.jaypeebrothers.com

People's Republic of China
People's Medical Publishing House
International Trade Department
No. 19, Pan Jia Yuan Nan Li
Chaoyang District
Beijing 100021, P.R. China
Tel: 8610-67653342
Fax: 8610-67691034
www.pmph.com/en

Contents

SECTION IV Vascular Access

SECTION VIII Upper Extremity Diseases

The e-book edition can be found on our online platform, Ssparkl. See our website www.pmph-usa.com for details.

Contributors

Mark A. Adelman, MD
New York University Langone Medical Center
New York, New York

Nicholas D. Andersen, MD
Duke University Medical Center
Durham, North Carolina

Frederic Baumann, MD
Miami Cardiac & Vascular Institute
Baptist Hospital
Miami, Florida

Kyla M. Bennett, MD
University of Wisconsin Hospital
Madison, Wisconsin

Ehsan Benrashid, MD
Duke University Medical Center
Durham, North Carolina

Thomas C. Bower, MD
Mayo Clinic
Rochester, Minnesota

Col. (ret.) Mark W. Bowyer, MD
Uniformed Services University of Health Sciences
Bethesda, Maryland

Armando Cardenas, MD
Northwestern University Feinberg School of Medicine
Chicago, Illinois

Rabih A. Chaer, MD, MSc
University of Pittsburgh Medical Center
Pittsburgh, Pennsylvania

David W. Chang, MD
University of Chicago Medicine & Biological Sciences
Chicago, Illinois

Kristofer M. Charlton-Ouw, MD
University of Texas Medical School at Houston
Memorial Hermann Heart & Vascular Institute
Texas Medical Center
Houston, Texas

Kenneth J. Cherry, MD
University of Virginia
Charlottesville, Virginia

Matthew A. Corriere, MD, MS
Wake Forest University School of Medicine
Winston-Salem, North Carolina

Jeffrey D. Crawford, MD
Oregon Health & Science University
Portland, Oregon

Robert S. Crawford, MD
University of Maryland School of Medicine
Baltimore, Maryland

David C. Cron, BS
University of Michigan Medical School
Ann Arbor, Michigan

Michael D. Dake, MD
Stanford University School of Medicine
Stanford, California

Victor J. Davila, MD
Mayo Clinic Arizona
Phoenix, Arizona

Richard H. Dean, MD
Wake Forest University Health Sciences
Winston-Salem, North Carolina

Brian G. DeRubertis, MD
David Geffen School of Medicine at UCLA
Los Angeles, California

Kush R. Desai, MD
Northwestern Feinberg School of Medicine
Chicago, Illinois

Tina R. Desai, MD
Stanford University School of Medicine
Stanford, California

Gregory Dumanian, MD
Northwestern University Feinberg School of Medicine
Chicago, Illinois

Raymond E. Eid, MD
University of Pittsburgh Medical Center
Pittsburgh, Pennsylvania

Michael J. Englesbe, MD
University of Michigan Medical School
Ann Arbor, Michigan

Mark K. Eskandari, MD
Northwestern University Feinberg School of Medicine
Chicago, Illinois

Ronald Fairman, MD
Hospital of the University of Pennsylvania
Philadelphia, Pennsylvania

Mark A. Farber, MD
University of North Carolina at Chapel Hill School of Medicine
Chapel Hill, North Carolina

Peter L. Faries, MD
Icahn School of Medicine at Mount Sinai
New York, New York

Cindy Felty, C-ANP
Mayo Clinic
Rochester, Minnesota

Ripal T. Gandhi, MD
Miami Cardia & Vascular Institute
Baptist Hospital
Miami, Florida

David L. Gillespie, MD
Cardiovascular Care Center
Southcoast Health System
Fall River, Massachusetts

Julia Glaser, MD
Hospital of the University of Pennsylvania
Philadelphis, Pennsylvania

Marc H. Glickman, MD
Eastern Virginia Medical School
Norfolk, Virginia USA

Jennifer Grant, MD
Advocate Lutheran General Hospital
Park Ridge, Illinois

Roger T. Gregory, MD
Eastern Virginia Medical School
Norfolk, Virginia

Sung Wan Ham, MD
Keck School of Medicine
University of Southern California
Los Angeles, California

Daniel Han, MD
Icahn School of Medicine at Mount Sinai
New York, New York

Donald G. Harris, MD
University of Maryland School of Medicine
Baltimore, Maryland

Dirk Hentschel, MD
Brigham and Women's Hospital
Boston, Massachusetts

Karen J. Ho, MD
Northwestern University Feinberg School of Medicine
Chicago, Illinois

Andrew W. Hoel, MD
Northwestern University Feinberg School of Medicine
Chicago, Illinois

G. Chad Hughes, MD
Duke University Medical Center
Durham, North Carolina

Karl A. Illig, MD
University of South Florida Morsani College of Medicine
Tampa, Florida

Juan Carlos Jimenez, MD
David Geffen School of Medicine at UCLA
Los Angeles, California

Randolph Todd C. Jones, MD
New York University Langone Medical Center
New York, New York

William D. Jordan, Jr, MD
University of Alabama at Birmingham
Birmingham, Alabama

Joseph Karam, MD
Washington University School of Medicine
St. Louis, Missouri

Melina R. Kibbe, MD
Northwestern Feinberg School of Medicine
Chicago, Illinois

Christopher J. Kwolek, MD
Harvard Medical School
Boston, Massachusetts

Peter F. Lawrence, MD
David Geffen School of Medicine at UCLA
Los Angeles, California

Jeffrey H. Lawson MD, PhD
Duke University Medical Center
Durham, North Carolina

Charles C. Leithead, MD
University of Alabama at Birmingham
Birmingham, Alabama

Robert J. Lewandowski, MD
Northwestern University Feinberg School of Medicine
Chicago, Illinois

Timothy K. Liem, MD, MBA
Oregon Health & Science University
Portland, Oregon

Benjamin B. Lind, MD
Northshore University HealthSystem
Skokie, Illinois

Claire Matsumura and Jon S. Matsumura, MD
University of Wisconsin School of Medicine and Public Health
Madison, Wisconsin

Walter J. McCarthy, III, MD, MS
Rush University Medical Center
Chicago, Illinois

Mary McGrae McDermott, MD
Northwestern University Feingold School of Medicine
Chicago, Illinois

Matthew W. Mell, MD, MS
Stanford University School of Medicine
Stanford, California

Karthik Mikkineni, MD
Allegheny General Hospital
Pittsburgh, Pennsylvania

Lauren Mioton, MD
Northwestern University Feinberg School of Medicine
Chicago, Illinois

Samuel R. Money, MD, MBA
Mayo Clinic Arizona
Phoenix, Arizona

Courtney Morgan, MD
Northwestern University Feinberg School of Medicine
Chicago, Illinois

Satish Muluk, MD
Allegheny General Hospital
Pittsburgh, Pennsylvania

David L. Nahrwold, MD
Northwestern University Feinberg School of Medicine
Chicago, Illinois

Gustavo S. Oderich, MD
Mayo Clinic
Rochester, Minnesota

Kristine C. Orion, MD
Yale University School of Medicine
New Haven, Connecticut

Christopher D. Owens, MD, MSc
University of California, San Francisco
San Francisco, California

C. Keith Ozaki, MD
Brigham and Women's Hospital
Boston, Massachusetts

Godfrey Parkerson, MD
University of South Florida Morsani College of Medicine
Tampa, Florida

Federico E. Parodi, MD
Cleveland Clinic
Cleveland, Ohio

Juan C. Parodi, MD
University of Buenos Aires
Buenos Aires, Argentina

Marco G. Patti, MD
University of Chicago Medicine
Chicago, Illinois

William H. Pearce, MD
Northwestern University Feinberg School of Medicine
Chicago, Illinois

Constantino Peña, MD
Miami Cardiac & Vascular Institute
Baptist Hospital
Miami, Florida

Bruce A. Perler, MD, MBA
The Johns Hopkins School of Medicine
Baltimore, Maryland

Robert Jason T. Perry, MD
University of Virginia
Charlottesville, Virginia

Richard Pin, MD
Cardiovascular Care Center
Southcoast Health System
Fall River, Massachusetts

Aleksandra Policha, MD
New York University Langone Medical Center
New York, New York

David N. Ranney, MD
Duke University Medical Center
Durham, North Carolina

Reid A. Ravin, MD
Icahn School of Medicine at Mount Sinai
New York, New York

Norman M. Rich, MD
Edward Hebert School of Medicine USUHS
Bethesda, Maryland

Caron B. Rockman, MD
New York University Langone Medical Center
New York, New York

Heron Rodriguez, MD
Northwestern University Feinberg School of Medicine
Chicago, Illinois

Johnathon Rollo, MD
David Geffen School of Medicine at UCLA
Los Angeles, California

Thom Rooke, MD
Mayo Clinic
Rochester, Minnesota

Connie Ryjewski, APN
Advocate Lutheran General Hospital
Park Ridge, Illinois

Robert K. Ryu, MD
Northwestern Feinberg School of Medicine
Chicago, Illinois

Ulka Sachdev, MD
Ohio State University Wexler Medical Center
Columbus, Ohio

Hazim J. Safi, MD
University of Texas Medical School at Houston
Memorial Hermann Heart & Vascular Institute
Texas Medical Center
Houston, Texas

Luis A. Sanchez, MD
Washington University School of Medicine
St. Louis, Missouri

Harleen K. Sandhu, MD, MPH
University of Texas Medical School at Houston
Houston, Texas

Lewis B. Schwartz, MD
Advocate Lutheran General Hospital
Park Ridge, Illinois

Samir K. Shah, MD
Brigham and Women's Hospital
Boston, Massachusetts

Cynthia K. Shortell, MD
Duke University Medical Center
Durham, North Carolina

Amanda K. Silva, MD
University of Chicago Medicine & Biological Sciences
Chicago, Illinois

Jean Starr, MD
Ohio State University Wexler Medical Center
Columbus, Ohio

Raghuveer Vallabhaneni, MD
University of North Carolina at Chapel Hill School of Medicine
Chapel Hill, North Carolina

Frank J. Veith, MD
New York University Medical Center'
New York, New York
Cleveland Clinic
Cleveland, Ohio

Robert L. Vogelzang, MD
Northwestern Feinberg School of Medicine
Chicago, Illinois

Haimanot Wasse, MD, MPH
Northwestern Feinberg School of Medicine
Chicago, Illinois

Fred A. Weaver MD, MMM
Keck School of Medicine
University of Southern California
Los Angeles, California

John V. White, MD
Advocate Lutheran General Hospital
Park Ridge, Illinois

James S.T. Yao, MD, PhD
Northwestern University Feinberg School of Medicine
Chicago, Illinois

Kimberly C. Zamor, MD, MS
Northwestern University School of Medicine
Chicago, Illinois
Boston University School of Medicine
Boston, Massachusetts

Preface

This is the year we celebrate the 40th Annual Northwestern Vascular Symposium sponsored by the Division of Vascular Surgery, Feinberg School of Medicine, Northwestern University. This remarkable milestone would not be feasible without the continued efforts of Drs. Yao and Pearce as well as the rest of the Northwestern vascular surgery faculty. The genesis of the symposium was developed by Drs. Bergan and Yao with the intent of hosting renowned thought leaders in the field of vascular surgery to provide contemporary reviews of vascular surgery along with spirited discussions centered on the evolution of vascular and endovascular surgery. Over the years, the program has changed from a topic-oriented program to a more comprehensive overview as developed by Dr. Pearce.

Once again, this year we have brought together 50 national experts for our 2 ½ day annual meeting to address timely topics and controversies in vascular and endovascular surgery. As has been the tradition, presentations cover the full spectrum of vascular surgery including changes in management of extracranial cerebrovascular disease, new treatment options for lower extremity arterial occlusive disease, hemodialysis, improvements in techniques for complex venous disease, as well as developments in aortic stent graft repair in the chest and abdomen. In conjunction with the presentations are corresponding chapters found in this hardcover book with more in depth details and "pearls" from the experts.

Over the last 4 decades, our symposium has been held at iconic hotels in the heart of Chicago including the Drake and Fairmont, this year we have again chosen the InterContinental Hotel for our December Symposium as our venue given its prime location in the heart of Chicago along the Magnificent Mile. Please join us in celebrating this wonderful milestone in our Annual Symposium. It is our sincere hope that you will find the contributions in this book valuable to your practice of vascular and endovascular surgery. We thank you for your continued interest and support of our annual meeting.

—Mark K. Eskandari, MD
—William H. Pearce, MD
—James S.T. Yao, MD, PhD

Acknowledgments

We thank our esteemed authors who have once again thoughtfully contributed to this year's book. Their willingness to share their personal expertise and knowledge is what makes our book a success to other practitioners. Special thanks to Sara Minton, our executive course director, for her hard work in assembling and proofing the chapters and for keeping us on track with the deadlines of the Symposium. Without her, the symposium and book would not have been possible. We would also like to thank W.L. Gore & Associates, Incorporated for their continued generous educational grant which helps support the Symposium and printing of the book.

Mark K. Eskandari, MD   William H. Pearce, MD   James S.T. Yao, MD, PhD

1

40th Anniversary of the Northwestern Vascular Symposium—A Reflection

James S.T. Yao, MD, PhD

According to Webster's dictionary,[1] in ancient Greece, a symposium was an entertainment characterized by drinking, music and intellectual discussion. As it evolved, it became a conference focused on a subject with current significance. The Northwestern Vascular Symposium developed following the pursuit by leaders of the Society for Vascular Surgery (SVS) of better training for vascular surgeons and certification in vascular surgery. E. J. Wylie in his ISCVS-NA presidential address first pointed out the need for better training of vascular surgeons.[2] James DeWeese, who headed the Inter-Society Commission for Heart Disease Resources (ICHD) sponsored by the American Heart Association, also found inadequate vascular care in many hospitals in the United States.[3] In order to improve training and certification in vascular surgery, SVS engaged in negotiation with the American Board of Surgery (ABS) and the Resident Review Committee (RRC) for better training of vascular surgery in surgical residency. At the time, both RRC and ABS showed little interest. SVS and the International Society for Cardiovascular Surgery (ISCVS) set up a committee named Program Evaluation and Endorsement Committee (PEEC) to establish an approval process for one-year vascular fellowship programs. After 17 programs were approved, RRC and ABS decided to get involved and negotiations started, with many past presidents of SVS being involved in the negotiations. It took at least 13 years (1970–1983) of bitter negotiations before the first Certificate of Special Qualification in General Vascular Surgery was awarded to E. J. Wylie.[3]

With vascular surgery emerging as a surgical specialty, educational activities also increased. The first symposium in vascular surgery was sponsored in 1973 by Dr. Henry Haimovici of Montefiore Medical Center in New York. This symposium later became the well-known VEITH Symposium under the leadership of Dr. Frank Veith. Haimovici was a pioneer vascular surgeon. He served as president of the International Society of Angiology and later of ISCVS. A great writer, he wrote several classics including a complete textbook on vascular surgery.[4]

The idea of having a symposium at Northwestern was solely the idea of John Bergan. He strongly believed that vascular surgery was much different from general surgery.[5] He thought the best way to advance the field was to have a scientific exchange among national and international scholar-surgeons. Although I was new on the faculty, Bergan treated me equally in planning the meeting program. We each made a program and then we combined them after an in-depth discussion to finalize the program. The equal partnership exercised by Bergan led to the birth of the Bergan-Yao partnership in vascular surgery that lasted for 16 years (Figure 1-1). December was chosen for the date of the symposium because it is a good time to reflect on what has been done during the year and to chart for the future. With the support of a generous grant from the Scholl Foundation, the first Northwestern Vascular Symposium was held on December 2, 1976, at the Drake Hotel[5] with the topic of *Venous Problems.* It was a 2½ day meeting with a faculty of 33 national and international leaders, pathologists, physiologists and vascular surgeons to provide a multidisciplinary approach to the disease. The symposium represented the first meeting attended by international experts to address a much neglected subject.

We are honored to have had the opportunity to dedicate several symposia to outstanding vascular surgeons. The first symposium was dedicated to Geza de Takats, a Hungarian surgeon who moved to Chicago in 1925 and was invited by Dr. Allan Kanavel, Chairman of Surgery at Northwestern, to join the faculty. De Takats established the first vascular clinic at Northwestern and is considered to be the father of vascular surgery in Chicago. He served as president of SVS in 1953. The meeting was a great success with Chicago Mayor Richard J. Daley in attendance for the opening ceremony and the first day of the meeting. December 2, 1976, was proclaimed the Dr. Geza de Takats Day in Chicago (Figure 1-2). In 1995, we were honored to have Mayor Richard M. Daley, son of the first Mayor Daley, to join us in the symposium to honor yet another pioneer surgeon, Michael E. DeBakey (Figure 1-3). Table 1-1 lists the surgeons to whom symposia have been dedicated.

The format of the Symposium has changed over the span of 40 years. In the beginning, the topic of the symposium was often focused on a specific disorder. As new

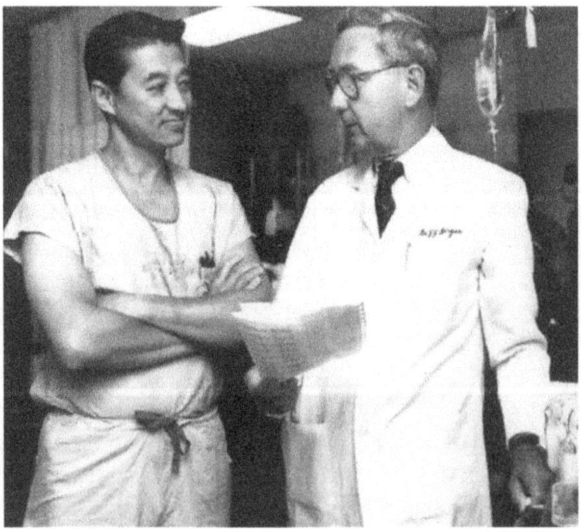

Figure 1-1. The Bergan-Yao team.

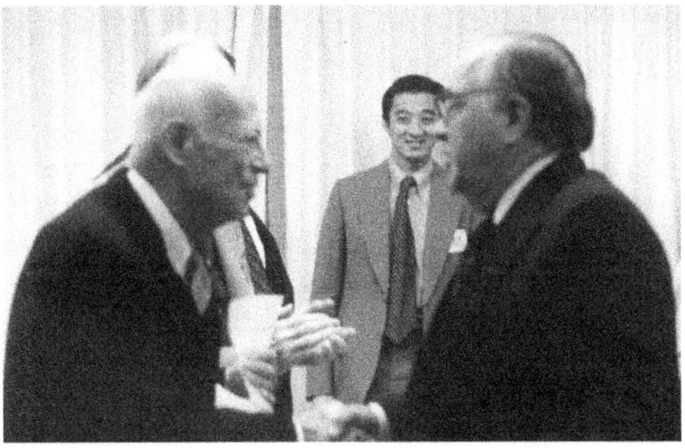

Figure 1-2. Geza de Takats, James Yao, Mayor Richard J. Daley.

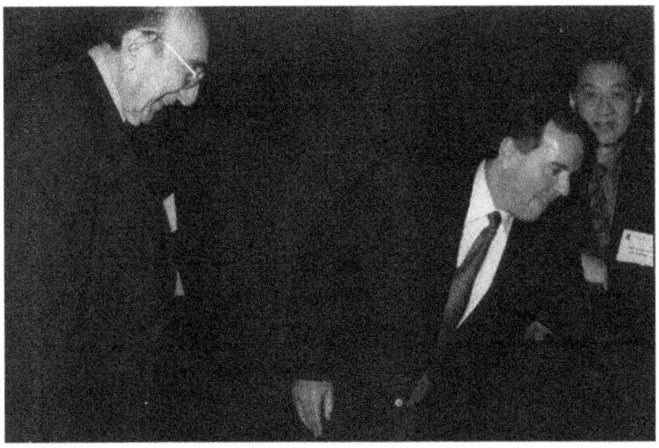

Figure 1-3. Michael DeBakey, Mayor Richard M. Daley, James Yao.

TABLE 1-1. FAMED VASCULAR SURGEONS HONORED BY NORTHWESTERN VASCULAR SYMPOSIUM

Year*	Name	Symposium
1982	Edwin J. Wylie	Cerebral Insufficiency
1993	Stanley Crawford	Aneurysm: New Findings and Treatment
1994	D. Emerick Szilagyi	Advances in Treatment of Ischemic Extremities
1995	Michael E. DeBakey	Arterial Surgery: Management of Challenging Problems
1997	Jesse Thompson	Techniques in Vascular and Endovascular Surgery
2002	James DeWeese	Trends in Vascular Surgery
2008	Robert Rutherford	Techniques and Outcomes in Endovascular Surgery

*Copyright year of the symposium book. The copyright date is often the year after the date of the symposium for which the book was published.

technology evolved, we changed the format to a review covering all aspects of vascular practice. This change was requested by participants of the symposium. In addition, we added morning breakfast meetings on Friday and Saturday with case presentations by our vascular fellows to reflect our interest in clinical surgery.

The Northwestern Vascular Symposium is well known for its ability to produce a book at the time of the symposium, to serve as a permanent record of the presentations at the meeting. The first book, *Venous Problems*, was published 2 years after the meeting, as old printing techniques were still in use. In 1978, Grune and Stratton, using the newly introduced computer typesetting technique, greatly reduce the printing time and the book, *Gangrene and Severe Ischemia of the Lower Extremity*, was distributed at the time of the meeting. In the ensuing years, from 1978 to 2014, we have successfully produced a book containing all presentations at the time of each meeting a total of 38 books published under the editorial leadership of the current Chief of the Division of Vascular Surgery. We are thankful for the many leaders in vascular surgery who have given up their time to join the faculty of the symposia and to prepare manuscripts for the accompanying books.

In 2010, we develop a new series of monographs based on previously published symposia. The series is called *Modern Trends in Vascular Surgery*, with five topics: *Carotid Artery Disease, Endovascular Technology, Venous Disorders, Aorta and Its Body Branches* and *Lower Extremity Ischemia*. We selected chapters published within the past 5 years that were of special interest in each of the categories. These were supplemented with a few new chapters to maintain continuity and ensure complete coverage of each topic. Table 1-2 shows the dates and titles of the books related to the Northwestern Vascular Symposium published over the last 40 years.

TABLE 1-2. BOOKS PRODUCED IN CONJUNCTION WITH THE NORTHWESTERN VASCULAR SYMPOSIUM

Copyright Date*	Title
Editors: John J. Bergan, James S. T. Yao	
1978	*Venous Problems*
1978	*Gangrene and Severe Ischemia of the Lower Extremities*
1979	*Surgery of the Aorta and Its Body Branches*
1980	*Operative Techniques in Vascular Surgery*
1982	*Aneurysms: Diagnosis and Treatment*
1983	*Cerebrovascular Insufficiency*
1984	*Evaluation and Treatment of Upper Extremity Disorders*
1985	*Surgery of the Veins*
1986	*Reoperative Arterial Surgery*
1987	*Vascular Surgical Emergencies*
1988	*Arterial Surgery: New Diagnosis and Operative Techniques*
1989	*Aortic Surgery*
1990	*Techniques in Arterial Surgery*
1991	*Venous Disorders*
Editors: James S. T. Yao, William H. Pearce	
1992	*Technologies in Vascular Surgery*
1993	*Longterm Results in Vascular Surgery*
1994	*Aneurysms: New Findings and Treatment*

(Continued)

TABLE 1-2. *(Continued)*

Copyright Date*	Title
1995	*The Ischemic Extremity: Advances in Treatment*
1996	*Arterial Surgery: Management of Challenging Problems*
1997	*Progress in Vascular Surgery*
1998	*Techniques in Vascular and Endovascular Surgery*
1999	*Practical Vascular Surgery*
2000	*Modern Vascular Surgery*
2001	*Current Techniques in Vascular Surgery*
2002	*Advances in Vascular Surgery*
Editors: William H. Pearce, Jon S. Matsumura, James S. T. Yao	
2003	*Trends in Vascular Surgery*
2004	*Trends in Vascular Surgery*
2005	*Trends in Vascular Surgery*
2006	*Trends in Vascular Surgery*
2007	*Trends in Vascular Surgery*
2008	*Vascular Surgery in the Endovascular Era*
Editors: Jon S. Matsumura, Mark D. Morasch, William H. Pearce, James S. T. Yao	
2009	*Techniques and Outcome in Endovascular Surgery*
Editors: Mark K. Eskandari, Mark D. Morasch, William H. Pearce, James S. T. Yao	
2010	*Vascular Surgery: Therapeutic Strategies*
2011	*New Findings in Vascular Surgery*
2011	*Contemporary Vascular Surgery*
Editors: Mark K. Eskandari, William H. Pearce, James S. T. Yao	
2013	*Current Vascular Surgery: 2012*
2014	*Current Vascular Surgery: 2013*
2015	*Current Vascular Surgery: 2014*
Modern Trends in Vascular Surgery (recompilation books published 2010–2011)	
Endovascular Technology	
Editors: Mark K. Eskandari, Mark D. Morasch, William H. Pearce, James S. T. Yao	
The Ischemic Extremity	
Editors: Heron E. Rodriguez, William H. Pearce, James S. T. Yao	
Surgery of the Aorta and Its Body Branches	
Editors: Mark D. Morasch, William H. Pearce, James S. T. Yao	
Venous Disorders	
Editors: Melina R. Kibbe, William H. Pearce, James S. T. Yao	
Carotid Artery Disease	
Editors: Mark K. Eskandari, William H. Pearce, James S. T. Yao	

*Note: The copyright date is often the year after the date of the symposium for which the book was published.

A TRIBUTE TO JACK HOOVER AND DONALD LASS OF W. L. GORE & ASSOCIATES

The Northwestern Vascular Symposium and its compendium book could not have been possible without the support from an education grant from W. L. Gore & Associates. The grant is unrestricted funding and is designated to be used for postgraduate education for vascular surgeons. The 2½ day symposium program is formulated by members of the Division of Vascular Surgery. W. L. Gore & Associates is not involved nor consulted. We thank Mr. Robert Gore and Ms. Terry Kelly, Chief Executive Officer, for their foresight in the academic-industry alliance to promote advances in the field. More importantly, they assigned two outstanding business executives, Mr. Jack Hoover and Mr. Donald Lass, to work with us. As we cherish these four decades of academic-industry alliance, I, on behalf of past and present members of the Division of Vascular Surgery, pay tribute to Jack and Don.

John T. (Jack) Hoover (Figure 1-4) was born April 22, 1929, an only child. He graduated from Penn State University in 1951 with a BS in chemistry. Jack then served in the US Army from 1951 to 1953. He first worked as a shift supervisor for Squibb in New Brunswick. In 1955, he started working for American Cyanamid and won salesman of the year twice then became regional manager. In 1970, he was working for ICI America and met Bill and Bob Gore. He then was recruited by W. L. Gore in 1975 to develop the medical division. Under the leadership of Jack Hoover, W. L. Gore outperformed all other graft companies. Jack retired in 1992 but remained on the Board until the end of 2010.

Donald Lass (Figure 1-5) was born December 12, 1946, and raised in Chicago. He attended Northern Illinois University in DeKalb from 1964 to 1968 and graduated with a BS in marketing. He then worked for Montgomery Ward and Company as a copy writer.

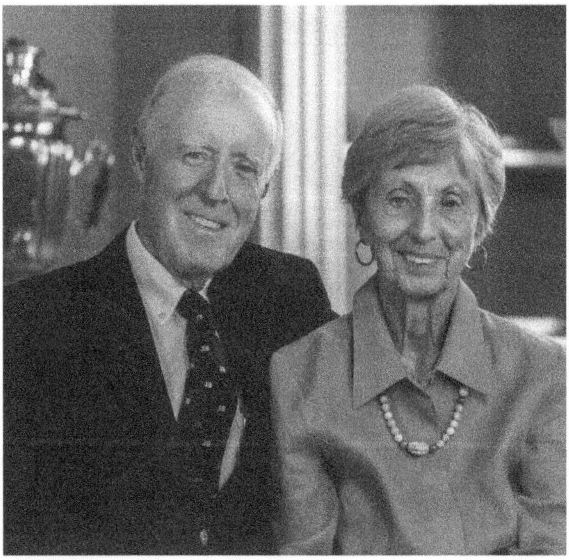

Figure 1-4. John T. and Beverly Hoover.

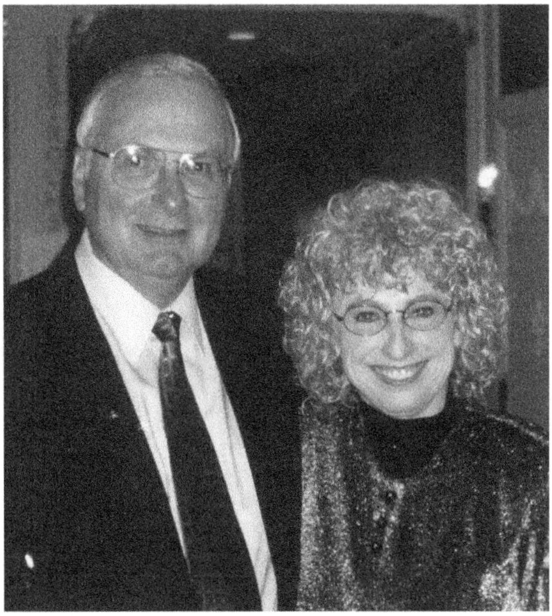

Figure 1-5. Donald and Diana Lass.

In 1968, he served in the US Army Reserve and, from 1968 to 1975, he sold pharmaceuticals for Lederle. In 1975, he was recruited by Jack Hoover to join W. L. Gore and became the first of many sales associates covering 17 states from the Appalachians to the Rockies and from Canada to Texas. Don spent 37 years at Gore and retired in 2011.

Both Jack Hoover and Don Lass are consummate sales representatives. They presented the facts of their product to you and never engaged in hard sell pressure techniques. They supported the idea of an education grant and believed in a close alliance between academic centers and industry as the main force to improve products for patients. Under their leadership, W. L. Gore has supported education programs in many academic centers. At no time did Hoover and Lass demand that we popularize their product.

In addition to the education grant to Northwestern, both Hoover and Lass recognized the need to develop young leaders in vascular surgery. When the concept of a traveling fellowship modeled after the well-known James IV Traveling Fellowship was brought up, they both gave their unconditional support.[6] The SVS E. J. Wylie Traveling Fellowship is supported by donations from W. L. Gore and Associates. The fellowship program has been a great success and young surgeons have benefited from the program. Three Wylie fellows have been elected to the office of president of SVS (Craig Kent, Peter Gloviczki and Julie Freischlag, the first female President of SVS).

EPILOGUE

I am fortunate to have been involved from the beginning of the Northwestern Vascular Symposium and I attended all but one of the meetings. The meeting that I missed I was in China for an invited visit and Don Lass became the only attendee with a perfect

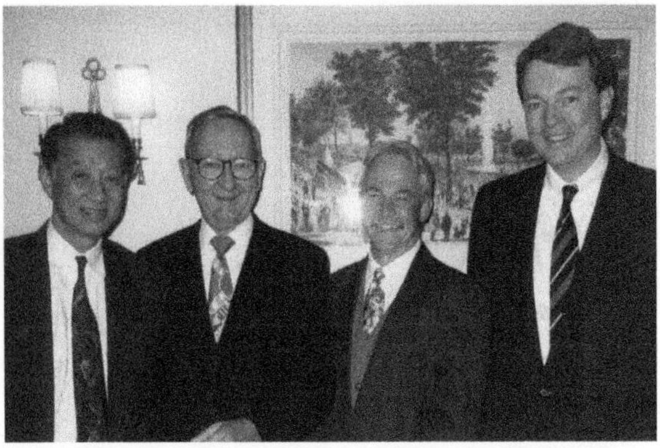

Figure 1-6. James Yao, John Bergan, William Flinn, Walter McCarthy.

score. Unfortunately, hip surgery in 2014 denied him the honor and now, in fact, there is no perfect attendance record.

The past 40 years have taught me that progress in surgical care is an ongoing process and it is largely driven by technology. Care of vascular disease is no longer just an operative craft and technology will play an important role in its future. Academic-industry cooperation is essential for future advances and, as demonstrated here, it is possible.

The success of the symposium is a team effort. I thank Bill Flinn and Walt McCarthy for their unrelenting support (Figure 1-6). After Bergan left the division, William Pearce returned and expanded basic science research. In 1990, when endovascular repair of abdominal aortic aneurysm was introduced, we asked Jon Matsumura to develop the technology. Mark Morasch, Mark Eskandari, Melina Kibbe and Heron Rodriquez were recruited to the Division and, at present, Mark Eskandari is the Chief of the Division. Under his leadership, three young faculty members have joined the Division: Karen Ho, Andy Hoel and Tadaki Tomita. All of these bright young vascular surgeons are leaving their marks on the symposium.

Finally, in the midst of the celebration of our 40 year anniversary, it is with much regret that I report to you that, of 38 speakers at the first symposium, we have identified only 14 faculty members who are still alive. We thank all of them for their valiant effort at the first symposium and assure them that the Northwestern Vascular Symposium will go on.

ACKNOWLEDGEMENT

We thank Janet Goldstein for preparation and editing of this manuscript and Sara Minton for administering the symposium. Both Janet and Sara are indispensable to the symposium.

REFERENCES

1. *Webster's New World Dictionary of American Language—Third College Edition*. New York: Macmillan General Reference, 1994.
2. Wylie EJ. Vascular surgery: A quest for excellence. *Arch Surg* 1970;101:645–648.

3. DeWeese JA. Accreditation of vascular training programs and certification of vascular surgeons. *J Vasc Surg* 1996;23:1043–1053.
4. Veith FJ, Ascher E. A tribute to Henry Haimovici September 7, 1907 – July 10, 2001. *J Vasc Surg* 2001;34:1135–1136.
5. Yao JST. 30th Anniversary of Northwestern Vascular Symposium. In Pearce WH, Matsumura JS, Yao JST, eds. *Trends in Vascular Surgery*. Evanston IL: Greenwood Academic; 2006. pp xvii–xxii.
6. Yao JST, Stoney RJ. The E. J. Wylie traveling fellowship. *J Vasc Surg* 1996;23:1088–1091.

2

The Evolution of Vascular Surgery

A Forty-Year Perspective

Richard H. Dean, MD

It is a humbling privilege to participate in the symposium celebrating the 40th anniversary of the founding of the Northwestern University (NWU) Vascular Surgery Fellowship and to provide commentary on my perspectives regarding the discipline of vascular surgery over the intervening 40 years. Dr. Paul Stanton, from the Georgia Baptist Surgical Residency, and myself, from the Vanderbilt University Surgical Residency, shared the unique experience of being its first two fellows in 1974. Paul spent his year at the Veterans Administration Hospital while I worked at the Wesley Pavilion and the "Vascular Laboratory" for my entire year as a Northwestern University Research Instructor in Surgery. We both found these sites and related experiences as ideal foundations from which to launch our professional careers. Among my fondest memories of that year, however, were the daily round trips from my home in Wilmette, Illinois to the Wesley Pavilion, riding "shot-gun" beside the driver, Jimmy Yao. Without question, we could have solved all of the world's problems during those trips, if only the proper audiences had accompanied us. The other benefit of being chaperoned by Jimmy was that when he decided it was time to go home, I had to go as well. Those memories are only surpassed by the privilege of having Jimmy as a lifelong supporter and as a deeply cherished personal friend from that year forward.

Although I could fill several pages of this narrative with stories of my year at Northwestern with Jimmy Yao and John Bergan, I feel confident that many here today could also similarly reminisce. In contrast, I will take the prerogative to focus my comments and perspectives on how the discipline of vascular surgery and its fellowships have evolved from the 1974 era. I will include my perspective on the important events in our specialty's maturation since that time, and, take advantage of this opportunity to voice my opinion on important constructs for our specialty's future.

My first admonishment regarding this missive is to remind all that this is not a history, requiring references and supporting data; but, instead, it is based on my personal views molded by perspectives from the platforms of my professional career. These platforms began as a surgical resident at Vanderbilt University, followed by the Vascular Fellowship at Northwestern University, then as the first Vascular Surgery Program Director at Vanderbilt and at Wake Forest University, The Chair of Surgery at Wake Forest, a Society for Vascular Surgery (SVS) officer, an American Board of Surgery (ABS) member and examiner, and, finally, a view from the "Dark Side" as the President & CEO of Wake Forest University Health Sciences and Director of its Medical Center. Without question, each of these experiences provided unique perspectives regarding the evolution and maturation of our discipline within the broader family and network of all surgical specialties. It is these experiences and their attendant influence on my perspectives that form the context of this narrative.

THE NORTHWESTERN UNIVERSITY VASCULAR SURGERY FELLOWSHIP AND SYMPOSIUM

A variety of vascular surgery fellowships had existed for several years prior to the formation of the Northwestern University fellowship in 1974. Leaders of such programs included icons of our specialty such as Dr. Jack Wiley in San Francisco, Dr. Clement Darling in Boston, Dr. Andrew Dale in Nashville and Dr. Jesse Thompson in Dallas, to mention but a few. Criteria for such programs were varied and were primarily governed by the individual program's leader. Most programs were designed to provide the trainee with a rich exposure to the operative management of vascular disease not present in most general surgery residencies. In contrast to that norm, essentially all vascular surgery procedures at Vanderbilt were actually performed by the Chief Resident. Thereby, I had received a rich operative experience, even performing 34 renal artery reconstructions as a chief resident. To me, the enticing attraction of the newly announced Northwestern University program, starting July 1, 1974 under the leadership of Drs. John Bergan and Jimmy Yao, was the intent to provide me with an experience as a teaching assistant to chief residents in the operating room; to marry that opportunity with the chance to participate in advancing knowledge of Doppler ultrasound in the evaluation of occlusive vascular disease under the mentorship of Jimmy Yao; and, to explore personal interests in the study of hyperlipidemia in animal models. In short, I was most interested in a program that challenged one's thoughts and provided significant opportunities to further his or her understanding of the vascular diseases being considered for surgical management. Thereby, the planned Northwestern University Vascular Surgery Fellowship was the perfect match for me. Without question, over its 40-year duration, it has remained a rich breeding ground for excellent vascular surgeons and individuals who aspire to an academic career. To date, seventy-eight (78) vascular fellows have been trained at Northwestern and approximately 40% of these have sustained academic careers. Remarkably, thirteen of these graduates have held offices in regional or national surgical organizations.

I recall one memorable moment during the 1978 Northwestern University Vascular Surgery Symposium. This moment occurred immediately following my presentation on renovascular hypertension when a question was asked by a patron saint of vascular surgery and Emeritus Professor of Surgery at Northwestern, namely Gesa deTakis. Then in his 80s, Dr. deTakis asked such a penetrating question based on contemporary knowledge of "my field" that I could hardly respond at his level of knowledge and insight into my chosen field of career interest. To this day, I marvel at the depth of his intellect and contemporary knowledge of then current events, even at that late date in his life.

EMERGENCE OF THE DISCIPLINE OF VASCULAR SURGERY AND ITS TRAINING PROGRAMS

The origins of vascular surgery have many progenerators. First, one must remember that many of my generation of surgical residents were trained by leaders that selected their specific specialty of general surgery after all their formal training was concluded. Dr. H. William Scott, Jr., Chair of Surgery at Vanderbilt during my residency, had the same year of neurosurgical training that his peers received who subsequently selected Neurosurgery as their focused career interest. Actually, Dr. Scott did one of the earliest procedures to correct the "subclavian steel" syndrome and had research interest in hyperlipidemia and experimental atherosclerosis but spent many years, including the six years of my general surgery residency, mostly doing vagotomy and antrectomies for peptic ulcer disease and jejuno-ileal bypasses for morbid obesity. The same official training that produced a Dr. Scott birthed surgeons such as Dr. Michael DeBakey and other noted cardiac surgeons that continued to dabble in general surgery and to consider noncardiac vascular surgery as within their domain. This all-encompassing view of cardiovascular surgery was the environment that spawned the partnering of two different societies for our annual meetings at the time of my training and career launch, namely, the North American Chapter of the International Society of Cardiovascular Surgery and the Society of Vascular Surgery. Several of the leaders in vascular surgery during the 1960s and 1970s were also recognized as leaders of American Surgery, as witnessed by their leadership roles in the American Board of Surgery and the American College of Surgery.

With the exception of sites with leaders such as those mentioned above, few surgical programs had a distinct and separate vascular surgery service before the 40-year era we now celebrate. In 1980 the Society of Vascular Surgery (SVS) initiated sponsorship, evaluation, and approval of vascular surgery fellowship programs through its Program Evaluation and Endorsement Committee (PEEC) as proposed by Dr. Bill Blaisdall in his 1979 SVS Presidential Address. Through its sponsorship, surgical practices devoted only to vascular surgery began to populate metropolitan areas throughout the country, thus elevating vascular surgery as a legitimate discipline of surgery. I argue that prior to the mid-1970s, most vascular surgery procedures performed in private practice and at academic medical centers were undertaken by cardiac surgeons, or self-taught general surgeons with at least a passing interest in vascular surgery. From my perspective, the engagement of the SVS and its ultimate creation of the PEEC for oversight and approval of vascular surgery training programs strengthened a movement that attracted many who previously would have chosen cardiac surgery careers. I, for one, had switched during the fall of my general surgery chief residency year from a scheduled position as a cardiac surgery resident at Vanderbilt to pursue an enlightened academic career plan of vascular surgery through the newly approved Northwestern University Vascular Surgery Fellowship program in 1974.

The growth of vascular surgery fellowship programs and the increasing numbers of their graduates both in private practice and in academic surgery throughout the country then led to the realization of a need for standardizing such programs under the Accreditation Council for Graduate Medical Education (ACGME) and the provision of certification of their graduates' qualifications by the ABS. In 1983, the ABS instituted examinations for individuals seeking a certificate of "Special Qualifications in General Vascular Surgery." The initial criteria for sitting for the examination were that the applicant held ABS certification and met entry criteria for vascular surgery cases volume ("grandfather category") or had completed a PEEC-approved program and met case volume criteria for their initial year of practice. Commensurate with the ABS action, the ACGME approved its Residency Review Committee (RRC) for Surgery's proposed guidelines for approval of vascular surgery training programs. By 1984, the SVS had transferred the responsibility to the RRC for Surgery for review and approval of all active and future vascular surgery training programs.

I felt privileged to be one of the examiners for the first ABS sponsored oral certifying examination for Special Qualifications in Vascular Surgery in 1985. That initial oral examination was primarily composed of "grandfathered" applicants, and, was a fascinating experience. In many ways, it must have paralleled the experiences of those ABS examiners who conducted the first oral examination for certification in general surgery in 1938. If nothing else, to me, that experience underscored the need and value of standardization of vascular surgery training programs. On the one hand, many of the examinees had deep knowledge in certain areas but had major gaps or shallow knowledge in other topics related to vascular disease and its management. Subsequently, when I matched up these examinees having only "focused" knowledge with their site of training, I was initially shocked that highly reputed surgeons had trained these candidates. But, on reflection, such training occurred before program standardizations and approvals. Their program content simply reflected only the interest and biased variety of vascular conditions referred to the reputed senior surgeon to whom the trainee was attracted.

MOUNTING STORMS AND CONFLICTS

The maturation of vascular surgery as a discipline and the attendant desire to be recognized as a primary surgical specialty with its own oversight and management led to a severe schism within the leadership ranks of vascular surgery. On the one hand, a subgroup of program leaders insisted that breaking away from the American Board of Surgery and forming an independent American Board of Vascular Surgery, much as Cardiac surgery had done several decades before, was the only way to obtain true maturation as a "primary" specialty of surgery. Others, including myself, believed that there was an opportunity to obtain "self-governance" within the American Board of Surgery umbrella. For the better part of a decade, a few individuals in leadership positions within the SVS pursued their mission to achieve total separation from the ABS, thus creating a polarized environment throughout our discipline.

This conflict led to heated internal debate within the SVS into which most members were drawn. At one point, I perceived that it had become so politicized that prominent program directors and SVS leaders in our field were essentially ordered to support secession or be branded as traitors to the cause of vascular surgery and risked being banished as outsiders by those leading the march to total secession.

During the early phase of this movement toward separation from the ABS, in the mid-late 1990s, I was privileged to serve on an ad hoc committee of the SVS Council to discuss the emerging problem with the ABS and the issue of having nonvascular surgeons on the RRC evaluate vascular surgery fellowship programs. In no small way this was brought about when one fellowship program had been cited and warned of potential probation by the RRC based on an inadequate case volume reported by his fellows related to open aortic procedures (note that the minimum experience had been set at ten such cases per trainee by the RRC). In hindsight, I perceive that this ad hoc committee was the initial foray to launch the movement toward subsequent plans for separation. At its peak, leaders of this plan for succession had incorporated their own "American Board of Vascular Surgery" and sought recognition as a separate board by the American Board of Medical Specialties (ABMS). This recognition was never realized.

Having been a member of the American Board of Surgery during this period (1993–1999), I had the opportunity to witness both the internal conflict within our discipline as well as the polarized views within the ABS itself. As mentioned above, the ABS attempted to evolve its relationship with the vascular community by creating the ABS Committee on Vascular Surgery, developing an examination to award a Certificate of Special Qualifications in Vascular Surgery, and consideration of other means to appease the erupting cavern between the ABS and the vascular surgery group pushing for "independence."

In my opinion, this conflict reached its pinnacle for the ABS as it planned its 1999 Winter Retreat meeting. At that time, there were two vascular surgeons on the ABS. I was completing my 6-year tour, having been appointed through the Southern Surgical Association. The other "vascular" member was Dr. Pat Claggett of Dallas, Texas who had joined the ABS as the nominee from the SVS in 1997. Pat was then assigned as the Chair of the ABS sub-board, formally named the "Vascular Surgery Committee" of the ABS. The primary topic for this three-day ABS retreat was the "the vascular surgery issue." For this focused retreat, the ABS invited Dr. Bill Baker of Loyola (Chicago), representing the vascular community, and asked me to also address the Board to give my views on the topic. At this point, I was a suspect commentator. On the one hand, I was no longer practicing vascular surgery as I had just assumed the full-time position as Director of our Medical Center and V.P. of Health Affairs of WFU. On the other hand, I had *only* practiced vascular surgery in my clinical career and had been a vascular surgery program director. In some ways, I felt myself to be neither fish nor fowl. From this vantage point, however, I felt I had no party to represent other than my personal views on both the ABS's past approaches to subspecialization and my negative view of the succession initiative. With this backdrop, I provided my views on this matter. The narrative text of that speech is provided below.

To say the least, I was pleased that my presentation was positively received by most members of the Board and served as a moment from which the ABS evolved its approach to solve the "vascular surgery issue" through creating a Board of Vascular Surgery under the ABS umbrella. The consequence of that decision has led to the transfer of oversight and management related to vascular surgery certification to the Vascular Surgery Board and began a new era in the ABS's approach to other specialties by also forming self-managing Boards of Pediatric Surgery, Surgical Oncology, and Critical Care under its umbrella.

Presentation to the American Board of Surgery at its January, 1999 Retreat

By: Richard H. Dean, MD

Thanks for asking me to provide my views on this critical debate, the conclusions from which will define, from my perspective, a significant component of this body's future.

I realize that I may have been asked to comment on this topic as I am seen by many of you as a vascular surgeon and might argue the views of that discipline. But, I must remind you that I am now considered a twice-removed foreigner to my former colleagues. Twice removed, in that first, I stepped away as head of Vascular Surgery at Vanderbilt to head Surgery at Wake Forest that housed all surgical specialties – actually, after I arrived, Ophthalmology lobbied and rejoined my re-nomenclatured Division of Surgical Sciences. Then I went completely to the dark side when I accepted the position of Director of the Medical Center, head of WFU Health Sciences and stopped operating. Nonetheless, functioning on a daily basis outside the sphere of surgery gives me a little different perspective from which to comment on what I believe to be a critical fork in the road facing the ABS.

I would like to approach my thoughts by offering a few questions and a few comments on ABS's history. My first question is this: "Is this body The American Board of Surgery or should it actually be named the American Board of General Surgery?" I argue that when one looks at its historical past, it has chosen (maybe without thought) to maintain absolute control over its past domain, despite the sequential emergence of multiple mature sub-disciplines of Surgery. Several of these disciplines, including cardiac surgery and others, extracted themselves over vigorous attempts by the ABS to prevent their maturation to adulthood, and, thereby, caused their complete severance and their creation of independent Boards.

In other words, at each step in our past, the ABS has attempted to control disciplines that have matured to full-fledged adulthood by any appropriate and measurable parameter. Instead of recognizing that evolution, in the past the Board has attempted to maintain its complete control even though those "in control" were generalists and not engaged in the forefront of the particular sub-specialty's maturation. The consequence of that "control mentality" has been to have the ABS sequentially loose its overarching strategic domain as a cost of its insistence in controlling the "operational" aspects of certification for maturing specialties.

To me, those past behaviors and the current issue have similarity to another relationship about which most of us have experience; namely, the maturation of children and their evolving relationship to their parents. I ask myself, what happens when a parent attempts to control their child beyond a certain age and maturity? Well, they become a permanent dependent or they rebel and divorce themselves completely from the family. My point is that the ABS should not stop emerging specialties from their maturation. Instead, the ABS should embrace such maturation and alter its relationship to such emerging specialties to allow them to become operationally independent while remaining a family member and becoming a "partner" in addressing strategic issues that might affect the entire family. I think our history as the ABS gives ample evidence that the controlling parent mentality is not a prescription for success and has been shown to be a losing battle both in family life and in the life of the continuously evolving disciplines of Surgery.

If we cannot act in such an enlightened mind-frame with this issue of Vascular Surgery, then we must also accept the fact that we will continue to repeat the same short-sighted view in the future with other specialties such as trauma surgery, oncologic surgery, etc. I believe we must address this issue now and address it with a more encompassing approach than our history would predict.

In short, I believe that the Board needs to define thresholds of maturation that when reached, open formal engagement by that discipline within the ABS, much as has been the case for Vascular Surgery. Such thresholds should be monitored with approved metrics to remove at least some of the politics from the process. Then, when the discipline has evolved to a point of having its own RRC-approved residency programs, as has Vascular Surgery, it should be considered an adult and should be provided a level of self-governance within the overall body of the ABS. Such is the case within the realm of medicine where essentially all of the medical specialties are still under the strategic umbrella of the American Board of Internal Medicine while being provided control over their discipline's unique affairs.

In closing, unless we approach this issue in such a way, the ABS will continue to fight this issue with each of the emerging disciplines as they reach "adulthood."

In short, we should consider creating a formal structure within the overarching umbrella of the ABS within which Vascular Surgery can manage its own affairs within the family. We already have a Vascular Surgery Committee, but it is time to evolve that structure to a high level of self-management and set the framework for those countless areas of surgery that will be birthed and mature in the future. Although I suggest such a structure be a "Board" of the ABS; or, if this is a "bridge too far," then it should be something like the Vascular Surgery Council of the ABS. To me, the most important declaration is to define and establish its self-management role rather than just giving it a title and maintaining all functional control outside its purview.

Again, thanks for the opportunity to provide a voice from the "dark side" of administration, a voice, however, that hopefully still maintains the genetic code of a surgeon.

Without question, the ABS now has adopted an enlightened philosophy of inclusion and self-management by newly emerging yet mature surgical specialties rather than continuing its failed prior philosophy of control and confinement. Their former strategy did not succeed in its past and is unlikely to succeed in its future. From my perspective, the ABS will never revert to its prior mentality of protectionism and suppression of disciplines in an effort to maintain its control over its domain.

We all should also recognize and applaud those members of Vascular Surgery's leadership who held our discipline together during that tumultuous era in our history despite its personal cost and conflict with other nationally recognized vascular surgeons. In doing so, they succeeded in realizing the vision of Vascular Surgery as being a mature adult in the family of Surgery.

PERSPECTIVES ON THE EVOLUTION OF TRAINING PROGRAMS

Over my 40-year perspective of this narrative, vascular surgery has attained the full status as an independent department in many academic health centers. For example, the first distinct vascular surgery service was not formed at Wake Forest until 1987. Its RRC-approved vascular surgery training program began shortly thereafter, in 1992. It now is an independent Department of Vascular and Endovascular Surgery along with eight other mature specialties of surgery. The point between a time when most vascular surgery was performed by general surgeons or cardiac surgeons and the current era when all open vascular surgery and most endovascular procedures are performed by board-certified vascular surgeons has not been one of cordial transformation in many academic health centers. I was fortunate to have been trained at two institutions that were led by enlightened surgical leaders, namely Dr. H.W. Scott, Jr. at Vanderbilt and Dr. John Beale at Northwestern, who recognized the need and value of embracing vascular surgery as a defined discipline with its own clinical service and training program. Battles waged by cardiac surgery and general surgery to maintain engagement in vascular surgery were not waged at either of these two places during this time period.

Traditionally, training in vascular surgery only followed completion of a general surgery residency, and one could not sit for certification in vascular surgery until he/she had successfully passed their ABS examinations in general surgery. Also, there are at least two unique 4 years +2 years programs approved (years general surgery + years vascular surgery training) that provide a particularly rich vascular experience to the general surgery resident from which a graduate may also sit for both general surgery and vascular surgery boards. Recently, however, additional alternate residency tracks for individuals planning a vascular surgery career have been approved by the RRC with 3 years + 3 years and a 0 + 5 years options available for implementation. Although each of these alternates to the traditional 5 years + 2 years track have proponents and may provide adequate training for narrowly defined careers, they qualify for certification in vascular surgery alone, and graduates have no standing as applicants for certification in general surgery.

The 3 years + 3 years and 0 + 5 years alternative paths have only been available since my departure from active practice and fellowship oversight. Nevertheless, I feel compelled to offer my perspective regarding the added alternatives to the more traditional 5 year + 2 year path and its opportunity for "dual" certification. I recognize that with the addition of catheter-based management of vascular disease comes an opportunity for a physician to develop a career solely related to such minimally invasive techniques as witnessed by the numbers of interventional radiologists and cardiologists performing such procedures on patients with peripheral and cerebrovascular disease. That having been said, I continue to maintain that a board-certified vascular surgeon should be well educated regarding all aspects of the disease they plan to manage and should be trained and competent in all aspects of medical and surgical management of such patients, irrespective of their age or co-existent medical and/or surgical problems. To say the least, the training I received in the performance of complex pancreatic or other nonvascular intra-abdominal and retroperitoneal procedures and senior experiences in pediatric surgery during my general surgery residency served me well in my development of new techniques for management of renal and juxta-renal aortic diseases and vascular disorders in children. With this background, I am encouraged that most vascular surgery training programs continue to provide the traditional path of 5 years + 2 years to dual general surgery and vascular surgery certification.

TIME LIMIT CONTROLS ON TRAINING

I provide my perspective regarding the 80-hour workweek for residents with the realization that I am a creature of a prior generation of surgeons where all responsibility for the patient's outcome following a surgical intervention rested on the shoulders of the surgeon. There were no committee management teams beyond the operating surgeon and the residents. Instead, I used advisory consultants who were solicited as needed. I must admit that I now perceive that the surgeon may only be responsible for the operation; the management of morbidities and complications not directly related to the procedure are charged to the respective team members who represent disciplines relevant to the patient's nonprocedure-related care. I agree that such teams have significantly standardized and reduced negative variations in care and the associated adverse outcomes of care. I still contend that a committed and knowledgeable surgeon surrounded by excellent residents and nursing staff and available consultants, as appropriate, set a high bar of excellence that cannot be surmounted by the current systems.

To coin a phrase from the institution from which I received my Bachelors of Arts degree, the Virginia Military Institute, where old codgers like me would come back talking about the "Old Corps," I am from the generation of surgical residents that worked a 125 hours per week average schedule. Also, I was reared in a general practitioner's family in a small town where evening office hours and middle of the night home visits were the norm. Thereby, one should not be surprised that, from my perspective, the institution of constrained commitments to the patient through "the 80-hour work week" for residents, and the distribution of postoperative care among multiple specialties has begun a sequential erosion of the primacy of a physician's commitment to his/her profession.

Unfortunately, I am a realist and both understand and agree with the need for standardization of care. I also must admit that the erosion of the surgeon's role in the total care of a patient has been the result of our collective neglect or even dismissal without action regarding the wide variations in care and outcome in our past. Without question, it has been our unwillingness to police our own ranks in a timely fashion that has led to much of the regulatory revisions in training and in the practice of medicine throughout our country.

CATHETER-BASED ENDOVASCULAR PROCEDURES

At many institutions, interventional radiologists and cardiologists at have threatened the vascular surgeon's domain since the arrival of catheter-based endovascular procedures. Unlike cardiac surgeons, however, we should be proud of the response of vascular surgery to these incursions. In short, vascular surgery has maintained its "territorial" integrity by espousing to be the only disease-oriented discipline and by embracing the newly birthed discipline of vascular medicine as a component of vascular surgery. This position was significantly enhanced when the first endovascular stented grafts were inserted and championed by a vascular surgeon, namely, Dr. Juan Parodi of Brazil. The addition of training in the use of endovascular techniques in most vascular surgery training programs has further cemented our position amongst the competing disciplines. I often wonder how the world of cardiac surgery might have evolved differently and how many fewer stenotic coronary artery dilatations and stents might have been performed, if the discipline of cardiac surgery had similarly adopted our holistic approach to the patient in the early period of that discipline's maturation and had included the evaluation and medical management of ischemic heart disease in its repertoire as well.

In relation to this last comment, I provide the following short vignette of my experience at Vanderbilt as the NIH-funded Principle Investigator of the longitudinal study of hypertensive patients with renovascular disease (RVD) and the randomized, prospective study comparing medical versus surgical intervention for renovascular hypertension (RVH).

Realizing how many atherosclerotic RVD patients with uncontrolled hypertension and angina pectoris were being presented to me for renal revascularization, in the late 1970s, I wanted to insert coronary angiography as a standard diagnostic study of all patients with atherosclerotic RVD. I was challenged by Dr. John Oates, Chairman of Medicine and the senior medical physician engaged in our SCORE in Hypertension. His point was that such a study was not clinically indicated since there had been no difference in the operative mortality of patients undergoing renal revascularization in the 1960s and early 1970s when comparing patients with and without preoperative angina pectoris. Indeed, the operative mortality had been ~1% for both. His logic was that removal of the cardiac afterload by resolving their uncontrolled hypertension would resolve their clinical manifestation of coronary artery disease. He did agree to our undertaking a systematic preoperative angiographic study of the coronary arteries in all patients, independent of clinical symptoms as a clinical research study, but only after determining whether the study was clinically required and whether or not coronary intervention was required based on clinical parameters rather than "to be defined" angiographic parameters (excluding severe main left coronary artery narrowing). The outcome of this "faux research" study of the coronary arteries showed a significant incidence of clinically silent but angiographically significant coronary artery disease. Further, we found no correlation between the presence of the asymptomatic CAD and perioperative mortality or follow-up heart-related deaths when such CAD was left undisturbed by intervention. Admittedly, these patients were not consistently followed long-term for cardiac events, and these observations were not published.

I often wonder what the impact of a randomized trial of medical versus interventional treatment of the asymptomatic but anatomically severe CAD might have revealed and what impact such information might have had on the entire history and explosive expense related to interventions for CAD in the current era of empiric stenting of such lesions.

LEST WE FORGET ABOUT THE PAST

My final commentary on the evolution of vascular surgery over the last 40 years is an admonition not to forget knowledge gained during earlier eras when adopting new techniques to manage atherosclerotic occlusive vascular disease. This admonition is driven by my observations of current events surrounding the area of my prior academic and clinical interest, namely the evaluation and treatment of renovascular hypertension (RVH). Specifically, my perception is that well-defined progress in knowledge regarding criteria for the diagnosis of RVH has disappeared from contemporary evaluation and management of RVD. Unfortunately, this amnesia regarding prior knowledge may even have infected the intellect of study sections at the National Heart, Lung and Blood Institute (NHLBI). I refer to the NHLBI's sponsorship of the broadly acclaimed multicenter randomized, prospective trial of medical management alone versus intervention with percutaneous transluminal angioplasty plus stenting

(PTA+S) of patients with anatomically significant renal artery stenosis and severe hypertension.[1]

In the above-referenced study, patients with anatomically significant renal artery lesions were entered into the trial without any assessment of the functional significance of the renal artery lesion. Not to my surprise, no statistical difference in renal function or hypertension responses was noted during follow-up of these two trial arms. Why was this outcome not surprising? The reason lies in a 1973 report by Dr. John Foster, with whom I was a co-author, who published the results of the angiographic study of 1070 hypertensive patients; and, the performance of functional studies on the subset who had anatomically significant renal artery stenosis.[2] The functional studies consisted of renal vein renin assays (RVRA) and split renal function studies (SRFS). As shown in Table 2-1, only 114 (38%) of the 297 patients with significant atherosclerotic renal artery lesions were shown to have RVH based on the results of functional studies (Table 2-1).

Note that a subsequent report from Vanderbilt[3] showed that 93% of patients with renal artery stenosis, positive RVRA and/or SRFS, and a successful renal revascularization procedure were cured or had significant improvement of their hypertension. Further, we subsequently published data showing that we only witnessed significant postoperative renal function improvement in the revascularized kidney when the preoperative split renal function study was positive for creatinine hyperconcentration in the urine from the affected kidney.[4]

So, in reference to the recent NHLBI-funded multicenter trial, less than 40% of the randomized patients may have had a causal relationship between their anatomic renal artery lesion and their co-existent hypertension. Thereby, greater than 60% of the patients in the interventional arm of the trial may have been subjected to the potential negative impact of PTA+S without any expectation of benefit.

I recognize that SRFS have not been performed in any medical center for over twenty years and that RVRAs are rarely accurate when performed infrequently and without stringent controls. Therefore, nationwide, there is no reliable functional study currently available to prove the presence of RVH. My point, however, is that until a reliable substitute for the above-described functional studies is found, a study such as the multicenter trial mentioned above is suspect. Nevertheless, I appreciate the fact that the results of that study will appropriately curtail irrelevant and expensive interventions using minimally invasive techniques such as PTA+S to treat likely "asymptomatic" renal artery lesions.

Separately, I feel compelled to mention that PTA+S, though obviously much less invasive than surgical revascularization, has not had comparatively equal success in the frequency of hypertension benefit or retrieval of renal function when compared to open operative revascularization. Comparison of the results obtained through use

TABLE 2-1. RESULTS OF THE EVALUATION OF 1,070 HYPERTENSIVE PATIENTS

Result	Renal Arteriogram	Renovascular Hypertension[a]
Normal	610 (57%)	0
Renal artery stenosis due to:		
Atherosclerosis	297 (43%)	114 (38%)
Fibromuscular Dysplasia	116	62 (53%)

[a] Positive split renal function studies and/or positive renal vein renin assays.

of these two interventional modalities at Wake Forest clearly demonstrated a higher benefit rate in hypertension response and renal function retrieval from operative renal revascularization.[5,6] Unfortunately, a prospective, randomized trial comparing these two modalities has never been undertaken.

At a more fundamental level, I implore all who are constructing or evaluating the scientific merit of clinical trials to cull, be knowledgeable of, and incorporate prior scientific findings still pertinent to the study or treatment of vascular lesions wherever they may reside. In this instance, the current randomized study only showed what was known in the 1950s and 1960s during which time similar empiric interventions on RVD without functional evaluation led to similar negative outcomes and led to a temporary period of disillusion regarding the value of renal revascularization. But that period was followed by the development of the functional studies mentioned above. With the disappearance of those functional studies from contemporary evaluation, our discipline is in dire need for their less invasive but accurate predictors of benefit in order to reestablish the credibility of interventional management of RVH.

In closing, I must admit that the era in which vascular surgery finds itself in the 2nd decade of the 21st century is profoundly different from the 8th decade of the 20th century. Nevertheless, many of the same challenges of prior eras remain equally relevant today. The discipline must continue to defend its holistic view of its role in the diagnosis and management of vascular disease and resist the ever-present temptation of accepting the "interventionalist's" mentality, both within our specialty and beyond. An excellent technical vascular surgeon with whom I once interacted provided the most notable example of such a mindless approach. To quote him, "*If I am referred a patient with a lesion that I know I can fix, I do so. Both the patient and the referring physician are happy.*" We must remember that vascular disease is endemic to our population and resist the mentality that surgery or catheter-based intervention is the answer to all such anatomic lesions. Finally, while we must continue to challenge dogma and practices of the past, we should not forsake prior knowledge and then presume its rediscovery is an advancement of the science of our discipline.

REFERENCES

1. Cooper CJ, Murphy TP, et al. Stenting and medical therapy for atherosclerotic renal-artery stenosis. *N Eng J Med*. 2014; 370:13–22.
2. Foster JH, Dean RH, Pinkerton JA, et al. Ten years' experience with the surgical management of renovascular hypertension. *Ann Surg*. 1973;177;755.
3. Dean RH. Renovascular hypertension. *Curr Prob Surg*. 1985; Feb;22:6–67.
4. Dean RH, Englund R, Dupont WD, et al. Retrieval of renal function by revascularization: study of preoperative outcome predictors. *Ann Surg*. 1985;202:367–375.
5. Cherr GS, Hansen KJ, Craven TE, et al. Surgical management of atherosclerotic renovascular disease. *J Vas Surg*. 2002;5(1):6–13.
6. Corriere MA, Pearce JD, Edwards MS, et al. Endovascular management of atherosclerotic renovascular disease: early results following primary intervention. *J Vasc Surg*. 2008;48(3):580–88.

3

Historical Events of SVS Based on the Interview Program: Administrative and Management Issues

Walter J. McCarthy, III, MD, MS, James S.T. Yao, MD, PhD, Roger T. Gregory, MD, Norman M. Rich, MD, and The History Project Work Group of SVS

In an effort to preserve the history of vascular surgery as a distinct specialty and establish the history of the Society for Vascular Surgery (SVS), a committee (the History Project Work Group) was formed to conduct interviews with leaders and contributors in vascular surgery. The work group is chaired by James S. T. Yao with nine members (Norman Rich, Roger Gregory, William Baker, Kenneth Cherry, Melina Kibbe, Peter Lawrence, Mark Eskandari, Walter McCarthy, William Pearce) and Calvin Ernst as consultant. Members of the Work Group conducted one- to two-hour interviews that were recorded in high-D digital videography disc (DVD) to be made available in hard copy or accessed via the internet by computer and/or a variety of hand held devices. The scope of the current project and what we have learned have been reported recently.[1–4] Since September 2011, the committee has conducted 80 interviews with 40 past presidents of SVS and American Association for Vascular Surgery (AAVS, formerly International Society for Cardiovascular Surgery-North American chapter [ISCVS-NA]), 5 recipients of innovative awards, 20 honorary members of SVS, and 15 selected members of SVS (Table 3-1). To highlight the historical events, short clips were taken from these interviews. These highlights can be shown in short clips of no more than 5 minutes or compiled and used to reconstitute the historical events of SVS as it developed chronologically. This compilation "History DVD" will be uploaded to a You-Tube designated channel at the SVS website. Once uploaded, You-Tube will process the videos such that they can be viewed on a wide variety of mobile devices.

TABLE 3-1. LIST OF MEMBERS INTERVIEWED AND THEIR DESIGNATED SUBTITLES

No.	Date of Interview	Interviewee	Interviewer	Subtitle
1.	9/26/11	Denton A. Cooley	R. Gregory	Pioneer cardiac and vascular surgeon
2.	11/18/11	Anthony M. Imparato	R. Gregory	Insight into carotid plaque morphology
3.	11/18/11	Frank C. Spencer	R. Gregory	The voice of reason
4.	11/18/11	Julius H. Jacobson	R. Gregory	Microvascular surgeon and philanthropist
5.	12/8/11	Norman M. Rich	R. Gregory	Military surgeon at war and peace
6.	12/8/11	James S.T. Yao	R. Gregory	International star of vascular surgery
7.	12/8/11	Ronald J. Baird	W. McCarthy	Our northern cardiovascular partner
8.	12/9/11	Leonel Villavicencio	R. Gregory	The Mexican maestro
9.	12/9/11	Richard H. Dean	M. Eskandari	Young vascular surgery advocate
10.	1/11/12	William F. Blaisdell	N. Rich	A true pioneer in vascular surgery
11.	1/20/12	John F. Connolly	P. Lawrence	American ambassador in vascular surgery
12.	2/20/12	Wiley F. Barker	P. Lawrence	A true leader in vascular surgery
13.	3/1/12	Jonathan B. Towne	W. McCarthy	Statesman for vascular surgery
14.	3/15/12	Ramon Berguer	W. Baker	World expert in vertebral surgery
15.	3/26/12	Craig D. Miller	W. McCarthy	Pioneer vascular surgeon in thoracic aorta
16.	4/27/12	Ronald J. Stoney	N. Rich	Master technical vascular surgeon
17.	5 /1/12	Juan C. Parodi	M. Kibbe, J. Yao	Inventor of endovascular graft
18.	5/25/12	Thomas J. Fogarty	R. Gregory, M. Kibbe, J. Yao	Inventor, entrepreneur and philanthropist
19.	5/25/12	William H. Pearce	R. Gregory	Research investigator in vascular surgery
20.	5/31/12	Ben Eiseman	N. Rich, W. Pearce	Surgeon for all seasons
21.	6/1/12	Jack L. Cronenwett	W. Baker	Visionary leader in vascular surgery
22.	6/6/12	Craig K. Kent	P. Lawrence	Vascular scientist
23.	6/7/12	Lazar J. Greenfield	P. Lawrence	Inventor of medical device
24.	6/7/12	Thomas S. Riles	R. Gregory	Simulation expert in vascular surgery
25.	6/7/12	Richard M. Green	N. Rich	Vascular surgeons for mentors
26.	6/7/12	Anthony D. Whittemore	N. Rich	Vascular surgeon providing leadership in hospital affairs
27.	6/7/12	Wesley S. Moore	R. Gregory	Coined the magic word, "Endovascular"
28.	6/8/12	G. Patrick Clagett	W. McCarthy	Innovative clinical vascular surgeon
29.	6/8/12	Herbert Dardik	M. Kibbe	Defying the norm
30.	6/19/12	William H. Baker	W. McCarthy	Master carotid surgeon
31.	6/21/12	Christopher K. Zarins	M. Kibbe	Creator of new knowledge
32.	6/25/12	Robert L. Kistner	W. McCarthy	Pioneer venous valve surgeon

No.	Date of Interview	Interviewee	Interviewer	Subtitle
33.	7/17/12	George P. Noon	R. Gregory	Modest surgeon to mentors and giants
34.	7/17/12	Jimmy F. Howell	R. Gregory, J. Yao	Master cardiovascular surgeon
35.	7/17/12	Kenneth L. Mattox	R. Gregory, J. Yao	Trauma top knife
36.	7/26/12	Thomas F. O'Donnell	W. Baker	Venous expert turns CEO of medical center
38.	7/27/12	Hassan Najafi	W. Baker	Complete cardiovascular surgeon
39.	9/5/12	Norman R. Hertzer	W. McCarthy	Leader in outcome study
40.	9/11/12	Alexander W. Clowes	M. Kibbe, W. Pearce	Career investigative surgeon
41.	10/1/12	Richard F. Cambria	W. Pearce	Leader in thoracic vascular surgery
42.	10/1/12	Anton N. Sidawy	W. Baker	Scholarly academic surgeon
43.	10/17/12	Allan D. Callow	P. Lawrence, N. Rich	Carotid surgeon and philanthropist
44.	11/15/12	Jan Brunkwall	N. Rich	Leading endovascular surgeon
45.	11/15/12	Roger M. Greenhalgh	R. Gregory	Born to be a surgeon
46.	11/15/12	James May	R. Gregory	First endovascular surgeon in Australia
47.	11/16/12	Larry H. Hollier	R. Gregory	Surgeon, teacher, and CEO
48.	11/16/12	K. Wayne Johnston	N. Rich	Distinguished Canadian surgeon and leader
49.	11/16/12	Jonathan D. Beard	R. Gregory	Hemodynamic innovator and leader
50.	11/28/12	Jock H. Wheeler	W. McCarthy	Gentleman, dean and superb surgeon
51.	11/28/12	Roger T. Gregory	W. McCarthy	Multitalented vascular surgeon
52.	11/28/12	Frank J. Veith	R. Gregory	Educator, devoted advocate for vascular surgery
53.	3/6/13	John L. Ochsner	R. Gregory	Rex in vascular surgery
54.	4/4/13	Edward B. (Ted) Diethrich	R. Gregory, J. Yao	Public educator and innovator in vascular surgery
55.	4/19/13	Gregorio A. Sicard	W. McCarthy	Expert in open and endovascular surgery
56.	4/30/13	John A. Mannick	W. Baker, W. McCarthy	Lifelong academic vascular surgeon
57.	5/12/13	Frank W. Logerfo	M. Kibbe	Lifelong basic science researcher
58.	5/30/13	James C. Stanley	W. McCarthy, J. Yao	Defender of vascular surgery as an independent surgical specialty
59.	5/30/13	John P. Harris	M. Kibbe	Leader in Australian vascular surgery
60.	5/30/13	Stephen W.K. Cheng	P. Lawrence	Leader in Asian vascular surgery
61.	5/30/13	Jan D. Blankensteijn	W. McCarthy, J. Yao	European leading endovascular surgeon

(Continued)

TABLE 3-1. *(Continued)*

No.	Date of Interview	Interviewee	Interviewer	Subtitle
62.	5/30/13	Jean-Baptiste Ricco	W. McCarthy, J. Yao	President of European Society for Vascular Surgery
63.	5/31/13	Frans L. Moll	K. Cherry, J. Yao	Leader in endovascular surgery in Holland
64.	5/31/13	Enrico Ascher	K. Cherry, J. Yao	Brazilian-American leading vascular surgeon (from Brazil, living in New York)
65.	5/31/13	J. Fernandes e Fornandes	K. Cherry, J. Yao	Leading vascular surgeon in Portugal
66.	5/31/13	Anatoly V. Pokrovsky	N. Rich, J. Yao	Russian pioneer in cardiovascular surgery
67.	8/1/13	Jerry Goldstone	W. McCarthy	A pragmatic vascular surgeon
68.	8/19/13	Robert B. Smith	W. Pearce, J. Yao	Ultimate gentleman vascular surgeon from Atlanta
69.	3/14/14	Peter Gloviczki	M. Eskandari, J. Yao	A magical surgeon
70.	6/5/14	Christos Liapis	N. Rich	
71.	6/5/14	William Maloney	J. Yao, J. Towne, J. Goldstone, N. Rich	Executive Director, SVS-AAVS
72.	6/5/14	Piergiorgio Cao	N. Rich	
73.	6/6/14	Jacob Buth	R. Gregory, J. Yao	
74.	6/6/14	Takis Balas	N. Rich, J. Yao, R. Gregory	Senior surgeon in Greece
75.	6/6/14	Robert Zwolak	R. Gregory, J. Yao	Our man in Washington
76.	6/6/14	Oliver Goeau Brissonnier	N. Rich, J. Yao	
77.	2/6/15	Julie Freischlag	W. McCarthy, M. Kibbe	First woman president of SVS
78.	6/18/15	Timothy Chuter	R. Gregory, J. Yao	Innovative endovascular genius
79.	6/19/15	John Wolfe	R. Gregory, J. Yao	Academic English vascular surgeon
80.	6/19/15	Jean Pierre Becquemin	W. McCarthy, J. Yao	

In the beginning of the Society for Vascular Surgery (SVS), the Vascular Annual Meeting (VAM) was the most important function of the Society. The annual meeting brings members and guests together for an exchange of information. The first annual meeting was held June 8, 1947, at the Dennis Hotel, Atlantic City. In the beginning, the VAM was always held in early June at the same time as the AMA meeting at Atlantic City. Presentations in the first two years were on venous problems. The first presentation on arterial disease was in 1948 by Linton on popliteal aneurysm.

In 1951, the International Society of Cardiovascular Surgery, North American Chapter (ISCVS-NA) was formed. The majority of members were practicing vascular surgeons and soon it became the sister vascular society of SVS.

As time progressed, many critical issues emerged. Table 3-2 lists some of the notable events. Quite often, these issues needed to be addressed by SVS as well as by ISCVS-NA. In 1975, SVS and ISCVS-NA decided to form a joint council to address issues that may affect both Societies. They hired Mr. William Maloney to manage the annual meeting and to coordinate the business of each society. From 1975 until the merger of SVS and American Association for Vascular Surgery (AAVS, formerly ISCVS-NA) in 2003, Mr. Maloney worked closely with the presidents of both societies.

TABLE 3-2. NOTABLE EVENTS IN ADMINISTRATION AND MANAGEMENT OF SVS

1946	31 general surgeons with interest in vascular surgery founded the Society for Vascular Surgery (SVS)
1947	First annual meeting of SVS, June 8th, Dennis Hotel, Atlantic City
1951	The birth of International Society for Cardiovascular Surgery • North American chapter (ISCVS-NA) emerges as a sister vascular society of SVS
1951	International Society of Angiology
1957	International Cardiovascular Society
1966	Vietnam Vascular Registry by Norman Rich
1967	Joint Annual meeting of SVS and ISCVS-NA started
1970	Cardiac surgery became an independent surgical specialty
1971	Support of granting certificate to qualify surgeon from thoracic surgery representative, Hassan Anafi
1972	The vascular Credentials Committee renamed Program Evaluation and Endorsement Committee (PEEC)
1975	Joint Council
1975	Mr. William Maloney of PRRI (Professional Relation Research Institute) hired as Executive Director to oversee the business of SVS and ISCVS-NA
1975	John Mannick, James Yao and Alexander Clowes: Strategy planning for finding support for research 1. Cofounding with NHLBI/NIH of mentored research (KO8), clinical study (K23) grants to be supported by the von Liebig Foundation; 2. $3,000,000 matching grant from an anonymous donor; 3) $500,000 to support the Research Initiatives meeting (since renamed Joan and Julius Jacobson Research Initiatives meeting)
1978	E.J. Wylie traveling fellowship
1980	American Venous Forum founded
1984	Journal of Vascular Surgery • Founding editor: Michael DeBakey • Senior editor: Jesse Thompson
1984	Rutherford's *Textbook of Vascular Surgery*, now in the 8th edition, was first published. It is currently sponsored by SVS, who will have the right to appoint the editor.
1994	Association of Program Directors founded
1996	American Board of Vascular Surgery
1996	The 50th anniversary of SVS celebration: • The Celebration Committee • Calvin Ernest (Co-Chair) • James S. T. Yao (Co-Chair) • Members: Jesse Thompson, Allan Callow, Wiley Barker, James DeWeese, Harris B. Shumacker ,Jr. Of the 31 founders, only Michael DeBakey and Shumacker were still alive and well (Figure 6) A special issue of Journal of vascular surgery edited by Ernst and Yao was published

(Continued)

TABLE 3-2. *(Continued)*

2000	International Society of Cardiovascular Surgery-North American Chapter (ISCVS-NA) name changed to American Association for Vascular Surgery (AAVS)
2002	Political Action Committee (PAC)
2003	Merger of SVS and AAVS
2004	Administrative Structure of the new organization: • International Relations Committee • International Scholar Program • Chapters with other countries • Rutherford's *Textbook of Vascular Surgery* was given official sponsorship by SVS, editors to be appointed by SVS • Vascular Specialist—Official newspaper of SVS • SVS volunteers serve wounded soldiers • *The Pulse*—Newsletter of SVS • Quality Performance Initiatives • NSQIP: National Surgical Quality Improvement Program • Electronic media and SVS • History projects • Use of YouTube and the SVS website to disseminate information

In the early 1970s, several leading surgeons were concerned about the inadequacy of vascular training in the general surgical residency. The driving force for better training in vascular surgery that would result in better care for patients was from E. J. Wylie and James DeWeese. In his presidential address, Wylie called for one year of vascular fellowship training. The Inter-Society Council of the American Heart Association report on vascular care, in which U.S. hospitals were surveyed by Jim DeWeese's committee, which included Bill Blaisdell and John Foster as members, also found inadequacy of vascular training leading to poor vascular care of patients. Both Wylie and DeWeese agreed that a one-year fellowship in vascular surgery training was the only way to improve vascular care. When this idea was presented to the American Board of Surgery (ABS), there was little interest in the proposal. Under the leadership of several former presidents of SVS, the SVS Vascular Credential Committee was renamed the Program Evaluation and Endorsement Committee (PEEC). The PEEC then began site visits to approve one-year vascular fellowship programs. When the program was in place, the Residency Review Committee (RRC), with representation from ABS, American Medical Association, and American College of Surgeons, joined in and negotiations with ABS began. In his interview, Ron Stoney recalled the bitter negotiations with the governing agency. It took 12 years for Wylie to be awarded the first certificate in vascular surgery in recognition of his efforts.

The idea of a traveling fellowship modeled after the James IV traveling fellowship was hatched in a dinner with Jack Hoover and Don Lass of W. L. Gore and Associates in 1978. John Bergan and James Yao were present. It was agreed that the person-to-person contact was unique and would broaden the horizons of vascular surgery. At present three Wylie fellows have been elected president of SVS (Craig Kent, Peter Gloviczki and Julie Freischlag, first woman President of SVS).

In 1980, 20 members of SVS (Robert Barnes, John Bergan, John Cranley, W. Andrew Dale, Ralph DePalma, James DeWeese, Lazar Greenfield, Robert Hobson, Michael Hume, George Johnson, Robert Kistner, John Porter, Seshadri Raju, Norman Rich, Charles Rob, Joseph Sladen, D. E. Strandness, David Sumner, Leonel Villavicencio, and James S.T. Yao) founded the American Venous Forum (AVF) so that members of

SVS could donate to the Society under the tax exempt status. AVF operates independently and posts no financial burden to SVS. AVF and *Journal of Vascular Surgery (JVS)* have joined together to publish a new journal, *Journal of Vascular Surgery: Venous and Lymphatic Disorders*. The first issue was published in January 2013.

Michael DeBakey conceived the idea to have a journal published by SVS and approached the joint council about it. It was decided that DeBakey would be founding editor and under him would be two senior editors, Emerick Szilagyi and Jesse Thompson. Szilagyi was known to be the conscience of vascular surgery. John Ochsner chaired a publication committee to select a publisher and, under Ochsner's guidance, CV Mosby was selected with a generous financial package. The *Journal of Vascular Surgery* made its official appearance in January 1984.

In 1984, at the Joint Council meeting, Allan Callow suggested the establishment of a Lifeline Foundation to support research. It was decided a small asset of SVS would be used to support young members for basic science research. The Foundation was registered as a 501C(3) tax exempt organization to allow donations to the Foundation by members or others. During the time when John Mannick was president of Lifeline Foundation, he together with Alec Clowes and James Yao, developed a strategy to increase funding support for Lifeline Foundation. The group visited Claude Lenfant, director of NIH, to establish research support for young vascular surgeons. The group also worked with the von Liebig Foundation for cofunding support of NIH KO-8 and K-23 grants. In addition, the group initiated the $3 million matching grant sponsored by an anonymous donor as well as a $500,000 donation by Julius Jacobson to support the Research Initiatives meeting, which was renamed the Joan and Julius Jacobson Research Initiatives meeting.

The first Research Initiatives meeting, a joint meeting with NIH staff and investigators, was planned by Robert Barnes and D. E. Strandness along with John Watson, Chief of Devices and Technology, NHLBI. The meeting was in workshop format and covered a variety of vascular disease problems. The success of the meeting got the attention of Claude Lenfant and future meetings were planned. In 1988, the first jointly sponsored meeting was held in Bethesda on February 19–20 after which an annual joint meeting on specific topics was held at Bethesda in the month of February. In recent years, the Vascular Research Initiatives Conference has merged with the annual meeting of the Council on Atherosclerosis, Thrombosis and Vascular Biology of the American Heart Association.

In 2000, the name International Society for Cardiovascular Surgery-North American chapter (ISCVS-NA) was changed to American Association for Vascular Surgery (AAVS) because the word "International" gave the wrong representation of the organization. It was often mistakenly thought that the society was an international body rather than an organization with the majority of its members being clinical practicing surgeons in the United States. Similarly, government agencies preferred to deal with one body representing all vascular surgeons rather that two separate organizations. Thus, the merger of SVS and AAVS was accomplished in 2003. Jack Cronenwett representing the SVS and Tom Riles of AAVS worked in harmony to shepherd the merger of these two societies.. Both are happy with the outcome and as one would say, "UNITED, WE STAND." In 2004, the structure of the combined organization was established. This included publications, committees dealing with international relations, chapters in other countries, service to the military, and quality improvement initiatives. The structure remains relatively unchanged to this day.

In 2002, the leadership of SVS established the Political Action Committee to deal with government agencies on healthcare issues related to vascular surgery. Members serving in the beginning were Hugh Trout, Tom Riles, and Robert Zola, under the direction of William Pearce, then President of AAVS. The committee worked to promote the Screening Abdominal Aortic Aneurysms Very Efficiently (SAAAVE) act, which was signed into law by President Bush on February 8, 2006. They have raised $100,000 per year to support political campaigns and have worked on reimbursement and healthcare issues.

SVS has grown significantly since the beginning. The responsibility of the society is no longer just planning of the annual meeting. As you can see in this article, the society has faced many issues. These include reimbursement, medical-legal issues, finance, philanthropy, research, education, training, and certification. It is of interest to note the high number of issues in administration and management that the SVS has had to deal with. As Anton Sidawy said in his interview "SVS is not a society. It is now an institution." In addition, several vascular surgeons have held high administrative positions in their own institutions (Table 3-3). They were interviewed with the intention of finding how vascular surgery fares in the hospital structure and how our position as a leader in the hospital structure can be improved. With "Obama-care" in place, learning how to adjust to new systems of hospital care is of great importance to vascular surgeons.

COMMENTS

It has been said that oral history is history come alive and that has been our experience. After the completion of 80 interviews, we concluded the interview program described here has given a different dimension to recording the history of SVS. Unlike a written history, the oral history offers several advantages: (1) In audiovisual recording, facial expression and body language of the interviewee can be seen instantly; these subtleties may help to interpret the answers. (2) The interview process is interactive and the interviewee can ask questions if desired. (3) Current videotape technology produces a superb image and a short clip can be recorded instantly. We found viewers are interested in short clips to highlight historical events. Also, we found the interview

TABLE 3-3. EXAMPLES OF VASCULAR SURGEONS WHO HAVE ACHIEVED HIGH ADMINISTRATIVE POSITIONS IN THEIR HOSPITALS OR UNIVERSITIES

Vascular Surgeon	Position Achieved	Hospital/Medical School
Richard Dean	President	Wake Forest University Health Science
Larry Hollier	Dean	LSU School of Medicine
Thomas O'Donnell	President	New England Medical Center
Anthony Whittemore	Chief Medical Officer/Senior Vice President for Clinical Affairs	Brigham & Women's Hospital
Jock Wheeler	Dean	Eastern Virginia Medical School
Julie Freischlag	Vice Chancellor for Human Health Sciences and Dean of the School of Medicine	University of California, Davis

program to have educational value in terms of advice to young surgeons, the influence of mentorship, and tips for research planning. Finally, the audio recorded interview can be transcribed and edited to produce a book on leaders and contributors as a permanent record. We highly recommend that academic centers record their history as we described here. As Abraham Lincoln said, "We cannot escape history. Nothing has really happened until it has been recorded."

ACKNOWLEDGMENT

The authors express their deep appreciation for the editorial expertise of Jan Goldstein.

REFERENCES

1. Yao JST, Gregory RT, Rich NM, et al. Interviews with pioneers of vascular surgery*J Vasc Surg*. 2012;56:e52–e57
2. Yao JST, Gregory RT, Rich NM, History Project Work Group of the Society for Vascular Surgery. Interviews of leaders and contributors in vascular surgery. In Eskandari MK, Pearce WH, Yao JST, eds. *Current Vascular Surgery 2012*. Shelton CT: People's Medical Publishing House-USA, 2013, pp. 1–8
3. Gregory RT, Yao JST, Rich NM and the History Project Work Group of the Society for Vascular Surgery. Interviews with Pioneers of Vascular Surgery: Observations and Lessons Learned. In Eskandari MK, Pearce WH, Yao JST, eds. *Current Vascular Surgery 2013*. Shelton CT: People's Medical Publishing House-USA, 2014. pp 1–9
4. Yao JST, Gregory RT, Rich NM and the History Project Work Group of the Society for Vascular Surgery. Interviews with Leaders and Contributors of Vascular Surgery: A Summation. In Eskandari MK, Pearce WH, Yao JST, eds. *Current Vascular Surgery 2014*. Shelton CT: People's Medical Publishing House—USA, 2015, pp. xxxi–xxxix

4

Historical Events of SVS Based on the Interview Program: Innovations in Vascular Surgery

Roger T. Gregory, MD, James S.T. Yao, MD, PhD, Walter J. McCarthy, III, MD, MS, Norman M. Rich, MD, and The History Project Work Group of SVS

Before we describe the development of operative treatment, we need to review what has been done in the past. In general, there are three eras, which are described below.

ERA I: ANTIQUITY AND REPARATIVE SURGERY

Vascular surgery, like general surgery, began in antiquity with the Greeks or Romans. Early interest was focused on anatomy and, in Era I, operative treatment was often indirect with ligation being a common procedure. In 1543, Andreas Vesalius published his seven-volume book on human structure (*De Humani Corporis Fabrica*). Later interest was directed to the discovery of circulation as described by William Harvey in *Exercitatio Anatomica de Motu Cordis et Sanguinis in Animalibus* in 1628.

Most likely, vascular surgery began in 1546 when Ambroise Pare (Figure 4-1) used mass ligation to stop arterial bleeding. There are other reports that the great surgeon of ancient India, Sushruta, first practiced ligation of blood vessels.[1] For treatment of aneurysm, proximal or distal ligation or both was common (Figure 4-2). Sympathectomy, advocated first by Leriche in 1917, was the only method to increase limb blood flow.

Early ground breaking operative procedures and discoveries are listed in Table 4-1. Ligation was a common procedure for treatment of aneurysm and the case

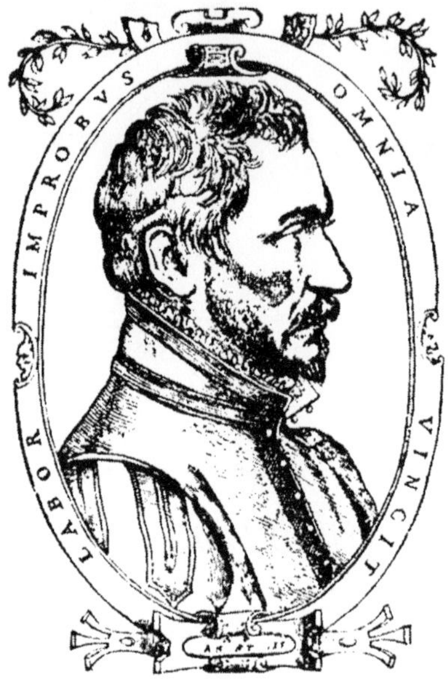

Figure 4-1. Ambroise Pare, the first to stop bleeding using mass ligation technique.

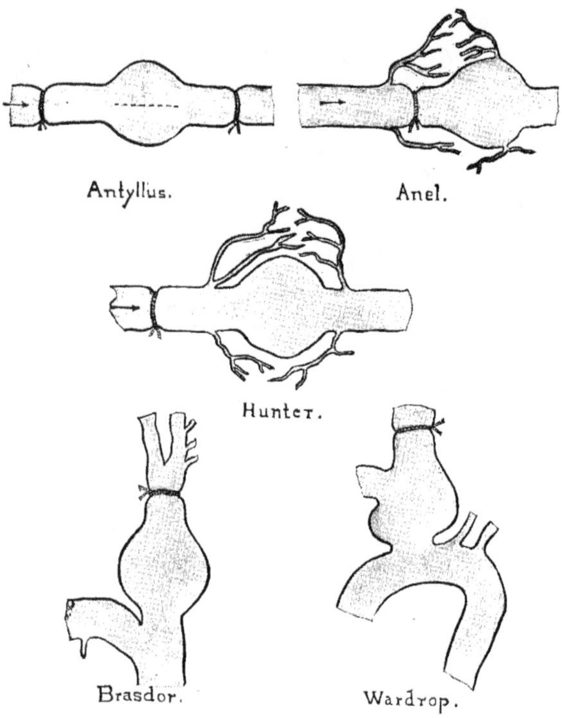

Figure 4-2. Ligation of aneurysm by different surgeons.

TABLE 4-1. LANDMARK HISTORICAL EVENTS IN THE ANTIQUITY PERIOD

1728	Ligation of femoral artery – John Hunter
1759	Arterial repair aided by a pin – Hallowell
1817	Ligation of abdominal aorta – Astley Cooper
1888	Endoaneurysmorrhaphy – Rudolph Matas
1896	First arterial anastomosis in human – John B. Murphy
1899	Description of the full thickness of arterial anastomosis – Julius Doerfler
1906	Triangulated suturing technique – Alexis Carrel (received Nobel Prize in 1912)
1915	The invention of heparin – Jay McLean
1920	The first arteriogram (trans lumbar aortogram) – Reynaldo dos Santos

by John Hunter is best known. The specimen showing the popliteal aneurysm is still on display at the museum in London (Figure 4-3). During the early time period, the teaching was to avoid trauma to the intima, which could explain why J. B. Murphy chose to use the invaginated technique for anastomosis. Later, Doerfler and Alexis Carrel used full thickness of the arterial wall for anastomoses and Carrel was awarded the Nobel Prize for the triangulated suturing technique (Figure 4-4).Two nonsurgical discoveries helped the growth of vascular surgery: Heparin, discovered by Jay McClean, and the arteriogram, developed by Reynaldo dos Santos. Ronald Baird gave

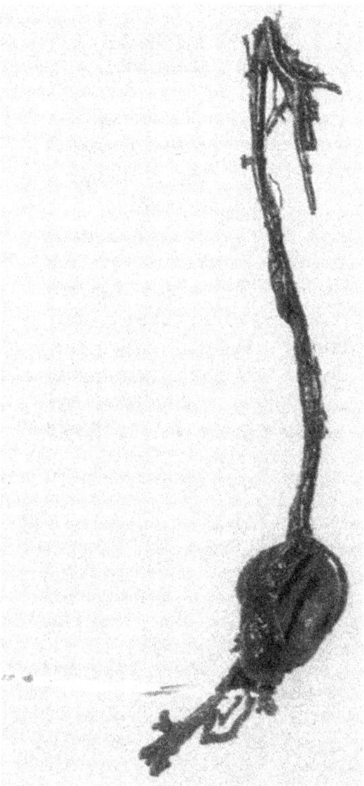

Figure 4-3. Hunter's ligation of femoral artery for popliteal aneurysm.

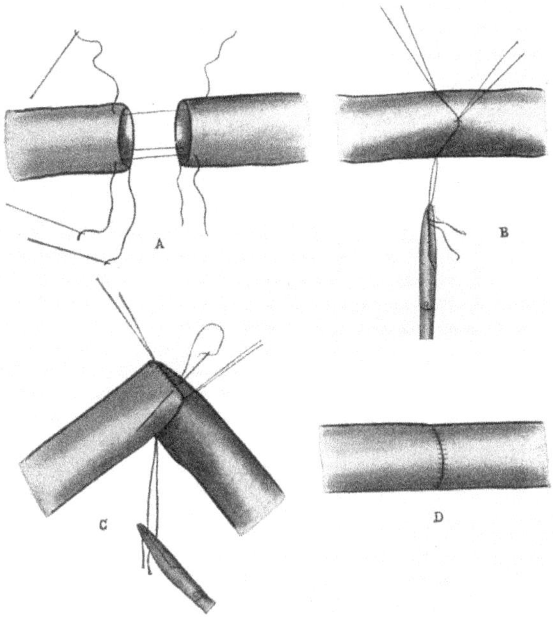

Figure 4-4. Alexis Carrel won the Nobel Prize for triangulated suturing technique and organ transplantation.

his Presidential address on Heparin and the clip of his interview videotape told the story.

During World War II from 1939 to 1945, DeBakey and Semeone reported the high incidence of amputation as a result of ligation. In an interview with Bill Blaisdell during the 50th anniversary celebration of SVS, DeBakey stated that the formation of the Society for Vascular Surgery was partly due to the concern about the high amputation rate during World War II. DeBakey further emphasized that vascular surgery should be a surgical specialty.

ERA II: DIRECT AND RECONSTRUCTIVE ARTERIAL SURGERY

After the report on thromboendarterectomy by Dos Santos, surgeons began to operate directly on arteries (Table 4-2). One of the world's most respected surgeons, Denton Cooley, repaired a ruptured thoracic aortic false aneurysm while he was a surgical resident at Hopkins in 1949. This made him the first surgeon to repair a ruptured thoracic aorta false aneurysm. In 1951, Edwin J. Wylie was the first American surgeon to use thromboendarterectomy in treatment of occlusive arterial disease. In his interview, Ron Stoney, partner of Wylie, talked about the friendship and respect between Dos Santos and Wylie.

TABLE 4-2. EVOLUTION OF OPERATIVE MANAGEMENT

1946	Thromboendarterectomy – A direct surgical technique on the artery to remove the atherosclerotic plaque – Cid dos Santos
1949	Femoral popliteal vein graft – Jean Kunlin
1949	First repair of a ruptured thoracic aortic false aneurysm – Denton Cooley
1950	Arterial repair in Korean War – Frank Spencer
1951	Aortic homograft for aortic aneurysm – Charles DuBost
1951	Edwin J. Wylie was the first American surgeon to use thromboendarterectomy in treatment of occlusive arterial disease
1953/1954	Carotid endarterectomy performed by Michael DeBakey and H. H. G. Eastcott
1953	Michael DeBakey perfected and popularized the use of Dacron graft Seldinger performed catheter arteriogram
1955	Semi-closed femoral endarterectomy – a serious attempt of endovascular surgery – Jack Cannon and Wiley Barker
1960	Michael DeBakey observed that the distribution of atherosclerotic lesions in arteries is often segmental in nature, a pathologic pattern that favors the use of bypass graft
1963	First axillo-femoral bypass – William Blaisdell
1964	First coronary vein bypass graft – Jimmy Howell and Edward Garrett
1966	Embolectomy – Thomas Fogarty Prosthetic graft – Arthur Voorhees
1967	Bypass to isolated popliteal artery – John Mannick Bypass to anterior or post-tibial arteries – Jimmy Howell
1970s	Decade of development of noninvasive tests and vascular diagnostic laboratory –Doppler ultrasound and duplex scan – Eugene Strandness –Hemodynamics for surgeons – David Sumner –Ankle-brachial index (ABI) – James Yao
1971	Discovery of Gore-Tex graft – Ben Eiseman
1974	The success of the cone-shaped filter – Lazar Greenfield
1975	First femoropopliteal Gore-Tex graft in America – Roger Gregory
1978	Percutaneous transluminal angioplasty – Andreas Gruentzig
1979	Balloon expansion stent – Julio Palmaz
1984	Self-fixing synthetic endovascular graft – Nicholay Vodolos
1988	Voluntary care of wounded soldiers at Walter Reed or Landstuhl, Germany
1992	Endovascular graft for aortic aneurysm – Juan Parodi EVT (endovascular graft) – Wesley Moore
1994	Outcome research – Norman Hertzer

The decade of the 1950s was the breakthrough period with the introduction of three signature operations: femoral popliteal vein graft by Kunlin; aortic homograft for aortic aneurysm by DuBost; and carotid endarterectomy performed by DeBakey and Eastcott in 1953 and 1954, respectively. It must be emphasized that the procedure by Eastcott was a transection of the diseased segment followed by reanastomosis of the two ends of the artery. In 1953, one of the major advances was the catheter arteriogram via the femoral artery and, with selective examination of different vascular beds, we were able to extend the operative approach to the superior mesenteric artery. Bypass graft to renal, mesenteric, tibial, and plantar arteries is now possible. In 1960, DeBakey observed that the distribution of atherosclerotic lesions in arteries is often segmental in nature, a pathologic pattern that favors the use of bypass graft. DeBakey's contributions to vascular surgery are legendary and too numerous to mention in this chapter. With the recruitment of Denton Cooley, Stanley Crawford, Arthur Bell, George Morris, and Edward Garrett, he single handedly transformed Houston into a major center for cardiovascular surgery.

In 1950, the dilemma of repair of an injured artery versus ligation was well illustrated by Frank Spencer serving in the Korean War. When he was told the rule book stated that ligation was required in all injured arteries, Spencer said in his interview, "This is an interesting situation, if you succeed in repair of an artery you got a decoration and if you failed you got court-marshaled."

Edwin Wylie was the first American surgeon to use thromboendarterectomy in treatment of occlusive arterial disease. In 1955, Cannon and Barker introduced the semi-closed endarterectomy, an initial attempt at endovascular surgery.

In his recollections about the development of vascular surgery, Charles Rob cited prosthetic graft for replacement of aorta and the femoral embolectomy catheter as the two most important inventions in vascular surgery since World War II. Fogarty described how he constructed the embolectomy catheter and how, interestingly, the paper on this technique was rejected by a few surgical journals before it was accepted by Loyal Davis of *Surgery, Gynecology, and Obstetrics* for the Surgeon at Work section.

Robert Smith, a close colleague of Voorhees, talked about the first use of prosthetic graft (vinyon-N) in an emergency operation for ruptured aortic aneurysm by Blakemore. When Blakemore asked for homograft but none was available, Voorhees left the operating room and went to the laboratory to construct a vinyon-N tube for use as a graft. The patient died of exsanquination 2 days later but the graft was patent. The successful use of prosthetic graft by the Blakemore-Voorhees team has inspired many surgeons to work with their industrial partners to develop the ideal prosthetic graft. The Dacron graft emerged as the graft of choice for replacement of aortic aneurysm.

In 1963, Wesley Moore told the story of how an ax-fem graft was developed while he was at the VA hospital in a case with Bill Blaisdell. The patient suffered a cardiac arrest during induction for redo of acute thrombosis of an aortofemoral graft done two days earlier. The patient was not a candidate for redo aortic graft operation, and it was the quick thinking of Bill Blaisdell to use the axillary artery as the inflow to the femoral artery that saved the patient. The ax-fem graft was a game-changing idea. The success of the ax-fem graft opened a new field in reconstructive surgery for revascularization in high risk patients and extra-anatomical bypass was born.

When infra-inguinal femoral bypass was first introduced, the distal anastomosis was often at the above-knee popliteal artery. As time progressed, distal anastomosis extended to the tibial or peroneal artery. John Mannick's discussion of his experience with bypass to isolated popliteal arteries is interesting. In addition to being the first to perform coronary bypass, Edward Garrett and Jim Howell were also the first to report bypass to anterior tibial and peroneal arteries.

In the decade of the 1970s many vascular surgeons were pursuing the study of non-invasive testing for diagnosis and objective assessment of vascular disease. Leading the field was D. E. Strandness of the University of Washington, Seattle group. Initially, indirect tests using plethysmography were common. With the Doppler ultrasound and duplex scan in conjunction with flow velocity recording directly over the stenotic lesion, the degree of stenosis could be estimated. In addition, the use of a Doppler made recording of ankle systolic pressure a simple procedure. The ankle/brachial index has been shown to be correlated with the degree of ischemia. For more information, the book "Hemodynamics for Surgeons" written by Strandness and David Sumner provides many answers.

Unlike arterial disease, operative management is seldom practiced in patients with venous problems. The placement of a vena cava filter is the exception. Lazar Greenfield recalled his experience on working with a petroleum engineer who encountered similar problems in their oil pipes and used a cone-shaped filter to trap the oil sludge and maintain the flow of oil. Greenfield emphasized the importance of learning from other disciplines when facing a similar problem.

ERA III: ENDOVASCULAR SURGERY

The late 1980s saw the development of minimally invasive catheter-based technology—endovascular surgery. Dr. N. L. Vodolos, a Russian surgeon in the Ukraine, has claimed to be the first to implant an endograft in a patient in 1984.[2] Despite this great success, there was no impact on the practice of vascular surgery in Russia. In contrast, the publication of five successful endovascular grafts by Parodi heralded the endovascular revolution in America.

Juan Parodi had been working on endovascular graft replacement since 1976 when he was a surgical resident at the Cleveland Clinic. However, it was not until 1988, when he began to work with Julio Palmaz, that his technique could be applied to treatment of aortic aneurysms. In 1990, a good friend of the President of Argentina, who had prohibitive surgical risks for the usual open procedure, underwent the endovascular graft procedure, which went well. Parodi performed the endovascular graft procedure on four more patients and all went well without problems. His paper describing these five cases was rejected by *Journal of Vascular Surgery* but later published in *Annals of Vascular Surgery*. Greg Sicard told the story in his interview, stating that John Bergan was instrumental in publishing the paper in *Annals*. When the article was published in *Annals*, John Bergan wrote an editorial comment predicting that there would be opposition, stating "In vascular surgery no change for the better has occurred that wise and good men have not opposed." The paper became a landmark publication and initiated a drastic change in the training and practice of vascular surgery. While Parodi conceived the idea of endovascular graft, others like Lazarus of Utah also were working on endografts with Wesley Moore and Endovascular Technologies (EVT) in a clinical trial. They performed the first endovascular graft implantation at UCLA Medical Center on February 10,1993. Since then, the endovascular revolution has swept vascular practice in America. The Society for Vascular Surgery (SVS) was busy providing retraining courses for endovascular technology, the endovascular graft registry under Rodney White started to track long term results and vascular fellowships were extended by a year to include training of endovascular technology. Finally, operating rooms were remodeled to include specialized equipment to accommodate endovascular surgery. In a short period, vascular surgery adjusted and continued to provide vascular care to patients. Vascular surgery has become a hybrid specialty and vascular surgeons must be equipped to provide open surgery or endovascular technology to patients.

Finally, no matter what you attempt to do, the outcome of your operative treatment is everything. The importance of outcome studies was stressed by Norman Hertzer in his Presidential address and has become an important element in the practice of vascular surgery.

COMMENTS

In all surgical specialties, operative treatment is always changing and in vascular surgery there is no exception. Operating, in a strict sense, is nothing but a craft requiring manual dexterity. It did not take long for technology to move in to further the development of this craft. As Francis Moore once said, "Advances in surgery have resided largely in the growth of effective technology." As vascular surgery progressed from ligation to direct reconstructive surgery, technology made a major step to develop surgery within the artery, i.e., endovascular surgery as defined by Wesley Moore.

At present, the distinction between a vascular surgeon and a general surgeon is clear partly due to vascular surgeons having acquired endovascular skills. Vascular surgery is now a matured surgical specialty. As we review the 80 interviews with leaders and contributors, we have a colorful past and, most important, we have expertise in every part of the vascular system.

ACKNOWLEDGEMENT

The authors express their deep appreciation for the editorial expertise of Jan Goldstein.

REFERENCES

1. Yao JST, Gregory RT, Rich NM, et al. Interviews with pioneers of vascular surgery. *J Vasc Surg.* 2012;56:e52–e57.
2. Svetlikov AV. Unknown pages in the history of vascular stent grafting. *J Vasc Surg.* 2014;59:865–8.

5

The American College of Surgeons Makes History Come Alive

David L. Nahrwold, MD

Historians and filmmakers have made history come alive to a receptive public. Even professional organizations have been stimulated to examine and record their histories. The vascular surgery community is in the vanguard. The work of The Society for Vascular Surgery to preserve its history and that of its illustrious members is admirable.

The American College of Surgeons (ACS), founded in 1913 by a group of surgeons led by Chicago surgeon Dr. Franklin Martin, has changed the face of health care and influenced the medical profession for more than 100 years (Figure 5-1). Fortunately, records of its activities and information about its leaders have been preserved and presented periodically for serious reflection and learning as well as for our pleasure. The Murphy Memorial Building, on Erie Street in Chicago, was opened in 1926. The records of the College were kept in the basement and the attic of the Murphy until the late 1990s. Through the efforts of Dr. C. Rollins Hanlon, former director of the College, these valuable materials were moved into the current headquarters of the ACS on St. Clair Street in Chicago and housed in a large archives room. Ms. Susan Rishworth was hired in 2000 to catalogue and manage the collection. After her retirement, Mr. Adam Carey became the College's archivist in 2014.

Included in the collection are complete sets of the minutes of the meetings of the Board of Regents and the Board of Governors of the College. Until the mid-1950s stenographers recorded everything said at each meeting, verbatim, in short-hand. After the meetings their recordings were collated and typed as a verbatim narrative that read like the record of a deposition. These records were paired with all the supporting material the Regents were provided for the meeting, such as reports of committees, position papers prepared by staff, reports from other organizations such as the American Board of Surgery and the American Surgical Association, and updates on congressional activity such as the debate over the social security act in the 1930s.

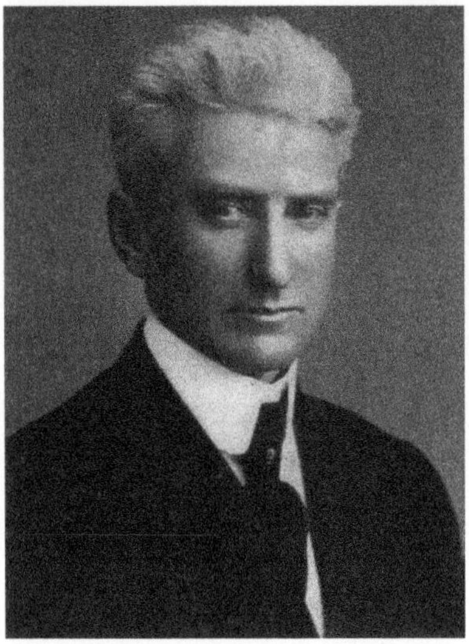

Figure 5-1. Dr. Franklin H. Martin, founder of the American College of Surgeons.

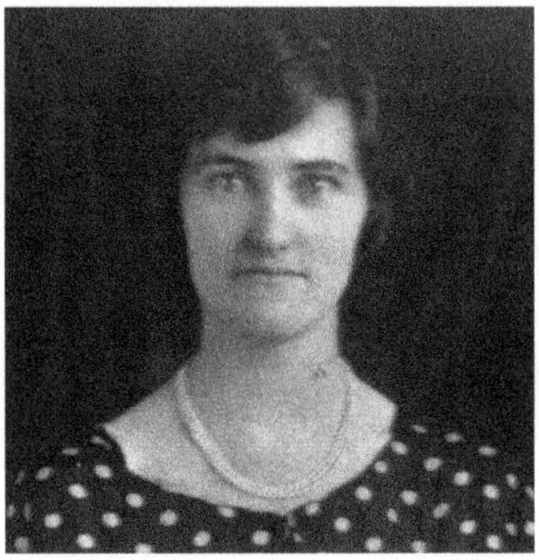

Figure 5-2. Miss Eleanor K. Grimm, Chief Administrative Officer, American College of Surgeons.

The minutes bring out the personalities of the officers and regents, and record important events. For example, the minutes of the meeting of June 10, 1956 state that Dr. Isidor Ravdin was in Washington, where he participated in ane operation on President Eisenhower. Banter between many of the distinguished surgeons is interesting and revealing.

Among the resources in the archives are 26 three-ring binders compiled by Miss Eleanor Grimm. Miss Grimm, at age 23, was hired by Dr. Martin as a stenographer in 1913 soon after the College was founded. She became his personal secretary, remaining so until Martin's death in 1935, but she also edited the College's publications, and by the time Martin died she was functioning as the chief administrative officer of the College, a position she held until she retired in 1950 (Figure 5-2).

In the late 1940s the Board of Regents asked the College's director of public relations to write a history of the organization. Ms. Grimm was called out of retirement to compile a historical record to facilitate the project. She dictated material about all the activities and programs of the College and information about its staff and leaders using a wire recorder. The recordings were transcribed and supported by documents, tear sheets from publications, and her personal notes, filling 26 loose-leaf binders. The director of public relations resigned from the College before writing the history, but Dr. Loyal Davis, who was editor of the College's journal, *Surgery, Gynecology, and Obstetrics* and chair of surgery at Northwestern, stepped in to write it, using Miss Grimm's notebooks as primary source material. His work, *Fellowship of Surgeons: A History of the American College of Surgeons*, was published in 1960 and reprinted seven times.[1] For many years Davis's book was given to each initiate during the convocation at the Clinical Congress. The book was a success because the College kept its records, which culminated in a book because a loyal employee, who had been present at the beginning, organized them and added to them.

Dr. George Stephenson, who worked for the College in many important roles from 1950 until his death in 1998, was also by virtue of his tenure and age the College's unofficial archivist and historian. In 1990 the College published his work, *The American College of Surgeons at 75*.[2] Stephenson described it as a companion piece to Davis's book and a chronicle of College activities from 1955 to 1988.

The most recent history was released in 2012 as part of the College's centennial celebration. *The American College of Surgeons, A History of Surgery and Surgeons 1913–2013* was written by Drs. David Nahrwold and Peter J Kernahan.[3] The book recounts the entire history of the College and was given to attendees at the 2012 Clinical Congress as a centennial gift.

The main activities of the College during its first fifty years were the Hospital Standardization Program, through which hospitals were evaluated for approval; its program to approve residency programs in general surgery and the surgical specialties; the continuing education of surgeons through its annual Clinical Congress; and its promotion of ethical and competent surgeons. The most significant and enduring contribution of the College was its Hospital Standardization Program, which transformed poorly managed, dirty hospitals occupied by the poor and sick into spotless, full-service institutions where patients were diagnosed, treated, and often cured of their diseases.

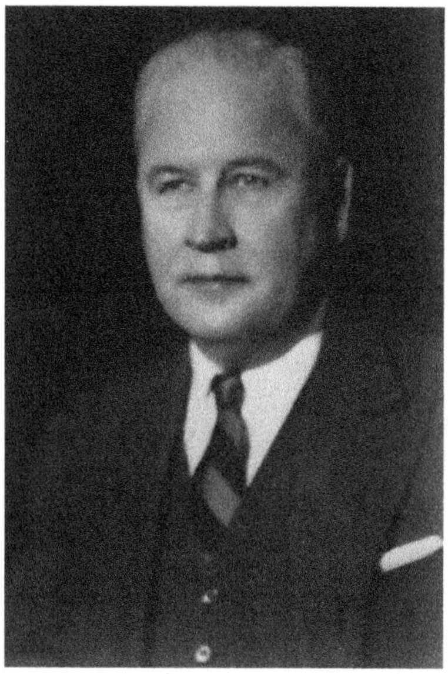

Figure 5-3. Dr. Arthur W. Allen, second President, the Society for Vascular Surgery.

The surgeon who preserved this program was Dr. Arthur W. Allen, chief of the East Surgical Service of the Massachusetts General Hospital. Jimmy Allen, as he was called by his friends, was a founder and in the second president of the Society for Vascular Surgery (Figure 5-3). Like a majority of the founding members, Allen was primarily a general surgeon, but he was interested in venous thromboembolic disease, as manifested by the title of his 1948 presidential address, "The Present Evaluation of the Prophylaxis and Treatment of Venous Thrombosis and Pulmonary Embolism."[4]

Allen was a Regent of the American College of Surgeons during his presidency of the Society of Vascular Surgery. A year later, in 1949, he was elected chairman of the Board of Regents, the most powerful office of the College. Allen and the College leaders were concerned about the excessive costs of the Hospital Standardization Program. Hospitals did not pay for their participation in the program; it was supported by the dues paid by the fellowship. Returning veterans complained that they were not receiving anything in return for their dues. Something had to be done. The College's director, Dr. Paul Hawley, had offered to transfer the program to the American Hospital Association (AHA), but the AMA vociferously opposed Hawley's proposal. Jimmy Allen stepped in and invited representatives of the ACS, AMA, AHA and the American College of Physicians (ACP) to a meeting on September 30, 1950. Chairing the meeting, Allen suggested that these organizations form a joint commission to take over the standardization program and accredit hospitals. The AMA and AHA representatives angrily rejected Allen's proposal, but he calmly guided them to agree to another meeting. After many contentious meetings, all led by Allen, the group finally agreed to form the Joint Commission on Accreditation of Hospitals, now known as the Joint Commission.[3] The founding of the Joint Commission was led by a surgeon who was a founder and president of the Society for Vascular Surgery.

In 2012, the College's centennial year, Dr. LaMar McGinnis, a past president of the College, prevailed on College staff to convene a group of surgeons interested in surgical history. With the support of Dr. David Hoyt, Executive Director of the College, a group met in April, 2020 and formed an entity within the College known as the Surgical History Group. An announcement in the June, 1913 *Bulletin* of *the American*

College of Surgeons invited all surgeons interested in history to attend a breakfast meeting at the Clinical Congress, which was held on October 8, 2013 in Washington, DC.[5] The featured speaker was John Schleicher, PhD, curator of the Orr collection of books at the University of Nebraska. The second meeting of the Surgical History Group was at the Clinical Congress in San Francisco in October, 2014, where the speaker was Dr. Craig A. Miller, who spoke about his new book, *The Big Z: The Life of Robert M. Zollinger, MD.*

The inaugural Clinical Congress session of the Surgical History Group was a panel discussion at the Clinical Congress in San Francisco on October 28, 2014. Panelists discussed the education and training of surgeons, the impact of professional organizations on American surgery, the influence of wars on surgery, and the partnership between surgeons and technology.

A poster session on surgical history and another panel discussion on factors shaping surgery over the 20th century were presented at the 2015 Clinical Congress.

An online history community was established by the College in 2014 on which ACS members post interesting historical documents and other material, announce events of interest, and use as a forum to discuss historically relevant issues and answer questions posted by the community leader, Dr. Kenneth Mattox. Postings and discussion by vascular surgeons would be most welcome. College communities can be accessed via the College's website under "member services."

Through the efforts of their members the Society of Vascular Surgery and the American College of Surgeons continue to preserve and bring alive the history of surgery and surgeons, hoping that future generations of surgeons will be inspired and motivated by the heritage left by their predecessors.

REFERENCES

1. Davis L. *Fellowship of Surgeons. A History of the American College of Surgeons.* Chicago: American College of Surgeons; 1960.
2. Stephenson GW. *American College of Surgeons at 75.* Chicago: American College of Surgeons; 1990.
3. Nahrwold DL, Kernahan PJ. *A Century of Surgeons and Surgery. The American College of Surgeons. 1913–2012.* Chicago: American College of Surgeon; 2012.
4. Shumacker HB. *The Society for Vascular Surgery.* Manchester, MA: The Society for Vascular Surgery; 1984.
5. Dr. LaMar McGinnis proposes forming club dedicated to surgical history. *Bull Am Col Surg.* 2013; 98:81.

6

Prevalence of Carotid Stenosis Varies by Race

Aleksandra Policha, MD and Caron B. Rockman, MD

In 2015, the United States population has grown to an astounding 321 million residents, making the U.S. the third most populous country in the world.[1] The population growth has been fastest among minorities, which now make up approximately one-third of the U.S. population.[2] According to the U.S. Census Bureau's estimation for 2011, almost 50% of American children under the age of 5 belonged to minority groups.[2] The fastest growing racial-ethnic groups are Hispanic Americans, now representing 17% of US population; black or African Americans accounting for 13%; and Asian Americans, American Indian and Alaskan natives representing 7%.[2] The Hispanic population is projected to more than double between 2000 and 2050, while the size of the Asian population is projected to increase by 79% during this time period.[2] As the ethnic minority population grows, health care, particularly preventive care, that caters to specific conditions with a high prevalence in each racial population would both improve quality of care and potentially lower costs. Epidemiologic studies of disease prevalence in different racial and ethnic groups represent the first line in shaping such customized health care.

Stroke remains one of the leading causes of mortality and morbidity in the United States, as well as worldwide. Stroke is the fifth leading cause of death and the primary cause of adult disability in the United States.[3] According to the American Heart Association (AHA), every 40 seconds someone in the United States suffers a stroke and each year approximately 795,000 Americans experience a new or recurrent stroke.[4] Stroke costs the nation $34 billion annually, including the cost of healthcare services, medications, and lost productivity.[4]

Multiple studies have demonstrated that stroke appears to be more common among certain racial populations.[5-15] For example, the Northern Manhattan Study (NOMAS) showed that both African-Americans and Hispanics had at least twice the incidence of stroke as compared with Caucasians.[6,8,16] Although the reasons for racial and ethnic differences in stroke incidence are not entirely clear, the disparate distribution of risk factor burden across racial groups must be considered a contributing factor. The Northern Manhattan Study showed that traditional atherosclerotic risk factors were more prevalent in certain racial groups.[6,8,16] Prevention of mortality, morbidity, and disability due to stroke requires a greater emphasis on the identification of individuals at high risk and efforts to modify the levels of risk factors in the affected population.

The prevalence of carotid artery stenosis (CAS), a treatable cause of ischemic stroke, has been shown to vary significantly by race.[16-21] Carotid artery disease is felt to be responsible for anywhere from 20% to 75% of cases of ischemic stroke in the United States.[22,23] The ability to actively treat significant carotid artery disease with either surgical or endovascular revascularization when clinically appropriate affords practitioners the potential ability to prevent future strokes. Perhaps more importantly, the presence of significant plaque at the carotid bifurcation serves as a marker for systemic atherosclerosis, and identifies patients who should be aggressively treated with pharmacological and lifestyle risk-reduction strategies. In this chapter, we summarize the existing literature on the incidence of stroke, the distribution of risk factor burden, and the variation of clinically significant CAS among different racial groups.

RATES OF STROKE ACROSS DIFFERENT RACIAL AND ETHNIC GROUPS

Cardiovascular diseases are the leading cause of the death in the United States, and it appears that disproportionate rates are seen in racial and ethnic minority populations.[24,25] Multiple studies in the literature document different rates of stroke in different racial and ethnic populations (Table 6-1).[6-16] The majority of these studies have demonstrated an increased risk of stroke in African-American and/or Hispanic patients as compared to Caucasian patients. The Northern Manhattan Study group reported that blacks had a 2.4-fold and Hispanics a twofold increase in stroke incidence compared with whites.[8] In their study, they also noted that atherosclerotic risk factors appeared to affect different ethnic groups in different ways.[6,8,16]

The incidence of stroke in the Native American population has been studied less frequently. The Strong Heart Study studied 4549 Native Americans, and reported that compared with US white and black populations, Native Americans have a higher incidence of stroke. The case-fatality rate for first stroke was also higher in Native Americans than in the US white or black populations in the same age range.[25]

The reasons for the increased risk of stroke in particular racial and ethnic populations are not entirely clear. A recent report from the REGARDS Investigators (Reasons for Geographic and Racial Differences in Stroke) encompassing more than 25,000 subjects reported that at age 45 years, incident stroke risk was nearly three times more likely in blacks than in whites.[26] Approximately half of the racial disparity in stroke risk was felt to be attributable to traditional risks factors including hypertension and socioeconomic factors. Therefore, the remaining half of the excess stroke risk in blacks was not explainable from these points of view. It is unclear whether they represent inherent differences in biology or genetic predisposition or are more reflective of different susceptibilities to atherosclerotic precursors or whether they are related to lifestyle and/or socioeconomic factors.

DISTRIBUTION OF STROKE RISK FACTORS ACROSS RACIAL GROUPS

We recently reviewed data from Life Line Screening (Independence, Ohio) on approximately 3.7 million individuals who underwent self-referred vascular screening tests at 20,000 sites between 2003 and 2008.[21] These individuals completed an extensive

TABLE 6-1. REPRESENTATIVE LITERATURE REPORTING DISPARITIES IN STROKE INCIDENCE AMONG DIFFERENT RACIAL-ETHNIC POPULATIONS

Author, Year	Data Source	Results
Howard, 1994[8]	National Longitudinal Mortality Study	Blacks had the highest relative risk of stroke mortality when compared to Whites and Hispanics.
Sacco, 1995[9]	Northern Manhattan Stroke Study	Atherosclerotic stroke was more prevalent in Hispanics and Blacks when compared to Whites. Extracranial atherosclerotic stroke was similar among the three races however intracranial disease was more frequent in Blacks and Hispanics.
Frey, 1998[10]	Barrow Neurological Institute stroke database (*n*=1716)	Prevalence of stroke types varied among Whites, Hispanics, and Native Americans. Lacunar stroke is more prevalent in Native Americans. Cardioembolic stroke is more prevalent in Whites. Hemorrhagic stroke is more prevalent in Hispanics. Native Americans had the lowest mean age stroke onset.
Sacco, 1998[11]	Northern Manhattan Stroke Study	The average annual age-adjusted incidence rate for stroke was greater for Blacks and Hispanics than for Whites. Among men, Blacks and Hispanics had a twofold increase in age-adjusted relative risk of stroke as compared with whites. Among women, Blacks and Hispanics were also found to have at least twice the incidence rates of stroke as whites.
Heuschamnn, 2008[12]	South London Stroke Register (*n*=2874, 63% whites and 28% black)	Total stroke incidence in the population decreased over the 10-year study. A similar decline in total stroke incidence was observed in Whites for men and women. In Blacks, total stroke incidence was reduced only in women. Total stroke incidence was higher in Blacks compared to Whites.
Lisabeth, 2008[13]	Brain Attack Surveillance in Corpus Christi (BASIC) project	There was no ethnic difference in the distribution of stroke type. Mexican American women had significantly elevated total stroke risk compared with non-Hispanic White women.
Cushman, 2008[14]	The Reasons for Geographic and Racial Differences in Stroke Study	Blacks had a greater age- and sex-adjusted mean 10-year predicted stroke probability than Whites.
Glymour, 2008[15]	Health and Retirement Study participants (*n*=20,661, reported first stroke 2175)	Black subjects had a 48% greater risk of first stroke incidence than Whites. Adjustment for adult socio-economic measures attenuated racial differences to a marginal degree.

(Continued)

TABLE 6-1. *(Continued)*

Author, Year	Data Source	Results
Rincon, 2009[16]	Northern Manhattan Stroke Study	The relative incidence rate for intracranial atherosclerotic stroke was higher among Blacks and Hispanics compared to extracranial atherosclerotic stroke.
Kleindorfer, 2010[17]	Greater Cincinnati/Northern Kentucky	Blacks had higher stroke incidence than Whites. When stratified by race and stroke subtype, this change was driven by a decrease in ischemic stroke incidence among Whites, whereas ischemic stroke incidence in Blacks was unchanged.
Howard, 2011[18]	Reason for Geographic And Racial Differences in Stroke national cohort study - REGARDS	The overall age-sex-adjusted black/white stroke incidence rate ratio (IRR) was 1.51: Black/white IRR was varied by age bracket with IRR of 4.02 for ages 45–54 and 0.85 for 85+.

Reproduced with permission from the *Journal of Vascular Surgery*.

Rockman, CB, Hoang H, Guo Y, Maldonado TS, Jacobowitz GR, Talishinskiy T. The prevalence of carotid artery stenosis varies significantly by race. J Vasc Surg 2013;57:327–37.

questionnaire, which included information on demographics, smoking, exercise, cardiovascular risk factors, comorbidities, and family history of atherosclerosis and vascular disease. Subjects who had a self-reported history of prior stroke or carotid artery intervention were excluded from the analysis. Of the 3,210,027 subjects included in our analysis, males comprised 35.6% (1,094,886) and females 64.4% (1,997,892). The great majority of subjects (85.6%) were between 51 and 80 years of age. Caucasians comprised 89.9% (2,845,936), African-Americans 3.1% (97,502), Hispanics 2.4% (75,240), Asians 2.0% (60,982), and Native Americans 2.8% (87,757) of the study population. The distribution of traditional atherosclerotic risk factors in the population varied significantly according to race ($p < 0.001$) (Figure 6-1). African-Americans had the highest prevalence of hypertension and diabetes, while Caucasians had the highest prevalence of hypercholesterolemia and a positive smoking history.

Other studies and national and regional surveys have similarly identified racial differences in cardiovascular risk factor prevalence. For example, in the 2003 Behavioral Risk Factor Surveillance System Survey (BRFSS), the prevalence of having two or more risk factors for heart disease and stroke (high blood pressure, high cholesterol, diabetes, current tobacco use, physical inactivity, and obesity) was highest among blacks (48.7%) and American Indians/Alaskan Natives (46.7%), and lowest among Asians (25.9%). The prevalence of having two or more cardiovascular risk factors was 35.5% among Caucasians and 39.6% among Hispanics.[27]

Cushman and colleagues evaluated the 10-year stroke risk by race and US region.[11] They found that African-Americans had a significantly higher age- and sex-adjusted mean Framingham Stroke Risk Score (FSRS) than Caucasians (11.3% vs. 9.7%). The FSRS predicts the 10-year probability of stroke based on nine stroke risk factors identified by the Framingham Heart Study Investigators: age, sex, systolic

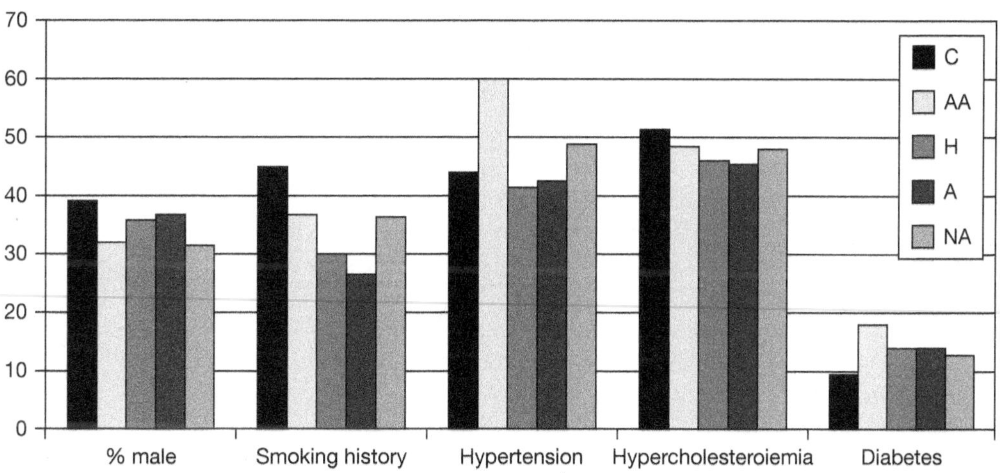

C = Caucasian

AA = African-American

H = Hispanic

A = Asian

NA = Native American

Figure 6-1. Prevalence of atherosclerotic risk factors in different racial groups. From Rockman CB, Hoang H, Guo Y, et al.[21] Reproduced with permission from Elsevier.

blood pressure, antihypertensive therapy, diabetes, current smoking, prior cardiovascular disease, atrial fibrillation, and left ventricular hypertrophy. This finding was true in all geographic regions and reflected a substantially worse risk factor profile in African Americans for all FSRS components (<0.0001 for each) except history of heart disease and atrial fibrillation, which were less common in African-Americans. Similarly, using data from the Third National Health and Nutrition Survey (NHANES III), Bravata et al.[28] found that in a population of noninstitutionalized Americans aged 40 years or older, with a self-reported stroke history, blacks had a higher prevalence of five risk factors independently associated with stroke: hypertension, treated diabetes, claudication, higher C-reactive protein, and inactivity. Whites had a higher prevalence of three risk factors: older age, myocardial infarction, and lower high-density lipoprotein cholesterol.

Less is known about the stroke risk factor burden among Hispanics and American Indians/Alaskan Natives. In the NOMAS, the proportion of strokes due to hypertension was reported to be greater among Caribbean Hispanics than among Caucasians.[29] In the San Antonio Heart Study, triglycerides, body mass index, and systolic and diastolic blood pressure were higher and high-density lipoprotein cholesterol level was lower in Hispanics than in non-Hispanic whites.[30] A recent study found metabolic syndrome to be more common among Hispanics than among whites or blacks or African Americans.[31] Even after adjustment for sociodemographic variables, metabolic syndrome was a better predictor of stroke risk among Hispanics than among whites. In NOMAS, hypertension, diabetes mellitus, hypercholesterolemia, heavy alcohol use, and current cigarette smoking were more prevalent in Hispanics than in whites.[29] Although the San Antonio Heart Study included Hispanics mostly of Mexican origin and NOMAS included Hispanics of Caribbean ancestry, the results appear similar.

DISTRIBUTION OF CAROTID ARTERY DISEASE ACROSS RACIAL GROUPS

There are fewer reports in the literature that deal with specific disparities in carotid artery disease among different racial and ethnic populations (Table 6-2).[16-20] Several of these have dealt with intima media thickness (IMT) as opposed to frank carotid plaque. As part of the Northern Manhattan Stroke Study, 526 stroke-free black, white and Hispanic residents were studied.[16] The maximal internal carotid artery plaque thickness (MICPT) was examined. The study reported that the mean MICPT was greater in whites and blacks than in Hispanics. After controlling for covariates including smoking, glucose, cholesterol, and hypertension, Hispanic race-ethnicity was still an independent determinant of less carotid plaque.

As part of the Insulin Resistance Atherosclerosis Study,[17] internal carotid artery (ICA) IMT and common carotid artery (CCA) IMT were assessed in 1020 non-diabetic participants, including blacks, Hispanics, and non-Hispanic whites. The study concluded that ethnic differences exist in CCA but not in ICA IMT in non-diabetic subjects. Blacks had significantly greater CCA IMT than non-Hispanic whites and Hispanics had significantly lesser CCA IMT than non-Hispanic whites; these differences remained significant after adjustment for traditional atherosclerotic risk factors.

Racial differences in carotid artery disease have been reported in non-U.S. populations as well. In a study from Amsterdam,[19] a hospital-based population of

TABLE 6-2. REPRESENTATIVE LITERATURE REPORTING DISPARITIES IN CAROTID ARTERY DISEASE AMONG DIFFERENT RACIAL-ETHNIC POPULATIONS

Author, Year	Data Source	Studied Ethnicities	Results
D'agostino, 1996[20]	The Insulin Resistance Atherosclerosis Study (n=1625)	White, Black, Hispanic	Blacks had significantly greater CCA IMT than non-Hispanic Whites Hispanics had significantly lower CCA IMT than non-Hispanic Whites. There were no significant differences in ICA IMT between Blacks or Hispanic versus non-Hispanic whites.
Sacco, 1997[19]	Northern Manhattan Stroke Study	White, Black, Hispanic	Average maximum ICA plaque thickness increased directly with age, and was greater in Whites and Blacks than Hispanics. After risk factor adjustment, Hispanic (versus non-Hispanic) race-ethnicity was still an independent determinant of less carotid plaque.
Wang, 2000[21]	Los Angeles County General Hospital	White, Hispanics, Blacks, Asians	There were significant differences in the degree of carotid stenosis among ethnic groups. Caucasian patients showed a statistically higher likelihood of having a severe or critical level of stenosis.
Wolma, 2009[22]	Academic Medical Centre, Amsterdam	White, Black, Asian, other	White patients have a higher odds ratio to have carotid artery stenosis. In Black and in Asian patients the association with carotid artery stenosis was substantially lower.
Mackinnon, 2010[23]	Family practices in South London, St. George's University of London	White, black	CCA IMT was higher in Black compared to White individuals. Carotid bifurcation and ICA IMT were also increased in Black subjects. In contrast, carotid plaque was more common in White individuals.

CCA = common carotid artery

ICA = internal carotid artery

IMT = intima media thickness

668 patients including whites, blacks and Asians was analyzed. The authors concluded that there is an association between white race and the presence of CAS. Not only in black but also in Asian patients, the association with CAS was substantially lower, even after adjusting for age, gender, hypertension and smoking. In the United Kingdom,[20] an additional study analyzed CCA and ICA IMT and plaque in 306 healthy black and 281 healthy white patients. The CCA IMT was higher in black as compared with white individuals after controlling for both cardiovascular risk factors and socioeconomic status. However, the presence of actual carotid artery plaque was noted to be more common in white individuals (OR 2.9, 95% CI 1.41-5.96).

Wang and colleagues conducted a study at Los Angeles County General Hospital, whereby they examined the degree of clinically significant carotid artery stenosis in a multiethnic patient population.[18] Carotid artery ultrasounds performed in 1006 hospitalized patients were reviewed. The indications for the examinations were variable, with 31% performed for stroke, 15% for TIA, 4% for amaurosis fugax, and 16% for syncope; thus, many of these patients had symptomatic cerebrovascular disease. The authors noted that 21.5% of Caucasian patients had greater than 59% stenosis, as compared with 10.1% of Hispanics, 8.7% of Blacks, and 10.7% of Asians (p<.001). The indications for ordering the test, patient age and gender did not vary significantly by race. When critical carotid stenosis was examined, 9.2% of Caucasians had greater than 79% stenosis, as compared with 4.3% of Hispanics, 2.9% of blacks, and 2.8% of Asians (p<.001). The authors concluded that significant differences in the degree of carotid stenosis exist among ethnic groups; Caucasian patients had a statistically higher likelihood of having severe or critical levels of stenosis.

Using Life Line Screening data, our group recently evaluated the prevalence of carotid artery stenosis by race in individuals undergoing self-paid vascular screening studies.[21] In both sexes, the prevalence of CAS increased with increasing age, although the proportion of patients with CAS in each age category was higher in male subjects than in female subjects. Overall, males between the ages of 81 and 100 had an 11% prevalence of CAS, while females in this age category had a 7.8% prevalence of CAS. In analysis of the relationship between age, race and CAS in male subjects, it was noted that in males of all ages, Native Americans had the highest rate of CAS, and Caucasians had the second highest rate (Figure 6-2, Table 6-3). Male African-American subjects had either the lowest or second lowest rate of CAS in all age groups except the youngest 40- to 50-year-old cohort. Female African-American subjects, on the other hand, did not appear to have the same degree of protection against CAS as did male African-American subjects, when compared to other races (Figure 6-3, Table 6-3). In female subjects of all ages, Native American subjects again had the highest rates of CAS, and Caucasian subjects had the second highest rates.

Similar analysis was performed for more severe CAS, equivalent to ≥80% by standard Duplex ultrasound criteria. The prevalence of severe CAS increased with increasing age. Males between the ages of 81 and 100 had a 5.7% prevalence of severe CAS, while females in this age category had a 3.6 % prevalence of severe CAS. In analysis of severe stenosis, it was noted that there was little change in the results of the analysis with regard to race (Table 6-4). In males of all ages, Native Americans again had the highest rate of severe CAS, and Caucasians had the second highest rate. Male African Americans had the lowest rate of severe CAS in age groups over 60 years, while female African-American subjects did not have the lowest prevalence of severe CAS in any age group, as compared to females of other races. In female patients of all ages, Native American subjects again had the highest rate of severe CAS, and Caucasians had the second highest rate.

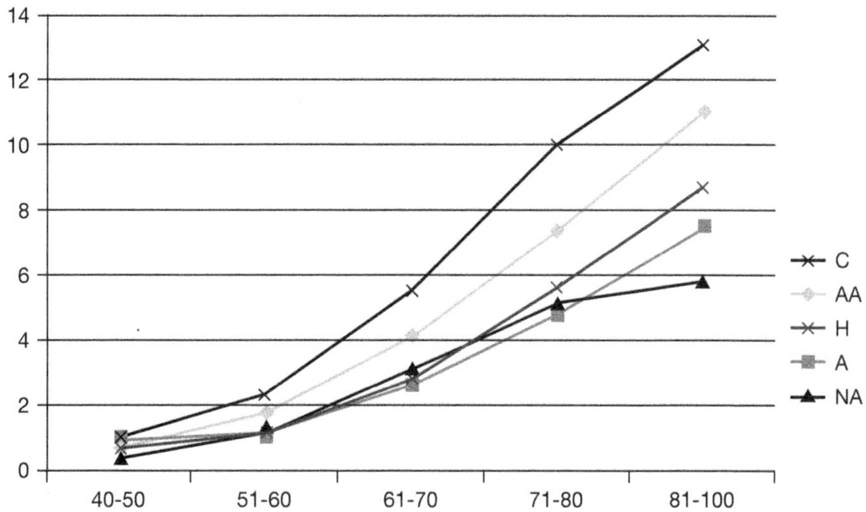

C = Caucasian
AA = African-American
H = Hispanic
A = Asian
NA = Native American

Figure 6-2. Relationship between race, carotid artery stenosis (□ 50%) and age in male subjects. From Rockman CB, Hoang H, Guo Y, et al.[21] Reproduced with permission from Elsevier.

TABLE 6-3. PREVALENCE OF CAROTID ARTERY STENOSIS (≥50%) AMONG MALES AND FEMALES OF DIFFERENT RACIAL GROUPS

Males	Age	Caucasian	Asian	African American	Hispanic	Native American
	40–50	0.7	0.4	0.9	0.7	1.0
	51–60	1.8	1.1	1.1	1.2	2.3
	61–70	4.1	3.1	2.6	2.8	5.5
	71–80	7.3	5.1	4.8	5.6	10.0
	>81	11.0	5.8	7.5	8.9	13.0
Females	40–50	0.9	0.9	0.8	0.8	1.1
	51–60	1.7	1.1	1.3	1.1	2.6
	61–70	3.4	2.2	2.6	2.3	4.7
	71–80	5.7	3.5	4.3	4.5	6.7
	>81	7.8	4.6	6.9	6.6	8.4

Reproduced with permission from the *Journal of Vascular Surgery*.

Rockman, CB, Hoang H, Guo Y, Maldonado TS, Jacobowitz GR, Talishinskiy T. The prevalence of carotid artery stenosis varies significantly by race. J Vasc Surg 2013;57:327–37.

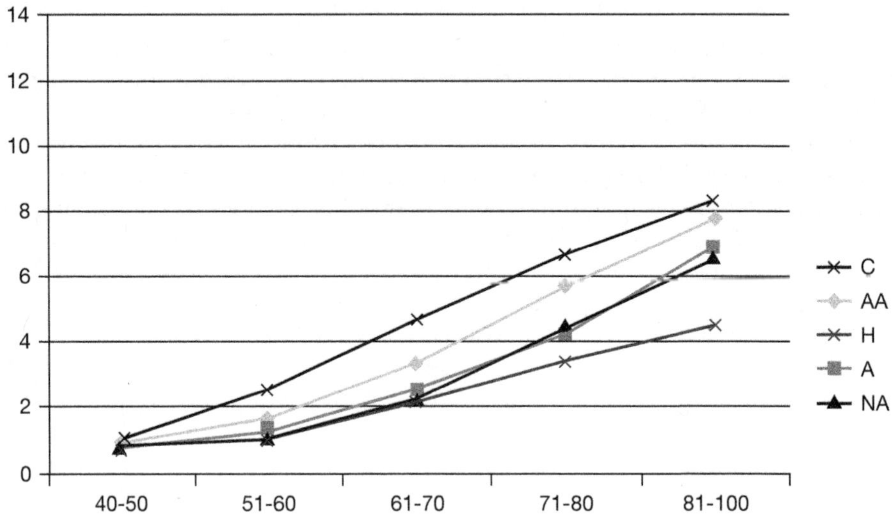

C = Caucasian

AA = African-American

H = Hispanic

A = Asian

NA = Native American

Figure 6-3. Relationship between race, carotid artery stenosis (≥ 50%) and age in female subjects. From Rockman CB, Hoang H, Guo Y, et al.[21] Reproduced with permission from Elsevier.

TABLE 6-4. PREVALENCE OF SEVERE CAROTID ARTERY STENOSIS (≥ 80%) AMONG MALES AND FEMALES OF DIFFERENT RACIAL GROUPS

Males	Age	Caucasian	Asian	African American	Hispanic	Native American
	40–50	0.2	0.2	0.1	0	0.2
	51–60	0.7	0.5	0.4	0.4	1.1
	61–70	1.9	1	1.2	1.4	2.6
	71–80	3.6	2.2	2.5	2.6	5.1
	>81	5.7	3.6	4.5	4	6.7
Females	40–50	0.2	0.2	0.1	0.2	0.3
	51–60	0.6	0.4	0.3	0.2	0.9
	61–70	1.4	1	0.8	0.8	2.1
	71–80	2.5	2	1.9	1.5	3
	>81	3.6	3.1	3.1	1.8	3.9

Reproduced with permission from the Journal of Vascular Surgery.

Rockman, CB, Hoang H, Guo Y, Maldonado TS, Jacobowitz GR, Talishinskiy T. The prevalence of carotid artery stenosis varies significantly by race. J Vasc Surg 2013;57:327–37.

In univariate analysis using the Caucasian population as the standard comparison group, we nßoted that African American, Asian, and Hispanic subjects were significantly less likely to develop CAS (≥ 50%), with unadjusted odds ratios of 0.64, 0.52, and 0.56, respectively (Table 6-5). Conversely, Native American subjects were 1.6 times as likely to develop CAS as compared to Caucasian subjects. Similar analysis of more severe carotid artery stenosis (≥ 80%) revealed similar unadjusted odds ratios (Table 6-5). When stratified by gender, it was noted that the unadjusted odds ratios for developing carotid artery stenosis in Hispanics, Asians and Native Americans as compared to Caucasians were essentially equivalent in male and female subjects of those races. However, African American males were less likely to develop CAS than African American females, with unadjusted odds ratios as compared to Caucasian males and females of 0.55 and 0.7, respectively (Table 6-6).

Multivariate analysis was performed, adjusting for smoking history, diabetes, hypercholesterolemia, hypertension and age. The adjusted odds ratios for the development of carotid artery stenosis as compared to Caucasian patients were again markedly reduced in African American, Hispanic and Asian subjects, and significantly increased in Native American subjects (Table 6-7). When comparing the unadjusted and adjusted odds ratios in each individual racial cohort, it was noted that the adjusted odds ratio for Native Americans was decreased as compared to

TABLE 6-5. UNADJUSTED ODDS RATIOS COMPARING OTHER RACES TO CAUCASIANS WITH REGARD TO THE PREVALENCE OF CAROTID ARTERY STENOSIS

Racial Group	Odds ratio for carotid stenosis > 50%	95% CI	Odds ratio for carotid stenosis > 80%	95% CI
Caucasian	1		1	
African American	0.64	0.61–0.67	0.59	0.55–0.63
Hispanic	0.56	0.53–0.59	0.48	0.44–0.52
Asian	0.52	0.49–0.56	0.46	0.42–0.50
Native American	1.6	1.56–1.65	1.7	1.61–1.75

Reproduced with permission from the *Journal of Vascular Surgery*.

Rockman, CB, Hoang H, Guo Y, Maldonado TS, Jacobowitz GR, Talishinskiy T. The prevalence of carotid artery stenosis varies significantly by race. J Vasc Surg 2013;57:327–37.

TABLE 6-6. UNADJUSTED ODDS RATIOS COMPARING OTHER RACES TO CAUCASIANS WITH REGARD TO THE PREVALENCE OF CAROTID ARTERY STENOSIS, STRATIFIED BY GENDER

	Caucasians	African-Americans	Hispanics	Asians	Native Americans
Females					
Odds ratio	1	0.7	0.57	0.52	1.63
95% CI		0.67–0.74	0.54–0.61	0.48–0.56	1.57–1.69
Males					
Odds ratio	1	0.55	0.55	0.54	1.65
95% CI		0.51–0.59	0.51–0.6	0.51–0.59	1.57–1.74

Reproduced with permission from the *Journal of Vascular Surgery*.

Rockman, CB, Hoang H, Guo Y, Maldonado TS, Jacobowitz GR, Talishinskiy T. The prevalence of carotid artery stenosis varies significantly by race. J Vasc Surg 2013;57:327–37.

TABLE 6-7. ADJUSTED ODDS RATIOS COMPARING OTHER RACES TO CAUCASIANS WITH REGARD TO THE PREVALENCE OF CAROTID ARTERY STENOSIS (ADJUSTED FOR SMOKING, DIABETES, HYPERCHOLESTEROLEMIA, HYPERTENSION AND AGE)

Racial Group	Unadjusted Odds Ratio	95% CI	Adjusted Odds Ratio	95% CI
Caucasian	1		1	
African American	0.64	0.61–0.67	0.65	0.62–0.68
Hispanic	0.56	0.53–0.59	0.74	0.70–0.78
Asian	0.52	0.49–0.56	0.69	0.65–0.73
Native American	1.6	1.56–1.65	1.3	1.25–1.34

Reproduced with permission from the *Journal of Vascular Surgery*.

Rockman, CB, Hoang H, Guo Y, Maldonado TS, Jacobowitz GR, Talishinskiy T. The prevalence of carotid artery stenosis varies significantly by race. J Vasc Surg 2013;57:327–37.

the unadjusted odds ratio; likely indicating a clinically significant effect of increased overall medical comorbidities in this group. Thus, approximately half of the increased prevalence of CAS in Native American subjects can be attributed to medical comorbidities, while the other half is presumably related to lifestyle or genetic factors. The unadjusted and adjusted odds ratios for African American subjects were essentially unchanged, likely indicating a relatively minor overall effect of aggregate concomitant atherosclerotic disease. Adjusted odds ratios for Asian and Hispanic subjects were less favorable than the unadjusted odds ratios, likely indicating a beneficial effect of fewer aggregate concomitant atherosclerotic precursors in these cohorts.

Multivariate analysis was utilized to determine the effects of traditional atherosclerotic risk factors upon the development of CAS in the different racial groups. In all races, increasing age was noted to be the most significant risk factor, with an adjusted odds ratio of 5.9 for subjects over the age of 70 years. A positive smoking history, diabetes, hypertension, and hypercholesterolemia all were significant independent predictors of CAS, with adjusted odds ratios of 1.9, 1.6, 1.6, and 1.4, respectively. The associations of traditional risk factors with the presence of CAS were nearly identical across all racial groups (Table 6-8).

Our results echo those of the Los Angeles County General Hospital study[18] discussed above: Caucasians appear to be more predisposed towards extracranial atherosclerotic occlusive disease than most other racial groups including African-American, Hispanic, and Asian populations. In our study, we described an asymptomatic screening cohort, as opposed to hospitalized patients with symptomatic cerebrovascular disease; thus, our results are likely more reflective of the true prevalence of occult carotid artery atherosclerosis in the general US population.

This information adds evidence to the hypothesis that the increased stroke rate in African-American patients and other racial groups is likely not related to an increased prevalence of extracranial cerebrovascular disease. In accordance with this, data from the NOMAS showed that among blacks, compared with whites, the relative rate of intracranial atherosclerotic stroke, extracranial atherosclerotic stroke, lacunar stroke, and cardioembolic stroke was 5.85, 3.18, 3.09, and 1.58, respectively.[32] Similarly, among Hispanics, compared with whites, the relative rate of intracranial atherosclerotic stroke, extracranial atherosclerotic stroke, lacunar stroke, and cardioembolic stroke was 5.00, 1.71, 2.32, and 1.42, respectively.[32] Thus, although the incidence of extracranial carotid disease may be greater in Caucasians, other factors account for the higher incidence of

TABLE 6-8. ADJUSTED ODDS RATIOS FOR OTHER ATHEROSCLEROTIC RISK FACTORS AND THEIR EFFECTS UPON THE DEVELOPMENT OF CAROTID ARTERY STENOSIS IN DIFFERENT RACES

Risk Factor	Asians	Hispanics	African-Americans	Native Americans	Caucasians
Smoking history	1.86	1.86	1.86	1.86	1.87
Diabetes	1.56	1.56	1.57	1.57	1.6
Hypercholesterolemia	1.44	1.44	1.43	1.43	1.44
Hypertension	1.61	1.61	1.61	1.61	1.64
50 and older	1.74	1.74	1.74	1.74	1.78
60 and older	3.35	3.35	3.35	3.33	3.39
70 and older	5.89	5.88	5.89	5.82	5.9
80 and older	9.42	9.4	9.4	9.2	9.4

Reproduced with permission from the *Journal of Vascular Surgery.*

Rockman, CB, Hoang H, Guo Y, Maldonado TS, Jacobowitz GR, Talishinskiy T. The prevalence of carotid artery stenosis varies significantly by race. J Vasc Surg 2013;57:327–37.

all forms of ischemic strokes in other racial/ethnic groups. Likewise, racial and ethnic differences in the incidence of hemorrhagic stroke were observed in the NOMAS patient population.[8] Incidence rates among Hispanic men were greater than those among black men and were almost three times those of white men (RR = 2.9).[8] Meanwhile, black women had the highest rate of intracerebral hemorrhage, over three times that of white women, while Hispanic women had twice the intracerebral hemorrhage rate of white women. The greatest subarachnoid hemorrhage incidence rate was found in black men, however, the small sample sizes precluded any meaningful comparisons or conclusions.[8]

To summarize, the prevalence of carotid artery stenosis varies significantly by race. Native American and Caucasian patients have the highest prevalence of CAS, while African American males and Asian females appear to have the lowest rates. When adjusting for age and other atherosclerotic risk factors, African-American, Asian, and Hispanic racial groups are approximately 30% less likely to have significant CAS, while Native Americans are 30% more likely to have CAS than Caucasians. The effects of other traditional atherosclerotic risk factors upon the development of CAS appear to be similar among different races. Increasing age appears to be the most significant factor in the development of carotid artery stenosis, across all races. Interestingly, the racial and ethnic differences in the incidence of CAS do not mirror the rates of ischemic stroke in these patient populations, suggesting that other factors, such as inherent biological differences, genetic predisposition, differences in lifestyle, socioeconomic factors and access to health care, play a significant role in the etiology of stroke. As the minority population in the United States continues to increase, knowledge of these etiological factors will guide future public health decisions.

REFERENCES

1. Commerce USDo. United States Census Bureau U.S. and World Population Clocks. 2015; Available from: http://www.census.gov/main/www/popclock.html
2. Commerce USDo. United States Census Bureau. 2015; Available from: https://www.census.gov/

3. American Heart Association and American Stroke Association. 2015; Available from: http://www.strokeassociation.org/STROKEORG/Professionals/CommunityResourcesandPatientEd/Stroke-Resource-Center
4. Mozaffarian D, Benjamin EJ, Go AS, et al. Heart Disease and Stroke Statistics-2015 Update. A Report From the American Heart Association. *Circulation.* 2015;131:e29–e322
5. Howard G, Anderson R, Sorlie P, et al. Ethnic differences in stroke mortality between non-Hispanic whites, Hispanic whites, and blacks. The National Longitudinal Mortality Study. *Stroke.* 1994;25(11):2120–5.
6. Sacco RL, Kargman DE, Gu Q, Zamanillo MC. Race-ethnicity and determinants of intracranial atherosclerotic cerebral infarction. The Northern Manhattan Stroke Study. *Stroke.* 1995;26(1):14–20.
7. Frey JL, Jahnke HK, Bulfinch EW. Differences in stroke between white, Hispanic, and Native American patients: the Barrow Neurological Institute stroke database. *Stroke.* 1998;29(1):29–33.
8. Sacco RL, Boden-Albala B, Gan R, et al. Stroke incidence among white, black, and Hispanic residents of an urban community: the Northern Manhattan Stroke Study. *Am J Epidemiol.* 1998;147(3):259–68.
9. Heuschmann PU, Grieve AP, Toschke AM, et al. Ethnic group disparities in 10-year trends in stroke incidence and vascular risk factors: the South London Stroke Register (SLSR). *Stroke.* 2008;39(8):2204–10.
10. Lisabeth LD, Smith MA, Sanchez BN, Brown DL. Ethnic disparities in stroke and hypertension among women: the BASIC project. *Am J Hypertens.* 2008;21(7):778–83.
11. Cushman M, Cantrell RA, McClure LA, et al. Estimated 10-year stroke risk by region and race in the United States: geographic and racial differences in stroke risk. *Ann Neurol.* 2008;64(5):507–13.
12. Glymour MM, Avendano M, Haas S, Berkman LF. Lifecourse social conditions and racial disparities in incidence of first stroke. *Ann Epidemiol.* 2008;18(12):904–12.
13. Rincon F, Sacco RL, Kranwinkel G, et al. Incidence and risk factors of intracranial atherosclerotic stroke: the Northern Manhattan Stroke Study. *Cerebrovasc Dis.* 2009;28(1):65–71.
14. Kleindorfer DO, Khoury J, Moomaw CJ, et al. Stroke incidence is decreasing in whites but not in blacks: a population-based estimate of temporal trends in stroke incidence from the Greater Cincinnati/Northern Kentucky Stroke Study. *Stroke.* 2010;41(7):1326–31.
15. Howard VJ, Kleindorfer DO, Judd SE, et al. Disparities in stroke incidence contributing to disparities in stroke mortality. *Ann Neurol.* 2011;69(4):619–27.
16. Sacco RL, Roberts JK, Boden-Albala B, et al. Race-ethnicity and determinants of carotid atherosclerosis in a multiethnic population. The Northern Manhattan Stroke Study. *Stroke.* 1997;28(5):929–35.
17. D'Agostino RB, Jr., Burke G, O'Leary D, et al. Ethnic differences in carotid wall thickness. The Insulin Resistance Atherosclerosis Study. *Stroke.* 1996;27(10):1744–9.
18. Wang MY, Mimran R, Mohit A, et al. Carotid stenosis in a multiethnic population. *J Stroke Cerebrovasc Dis.* 2000;9(2):64–9.
19. Wolma J, Nederkoorn PJ, Goossens A, et al. Ethnicity a risk factor? The relation between ethnicity and large- and small-vessel disease in White people, Black people, and Asians within a hospital-based population. *Eur J Neurol.* 2009;16(4):522–7.
20. Mackinnon AD, Jerrard-Dunne P, Porteous L, Markus HS. Carotid intima-media thickness is greater but carotid plaque prevalence is lower in black compared with whitesubjects. *AJNR.* 2010;31(10):1951–5.
21. Rockman CB, Hoang H, Guo Y, et al. The prevalence of carotid artery stenosis varies significantly by race. *J Vasc Surg.* 2013;57:327–37.
22. Endarterectomy for asymptomatic carotid artery stenosis. Executive Committee for the Asymptomatic Carotid Atherosclerosis Study. *JAMA.* 1995;273(18):1421–8.
23. Rockman CB, Jacobowitz GR, Gagne PJ, et al. Focused screening for occult carotid artery disease: patients with known heart disease are at high risk. *J Vasc Surg.* 2004;39(1):44–51.

24. Kurian AK, Cardarelli KM. Racial and ethnic differences in cardiovascular disease risk factors: a systematic review. *Ethn Dis.* 2007;17(1):143–52.
25. Zhang Y, Galloway JM, Welty TK, et al. Incidence and risk factors for stroke in American Indians: the Strong Heart Study. *Circulation.* 2008;118(15):1577–84.
26. Howard G, Cushman M, Kissela BM, et al. Traditional risk factors as the underlying cause of racial disparities in stroke: lessons from the half-full (empty?) glass. *Stroke.* 2011;42(12):3369–75.
27. Centers for Disease Control and Prevention (CDC). Racial/ethnic and socioeconomic disparities in multiple risk factors for heart disease and stroke: United States, 2003. MMWR Morb Mortal Wkly Rep. 2005;54:113–117.
28. Bravata DM, Wells CK, Gulanski B, et al. Racial disparities in stroke risk factors: the impact of socioeconomic status. *Stroke.* 2005;36:1507–1511.
29. Sacco RL, Boden-Albala B, Abel G, et al. Race-ethnic disparities in the impact of stroke risk factors: the northern Manhattan Stroke Study. *Stroke.* 2001;32:1725–31.
30. Mitchell BD, Stern MP, Haffner SM, et al. Risk factors for cardiovascular mortality in Mexican Americans and non-Hispanic whites: San Antonio Heart Study. *Am J Epidemiol.* 1990;131:423–433.
31. Boden-Albala B, Sacco RL, Lee HS, et al. Metabolic syndrome and ischemic stroke risk: Northern Manhattan Study. *Stroke.* 2008;39:30–5.
32. White H, Boden-Albala B, Wang C, et al. Ischemic stroke subtype incidence among whites, blacks, and Hispanics: the Northern Manhattan Study. *Circulation.* 2005;111:1327–1331.

7

Recommendations for Carotid Treatment among the Elderly

Kristine C. Orion, MD and Bruce A. Perler, MD, MBA

Stroke is the fourth leading cause of death, the second leading cause of cognitive decline, and the leading cause of adult disability in the United States, with similar epidemiologic findings in much of the Western world. The American Heart Association reports that 795,000 strokes occur annually in the United States, including 610,000 first time and 185,000 recurrent strokes. Currently, stroke is responsible for an estimated 137,000 deaths per year in this country or 5% of total annual mortality. Of those strokes that are not fatal, at least 15–20% are severely disabling and another 15–20% of stroke survivors will eventually experience a subsequent incapacitating event in the future. From a financial perspective, according to the Centers for Disease Control, the direct healthcare costs of stroke and the financial cost of days of missed work account for more than $34 billion annually.

Nearly 80% of cerebrovascular accidents are ischemic in origin. Carotid artery disease is the most frequent cause with embolization of plaque and/or thrombus from the carotid artery bifurcation, common carotid (CCA), or internal carotid (ICA) artery to the brain. Alternatively, among patients with very severe carotid stenoses, stroke can result from markedly reduced cerebral flow causing a low flow state leading to cerebral infarction. It is clear that many strokes are therefore completely preventable through the timely diagnosis of clinically significant carotid artery disease and the safe performance of carotid endarterectomy (CEA) or carotid artery stenting (CAS).

INDICATIONS FOR CAROTID INTERVENTION

CEA was first performed in the 1950s. After several natural history studies demonstrated the etiologic relationship between carotid artery stenosis, primarily due to atherosclerosis, and ischemic stroke, the procedure experienced remarkable growth over the next three decades with more than 100,000 operations performed annually in the United States by the early 1980s. As the procedure became more widely known and performed by an increasing number of surgical practitioners, however, several published reports documented unacceptably high rates of perioperative stroke and mortality in many centers, clearly negating the benefit of the procedure. This led to a backlash in the medical and neurologic communities and a marked reduction in referral of patients for carotid surgery and substantial drop-off in the volume of procedures performed in this country.

Subsequently, however, the completion of several randomized, prospective clinical trials in the 1990s, including patients with symptomatic and asymptomatic carotid disease, provided level I evidence confirming the safety and efficacy of CEA and best medical therapy compared to best medical therapy alone in terms of stroke prevention both in symptomatic and asymptomatic patients (Table 7-1).

CEA: Symptomatic Disease

The North American Symptomatic Carotid Endarterectomy Trial (NASCET) demonstrated a clear benefit of CEA and best medical management compared to best medical management alone for symptomatic patients with high-grade (70–99%) ICA stenoses.[1] In the same year, the European Carotid Surgery Trial (ECST) demonstrated a similar but smaller benefit in symptomatic patients with 70–99% ICA stenoses.[2] Analysis of a second cohort of symptomatic patients with moderate (50–69%) stenoses in the NASCET trial demonstrated a smaller but statistically significant benefit as well.[3] Today, there continues to be a consensus that the patient with a ≥50% symptomatic ICA stenosis is optimally served by CEA (Table 7-1).

CEA: Asymptomatic Disease

Similarly, Level I evidence derived from randomized prospective clinical trials clearly established the indications for CEA among patients with asymptomatic ICA stenoses. The Asymptomatic Carotid Atherosclerosis Study (ACAS) demonstrated a significant benefit of CEA and best medical management compared to best medical management alone for patients with asymptomatic 60–99% stenoses.[4] The inclusion criteria were similar, and the ACAS findings were confirmed, in the Asymptomatic Carotid Surgery Trial (ACST) in Europe.[5] In fact, based upon this evidence, the recently published Society for Vascular Surgery (SVS) Clinical Practice Guidelines noted that CEA "should be considered" for

TABLE 7-1. CAROTID ENDARTERECTOMY VERSUS BEST MEDICAL THERAPY: RANDOMIZED TRIALS

Trial	Perioperative			*P*
	Indication	CVA / Death	Risk Reduction	
NASCET	Sx: ≥70%	5.8%	16.5% / 2yrs	<0.001
	Sx: 50–69%	6.7%	10.1% / 5yrs	<0.05
ECST	Sx: 70–99%	7.5%	9.6% / 3 yrs	<0.01
ACAS	Asx: ≥60%	2.3%	5.9% / 5 yrs	0.004
ACST	Asx: >60%	3.1%	5.4% / 5 yrs	<0.0001

Sx: Symptomatic

Asx: Asymptomatic

NASCET: North American Symptomatic Carotid Endarterectomy trial; ECST: European Carotid Surgery Trial; ACAS: Asymptomatic Carotid Atherosclerosis Study; ACST: Asymptomatic Carotid Surgery Trial.

asymptomatic patients with ≥60% stenoses if the patient can be assumed to have at least a 3-5-year life expectancy and if the perioperative stroke/death rate is ≥3% (Table 7-1).[6]

However, this recommendation with respect to asymptomatic carotid disease has most recently been challenged by respected leaders in the field. Specifically, it has been argued that in light of recent significant improvements in the medical management of cardiovascular disease in general and cerebrovascular disease in particular, most, if not all, patients with asymptomatic ICA stenoses should be treated medically without intervention. This challenge to the evidence derived from randomized, prospective clinical trials, while not illogical on its surface, is not really supported by the predominance of the evidence. Specifically, while there has been a measurable improvement in the outcome of patients with asymptomatic carotid disease managed in contemporary practice with modern medical therapy, including the aggressive use of anti-platelet agents and statin medications, the outcome of CEA has also significantly improved compared to the surgical results in these trials not only as a result of better trained carotid surgeons, but perhaps most importantly because of the benefits of the same improved medical therapy. For example, in a series of nearly 1,600 patients undergoing CEA at the Johns Hopkins Hospital, we reported a significantly lower 30-day mortality and 30-day stroke rate among patients undergoing CEA while taking statins compared to patients who were not on these medications at the time of surgery. In fact, through multivariable analysis, we demonstrated that statins were associated with a threefold reduction in the rate of stroke ($p = .019$) and fivefold reduction in the rate of mortality ($p = .049$) at 30 days.

ASYMPTOMATIC DISEASE: PLAQUE CONSIDERATIONS

Although the ACAS and ACAS studies concluded that CEA was indicated for patients with a >60% ICA stenosis, the clinical benefit when compared to medical management was relatively narrow so that a higher degree of stenosis, generally >80%, seems a more appropriate criterion to consider performing CEA upon an asymptomatic patient in the absence of other confounding issues such as plaque morphologic considerations. It is clear, however, that the risk of subsequent strokes among patients managed medically increases with increasing degrees of stenosis. For example, the Asymptomatic Carotid Stenosis and Risk of Stroke (ACSRS) study evaluated the correlation between severity of stenosis and ischemic events.[7] Among 1,115 patients followed for up to 7 years, the incidence of ischemic strokes increased progressively with increasing severity of ICA stenosis. Specifically, using NASCET Duplex criteria, the hemispheric stroke rate was 3.4% among those with 50–69%, 3.2% among those with 70–89%, and 11.9% among those with 90–99% ICA stenoses.[7] Using the European method of stenosis grading, the ACSRS Study found a directly linear correlation between the degree of stenosis and stroke risk.[7] These findings have been corroborated by other investigations, demonstrating a relationship between the severity of ICA stenosis and future ischemic neurologic events.

In addition to the severity of the stenosis, progression of stenosis also has been correlated with future stroke risk among asymptomatic patients. In one report, for example, there was a twofold increased incidence of stroke among patients who experienced progression in the degree of carotid stenosis.[8]

Furthermore, increasing evidence demonstrates that the character of the plaque has significant prognostic value in predicting future stroke risk and therefore is an important criterion to consider in the selection of asymptomatic patients for intervention. Echolucency, ulceration, or evidence of intra-plaque hemorrhage are signs of the vulnerable or potentially unstable plaque. In a recent study, plaques were removed from 158 symptomatic patients at the time of CEA and analyzed. Multivariate stepwise analysis demonstrated that a large lipid core (OR 4.00, $p = 0.042$) and a low gray scale median (OR 6.21, $p = 0.003$) were independently associated with recurrent cerebral events.[9] Likewise, intra-plaque hemorrhage detected with duplex ultrasound or magnetic resonance (MR) imaging has been associated with plaque instability and may be a marker of patients who might benefit from carotid intervention. Other objective indicators of potential plaque instability and future stroke risk include microemboli seen on transcranial Doppler examinations and so called silent infarcts seen on CT or MR scans, indicative of previous microemboli. Both criteria are also highly correlated with future stroke risk, and therefore identify patients who might better be served by timely carotid intervention.

CAROTID ANGIOPLASTY AND STENTING

For nearly 60 years CEA has been the conventional standard of care for patients with clinically significant carotid artery disease in need of intervention. However, there has been a dramatic evolution in the management of vascular disease in recent years with as many as 70% to 80% of traditional open operations replaced by less invasive endovascular interventions. Within that context carotid angioplasty and stenting (CAS) has emerged as another option to treat patients with clinically significant carotid artery disease. In fact, in the early years of the clinical performance of CAS it was purported that this endovascular approach, as a less invasive therapy, would be most ideal for high-risk patients such as the elderly patient population. Early clinical experience ironically demonstrated, however, that the risks of CAS were significantly higher among the very elderly than when performed among younger patients.

COGNITIVE DECLINE

The prevention of stroke is the universally accepted indication, or goal, of medical management, as well as CEA or CAS, among patients with carotid artery disease. However, it is clear that many individuals experience cerebral infarctions in the absence of a clinically recognizable neurologic deficit. These so-called silent cerebral infarcts may be manifested as transient ischemic attacks, but in most cases are completely asymptomatic, at least clinically. However, silent cerebral infarctions are being increasingly recognized as an important potential cause of long-term cognitive decline.

The prevalence of cognitive impairment is 25% among adults aged 65 and older and occurs in two-thirds of those aged 85 and older. In light of the rapid growth in the elderly segment of our population, it seems clear that dementia may become an epidemic problem in our society and place a substantial burden on our healthcare system in the future. It has been demonstrated that at least 25% of older individuals have evidence on imaging studies of previous silent cerebral infarcts. While the performance of CEA or CAS among the elderly in most cases would be undertaken to prevent clinical strokes, it is not unreasonable to consider the secondary benefit of such interventions to be the prevention of cognitive decline in this patient population with asymptomatic carotid artery disease. Evidence is growing to support this indication for intervention among the elderly.

In the Cardiovascular Health Study, for example, 4,006 right-handed men and women 65 or older were evaluated. Thirty-two individuals with asymptomatic high-grade (≥75%) left and 29 high-grade (≥75%) right ICA stenoses underwent a Modified Mini-Mental State Exam. After adjusting for right-sided stenosis, high-grade left ICA stenosis was associated with cognitive impairment (OR 6.7) compared to persons with no ICA stenosis. The persistence of this association after correction for right-sided disease suggests that it is not due to underlying risk factors for atherosclerotic disease in general.[10] In another study, 70 patients with advanced carotid stenosis (≥70%) were compared with 70 control patients. Utilizing the Montreal Cognitive Assessment (MoCA) test, which is highly sensitive for subtle cognitive impairment, the individuals with carotid stenosis performed worse on visuospatial and executive function ($p = 0.018$), abstraction ($p < 0.001$) and delayed recall ($p < 0.001$).[11] Other research has demonstrated reduced attention and verbal memory loss among persons with severe carotid stenoses. Furthermore, the Korean Longitudinal Study on Health and Aging evaluated the possible association of early carotid atherosclerotic changes and cognitive function, and reported an independent association of carotid intima-media thickness with the development of mild cognitive impairment. In 348 subjects, 56 showed progression of cognitive decline at 5 years, and even after adjusting for conventional baseline risk factors, those patients with greater baseline carotid intima-media thickness had increased risk of cognitive deterioration.

It is widely held that mild cognitive impairment is a transitional stage between cognitive changes of normal aging and vascular dementia. This debility is not severe enough to constitute dementia but is clearly beyond the cognitive functioning deficit that is expected in normal aging. Even among patients who have never suffered a stroke, declining cognitive function can be lifestyle altering. In fact, in a recent poll conducted by the Associated Press among middle-aged Americans concerning their biggest health fears as they aged, memory loss was second on the list behind cancer, and in fact ahead of stroke or heart disease. Therefore, while preventing the development of cognitive decline cannot be proposed as an accepted indication for CEA or CAS, and certainly is not definitely evidence-based at this time, it is not unreasonable in formulating a treatment plan for the elderly patient population with asymptomatic carotid disease to consider the potential benefit of that intervention on the prevention of cognitive decline in some of those patients.

EPIDEMIOLOGY OF CEREBROVASCULAR DISEASE IN THE ELDERLY

More than 40 million people in the United States are over the age of 65 years. In fact, the elderly represent the fastest growing segment of our population and the most robust growth is among those aged 75 and older. It is projected that by 2035, at least 11 million people will be aged 85 years or older. Improvements in, and better access to, health care has resulted in an expectation that approximately half of our population will survive to at least 80 years of age. In fact, there are currently about 50,000 centenarians in this country.

The incidence of stroke increases exponentially with advancing age; both ischemic stroke and intracerebral hemorrhage double in each successive decade after the age of 55. The overall annual incidence of stroke per 100,000 population for individuals between the ages of 55 and 64 years is 262, which increases to 582 for those 65–74 years of age. It is 1382 for ages 75–84, and 1824 for individuals more than 85 years of age. While there are multiple possible causes for stroke, ischemic stroke is a major occurrence, and this stroke prevalence among the elderly is not unexpected when one considers the epidemiology of carotid artery disease among this demographic group.

It has been clearly demonstrated that the prevalence of carotid artery disease increases with advancing age and may be found in at least 10% of individuals age 80 and older. For example, in one community-based study utilizing duplex ultrasound examination, a ≥50% asymptomatic ICA stenosis was identified in 6.4% of individuals between the ages of 50 and 79. However, another recent analysis documented a prevalence of significant asymptomatic carotid stenoses in 7% of women and more than 12% of men over the age of 70.[7]

Not only does the prevalence of stroke increase significantly with advancing age, but also the morbidity of a cerebrovascular accident is especially severe among the elderly. Mortality after ischemic strokes increases with age and can be as high as 80% for those aged 75 and older. Approximately 65% of patients younger than 75 years of age will survive their initial stroke and be living 6 months later, whereas only 52% of those between 75 and 84 years of age will be alive 6 months after their initial event. Only 33% of adults 85 years of age and older will be alive 6 months later. In addition, it has been estimated that the financial cost of cerebrovascular accidents among patients older than 80 years exceeds $3 billion per year. Furthermore, since a substantial number of of post-stroke octogenarians and nonagenarians are institutionalized, the emotional and social consequences can be devastating.

Therefore, it can be logically argued that it is the elderly patient population who can most benefit from the safe performance of carotid interventions, yet it is this demographic group in whom aggressive carotid intervention has been most closely scrutinized, especially among those with hemodynamically significant, but asymptomatic, carotid stenoses. The authors believe the evidence is compelling to support the performance of carotid interventions among the elderly with the same selection criteria as those applied to younger persons. Specifically, it can be strongly argued that elderly patients with symptomatic significant carotid stenoses and those with asymptomatic high-grade and/or unstable/vulnerable plaques should be seriously considered for intervention if the patient is a good risk for the intervention and has a reasonable life expectancy that will allow the patient to benefit from the intervention. Furthermore, with infrequent exceptions, CEA represents the preferred intervention in this patient population.

OUTCOMES OF CAROTID ENDARTERECTOMY IN THE ELDERLY

Perioperative Results

Although very elderly patients have been excluded in several randomized clinical trials, and NASCET specifically only included patients aged 79 or younger, that study demonstrated that the benefit of CEA actually increased with increasing age.[12] The absolute stroke risk reduction during the 2-year follow-up period was

9.7% for those under 65 years, 15.1% for ages 65 to 74 years, and 28.9% for those 75–79 years of age. In other words, only three patients in the oldest group, versus seven patients in the 65–74 year age group, and 10 patients in the younger than 65 years age group would be required to undergo CEA to prevent a single ischemic event. Among patients with asymptomatic carotid disease, numerous studies have documented excellent postoperative results among patients over the age of 80 after CEA. For example, in a series of 360 CEAs performed upon 334 patients aged 80 or older, no difference was noted in the perioperative stroke/death rate between the asymptomatic octogenarians and younger patients (0.9% vs 1.4%; $p = 0.86$).[13] In addition, several recent large database analyses have also examined the influence of advanced age on the outcome. In a 2010 report from the SVS Vascular Registry, the 30-day rates of stroke and death were 0.91% and 2.52%, respectively among 4,169 patients aged 65 years or older undergoing CEA.[14] When comparing the combined outcome of in-hospital stroke, death, and myocardial infarction in 2,760 asymptomatic patients undergoing CEA aged >75 years or older to 1,389 patients younger than 75 years of age, there was no statistically significant difference. Likewise in a report from the Carotid Artery Revascularization and Endarterectomy (CARE) registry, the in-hospital mortality rate was only 0.7% among the elderly versus 0% in the younger group ($p = 0.006$).[15] In addition, in a recent analysis of the performance of CEA among Medicare beneficiaries, including 140,376 patients 80–89 years of age and 6,446 patients 90 years of age or older, the in-hospital morality was 1.5% while 30-day mortality was 2.2%. Nonagenarians experienced a 2.1% in-hospital mortality and a 3.3% 30-day mortality.[16]

Long-Term Results

As detailed in the SVS clinical practice guidelines, patients must survive for several years following CEA to justify the perioperative risks and realize the clinical benefits. Among asymptomatic patients, for example, the data indicate that one should anticipate a 3–5 year survival to justify the performance of CEA among asymptomatic patients.[6] Considerable evidence indicates that carefully selected elderly patients in fact experience sufficient survival to realize the benefits of CEA and most importantly experience stroke-free survival. In one report, for example, during eight years of follow-up, 87% of post-operative octogenarians survived and experienced no neurologic symptoms. In fact, the incidence of late stroke was only 2% compared to 17% of those octogenarians who had not undergone a CEA.[4] A recent report compared 69 asymptomatic octogenarians undergoing CEA plus best medical therapy to 54 octogenarians receiving best medical therapy alone. Freedom from cerebral ischemic events at 5 years was significantly superior for those elderly patients undergoing CEA (98% vs 84%; $p = 0.04$).[17] In another recent study from Italy, 269 octogenarians underwent 345 CEAs with an 86% 6-year overall survival rate and with a 76% stroke-free survival. These patients experienced a 1.4% perioperative mortality rate, which although higher than in younger patients, was still remarkably low and within acceptable cotemporary guidelines.[18]

These outcomes are not unexpected. The United States National Vital Statistics Report affirms that the average 80-year-old American has an expected 5-year survival of 70% and an overall life expectancy of nine years. These data indicate an expected 5-year survival in the average 90-year old American. These actuarial data and the preponderance of evidence accumulated to date suggest that elderly patients should be evaluated for the performance of CEA according to the same guidelines as younger patients, assuming there are not specific prohibitive medical contraindications.

OUTCOMES OF CAROTID ANGIOPLASTY AND STENTING IN THE ELDERLY

Perioperative Results

As noted above, it had been logically assumed that the endovascular approach of CAS would be particularly appropriate for elderly patients due to their presumed higher operative risk. However, initial investigations of carotid stenting documented unacceptably high rates of major adverse events, especially periprocedural stroke rates. In the lead-in phase of the Carotid Revascularization Endarterectomy Versus Stent Trial (CREST), the 30-day perioperative stroke rate increased progressively with increasing age; 1.3% among those 60–69, 5.3% among those 70–79, and 12.1% among those >80 years of age ($p = 0.0006$). In another analysis of 386 patients undergoing CAS, the 30-day stroke rate was 8.0% among octogenarians versus 2.7% among younger patients ($p = 0.02$) and the combined 30-day stroke, death, and myocardial infarction rates were 9.2% among octogenarians versus 3.2% among younger patents ($p = 0.02$).[19] In a recent report of a small group of nonagenarians undergoing CAS, the periprocedural rate of stroke or death was 18.2% among symptomatic and 10% (1 of 10) among asymptomatic patients.[20] The ALKK Carotid Artery Stent Registry found that the heightened in-hospital death rate in octogenarians was mainly driven by the increase in occurrence of ipsilateral major strokes. The 30-day stroke rate in CAS group as 11.3% vs 1.8% in CEA group ($p < 0.05$).[21]

In contradistinction to the disappointing CAS results reported in several series to date, the group from Northwestern reported comparable results among elderly patients undergoing CAS compared to younger patients, with a periprocedural stroke rate of 3.4% among patients ≥80 years of age.[22] One explanation for the increased neurologic complication rate among the most elderly patient population documented in many studies may relate to anatomic limitations seen in this patient population. When compared to individuals younger than 80 years of age, octogenarians have an increased incidence of arch elongation (56% vs 82%, $p = 0.008$), arch calcification (30% vs 59%, $p = 0.003$), common carotid artery origin stenosis (22% vs 47%, $p = 0.06$), common carotid artery tortuosity (38% vs 70%, $p = 0.009$), and internal carotid artery tortuosity (50% vs 74%, $p = 0.019$).[23] As experience with CAS grows, it is becoming clear that case selection depends not just on an assessment of clinical factors, but must carefully weigh anatomic considerations. The Northwestern experience may reflect judicious case selection.

LONG-TERM RESULTS

Limited data are available on the long-term outcomes among elderly patients undergoing CAS. However, the CAPTURE 2 trial evaluated 142 consecutive patients ≥80 years of age who underwent 153 CAS procedures. Patients with excessive vascular tortuosity or heavy concentric lesion calcification were excluded. At 6 months, eight patients had died (5.6%). At one year, an additional 15 deaths occurred but of the 114 surviving patients, 96.5% were free from any stroke. The Kaplan-Meier estimate of survival after CAS was 90% at 1 year and 76% at 3 years following CAS. The authors emphasized that any benefit of CAS may be eliminated if the periprocedural event rates are too high, so careful case selection is critical.[24]

CAROTID ENDARTERECTOMY VERSUS CAROTID ANGIOPLASTY AND STENTING: COMPARATIVE ANALYSIS

Several recent studies have directly compared the outcomes of CEA ad CAS in the elderly patient population. Whereas a minority of studies has suggested comparable outcomes of CEA and CAS among very elderly patients, the preponderance of evidence appears to favor CEA as a less risky option in this patient population. For example, in a review including 8 CAS and 33 CEA data sets, the pooled relative risk of stroke was 2.18 after CAS versus 0.63 after CEA, leading to an absolute higher risk for stroke of 3.46 for CAS. Although mortality and myocardial infarction rate were comparable, this analysis concluded that CAS is inferior to CEA in the octogenarian population based on stroke outcomes alone.[25] A comprehensive meta-analysis and meta-regression analysis reviewed 512,685 CEAs and 75,201 CASs reported in 44 publications. Advanced age, defined as >65 years, was associated with a more than 50% increased risk of stroke (2.4% vs 1.7%) in elderly patients undergoing CAS but not CEA. CEA had equivalent cerebrovascular outcomes in old and young age groups. Although there was increased perioperative mortality in the older patients versus young patients after CEA (0.5% vs. 0.4%), it is not clear whether this is clinically important.[26]

RECOMMENDATIONS

Cerebrovascular disease is one of the most important health problems in the United States and the Western world. Stroke is a major cause of death and disability and is responsible for an enormous financial burden on our healthcare system. Further, evidence is growing that atherosclerotic carotid artery disease may be an important cause of cognitive decline in older persons. Cerebrovascular disease is an especially prevalent and important problem in the elderly. The prevalence of cerebrovascular disease in general, and stroke in particular, increases exponentially with advancing age. In light of the rapid growth in the elderly segment of our population, the incidence of stroke can only be expected to rise significantly in the years ahead.

While only one of several potential causes of stroke, atherosclerotic disease of the carotid artery is one cause that is easily identifiable and treatable before stroke occurs. Furthermore, it seems clear that it is the elderly patient population that can most benefit from the timely identification of significant carotid disease and intervention.

The indications for CEA have been defined through the performance of several randomized clinical trials that have provided Level I evidence in both the symptomatic and asymptomatic patient populations. However, the very elderly were generally excluded from these investigations largely because of the concern that this patient population would not survive long enough to appropriately measure the long-term benefits of the studied treatments. What we learned from these trials, however, is that if a patient lives long enough, safely performed CEA provides superior stroke-free survival compared to best medical management. Therefore, it seems clear that if an elderly patient has appropriate indications for intervention, including either a significant symptomatic or severe and/or unstable-appearing asymptomatic stenosis, and if that patient's level of overall medical risk and/or comorbidity suggests reasonable life expectancy, that patient should be treated as aggressively as a younger patient with similar clinical indications.[6] In other words, age per se should not be a contraindication to intervention. Rather, it should be the physiologic age rather than the chronological age that the clinician must consider in developing a clinical plan for the individual patient.

On the other hand, the evidence to date suggests that age should be an important consideration in electing to treat the patient with CAS as opposed to the conventional CEA procedure. While carotid angioplasty and stenting techniques continue to evolve and improve rapidly, including but not limited to better cerebral protection methods and stent design, at the present time the evidence seems compelling that CAS has been associated with a higher rate of periprocedural stroke than CEA, and especially in the elderly patient population and often as the result of anatomic confounding factors. Because it is the primary purpose of carotid intervention to prevent stroke, and while there will always be exceptions and special circumstances, most elderly patients in need of intervention would be optimally served by CEA rather than CAS.

REFERENCES

1. North American Symptomatic Carotid Endarterectomy Trial Collaborators. Beneficial effect of carotid endarterectomy in symptomatic patients with high-grade stenosis. *N Engl J Med.* 1991;325:3445–53.
2. European Carotid Surgery Trial Collaborative Group. MRC European Carotid Surgery Trial: interim results for symptomatic patients with severe (70–99%) or with mild (0–29%) carotid stenosis. *Lancet.* 1991;337:1235–43.
3. Barnett HJM, Taylor DW, Eliasziw M, et al. Benefit of carotid endarterectomy in patients with symptomatic moderate or severe stenosis. *N Engl J Med.* 1998;339:1415–25.
4. Executive Committee for the Asymptomatic Carotid Atherosclerosis Study. Endarterectomy for asymptomatic carotid artery stenosis. *JAMA.* 1995;273:1421–8.
5. Halliday A, Mansfield A, Marro J, et al. Prevention of disabling and fatal strokes by successful carotid endarterectomy in patients without recent neurological symptoms: randomized, controlled trial. *Lancet.* 2004;363:1491–502.
6. Ricotta JJ, AbuRahma A, Ascher A, et al. Updated Society for Vascular Surgery guidelines for management of extracranial carotid disease: Executive summary. *J Vasc Surg.* 2011;54:832–6.
7. Nicolaides AN, Kakkos SK, Griffin M, et al. Severity of asymptomatic carotid stenosis and risk of hemispheric ischemic events: Results from the ACSRS Study. *Stroke.* 2005; 30:275-84.
8. Sabeti S, Schlager O, Exner M, et al. Progression of carotid stenosis detected by duplex ultrasonography predicts adverse outcomes in cardiovascular high risk patients. *Stroke.* 2007;38:2887–94.
9. Salem MK, Sayers RD, Brown MJ, et al. Patients with recurrent ischemic events from carotid artery disease have a large lipid core and low GSM. *Eur J Vasc Endovasc Surg.* 2012;43:147–53.

10. Johnston SC, O'Meara ES, Manolio T, et al. Cognitive impairment and decline are associated with carotid artery disease in patients without clinically evident cerebrovascular disease. *Ann Intern Med.* 2004;140:237–47.
11. Popovic IM, Lovrencic-Huzjan A, Simundic AM, et al. Cognitive performance in asymptomatic patients with advanced carotid disease. *Cogn Behav Neurol.* 2011;24:145–51.
12. Moon JH, Lim S, Han JW, et al. Carotid intima-media thickness is associated with the progression of cognitive impairment in older adults. *Stroke.* 2015;46:1024–30.
13. Miller MT, Comerota AJ, Txilinis A, et al. Carotid endarterectomy in octogenarians: does increased age indicate "high risk"? *J Vasc Surg.* 2005;41:231–7.
14. Jim J, Rubin BG, Ricotta JJ 2nd, et al. SVS Outcomes committee. Society for Vascular Surgery Vascular Registry evaluation of comparative effectiveness of carotid revascularization procedures stratified by Medicare age. *J Vasc Surg.* 2012;55:1313–20.
15. Rajamani K, Kennedy KF, Ruggiero NJ, et al. Outcomes of carotid endaterectomy in the elderly: report from the National Cardiovascular Data Registry. *Stroke.* 2013;44:1172–4.
16. Lichtman JH, Jones SB, Wang Y, et al. Postendarterectomy mortality in octogenarians and nonagenarians in the USA from 1993-1999. *Cerebrovasc Dis.* 2010;29:154–61.
17. Ballotta E, Toniato A, Da Roit A, et al. Carotid endarterectomy for asymptomatic carotid stenosis in the very elderly. *J Vasc Surg.* 2015;61:382–8.
18. Pruner G, Castellano R, Jannello AM, et al. Carotid endarterectomy in the octogenarian: outcomes of 345 procedures performed from 1995–2000. *Cardiovasc Surg.* 2003;11:105–12.
19. Stanziale SF, Marone LK, Boules TN, et al. Carotid artery stenting in octogenarians is associated with increased adverse outcomes. *J Vasc Surg.* 2006;43:297–304.
20. Wach MM, Dumont TM, Shakir HJ, et al. Carotid artery stenting in nonagenarians: are there benefits in surgically treating this high risk population? *J Neurointerv Surg.* 2015; 7:182–7.
21. Zahn R, Ischinger T, Hochadel M, et al. Carotid artery stenting in octogenarians: results from the ALKK Carotid Artery Stent (CAS) Registry. *Eur Heart J.* 2007;28:370–5.
22. Long GM, Kibbe MR, Eskandari MK. Carotid artery stenting in octogenarians: is it too risky? *Ann Vasc Surg.* 2005;19:812–6.
23. Lam RC, Lin SC, DeRubertis B, et al. The impact of increasing age on anatomic factors affecting carotid angioplasty and stenting. *J Vasc Surg.* 2007;45:875–80.
24. Chaturvedi S, Matsumura JS, Gray W, et al. Carotid artery stenting in octogenarians: periprocedural stroke risk predictor analysis from the multicenter Carotid ACCULINK/ ACCUNET Post Approval Trial to Uncover Rare Events (CAPTURE 2) clinical trial. *Stroke.* 2010;41:757–64.
25. Usman AA, Tang GL, Eskandari MK. Metaanalysis of procedural stroke and death among octogenarians: carotid stenting versus carotid endarterectomy. *J Am Coll Surg.* 2009;208:1124–31.
26. Antoniou GA, Georgiadis GS, Georgakarakos EI, et al. Meta-analysis and meta-regression analysis of outcomes of carotid endarterectomy and stenting in the elderly. *JAMA Surg.* 2013;148:1140–52.

8

The Use of Shunts for Carotid Endarterectomy

Kyla M. Bennett, MD and Cynthia K. Shortell, MD

Given that carotid endarterectomy (CEA) is a prophylactic procedure, in which the goal is to clear the internal carotid artery of atherosclerotic plaque that might otherwise serve as a nidus for a life- or lifestyle-threatening thromboembolic event, there is a general expectation that the procedure be performed with as little morbidity as is possible.[1] For this reason, many of the procedure- and anesthesia-related adjuncts that are used during CEA have been the subject of intense scrutiny, since even the slightest effect such an adjunct might have on the incidence of periprocedural morbidity has the potential to significantly alter the comparative effectiveness of the procedure in preventing atherosclerotic stroke relative to current medical therapy.

Of the many technical steps that are involved in performing CEA, perhaps none is as controversial as the utilization of an intraluminal shunt during the period of the procedure in which the internal carotid artery must be clamped in order to remove the atherosclerotic plaque. Such shunts are typically placed just prior to carotid cross-clamping, and are removed just prior to completion of the primary or patch closure of the arteriotomy. Although there are theoretical benefits to continued ipsilateral carotid arterial perfusion during endarterectomy, there is considerable debate as to whether these benefits are actually realized and are therefore sufficient to warrant the additional technical steps that must be taken to place an intraluminal shunt and the similarly theoretical risks associated with shunt insertion.

The controversy surrounding the need for intraluminal shunt placement is best evidenced by the wide variation in the actual practice patterns of vascular surgeons who frequently perform CEA. A review of the practices of 74 surgeons from a regional vascular surgery quality initiative highlights the considerable variability in the utilization of carotid shunts (Figure 8-1). Twenty-eight of the surgeons included in that review used a carotid shunt in over 95% of the CEAs that they performed, while a non-negligible number of surgeons used shunts rarely or never. The remainder of the surgeon participants in the quality initiative used shunts at a varying rate, presumably for specific indications based on intraoperative neurologic monitoring results or carotid artery stump pressure measurements.

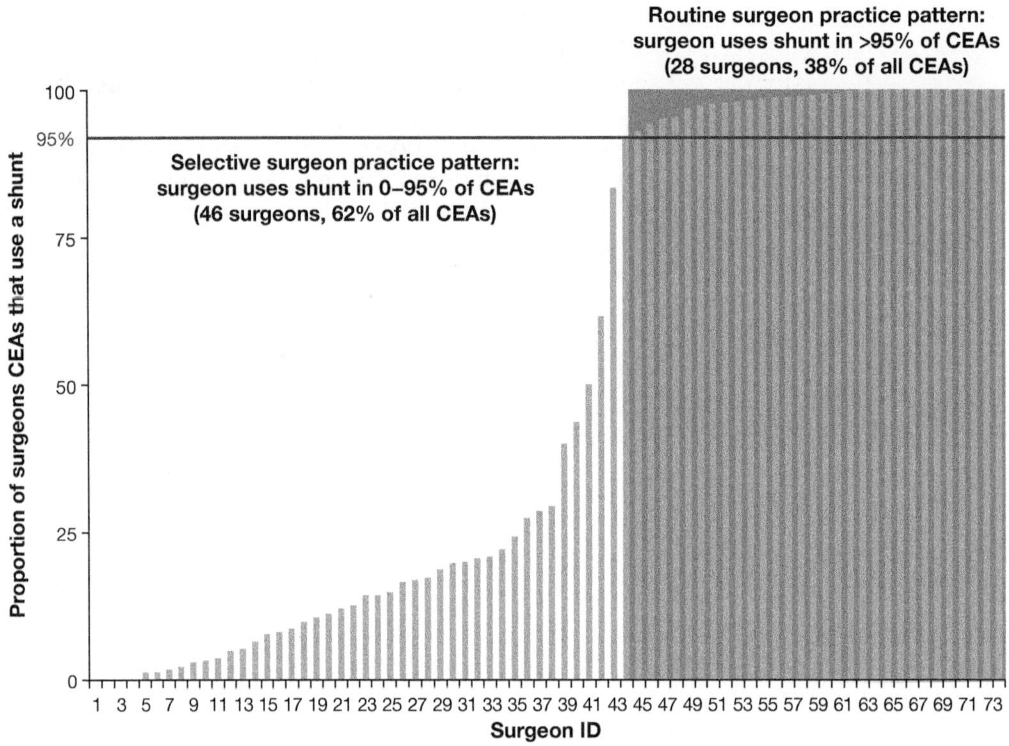

Figure 8-1. Surgeon practice patterns in shunt use in carotid endarterectomy (CEA). (Figure 2 from Goodney et al.[8] Used with permission from Elsevier.)

Given the considerable controversy in the need for shunting and the variability with which this procedural adjunct is actually used in practice, there is surprisingly little published evidence clearly supporting the need or lack of need for carotid shunting during CEA. The purpose of the current study is to review the available literature.

THEORETICAL ADVANTAGES AND DISADVANTAGES TO CAROTID SHUNTING

The primary theoretical advantage to carotid shunting during CEA is that the shunt permits continued ipsilateral carotid blood flow, and thus cerebral perfusion, during the period of the procedure in which the carotid artery is clamped. By extension, the use of a shunt during CEA should largely obviate the risk of intraoperative stroke that is due to clamp-induced cerebral ischemia. A multitude of single-center retrospective studies have demonstrated that the perioperative stroke rate among surgeons who routinely use shunts during CEA is consistently low, ranging from 0.7 to 3.6%.[2]

Although many surgeons use shunts routinely, other surgeons use them only for those patients who they believe to be at greatest risk for clamp-induced cerebral ischemia. Such patients typically include those with preoperative evidence of severe stenosis or occlusion of their contralateral carotid artery, or those patients who demonstrate evidence of neurologic or intravascular insufficiency at the time of carotid arterial clamping. Various modalities are available to guide the surgeon and anesthetist in deciding which patients might benefit from a shunt, including continuous electroencephalogram monitoring, transcranial Doppler ultrasonography, somatosensory evoked potential, cerebral oximetry monitoring, neurologic examination during regional anesthesia, and carotid stump pressure measurement.[2] Although no intraoperative neurologic or intravascular monitoring technique has been demonstrated to be superior to the others, alteration in one or more of the parameters measured with these techniques is used by many vascular surgeons as the criterion for using an intravascular shunt in order to reduce the risk of neurologic compromise secondary to clamp-induced hypoperfusion.[3] The use of some type of physiologic-based selection criterion in this manner results in an overall shunt placement rate of approximately 20% or less, and retrospective series that have detailed the results obtained with selective shunting protocols have yielded acceptably low perioperative stroke rates.[2]

The primary theoretical disadvantage to carotid shunt placement during CEA is that the instrumentation that is required to insert the shunt may potentially create atheroemboli or precipitate arterial dissection, placing the patient at risk of a thromboembolic cerebral ischemic event as well as other complications.[4,1] Given that the exact contributions of clamp-induced hypoperfusion and atheroembolism to cerebral ischemia during CEA is not currently known, opponents of carotid shunting fear that the potential harm associated with this procedural adjunct may outweigh its potential benefit.[4] Moreover, a number of published studies encompassing a large number of patients have shown that CEA can be performed without carotid shunts with an acceptably low incidence of perioperative stroke.[2]

DATA FROM PROSPECTIVE, RANDOMIZED TRIALS

To date, only a very few prospective, randomized trials have addressed the comparative outcomes of patients who undergo CEA with versus without intraoperative carotid shunting.

Palombo and colleagues prospectively studies 96 consecutive patients undergoing CEA for severe left internal carotid stenosis who were randomized to either receive or not receive a carotid shunt during endarterectomy. Patients with occlusion or severe stenosis of their contralateral carotid artery were excluded from the study. All of the procedures performed in this study were under general anesthesia and utilized the eversion technique. The outcome variables for their study were changes in the serum concentrations of several markers of cerebral ischemia immediately after (compared to immediately before) carotid clamping, and changes in neuropsychological testing 3 weeks after CEA (compared to preoperative testing). The authors found no significant differences between shunted and non-shunted patients in the preoperative or postoperative serum concentrations of the various markers of cerebral ischemia or in the preoperative or postoperative neuropsychological testing scores. The authors concluded that the choice of whether or not to use a shunt during CEA does not significantly influence the incidence of subtle cerebral damage, and that routine shunting is therefore without justification.

Gumerlock and colleagues performed a prospective randomized trial of intraoperative shunting on consecutive patients treated by an academic neurosurgical service between 1982 and 1986.[5] All patients in this study underwent preoperative bilateral carotid angiography, and all received general anesthesia with barbiturate induction intraoperatively. In addition, all patients included in this trial underwent primary closure of their carotid arteriotomy. Of the 63 CEA procedures which were randomized to intraoperative shunting, 32% had preoperative evidence of severe (>90%) contralateral carotid stenosis. Comparatively, only 19% of the 75 procedures randomized to the unshunted group had preoperative evidence of severe contralateral stenosis. The primary outcome for this study was the incidence of a new neurologic deficit within the first 24 postoperative hours. The incidence of such deficits was 0% in the shunted group, compared to 8% in the unshunted group (P = 0.02). The authors noted that none of the unshunted patients who sustained an early postoperative neurologic event demonstrated evidence of hemodynamically significant contralateral ICA stenosis preoperatively. Although the etiology of these neurologic events was therefore uncertain, the authors of the study concluded that shunt utilization during CEA resulted in fewer postoperative neurologic deficits.

Sandmann et al later published the results of a prospective randomized trial of shunt utilization in 503 patients undergoing CEA at an academic institution.[6] All of these procedures were performed under general anesthesia, and all patients received intraoperative neuromonitoring in the form of continuous electroencephalograms and somatosensory evoked potential monitoring. 157 of the procedures were performed by an attending surgeon, while 336 were performed by a surgeon-in-training. Technical factors precluded shunt utilization in 35 of the 250 patients who were originally randomized to the shunting group, while 10 of the 253 patients randomized to the no-shunt group ended up receiving a shunt due to significant neuromonitoring changes during carotid cross-clamping. In addition, 143 procedures required carotid reclamping due to technical issues found on intraoperative Doppler spectral analysis, and 200 procedures required an additional resection and end-to-end re-anastomosis of the ipsilateral artery to ensure adequate straightening.

The overall incidence of perioperative neurologic deficit did not differ significantly between patients who were primarily shunted (4.2%) and those who did not receive a shunt (3.3%). The highest incidence of perioperative stroke occurred in those patients who received a shunt secondarily (20%). The authors' primary conclusion was that intraoperative shunting should be used selectively based on the results of intraoperative neuromonitoring during carotid cross-clamping. This trial is subject to several criticisms, however. First is the considerable number of procedures which required carotid reclamping and/or additional arterial resection. Second is the fact that a small but important group of patients (those with significant changes in neuromonitoring during cross-clamping) who might be at greatest risk for perioperative neurologic compromise were essentially withdrawn from randomization by receiving a shunt secondarily due to these intraoperative changes.[6]

The most recent prospective randomized evaluation of shunt utilization during CEA was published by AbuRahma and colleagues in 2010.[7] In this single-center trial, 200 CEA patients were randomized to either a routine shunting group or a selective shunting group (in which a shunt was placed only if the patient's systolic carotid stump pressure measured less than 40 mm Hg during carotid cross-clamping. All of the patients in this trial received general anesthesia, and all arteriotomies were closed using prosthetic patch angioplasty.

Ninety-eight patients were randomized to the routine shunting group and 102 patients to the selective shunting group. Twenty-nine (28%) patients in the selective shunting group actually received an intraoperative shunt because their systolic stump pressure fell below the 40 mm Hg threshold. The two groups were similar with respect to their incidence of comorbid conditions, their indications for CEA, and their preoperative symptomatology. Although the two groups were comparable in terms of their degrees of ipsilateral and contralateral stenosis, patients from the selective shunting group who received an intraoperative shunt had a significantly greater degree of contralateral carotid stenosis compared to patients from the selective shunting group who did not receive a shunt (56% versus 34%, P = 0.002). Patients from the routine versus selective shunting groups had similar mean internal carotid artery diameters, mean carotid cross-clamp times, mean operative times, and mean arteriotomy length.

The 30-day combined stroke/TIA rate for the two groups was statistically no different (2% in the routine shunt group versus 3% in the selective shunt group), as were the 30-day incidences of other non-neurologic complications. The authors of the study concluded that either approach to intraoperative shunting during CEA (routine or selective) is acceptable, and that both are associated with low stroke rates. The authors' study design did not allow for a prospective comparison of procedures that did or did not include an intraoperative shunt, however, and was therefore unable to evaluate the outcomes associated with a "routine non-shunt" approach to CEA.

Chongruksut et al subsequently published a systematic review of the four previously discussed prospective, randomized trials in 2014 as a part of The Cochrane Collaboration.[3] The authors of this review noted that the reporting of methodology in these studies was poor, with the blinding of outcome assessors and the report of prespecified outcomes being generally unclear. The authors found no significant difference in the rate of stroke or death at up to 30 postoperative days between procedures in which a routine shunt was placed compared to procedures in which no shunt was placed. In their systematic review of the literature, the authors could not find any evidence of a study being performed where selective shunting was compared to routine non-shunting. The authors of this review concluded that the body of published evidence is "too limited to either support or refute the use of routine or selective shunting in carotid endarterectomy." The authors also concluded that no specific method of neuromonitoring has been found to be clearly preferential over others for use in selective shunting strategies.[3]

RETROSPECTIVE ANALYSES OF LARGE MULTICENTER DATA SOURCES

Given the lack of conclusive randomized data, and the practical difficulties that are inherent in conducting a well-designed trial in which all of the many facets of the CEA procedure are standardized *except* for shunt use, two groups have attempted to use data from large, multi-center, vascular-specific databases in order to further compare the outcomes of patients who undergo CEA with or without shunting.

In 2012, Goodney and colleagues published a retrospective analysis of patients from the Vascular Study Group of New England (VSGNE) which attempted to determine the impact of shunt practice patterns on outcomes after carotid endarterectomy in patients with contralateral carotid artery occlusion.[8] The VSGNE comprises information about all vascular surgery patients who receive operation from 74 vascular surgeons at 12 different hospitals in New England. The information contained within the VSGNE database is prospectively collected, and periodic audits are performed against claims data in order to ensure that all vascular surgery patients at a contributing hospital are captured by the VSGNE.[8] The authors of this study examined all patients from the VSGNE database who underwent primary CEA from 2003 through 2009 and in whom preoperative carotid imaging was available (including either duplex ultrasound, computed tomography, or magnetic resonance imaging). Patients who underwent combined CEA and coronary artery bypass grafting were excluded from analysis, and those in whom the details of shunt placement and/or intraoperative monitoring were missing, were excluded from analysis.

The primary predictor variable in the analysis by Goodney et al was the presence or absence of contralateral carotid occlusion (CCO). Secondary predictor variables included the type of intraoperative shunt used (when patients received a shunt), and the shunt practice pattern of the operating surgeon. Surgeons were categorized as routine shunters if >95% of the CEA procedures that they performed included intraoperative shunting, or as selective shunters if ≥95% of the CEA procedures involved shunt placement. The authors also considered defined usage from the perspective of the patient/procedure as the unit of analysis, classifying patients as receiving no shunt, a routine shunt (if their surgeon performed shunting in >95% of their patients), or a shunt for indication (if their surgeon placed shunts only for specific indications such as intraoperative EEG/neurologic changes or low carotid stump pressures during carotid clamping). The primary outcome variable for this analysis was the 30-day postoperative incidence of stroke or death.

The authors compared crude 30-day stroke/death rates stratified by both the presence/absence of CCO and by surgeon shunting practice (no shunt, routine shunt, or shunt placed for indication) using observed-to-expected (O/E) ratios. The O/E ratios were calculated by dividing the observed 30-day stroke/death incidence by the predicted incidence for each of the six groups. The expected stroke/death ratio was generated through multivariable logistic regression models in which an assortment of variables was used to estimate a given patient's risk of that outcome. These variables included demographic characteristics, comorbid characteristics (including the presence of diabetes, renal dysfunction, coronary disease, or congestive heart failure), carotid disease-specific characteristics (including the degrees of ipsilateral and contralateral carotid stenosis and preoperative neurologic symptom status), preoperative medication use (including aspirin, clopidogrel, and/or statin use), and procedure-specific characteristics (including use of eversion endarterectomy, patch angioplasty, heparin reversal with protamine, use of completion arteriography, and type of intraoperative monitoring that was used to determine the need for shunt placement in patients who received a shunt for a specific indication). A total of 353 patients with CCO and 5,279 without CCO were included in the analysis by Goodney and colleagues.[8] The 30-day stroke/death rate for patients with CCO was 4.0%. When stratified by the different categories of shunt use, the incidence of stroke/death was 3.4% for patients with no shunt, 4.1% for patients who received a shunt by a surgeon who was classified as a routine shunter, and 4.8% for patients who received a shunt by a surgeon who used intraoperative shunts selectively for specific indications (P = 0.88). The O/E ratios and 95% confidence intervals for the different categories of shunt use were not statistically different [1.0 (0.3-2.4) for "no shunt", 1.0 (0.4-2.4) for "routine shunt", and 1.1 (0.3-3.0) for "shunt for indication"]. The 30-day stroke/death rate for patients without CCO was 1.9%. Among the cohort without CCO, the 30-day stroke/death rate was significantly higher in patients who had a shunt placed for indication (4.1%) when compared to patients who had with no shunt or with shunts placed as part of routine practice (1.9% and 1.7% respectively, P = 0.03).

The authors of the Goodney study also analyzed post-CEA outcomes from the context of surgeon practice pattern in shunt use. They found that 62% of the CEA procedures included for analysis were performed by selective surgeons and the remainder were performed by routine shunters. Of the surgeons who were classified as selective shunters, 87% used shunts in <30% of the procedures that they performed. Figure 8-2 depicts the 30-day stroke/death rates for patients with CCO by shunt use and surgeon practice pattern. The lowest observed incidence of stroke/death (1.5%) occurred when intraoperative shunts were used by surgeons who were classified as routine shunters, with the O/E ratio in this group being 0.4 (95% CI 0.2-0.8). Procedures performed by selective shunters in which no shunt was placed were associated with a stroke/death rate of 3.4% and an O/E stroke/death ratio of 0.9 (95% CI 0.7-1.2). The highest stroke/death rate was observed when an intraoperative shunt was used for a specific indication by a surgeon who was classified as a selective shunter [observed stroke/death rate of 7.6%, or O/E ratio of 1.7 (95% CI 1.2-2.1).

The authors of the VSGNE analysis concluded from these results that intraoperative shunt use is associated with a lower rate of postoperative stroke/death in patients with CCO, but only when the shunt is placed by a surgeon who routinely utilizes shunts during CEA. Patients who receive a shunt by a surgeon who does not routinely use shunts during CEA appear to be at an increased risk of postoperative stroke or death. In short, the authors advocate that surgeons should rely on their normal practice pattern when performing CEA on patients with CCO; if surgeons routinely utilize shunts for non-CCO patients, then they can expect to achieve optimal outcomes when also placing shunts in patients with CCO. On the other hand, surgeons who do not

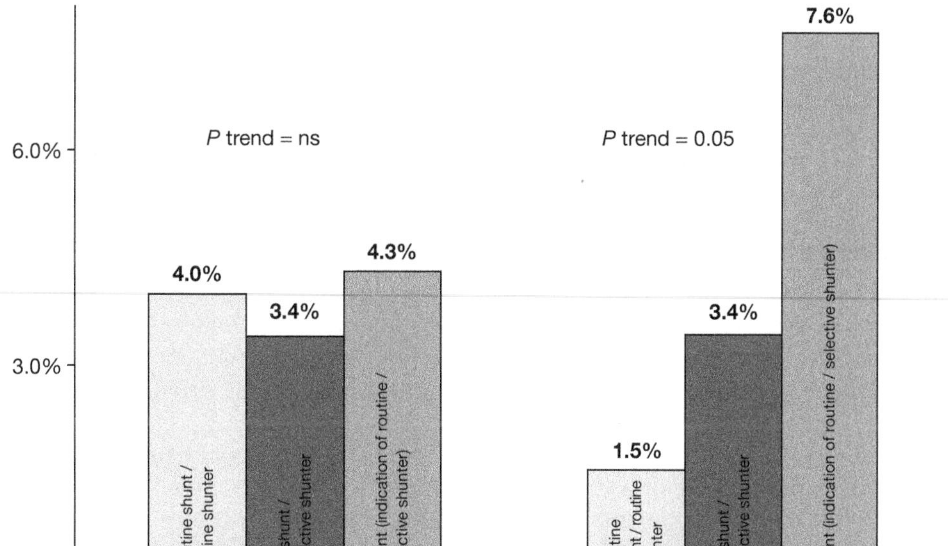

Figure 8-2. Predicted and observed 30-day stroke and death rate in patients with a contralateral carotid occlusion by shunt type and surgeon practice pattern (Figure 3 from page 8 of Goodney et al.[8] Used with permission from Elsevier.)

routinely utilize shunts for non-CCO patients should not use them for patients with CCO.

Our group has also attempted to determine the influence of shunt utilization on perioperative outcomes after CEA. We examined data from the 2012 American College of Surgeons National Surgical Quality Improvement Program (ACS-NSQIP) Procedure-Targeted Carotid Open database, which contains detailed disease- and procedure-specific information about patients undergoing CEA at one of 78 participating centers in the United States.[9,10] 3,153 CEA patients from this data source were included for analysis (1,130 of whom received an intraoperative shunt and 2,023 who did not). The patient- and procedure-related characteristics of these patients are shown in Table 8-1. In this analysis, a patient was considered to have a physiologic high-risk factor if they exhibited one or more of the following characteristics: class III or IV New York Heart Association congestive heart failure, left ventricular ejection fraction <30%, unstable angina within 30 days before surgery, or myocardial infarction within 30 days before surgery. Patients were considered to have an anatomic high-risk factor if they exhibited one or more of the following characteristics: previous ipsilateral CEA/carotid stenting, previous ipsilateral radical neck dissection, contralateral common carotid or ICA occlusion, prior radiation to neck, contralateral laryngeal nerve injury or palsy, and anatomic lesion at the second cervical vertebral level or higher. As can be seen from Table 8-1, patients from the 2012 Procedure-Targeted ACS-NSQIP data source who had a shunt placed during CEA were more likely to be female, were more likely to have occlusion of their contralateral ICA, were less likely to have received locoregional (versus general) anesthesia, and were more likely to have undergone patch angioplasty closure of their carotid arteriotomy when compared to patients in whom a shunt was not utilized during CEA. The overall combined 30-day incidence of postoperative stroke/TIA was 4.0% for patients with a shunt compared to 3.6% for patients without a shunt ($P = 0.55$), while the overall 30-day postoperative mortality rate was 1.3% for patients with a shunt compared to 0.6% for patients without a shunt ($P = 0.05$).

In an attempt to adjust for the fact that some surgeons place shunts only in those patients who they perceive to be at high risk for intraoperative cerebral hypoperfusion, we then performed a separate analysis using a subset of the entire ACS-NSQIP patient sample that was matched on the propensity for a patient to undergo CEA with an intraoperative shunt. For this analysis, a multivariate logistic regression model was created in order to estimate the likelihood that a patient would receive a shunt during CEA, with all of the variables listed in Table 8-1 being used as potential predictors of shunt placement. Our propensity matching algorithm resulted in a cohort of 1,072 patients with and without shunt placement who were well-matched for all known patient- and procedure-related factors (as evidenced by Table 8-2). Comparison of the propensity-matched cohort demonstrated no significant difference in either 30-day postoperative stroke/TIA (3.7% for patients with a shunt compared to 3.4% for patients without a shunt, $P = 0.64$) or mortality (1.1% in patients with a shunt compared to 0.7% for patients without a shunt, $P = 0.25$).

A final step in our analysis was to examine only those patients who had evidence of severe stenosis (80-99%) or occlusion of their contralateral ICA on preoperative imaging, a patient cohort which would theoretically have the most to gain from the use of an intraoperative shunting. Using similar propensity matching techniques as previously described, we created a cohort of 123 such patients with our without intraoperative shunt utilization. As before, the cohort did not differ significantly in any of the known patient- or procedure-related characteristics.

TABLE 8-1. PATIENT- AND PROCEDURE-RELATED CHARACTERISTICS OF ALL CEA PATIENTS FROM THE 2012 ACS-NSQIP PROCEDURE-TARGETED DATABASE, STRATIFIED BY USE OF INTRAOPERATIVE SHUNTING. (FROM BENNETT,[9] TABLE I, PAGE 98).

	All patients (N = 3153)	No shunt (N = 2023)	Shunt (N = 1130)	P value
Patient age, years, mean ± SD	71.4 ± 9.5	71.3 ± 9.5	71.5 ± 9.5	.77
Female	1215 (38.5)	746 (36.9)	469 (41.5)	.01
Physiologic high-risk factors	131 (4.2)	89 (4.4)	42 (3.7)	.36
Bleeding disorder	690 (21.9)	435 (21.5)	255 (22.6)	.49
Ipsilateral ICA stenosis ≥80%	2159 (68.5)	1377 (68.1)	782 (69.2)	.51
Type of preoperative symptoms				.19
Asymptomatic	1813 (57.5)	1173 (58.0)	640 (56.6)	
TIA or amaurosis fugax	756 (24.0)	494 (24.4)	262 (23.2)	
Cerebrovascular accident	584 (18.5)	356 (17.6)	228 (20.2)	
Contralateral ICA occlusion	149 (4.7)	73 (3.6)	76 (6.7)	<.001
Preprocedural antiplatelet	2772 (87.9)	1772 (87.6)	1000 (88.5)	.46
Preprocedural statin	2475 (78.5)	1598 (79.0)	877 (77.6)	.37
Preprocedural β-blocker	1777 (56.4)	1169 (57.8)	608 (53.8)	.03
Anatomic high-risk factors	397 (12.6)	253 (12.5)	144 (12.7)	.85
Locoregional anesthesia	408 (12.9)	358 (17.7)	50 (4.4)	<.001
Operative time, minutes, median (IQR)	116 (90–145)	117 (92–147)	113 (88–141)	.01
Patch angioplasty	2659 (84.3)	1615 (79.8)	1044 (92.4)	<.001

ICA, Internal carotid artery; *IQR*, interquartile range; *SD*, standard deviation; *TIA*, transient ischemic attack.

TABLE 8-2. PATIENT- AND PROCEDURE-RELATED CHARACTERISTICS OF PROPENSITY-MATCHED COHORT OF CEA PATIENTS FROM THE 2012 ACS-NSQIP PROCEDURE-TARGETED DATABASE, STRATIFIED BY USE OF INTRAOPERATIVE SHUNTING. (FROM BENNETT,[9] TABLE II, PAGE 99).

	No shunt (n = 1072)	Shunt (n = 1072)	*P* value
Patient age, years, mean ± SD	71.7 ± 9.4	71.4 ± 9.5	.50
Female	447 (41.7)	437 (40.8)	.64
Physiologic high-risk factors	40 (3.7)	40 (3.7)	1.0
Bleeding disorder	236 (22.0)	233 (21.7)	.88
Ipsilateral ICA stenosis ≥80%	747 (69.7)	742 (69.2)	.81
Type of preoperative symptoms			.69
Asymptomatic	605 (56.4)	615 (57.4)	
TIA or amaurosis fugax	249 (23.2)	254 (23.7)	
Cerebrovascular accident	218 (20.3)	203 (18.9)	
Contralateral ICA occlusion	53 (4.9)	50 (4.7)	.66
Preprocedural antiplatelet	949 (88.5)	945 (88.2)	.78
Preprocedural statin	815 (76.0)	837 (78.1)	.27
Preprocedural β-blocker	583 (54.4)	586 (54.7)	.89
Anatomic high-risk factors	122 (11.4)	126 (11.8)	1.0
Locoregional anesthesia	55 (5.1)	50 (4.7)	.35
Operative time, minutes, median (IQR)	115 (91–143)	114 (88–142)	.95
Patch angioplasty	983 (91.7)	986 (92.0)	.67

ICA, Internal carotid artery; *IQR*, interquartile range; *SD*, standard deviation; *TIA*, transient ischemic attack.

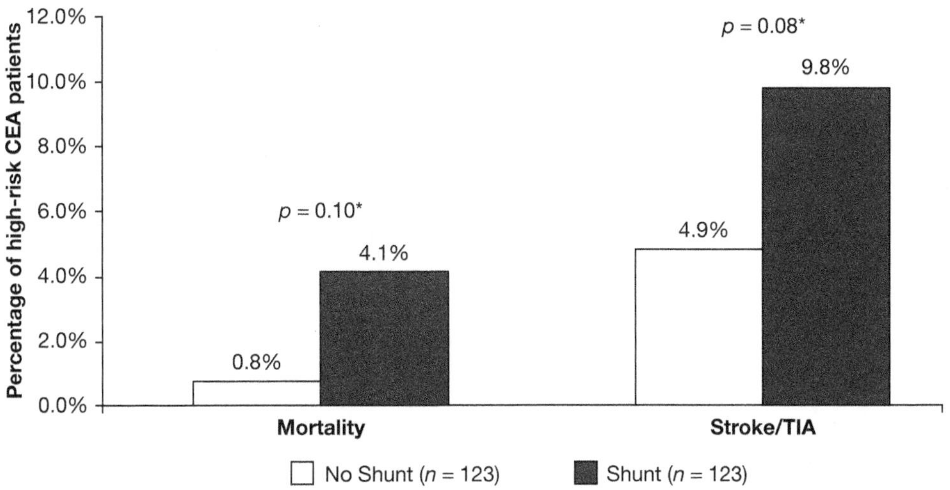

Figure 8-3. 30-day postoperative outcomes of a propensity-matched cohort of CEA patients from the 2012 ACS-NSQIP Procedure-Targeted Database with occlusion or severe stenosis of their contralateral ICA, stratified by the use of intraoperative shunting.

When analyzing the postoperative outcomes of these patients with severe stenosis or occlusion of their contralateral ICA (see Figure 8-3), we found that patients in whom a shunt was used during CEA sustained a two-fold higher 30-day incidence of postoperative stroke/TIA than patients who did not receive a shunt (although this difference did not reach statistical significance).

Our conclusion from this analysis of ACS-NSQIP data was that intraoperative shunt utilization during CEA appears to offer no identifiable benefit in terms of reducing the risk of either stroke or death, even in those patients who are at particularly high risk of perioperative cerebral hypoperfusion due to the presence of an occluded or severely stenosed contralateral ICA. Although our analysis is one of the largest to date to assess the impact of shunting on neurologic outcomes after CEA, we did face several important limitations. First, unlike the authors of the previously described VSGNE study, we were unable to control for surgeon practice pattern in our analysis since ACS NSQIP does not provide surgeon identifiers. In addition, we do not know whether patients received intraoperative neurologic monitoring during their CEA procedure (although we consider the use of locoregional anesthesia to be a reasonable proxy for the presence of such monitoring). Finally, as with the VSGNE study, our analysis was performed retrospectively. Even though we attempted to "mimic" randomization through the use of propensity matching techniques, both our analysis and that of Goodney et al. are unable to fully account for unknown but potentially confounding factors.

CONCLUSION

There is insufficient evidence to strongly support the routine use, selective use, or routine non-use of intravascular shunts during CEA. Data from prospective, randomized trials generally shows no difference in the incidence of perioperative neurologic complications after procedures performed with versus without shunts. However, a trial in which the three potential practice patterns of shunt use (routine use, selective use, routine non-use) has yet to be performed.

The results from two recent large vascular-specific databases are also somewhat conflicting in their conclusion with respect to the use of shunts during CEA. One study has shown that shunts may reduce the risk of perioperative stroke or death, but only when placed by a surgeon who routinely uses shunts. The other study showed no benefit to shunt use, even in patients who might be at higher risk for clamp-induced cerebral hypoperfusion due to severe stenosis or occlusion of their contralateral carotid artery.

In conclusion, the available evidence does not clearly support any one of the three possible shunt practice patterns. Advocates of each of these three practices have a wealth of data available that shows that their particular shunting practice is associated with an acceptably low incidence of perioperative stroke. The resolution of this controversy will likely not be achieved unless a comprehensive randomized trial that is of sufficient sample size and which includes three arms (routine shunt use, selective use based on a uniform neurologic or vascular monitoring parameter, routine non-shunt) is performed.

REFERENCES

1. Ott DA, Cooley DA, Chapa L, Coelho A. Carotid endarterectomy without temporary intraluminal shunt. Study of 309 consecutive operations. *Ann Surg*. 1980;191:708–14.
2. AbuRahma AF, Mousa AY, Stone PA. Shunting during carotid endarterectomy. *J Vasc Surg*. 54:1502–10.
3. Chongruksut W, Vaniyapong T, Rerkasem K. Routine or selective carotid artery shunting for carotid endarterectomy (and different methods of monitoring in selective shunting). *CDSR*. 2014, Issue 6. Art. No. CD000190.
4. Ferguson CG. Carotid endarterectomy: to shunt or not to shunt? *Arch Neurol*. 1986;43:615–7.
5. Gumerlock MK, Neuwelt EA. Carotid endarterectomy: to shunt or not to shunt. *Stroke*. 1988;19:1485–90.
6. Sandmann W, Kolvenbach R, Willeke F. Risks and benefits of shunting in carotid endarterectomy. *Stroke*. 1993;24:1098–99.
7. AbuRahma AF, Stone PA, Hass SM, et al. Prospective randomized trial of routine versus selective shunting in carotid endarterectomy based on stump pressure. *J Vasc Surg*. 2010;51:1133–8.
8. Goodney PP, Wallaert JB, Scali ST, et al. Impact of practice patterns in shunt use during carotid endarterectomy with contralateral carotid occlusion. *J Vasc Surg*. 2012;55:61–71.
9. Bennett KM, Scarborough JE, Cox MW, Shortell CK. The impact of intraoperative shunting on early neurologic outcomes after carotid endarterectomy. *J Vasc Surg*. 2015;61:96–102.
10. User guide for the 2012 ACS NSQIP procedure targeted participant use data file. American College of Surgeons National Surgical Quality Improvement Program; 2014. Available at: http://site.acsnsqip.org/wp-content/uploads/2014/01/ACS.NSQIP_2012.PT_PUF-.UserGuide.pdf. Accessed February 9, 2014.

9

Outcomes of Interventions for Carotid Stenosis Secondary to Radiation-Induced Stenosis and Restenosis After Carotid Endarterectomy

Reid A. Ravin, MD, Daniel Han, MD and Peter L. Faries, MD

Carotid endarterectomy (CEA) has a proven role in reducing the risk of stroke in patients with symptomatic carotid stenosis, and in asymptomatic patients with critical stenotic lesions. Carotid artery stenting with embolic protection (CAS) has also been shown to be safe and effective in treating carotid stenosis.[1,2] However, recent comparative randomized prospective trials have established CEA as first-line therapy for patients who require carotid intervention, because of the lower risk of periprocedural stroke.[3] Evidence still supports the selective use of CAS in those patients who are at higher risk of complications from CEA. One such cohort includes patients with "hostile necks" who have had external beam radiation (XRT) for malignancy with or without previous neck dissection. Although some controversy exists, observational studies have shown XRT patients are at higher risk for cranial nerve injuries, wound complications, and the increased use of interposition grafting during open carotid surgery.[4] Similar to the hostile necks encountered in previously irradiated fields, patients who have undergone previous carotid endarterectomy may also be at elevated risk of complications from re-operative carotid endarterectomy due to the loss of a clearly defined dissection plane. Given the acceptable safety profile of CAS with embolic protection, many practitioners routinely employ CAS as an alternative to CEA in patients with lesions secondary to restenosis and radiation-induced arteritis.

Despite the common use of CAS in patients with restenosis or XRT-related lesions, it is important to acknowledge that few of the randomized, prospective multicenter trials include patients without primary atherosclerotic lesions, and patients with restenotic and radiation-induced disease may have distinct outcomes. The few trials that include restenotic and XRT lesions frequently lump those patients in with primary atherosclerosis, without adequate numbers to perform rigorous subgroup analysis.[1,2] In-vitro, animal model, and observational data exists to suggest that restenosis and radiation arteritis exhibit unique pathophysiology, which may affect the natural history of the diseases and the outcomes of intervention.

RADIATION ARTERITIS

Radiation-induced arteritis was described over a century ago and has been increasing in prevalence due to iatrogenic use of external beam radiation for oncologic treatment. Initially, radiation exposure was thought to be a simple risk factor for atherosclerotic disease based on the observation that patients who have been exposed to radiation therapy for head and neck neoplasms had a moderately increased incidence of cerebral arterial disease. More recent studies have defined radiation arteritis as a distinct pathophysiologic process, and some progress has been made in understanding the molecular etiology of the disease.[5,6] Clinically, radiation arteritis manifests as a local rather than systemic process. Radiation-induced lesions can manifest throughout the field of exposure and are not limited to the more common sites of atherosclerotic disease, like areas of turbulent flow and bifurcation. The lesions themselves tend to be more concentric and of longer length than atherosclerotic lesions. In addition to lipid accumulation and intimal thickening, which are also seen in atherosclerosis, radiation arteritis tends to have more prominent fibrotic component, which is also characteristic of the skin and connective tissue in the irradiated field.[5]

The clinical manifestations of radiation arteritis are usually quite delayed, and major cardiovascular events can occur up to decades after treatment. Despite the characteristic patterns of disease described above, it can be difficult to definitively classify an individual lesion as radiation associated given the high prevalence of de novo atherosclerosis in the general population. This can make it difficult to establish radiation arteritis as a causative factor in an individual patient, as well as characterize the natural history of radiation arteritis as a distinct clinical entity. Patient suffering from radiation-induced arteritis have on average, less cardiovascular risk factors, and present at an earlier age than patients with primary atherosclerotic lesions, but there is significant overlap in cardiovascular risk factors among the populations suffering from atherosclerotic and XRT-related cerebrovascular disease.[7] There is, however, ample evidence to suggest that radiation-induced stenosis of the carotid artery is a clinically significant disease that, untreated, can progress to transient ischemic attacks (TIAs) and stroke at a rate similar to atherosclerotic disease.[4,5]

Several recent efforts have been made to describe the molecular pathophysiology responsible for radiation arteritis. There are long established in vitro, and in-vivo animal models for inducing radiation arteritis. For instance, Schiller et al. demonstrated that gamma radiation can be used to alter plaque composition and accelerate macrophage infiltration of atherosclerotic lesions in LDL receptor–deficient mice.[8] Until recently, however, the molecular physiology of radiation-induced vasculopathy has been unknown. Halle et al. hypothesize that radiation arteritis is caused by a combination of acute cytotoxic injury as well as an increase in oxidative stress, which causes a chronic inflammatory state.[6] The response of arteries to acute radiation injury includes upregulation of inflammatory cytokines and an increase in macrophage aggregation, as well as apoptosis of cells throughout the intima and media, which leads to further release of inflammatory signaling molecules. Despite the robust inflammatory response, these changes are likely insufficient to explain the increase in stenotic lesions seen in radiation-exposed vessels seen years after exposure.

The explanation for delayed manifestations of radiation arteritis may be due to a chronic increase in oxidative stress seen after radiation exposure. There is an initial large scale generation of oxygen free radicals after radiation exposure as well as a chronic overproduction of free radicals in irradiated tissues. The chronically elevated free-radical production may lead to the activation of a pro-inflammatory transcription factor known as NF-κB, which mediates many of the long-term effects of radiation arteritis.[6] These effects include the long-term production of inflammatory cytokines, inflammatory cell recruitment and foam cell formation. Future medical therapies may focus on the deactivation of NF-κB, and several medications including aspirin are already known to inhibit NF-κB.[6]

OUTCOMES OF CAROTID ENDARTERECTOMY IN XRT PATIENTS

Carotid Endarterectomy

CEA remains the first-line treatment for carotid artery occlusive disease. However, patients who have undergone XRT have a prominent fibrotic reaction that obliterates tissue planes and increases the difficulty of operative dissection. These hostile necks are frequently made even worse by previous neck dissections for cancer resections. Traditionally, patients with radiation arteritis have been considered to be high risk for carotid surgery given a higher rate of cranial nerve injury, wound complications, and anastomotic breakdown.[9] Major randomized trials have established that carotid endarterectomy needs to be done with <6% morbidity and mortality in symptomatic carotid stenosis and <3% in asymptomatic patients.[10] Prior to the wide application of carotid stenting, some authors questioned whether CEA could be performed with perioperative morbidity less than these cutoffs. More recent case series have shown acceptable perioperative results with carotid endarterectomy, and some groups are primarily recommending endarterectomy as the first-line approach in these patients.

Radiation arteritis remains a relatively uncommon cause of carotid stenosis and has been an exclusion criterion in many of the major randomized trials including the Carotid Revascularization Endarterectomy vs. Stenting Trial (CREST) as well as the Asymptomatic Carotid Atherosclerosis Study (ACAS). Despite being included in the Stenting and Angioplasty with Protection in Patients at High Risk for Endarterectomy (SAPPHIRE) study, as well as the North American Symptomatic Carotid Endarterectomy Trial (NASCET), the subgroup of patients with XRT did not reach sizes that were amenable to subgroup analysis.[1,2,11] The majority of the data on CEA after radiation therapy comes from small-institution specific case series, with few manuscripts including more than 40 patients, and the total number of patient outcomes reported in the literature are fewer than 500 cases. One of the larger case series on CEA after XRT comes from Tallarita et al. who looked at 27 patients who underwent 36 carotid endarterectomies after XRT.[12] The authors found that 5 of 36 (14%) reconstructions required interposition grafting, 22% had cranial nerve injury, and wound complications occurred in 14%. Cranial nerve injuries were even higher among the subgroup of patients who underwent XRT and previous radical neck dissection (28%), but due to the low numbers the difference did not reach statistical significance. Despite these relatively high morbidity rates, the series reported only one neurologic event in the patients undergoing CEA, and the procedures appeared durable with 87% freedom from restenosis and reintervention at 5 years. Leseche et al. also published a report on a series of 27 patients who underwent 30 carotid endarterectomies after previous neck radiation. Leseche also reports a relatively high use of interposition grafting (23%), but reported no cranial nerve injuries or wound infections.[13] Similar to Tallarita, Lescehe found the carotid reconstructions to be durable with a 10% restenosis rate and 6-24 months of follow-up. Kashyap et al. in their series of 24 patients undergoing carotid revascularization after radiation, report a cranial nerve injury rate of 23% and wound infection rate of 8%.[4] Notably, 15% of their patients required skin grafting with myocutaneous flaps to facilitate wound closure. Kashyap et al. reported good durability with a restenosis rate of 8% and no occlusions. Finally, Frego et al. published CEA results which included eight patients with previous neck radiation who were lumped in with other causes of hostile necks including patients with previous surgery and patients with inextensible necks.[10] The authors also noted a relatively high rate of cranial nerve injuries (21%) among all patients with hostile necks.

Almost all evidence on CEA after previous neck radiation comes from small retrospective reviews of single-institution databases. These case manuscripts are summarized in Table 9-1. Whatever prospectively gathered data exists from the NASCET trial and SAPPHIRE has not been used to perform a subgroup analysis for radiation-exposed patients.[1,2] Given that several studies cite a high rate of cranial nerve injury (CNI) and use of interposition-grafting, it is reasonable to assume some of the concerns about increased morbidity in previously irradiated necks are well founded. There is, however, no evidence to suggest that patients undergoing CEA for radiation arteritis have higher rates of restenosis, perioperative stroke, and other long-term deleterious outcomes.

TABLE 9-1. EVIDENCE ON CEA AFTER PREVIOUS NECK RADIATION FROM SMALL RETROSPECTIVE REVIEWS OF SINGLE-INSTITUTION DATABASES

Author (Year)	No. of Patients	No. of Procedures	Cranial Nerve Injuries (CNI) %	No. of Perioperative Neurologic Events
Kashyap (1999)[4]	24	26	23	0
Leseche (2003)[13]	27	30	0	0
Frego (2009)[10]	8	8	21	0
Tallarita (2011)[12]	27	29	22	0
Magne (2012)[14]	24	27	11	0

CAROTID ARTERY STENTING OUTCOMES AFTER RADIATION

CAS for carotid stenosis after radiation exposure has the substantial advantage over CEA of avoiding dissection in a hostile neck. given the unique pathophysiology of radiation arteritis, however, it is reasonable to question whether the results of CAS in atherosclerotic disease are generalizable to post-radiation patients. As with CEA after XRT, there is no subgroup-specific randomized trial data for CAS after radiation therapy despite these patients being included in several trials.[1,3] Given the elevated risk profile of XRT patients, many centers have routinely been offering CAS to these patients. Several mid-sized series have recently been published that examine the safety and durability of CAS in this select patient population.

The initial outcome data for CAS after XRT has been mixed, with some early case series reporting high rates of treatment failure. Protack et al. published a case series examining patients undergoing CAS after XRT that reported high rates of restenosis and stent occlusion.[15] The series included 23 patients undergoing CAS after XRT exposure, and after the duration of their follow-up, the XRT group had a 43% restenosis rate versus 13% for the atherosclerotic occlusive disease group. The authors defined restenosis as greater than 50% stenosis diagnosed on duplex ultrasound. None of the restenotic patients developed symptoms, and the authors ended up re-intervening on three of the XRT patients for critical lesions. It is of note that the authors did not use target lesion revascularization as an outcome measure, and one of the lesions that was re-intervened on was proximal to the original lesion. The authors also included one technical failure as a re-intervention, which was enough to alter the restenosis rate significantly in a relatively small series.

In their own institutional series, Favre et al. report rates or restenosis and stent thrombosis, which while higher than historical controls undergoing CAS for atherosclerotic disease, were less than those reported by Protack et al.[16] This represents the largest published series, with the authors including 135 patients who underwent 149 carotid artery stenting procedures for radiation-induced stenosis. They report promising early results with a combined stroke and death rate of 1.5% at 1 month, and a technical success rate of 98%. Over longer follow up (mean of 30 months), however, the authors noted an 18% anatomic failure rate, seven of which led to neurologic complications. The overall neurologic event–free survival rate in the series was 93.1% at 4 years, which compares favorably to the results of CAS for primary atherosclerotic lesions. The authors also state that statin use significantly decreased the number of anatomic failures in patients undergoing CAS after XRT. However, the effect of statin use on carotid stent-restenosis after XRT has not been investigated subsequently. Ting et al. report a restenosis rate similar to Favre in their series of 16 patients undergoing 18 CAS for radiation arteritis.[17] They had three instances of restenosis (17%) with a mean follow-up of 30 months. No new neurologic events were detected in that series.

In all of the case series previously mentioned, which are summarized in Table 9-2, the authors were reporting primary restenosis rates based on duplex ultrasound criteria, or in some cases duplex criteria followed by confirmatory angiogram. Sadek et al. report the results of a large retrospective database from our institutions, which included 28 patients who underwent XRT for radiation arteritis. Our review was unique in that we reviewed angiograms from reintervention attempts to determine the rate of target lesion revascularization (TLR).[19] The reported restenosis rates were

TABLE 9-2. OUTCOME DATA FOR CAS AFTER XRT: PRIMARY RESTENOSIS RATES

Author (Year)	No. of Patients	No. of Procedures	Restenosis >50%	All Reintervention %	Target Lesion Revascularization %
Protack (2007)[15]	23	23	43	13	NR
Harrod-Kim (2005)[18]	16	19	26	20	NR
Sadek (2009)[19]	19	19	4.5	4.5	0
Favre (2008)[16]	135	149	18	4.6	NR
Ravin (2015)[7]	43	43	9.4	7	0

4.5% at 12 months for XRT patients and 9.7% for the atherosclerosis patients. There was one TLR in the non-XRT group and no TLR among the XRT patients. One of the XRT patients who did develop restenosis developed it at a separate site distinct from the original lesion. Recently, our institution published another manuscript using the updated version of the database. In the more recent report, 43 XRT patients were included, and the restenosis rates for XRT and non-XRT CAS were 9.4% and 8.6%, respectively, with no significant difference.[7] These findings at our 50% restenosis cutoff are demonstrated by a Kaplan Meier graft in Figure 9-1. The reintervention rate for the XRT patient was 7%, and upon review of the angiograms, none of the reintervention constituted target lesion revascularization. One hypothesis for this apparent lack of target lesion revascularization among XRT patients is that the anatomic treatment failures are likely due to de novo lesions remote from the original disease. The pathophysiology of radiation arteritis may predispose patients to develope additional stenotic lesions in areas that were exposed in the radiation field. Few of the previously mentioned series reported the location of restenotic lesions, and it is unknown if any of those higher rates might be attributable to de novo lesions from radiation exposure.

Several manuscripts generated from our institutional database include anatomic detail about patients undergoing CAS for radiation arteritis. We also have included particle analysis of material captured in embolic protection filters, which allows us to quantify differences in the debris generated by CAS procedures.[7,19,20] Despite the aforementioned uncertainty about the pathophysiologic equivalency of atherosclerotic and XRT-related lesions, there were few measureable anatomic differences in the lesion characteristics of the two groups. There were no differences in length of lesion or size of stent used. Analysis of the extent of internal carotid artery (ICA) tortuosity by DeRubertis et al. revealed that there was increased tortuosity of the affected ICA; however, this finding was not borne out in more updated versions of the database.[7,20]

Particle analysis was performed on our cases by collecting used embolic protection filters and performing image analysis on the resulting debris. The software allows for quantification of the particles as well as size measurements. Our analysis revealed several significant differences in filters extracted from XRT and non-XRT patients. There was no difference in number of particles, but particles were larger on average, and a larger number of large particles were found in the XRT patients. The clinical significance of this, if any, is unknown, but the findings are at least suggestive that real pathophysiologic differences may exist in the plaque composition of patients with carotid lesions after XRT. Future studies will address the question further by performing histologic analysis of the captured debris.

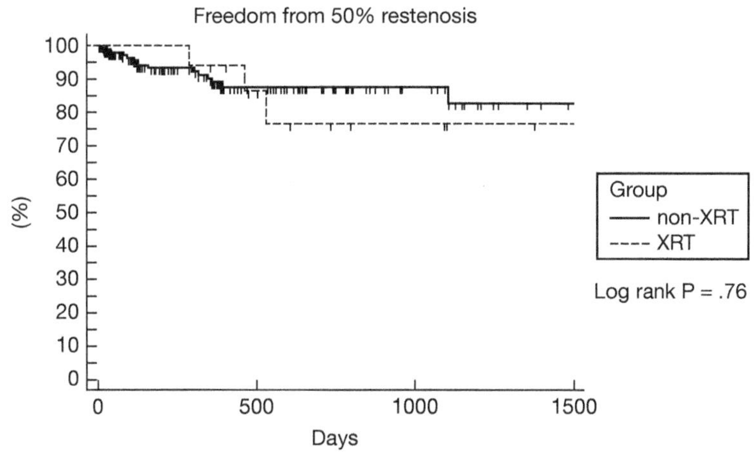

Number at risk (SE, %)

Group: non-XRT			
265	57 (3.1)	21 (3.1)	5 (5.6)
Group: XRT			
36	10 (9.1)	4 (12.2)	1 (12.2)

Figure 9-1. Restenosis rates for 43 XRT patients; 50% restenosis cutoff for a Kaplan Meier graft.

SUMMARY OF OUTCOMES CAS VERSUS CEA FOR RADIATION ARTERITIS

Carotid endarterectomy after XRT is challenging, and several sources have described higher rates of perioperative morbidity. However, few, if any of these studies have described an increased rate of major clinical endpoints including stroke, myocardial infarction (MI), or death in XRT patients undergoing CEA.[21] Based on this finding, as well as the largely anecdotal observation that most CNI are transient and of no clinical significance, some authors have challenged the belief that XRT patients are better served by treatment with carotid artery stenting.[19] Despite dissenting opinions, CAS still remains a widely applied alternative to CEA in patients who have undergone XRT. The advantage of CAS in XRT patients is readily apparent in that it completely avoids open surgery in a hostile neck. The outcomes of CAS for radiation arteritis seem acceptable with low rates of early or late neurologic events. However, several series have found elevated rates of restenosis and thrombosis in XRT CAS patients. These results were not duplicated in our institution's database, and we suggest that some of the late failures in the previously cited series may be to de novo lesions, which developed in the previously irradiated field. This propensity for de novo lesions to form within previously irradiated fields, is characteristic of radiation arteritis, which forms in response to oxidative stress induced by radiation damage, rather than at arterial branch points and other locations more typical of atherosclerotic disease. The diagnosis of in-stent restenosis can be difficult as the duplex criteria developed for native arteries has not been well validated in diagnosis of restenosis in stented arteries. Some authors have suggested that using the peak systolic velocities developed for native arteries leads to an overdiagnosis of in-stent restenosis in stented arteries.[22] This increased velocity in CAS arteries may be secondary to a loss of compliance in the stented arteries. These effects of velocity elevation most likely would be consistent across CAS performed for atherosclerosis and XRT; however, this has not been specifically investigated.

In-stent restenosis, which is usually due to neo-intimal hyperplasia in patients treated for atherosclerotic disease, may also be be responsible for restenosis in radiation-arteritis patients who have undergone CAS. However, the pathophysiology of these restenotic lesions has not been adequately studied in radiation arteritis patients, and there may be significant pathophysiologic differences. Additionally, the actual rate of restenosis and thrombosis in XRT patients undergoing CAS can only be estimated from the small retrospective series that have been published, and whether these patients are at higher risk of late restenosis remains an open question. Given the paucity of prospective data, and the conflicting nature of the retrospective data that exists, we feel both interventional and open surgical approaches are justifiable at this time.

CAROTID ARTERY STENTING FOR CAROTID RESTENOSIS

Unlike atherosclerotic carotid artery stenosis, which is prone to developing unstable plaque that can embolize, restenosis occurring within 24 months after revascularization is most often secondary to neointimal hyperplasia. Although statins have been shown to reduce overall mortality and stroke rates in patients with carotid artery stenosis, they seem to have little effect on rates of early restenosis following CEA, further reflecting a different underlying etiology.[23] Neointimal hyperplasia is a result of endothelial layer compromise that can occur during both CEA and balloon angioplasty during CAS. This injury exposes injured intima and media, which initiates platelet adhesion, fibrin deposition, and mesenchymal cell migration, ultimately leading to smooth muscle and intimal proliferation, effectively narrowing the revascularized lumen. The site of restenosis is most often at the level of the prior lesion, but can also occur at the proximal or distal clamp sites which may have been injured during CEA.[24]

Reported rates of restenosis following carotid revascularization with CEA and CAS vary significantly, ranging from 1% to 31%.[25] The clinical significance of carotid restenosis is often limited, however, as only 1–4% of patients progress to become symptomatic. While few would argue that symptomatic carotid restenosis necessitates reintervention, it is less clear when to intervene on asymptomatic carotid restenosis which makes up the majority of observed cases. It is important to note that there is a lack of consensus on the ultrasound velocity criteria used to define significant restenosis. The diagnosis of restenosis is further complicated in patients who have undergone prior carotid stenting, as velocities may be physiologically elevated within a noncompliant vessel wall that does not necessarily translate to a stenosis.[22]

The most commonly used threshold by several clinicians and investigators is a peak systolic velocity greater than 300 cm/sec to suggest a high-grade stenosis. A secondary analysis of the CREST trial was conducted by Lal et al. using this criteria for follow-up ultrasound scans at 1, 6, 12, and 24 months post-carotid revascularization.[26] At 2 years, the rates of restenosis were low for both CEA and CAS with just 62 of 1105 patients undergoing CEA and 58 of 1086 patients undergoing CAS meeting criteria for high-grade stenosis or occlusion. While mode of revascularization did not contribute to restenosis, female sex, diabetes, and hyperlipidemia were significant independent risk factors. Active smoking was an independent risk factor following CEA but did not contribute to the development of restenosis following CAS. These findings echoed similar reported results of increased risk of restenosis in women and diabetics, indicating that this cohort of patients may require closer monitoring.[27]

Similar to previously irradiated necks, prior CEA can cause significant scarring and loss of dissection planes, making anatomy harder to identify and increasing the risk of cranial nerve injuries. Almost every published study evaluating redo CEA confirms the higher rate of cranial nerve injury than initial CEA. For this reason, many clinicians advocate intervention with CAS for lesions with PSVs greater than 300 cm/sec, though redo-CEA is still routinely performed by some practitioners. Two recent meta-analyses evaluated patients undergoing CEA and CAS for carotid restenosis.[28,29] Tu et al. looked at 50 articles comprising 4,399 patients undergoing either CEA or CAS following prior CEA.[28] The authors noted no difference in 30-day perioperative mortality, stroke, or TIAs between the redo-CEA and CAS groups. As expected, the redo-CEA group experienced a statistically significant higher rate of cranial nerve injury within 30 days than the CAS group (5.9% vs. 0.1%). Interestingly, the redo CEA group also experienced a higher rate of perioperative MI (1.3% vs. 0.3%).

Fokkema et al. evaluated 13 studies with 1132 unique patients who underwent redo CEA or CAS following prior ipsilateral CEA.[29] Interestingly, a high number of patients evaluated in this study were noted to be symptomatic (40% of patients undergoing CEA, 30% of patients undergoing CAS). Similarly to Tu et al., the authors reported comparable perioperative stroke and death rate between CAS (2.3%) and CEA (2.7%). Cranial nerve injury rates were similar to other published rates—5.5% of patients undergoing CEA and 0.8% of patients undergoing CAS. The study also reported CAS-related complications with 1.9% of patients experiencing access site complications and 1.4% experiencing intraoperative bradycardia or arrhythmia.

Despite the lower risk of cranial nerve injury with CAS, redo CEA may still finds a role in the treatment of carotid restenosis. In addition, many of the reported cranial nerve injuries are noted to be transient with the majority of patients eventually regaining function. AbuRahma et al. analyzed 72 patients undergoing redo-CEA and 120 undergoing CAS for post-CEA stenosis.[30] In concordance with previous studies, the authors reported similarly low perioperative strokes of 3% for redo CEA and 1% for CAS. Cranial nerve injury rates were significantly higher in redo CEA patients at 14% and 0% in CAS patients. Only 1.4% of patients had a permanent cranial nerve injury.

One strategy to combat in-stent restenosis has been the use of drug-coated balloons (DCB) in the treatment of carotid stenosis. Piccoli et al. reported their results with the paclitaxel-coated InPact and Lutonix balloons in eighteen patients being treated for post CEA restenosis.[31] While the studied DCBs are typically recommended to be inflated for 3-4 minutes when used in the periphery, the authors used predilation of carotid lesions with DCBs for 30 seconds prior to routine stenting. One patient in their cohort experienced a TIA, and another patient died at 9 months from a myocardial infarction. At 18 months, no restenoses >50% were observed on duplex ultrasonography. While more studies are needed to determine the long-term efficacy, DCBs may limit the rate of in-stent restenosis and make CAS a more durable intervention for the treatment of post-CEA carotid restenosis.

CONCLUSION

Patients with restenosis after carotid endarterectomy and patients with XRT-induced carotid lesions pose a management challenge. The pathophysiology and natural history of these lesions is not well understood, and the challenges involved in operating on these patients are well documented. While technically possible with acceptable outcomes, carotid endarterectomy in the hostile neck appears to be associated with higher morbidity, particularly in regard to cranial nerve injury. Carotid artery stenting is a feasible alternative in XRT patients and in patients with restenosis following CEA. This technique completely obviates the need to re-enter a scarred neck and has Level One evidence supporting its perioperative safety. Some authors have raised concerns about restenosis rates in XRT patients undergoing CAS, although these elevated restenosis rates have not been consistently demonstrated. There is ample evidence to support the safety of CAS and CEA in patients with radiation-induced carotid lesions, as well as those patients with restenosis. Both approaches can be performed with excellent outcomes by experienced operators. It would be beneficial if future clinical trials that include XRT and restenosis patients attempted to perform sub-group specific analysis on outcomes for these challenging patients.

REFERENCES

1. Liakishev AA. [Protected carotid-artery stenting versus endarterectomy in high-risk patients. Results of SAPPHIRE trial.]. Russian. *Kardiologiia*. 2004;44:76.
2. Mas JL, Chatellier G, Beyssen B, et al. Endarterectomy versus stenting in patients with symptomatic severe carotid stenosis. *N Engl J Med*. 2006;355:1660–71.
3. Brott TG, Hobson RW, Howard G, et al. Stenting versus endarterectomy for treatment of carotid artery stenosis. *N Engl J Med*. 2010;363(1):11–23.
4. Kashyap VS, Moore WS, Quinones-Baldrich WJ. Carotid artery repair for radiation-associated atherosclerosis is a safe and durable procedure. *J Vasc Surg*. 1999;29:90–6; discussion 7–9.
5. Weintraub NL, Jones WK, Manka D. Understanding radiation-induced vascular disease. *J Am Coll Cardiol*. Mar 23 2010;55(12):1237–9.
6. Halle M, Gabrielsen A, Paulsson-Berne G, et al. Sustained inflammation due to nuclear factor-κ B activation in irradiated human arteries. *J Am Coll Cardiol*. 2010;55(12):1227–36.
7. Ravin RA, Gottlieb A, Pasternac K, et al. Carotid artery stenting may be performed safely in patients with radiation therapy-associated carotid stenosis without increased restenosis or target lesion revascularization: Results of a multicenter review. *J Vasc Surg*. 59(2):562.
8. Schiller NK, Kubo N, Boisvert WA, Curtiss LK. Effect of gamma-irradiation and bone marrow transplantation on atherosclerosis in LDL receptor-deficient mice. *Arterioscler Thromb Vasc Biol*. 2001;21(10):1674–80.
9. Melliere D, Becquemin JP, Berrahal D, Desgranges P, Cavillon A. Management of radiation-induced occlusive arterial disease: a reassessment. *J Cardiovasc Surg*. 1997;38(3):261–9.
10. Frego M, Bridda A, Ruffolo C, et al. The hostile neck does not increase the risk of carotid endarterectomy. *J Vasc Surg*. 2009;50(1):40–7.
11. Rothwell PM, Goldstein LB. Carotid endarterectomy for asymptomatic carotid stenosis: asymptomatic carotid surgery trial. *Stroke*. 2004;35(10):2425–7.
12. Tallarita T, Oderich GS, Lanzino G, et al. Outcomes of carotid artery stenting versus historical surgical controls for radiation-induced carotid stenosis. *J Vasc Surg*. 2011;53(3):629–36; e621–5.

13. Leseche G, Castier Y, Chataigner O, et al. Carotid artery revascularization through a radiated field. *J Vasc Surg*. 2003;38(2):244–50.
14. Magne JL, Pirvu A, Sessa C, Cochet E, Blaise H, Ducos C. Carotid artery revascularisation following neck irradiation: immediate and long-term results. *Eur J Vasc Endovasc Surg*. 2012;43(1):4–7.
15. Protack CD, Bakken AM, Saad WE, et al. Radiation arteritis: a contraindication to carotid stenting? *J Vasc Surg*. 2007;45(1):110–7.
16. Favre JP, Nourissat A, Duprey A, et al. Endovascular treatment for carotid artery stenosis after neck irradiation. *J Vasc Surg*. 2008;48(4):852–8.
17. Ting AC, Cheng SW, Yeung KM, et al. Carotid stenting for radiation-induced extracranial carotid artery occlusive disease: efficacy and midterm outcomes. *J Endovasc Ther*. 2004;11(1):53–9.
18. Harrod-Kim P, Kadkhodayan Y, Derdeyn CP, et al. Outcomes of carotid angioplasty and stenting for radiation-associated stenosis. *AJNR. Am J Neuroradiol*. 2005;26(7):1781–8.
19. Sadek M, Cayne NS, Shin HJ, et al. Safety and efficacy of carotid angioplasty and stenting for radiation-associated carotid artery stenosis. *J Vasc Surg*. 2009;50(6):1308–13.
20. Derubertis BG, Hynecek RL, Kent KC, Faries PL. Carotid tortuosity in patients with prior cervical radiation: increased technical challenge during carotid stenting. *Vasc Endovasc Surg*. 2011;45(7):619–26.
21. Fokkema M, den Hartog AG, Bots ML, et al. Stenting versus surgery in patients with carotid stenosis after previous cervical radiation therapy: systematic review and meta-analysis. *Stroke*. 2012;43(3):793–801.
22. Lal BK, Hobson RW,2nd, Tofighi B, et al. Duplex ultrasound velocity criteria for the stented carotid artery. *J Vasc Surg*. 2008;47(1):63–73.
23. AbuRahma AF, Srivastava M, Stone PA, et al. Effect of statins on early and late clinical outcomes of carotid endarterectomy and the rate of post-carotid endarterectomy restenosis. *J Am Coll Surg*. 2015;220(4):481–7.
24. Setacci F, Borrelli MP, De Donato G, et al. Reinterventions in vascular and endovascular carotid surgery. *J Cardiovasc Surg*. 2014;55(6):721–30.
25. Gagne PJ, Riles TS, Jacobowitz GR, et al. Long-term follow-up of patients undergoing reoperation for recurrent carotid artery disease. *J Vasc Surg*. 1993;18(6):991–98; discussion 999–1001.
26. Lal BK, Beach KW, Roubin GS, et al. Restenosis after carotid artery stenting and endarterectomy: a secondary analysis of CREST, a randomised controlled trial. *Lancet Neurol*. 2012;11(9):755–63.
27. Reina-Gutierrez T, Serrano-Hernando FJ, Sanchez-Hervas L, et al. Recurrent carotid artery stenosis following endarterectomy: natural history and risk factors. *Eur J Vasc Endovasc Surg*. 2005;29(4):334–41.
28. Tu J, Wang S, Huo Z, et al. Repeated carotid endarterectomy versus carotid artery stenting for patients with carotid restenosis after carotid endarterectomy: Systematic review and meta-analysis. *Surgery*. 2015;157(6):1166–73.
29. Fokkema M, Vrijenhoek JE, Den Ruijter HM, et al. Stenting versus endarterectomy for restenosis following prior ipsilateral carotid endarterectomy: an individual patient data meta-analysis. *Ann Surg*. 2015;261(3):598–604.
30. AbuRahma AF, Abu-Halimah S, Hass SM, et al. Carotid artery stenting outcomes are equivalent to carotid endarterectomy outcomes for patients with post-carotid endarterectomy stenosis. *J Vasc Surg*. 2010;52(5):1180–7.
31. Piccoli G, Biondi-Zoccai G, Gavrilovic V, et al. Drug-coated balloon dilation before carotid artery stenting of post-carotid endarterectomy restenosis. *J Endovasc Ther*. 2015;22(2):212–6.

10

Intrathoracic Subclavian Artery Aneurysm Repair

Nicholas D. Andersen, MD and G. Chad Hughes, MD

Although relatively uncommon, practitioners of aortic and vascular surgery should expect to encounter intrathoracic subclavian artery aneurysms (SAAs) with some frequency and be familiar with the natural history and treatment options for these lesions. The surgical approach to SAA repair is often complex and is challenged by the presence of congenital aortic arch anomalies, concomitant aortic pathology, prior aortic interventions, patient comorbid conditions, and/or hereditary connective tissue disease (CTD).[1] Conventional open intrathoracic SAA repair requires sternotomy or thoracotomy for access together with cardiopulmonary bypass and hypothermic circulatory arrest in many cases.[1–3] However, the advent of thoracic endovascular aortic repair (TEVAR) in 2005 provided an additional tool for the treatment of complex thoracic aortic pathology. In the present era, many SAAs can now be repaired by minimally invasive endovascular or "hybrid" open/endovascular techniques, which may allow for repair with reduced morbidity.[3,4] This chapter summarizes our current institutional approach to intrathoracic SAA repair using both open and TEVAR-based endovascular techniques.

EPIDEMIOLOGY

SAAs are rare entities that comprise 0.5% of all aneurysm repairs in the United States.[5] However, SAAs are perhaps 200 to 3,000 times more likely to occur in patients with other peripheral aneurysms or aortic pathology. Dent and colleagues reported SAA repairs were performed in 0.0007% (2 of 287,448) of individuals in the general hospital population, but in 0.13% (2 of 1,488) of individuals with aorto-iliac or peripheral arterial aneurysms.[6] There is likely even a stronger association between SAAs and thoracic aortic disease. At our institution, 925 patients underwent one or more thoracic aortic operations between 2005 and 2012, and 19 of these patients harbored a SAA meeting criteria for repair, yielding an incidence of SAA repair of 2.1% in individuals with thoracic aortic pathology requiring surgical repair. In addition, 53% (10 of 19) of SAA patients in our series had a history of prior aortic surgery, and 53% (10 of 19) underwent repair of concomitant thoracic aortic pathology at the time of SAA repair.[4]

The incidence of SAA may also be higher in patients with CTD as it was previously shown that 10% of SAA repairs occurred in patients with CTD.[7] In our series, 21% of SAA patients had CTD, and 4 of 45 patients with a confirmed diagnosis of CTD undergoing thoracic aortic surgery at our institution during the time period of the study harbored a SAA, for an overall incidence of 9% in this patient population.[4]

Lastly, SAAs often occur in conjunction with congenital aortic arch anomalies. Aneurysmal degeneration of an aberrant subclavian artery was first described by Burckhard F. Kommerell in 1936 and is commonly referred to as "Kommerell's diverticulum."[8] An aberrant right subclavian artery (RSCA) arising from a left-sided aortic arch occurs in 0.5% of the population and is the most common congenital anomaly of the aortic arch.[2] An aberrant left subclavian artery (LSCA) arising from a right-sided aortic arch is 10 times less common, and occurs in 0.05%–0.1% of the population.[9] Although rare, aberrant SAAs may be more unstable than native (non-aberrant) SAAs and were associated with a 19%–53% rate of rupture or dissection in prior comprehensive reviews.[2,10]

INDICATIONS FOR REPAIR

SAAs are repaired to prevent rupture or treat symptoms of thrombosis, embolization, pain, or local compression. A meta-analysis of 394 native SAAs found that symptoms were present in 84% of patients with, in order of decreasing frequency, local pain/pulsation, compression of neighboring structures, embolization, rupture, and thrombosis being the most common presenting symptoms. Rupture occurred in 9% of patients and carried a mortality rate of 19%. However, the authors were unable to identify a size threshold that was predictive of rupture. In addition, thrombosis was found to occur in smaller SAAs, ranging between 1.2 and 2.5 cm in size.[3] In 2004, Cina and colleagues reviewed all cases of aberrant SAAs occurring with a right-sided aortic arch and found that rupture occurred in SAAs ranging between 2 and 10 cm in size (average 5.8 ± 2 cm). The authors recommended SAA repair at a size of 3.0 cm, however, this recommendation was based only on the opinion that SAAs are easier to repair when small rather than statistical analysis.[10] Alternatively, Coselli and colleagues recommended SAA repair whenever feasible, regardless of size, given the high rate of complications.[1] In our practice, we elect to repair SAAs when symptomatic, in patients requiring operation for other aortic pathology, or at a size greater than 2.0 cm given the unpredictable natural history of SAAs and the documented risk of rupture and thrombosis at this size.

OPERATIVE TECHNIQUES

The following sections outline our operative techniques for open and endovascular-based SAA repair. The most important factors necessitating open repair include extensive thoracic aortic disease requiring concomitant open repair, CTD, or SAA anatomy not amenable to an endovascular approach. Failure of endovascular therapy is common in patients with CTD and we continue to recommend open aneurysm repair whenever feasible in these patients.[11] Alternatively, aberrant SAAs are well suited to repair by

TEVAR as the aneurysmal aberrant subclavian artery is the most distal branch vessel of the aortic arch. In the setting of an aberrant SAA with a concomitant native SAA, the aberrant and native subclavian arteries neighbor each other on the aorta and are easily treated by bilateral subclavian artery coverage with a single endograft.

OPERATIVE TECHNIQUES

Native Left SAA Repair – Endovascular Approach

An endovascular approach is utilized in patients with a native left SAA without concomitant aortic pathology requiring open repair (Figure 10-1). Selective LSCA revascularization (8 mm polytetrafluoroethylene graft) is performed at the time of the TEVAR procedure based on previously established indications and institutional protocols.[12] Proximal exclusion of the LSCA is accomplished by deployment of the aortic endograft with LSCA coverage. Distal SAA exclusion can be accomplished by ligation, coil embolization, or placement of an Amplatzer Vascular Plug (St. Jude Medical Inc., St. Paul, MN) via left brachial access.

Native Left SAA Repair – Open Approach

Open left SAA repair is most commonly required for patients undergoing concomitant extensive aortic replacement due to CTD or "mega aorta syndrome."[13,14] In patients with concomitant proximal (root/ascending/arch) aortic pathology, a total arch replacement (stage I elephant trunk procedure) is performed first using a modified Mt. Sinai/sidebranch technique.[14,15] If the LSCA arises proximally enough from the aortic arch such that it can be reached via sternotomy, then the aneurysmal segment of the LSCA is resected and the distal LSCA bypassed during total arch replacement

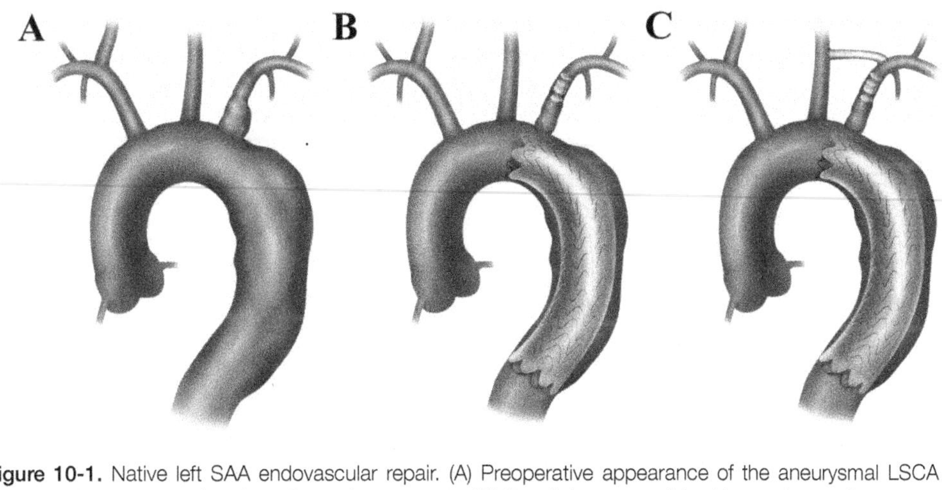

Figure 10-1. Native left SAA endovascular repair. (A) Preoperative appearance of the aneurysmal LSCA with a concomitant descending thoracic aortic aneurysm. (B) Repair is accomplished by endovascular coverage of the LSCA orifice and distal vascular plug occlusion proximal to the origin of the left vertebral artery. In the case shown, the thoracic endograft was used to treat a concomitant descending thoracic aortic aneurysm. (C) The LSCA was revascularized selectively via a left carotid-subclavian bypass for previously published indications.[12] From Andersen et al.[4] Reproduced with permission from the *Journal of Vascular Surgery.*

(Figure 10-2A). In patients in whom the LSCA arises too distally from the arch to be addressed via sternotomy, the left SAA is excluded by descending aorta to LSCA bypass at the time of 2nd stage open distal (descending/TAAA) aortic repair (Figure 10-2B, C).[16] Alternatively, for patients with only distal (descending/TAAA) disease requiring open repair, the LSCA may be addressed in a similar manner via the left chest at the time of open repair (Figures 10-3 and 10-4). Another option is the bilateral thoracosternotomy (clamshell) approach from which the proximal aorta, aortic arch

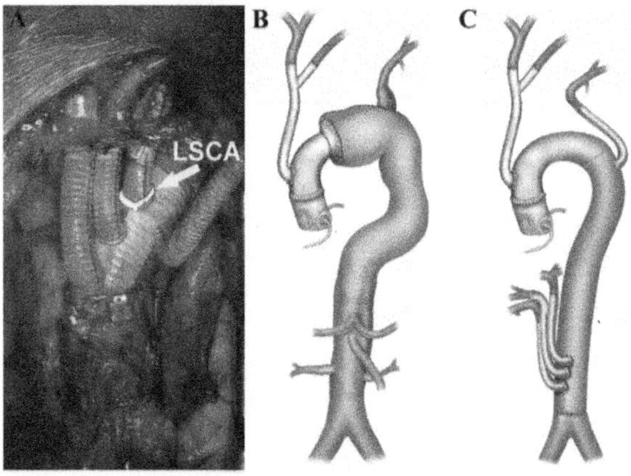

Figure 10-2. Native left SAA open repair. For patients with concomitant proximal (root/ascending/arch) aortic pathology, total arch replacement (stage I elephant trunk procedure) is first performed using a modified Mt. Sinai technique.[14,15] (A) For patients in whom the LSCA is accessible via a median sternotomy approach, the aneurysmal segment of the LSCA is resected and the distal LSCA bypassed at the time of total arch replacement. (B-C) For patients in whom the LSCA is not accessible via median sternotomy, the LSCA is bypassed from the new Dacron descending aorta at the time of 2nd stage open distal (descending/TAAA) aortic repair. From Andersen et al.[4] Reproduced with permission from the *Journal of Vascular Surgery.*

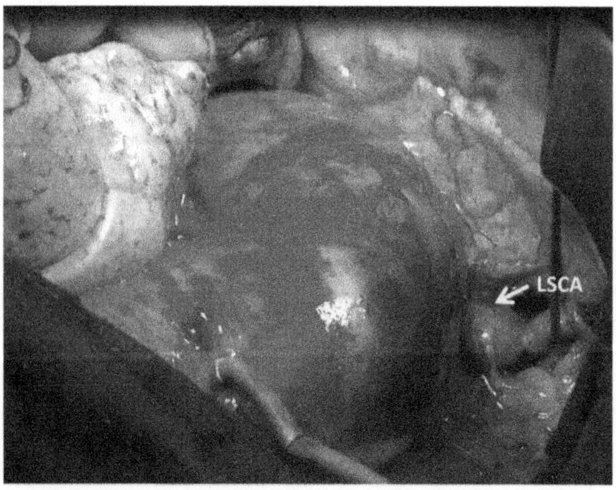

Figure 10-3. Native left SAA open repair via left thoracotomy. Appearance of the aneurysmal native left SAA as viewed from a left thoracotomy during concomitant open descending aortic replacement.

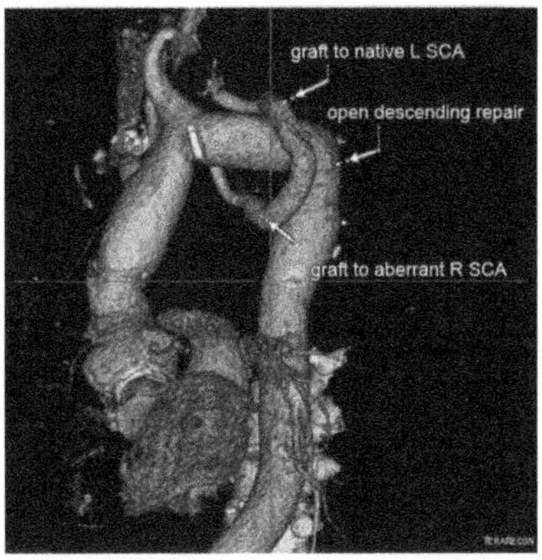

Figure 10-4. Native left SAA and aberrant right SAA open repair via left thoracotomy. Three-dimensional reconstruction CTA image demonstrating a patient in whom both a left SAA and aberrant right SAA were resected and bypassed via a left thoracotomy at the time of open descending aortic replacement.

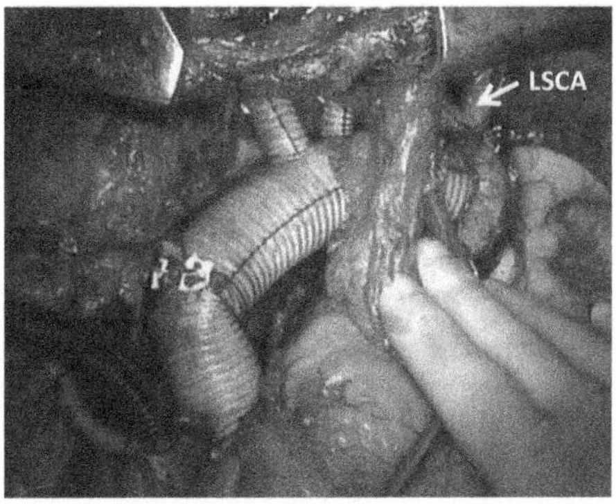

Figure 10-5. Native left SAA open repair via bilateral thoracosternotomy (clamshell) incision. Appearance of the bypassed native left SAA as viewed from a thoracosternotomy incision during concomitant open total arch replacement.

including the aneurysmal segment of the LSCA, and, if needed, proximal descending thoracic aorta can be replaced in a single operation (Figure 10-5).

Aberrant Left SAA Repair

Aberrant left SAAs (Kommerell's diverticulum) typically occur in patients with right-sided aortic arches and right descending thoracic aortas and are amenable to endovascular exclusion. Proximal exclusion of the aberrant LSCA is accomplished by endograft coverage of the LSCA orifice. Distal SAA exclusion is accomplished by coil embolization or vascular plug occlusion via left brachial access (Figure 10-6). In some cases, the aberrant LSCA may arise in close enough proximity to the native RSCA (Figure 10-7A) such that isolated endograft coverage of the LSCA orifice is not possible, and bilateral subclavian artery endograft coverage is required to achieve

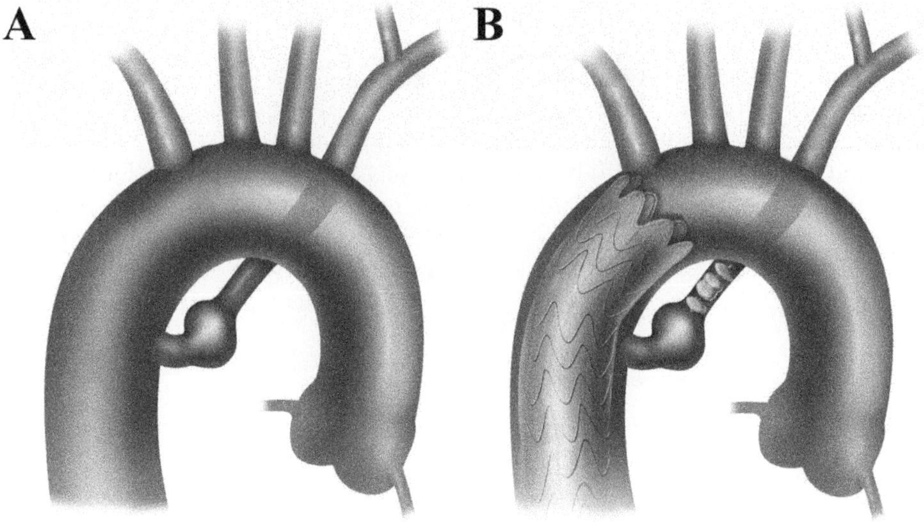

Figure 10-6. Aberrant left SAA (Kommerell's diverticulum) repair. (A) Preoperative appearance of an aberrant left SAA in a patient with a right-sided aortic arch and a right descending thoracic aorta. (B) Repair is accomplished by endovascular coverage of the LSCA orifice and vascular plug occlusion distal to the aneurysm. In the case shown, coverage of the RSCA or more proximal arch vessels was not required, although this may be necessary in some cases. From Andersen et al. Reproduced with permission from the *Journal of Vascular Surgery.*[4]

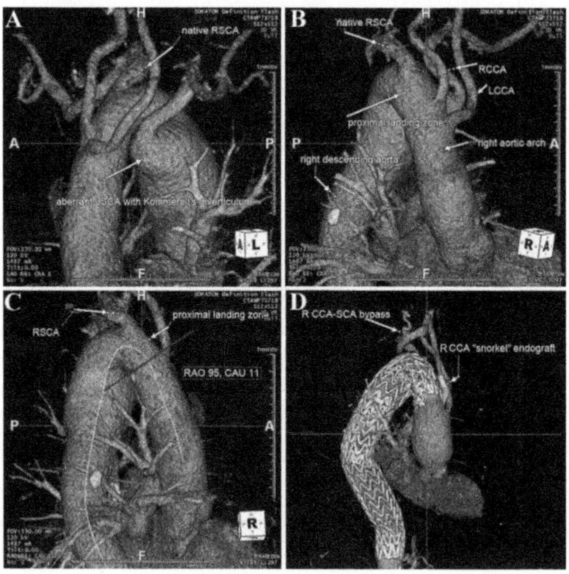

Figure 10-7. Aberrant left SAA (Kommerell's diverticulum) repair with bilateral SCA coverage. (A) Preoperative LAO view demonstrating a right aortic arch with an aberrant left SAA and native RSCA in close approximation. (B) Preoperative RAO view demonstrating the site of the intended proximal landing zone to include bilateral SCA coverage. (C) Steep RAO view is required to lay out the intended proximal landing zone. Note how the aberrant left SAA is unable to be visualized on this RAO imaging. (D) Postoperative three-dimensional CTA reconstruction imaging. The patient underwent endograft coverage of both SCAs with concomitant RSCA bypass and right common carotid artery snorkel stent placement to protect the orifice of the right common carotid artery.

adequate proximal landing zone (Figure 10-7B). As such, at least one subclavian artery will require revascularization, and bilateral subclavian artery revascularization is performed if indicated.[12] Of note, imaging of the aberrant left SAA with right arch/ right descending aorta for endovascular repair can pose challenges given the need for multiple imaging angles not typically utilized in standard TEVAR. For example, the aberrant left SAA is usually best seen in typical LAO angulation (Figure 10-7A), whereas the proximal and distal landing zones in the right arch and right descending aorta, respectively, are best seen in steep RAO imaging (Figures 10-7B–C) such that when the endograft(s) is deployed, the aneurysm is not visualized on the intraoperative image (Figure 10-7D).

Native Right SAA Repair

Native intrathoracic right SAAs without innominate artery involvement are uncommon and may be repaired by open bypass at the time of concurrent arch repair or interposition grafting via median sternotomy (Figure 10-8); a minimally invasive partial upper sternotomy approach is utilized if concomitant arch replacement is not required. More commonly, however, these aneurysms are associated with chronic dissection and innominate aneurysm and require replacement in conjunction with the innominate artery (Figure 10-9).

Aberrant Right SAA Repair

Aberrant right SAAs (Kommerell's diverticulum) are typically repaired using endovascular methods (Figure 10-10). Given the proximity of the aberrant RSCA to the other arch vessels, isolated endograft coverage of the RSCA orifice is generally

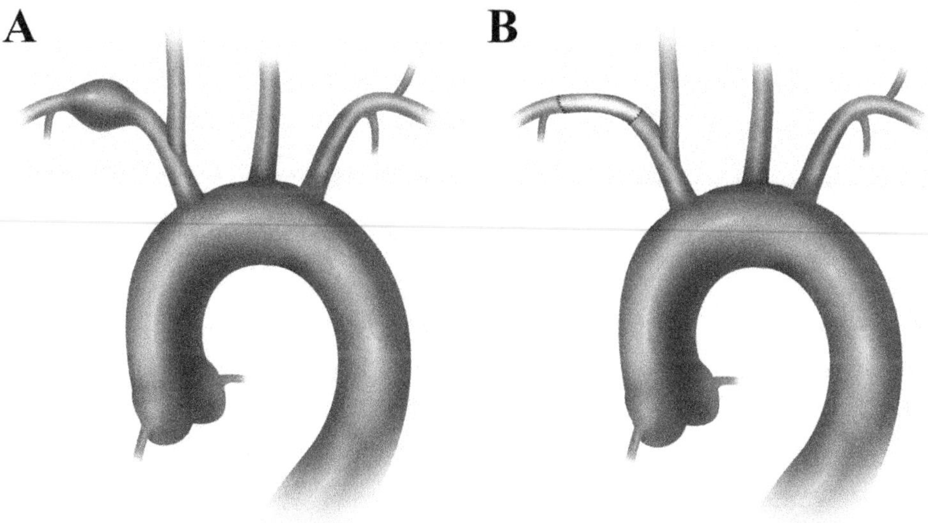

Figure 10-8. Native right SAA repair. (A) Preoperative appearance of a proximal native right SAA. (B) In the case shown, repair was accomplished by RSCA interposition grafting with aneurysm exclusion (endoaneurysmorrhaphy). From Andersen et al. Reproduced with permission from the *Journal of Vascular Surgery.*[4]

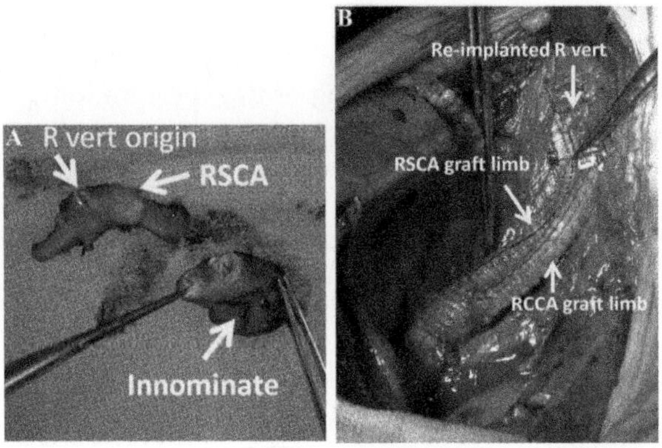

Figure 10-9. Native right SAA repair with innominate artery reconstruction. In this patient with a native right SAA and innominate artery aneurysm, reconstruction of the innominate artery with a branched graft was required. (A) Pathology photograph demonstrating the resected innominate artery with the intrathoracic RSCA, including the origin of the right vertebral artery. (B) Completion operative photograph demonstrating reconstruction of the innominate artery with a bifurcated graft to the RSCA and the right common carotid artery. Of note, the right vertebral artery was reimplanted in the anatomic position onto the distal RSCA graft limb.

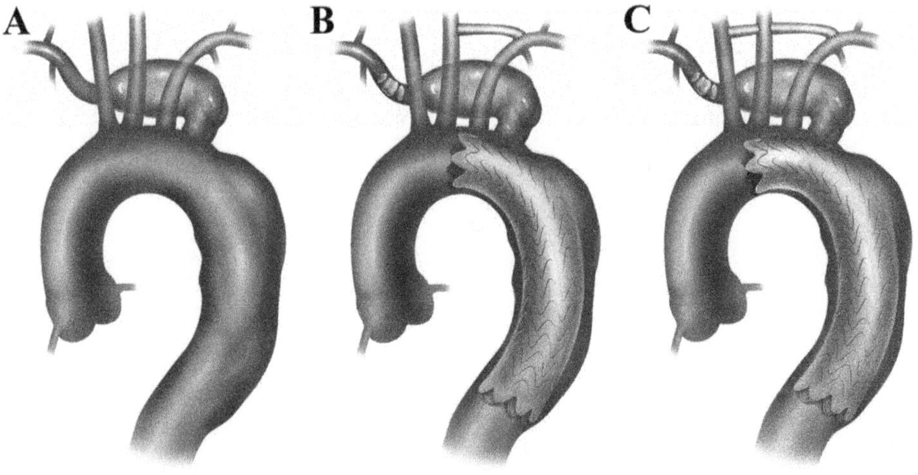

Figure 10-10. Aberrant right SAA (Kommerell's diverticulum) repair. (A) Preoperative appearance of an aberrant right SAA with a concomitant descending thoracic aortic aneurysm. (B) In the first scenario, repair was achieved via zone 2 endograft placement with bilateral SCA coverage and vascular plug occlusion of the aneurysm outflow. A left carotid–subclavian bypass was performed to revascularize at least one subclavian artery. (C) In the second scenario, zone 1 endograft placement was required to achieve adequate proximal seal, necessitating carotid-carotid bypass for LCCA revascularization in addition to LSCA revascularization. From Andersen et al. Reproduced with permission from the *Journal of Vascular Surgery.*[4]

not possible, and zone 2 – zone 0 (Ishimaru classification[17]) endograft coverage is required to achieve adequate proximal landing zone, yielding bilateral subclavian artery coverage in most cases. As such, at least one subclavian artery will require revascularization, and bilateral subclavian artery revascularization is performed if indicated.[12] For cases requiring zone 1 endograft coverage, a carotid-carotid bypass is performed to revascularize the left common carotid artery (LCCA) prior to LCCA coverage by the endograft. For cases requiring zone 0 endograft coverage, ascending aorta-based arch debranching is performed via median sternotomy to revascularize the right common carotid artery (RCCA) and LCCA prior to endograft coverage.[14,15,18]

OUTCOMES

In our previously published series spanning March 2005 to April 2012, nineteen patients underwent 20 operations to repair 22 (13 native, 9 aberrant) SAAs with an intrathoracic component.[4] Mean SAA diameter was 3.1 cm (range 1.6–6.0 cm). The mean patient age was 57 (range 24-80) years. 21% (n=4) of patients had a connective tissue disorder (two Loeys-Dietz, two Marfan). 36% (n=8) of SAAs were repaired by open techniques and 64% (n=14) via a TEVAR-based approach. Of the 12 patients with 14 SAAs repaired by TEVAR, repair was achieved by totally endovascular techniques in 17% (n=2) of patients and by hybrid techniques in 83% (n=10) of patients. All TEVAR cases required proximal landing zone in the aortic arch (zone 0-2) and revascularization of at least one arch vessel in 83% (10 of 12) of patients. Concomitant repair of associated aortic pathology was performed in 50% (n=10) of operations.

30-Day/In-Hospital Outcomes

All patients survived to hospital discharge. One patient died after hospital discharge but within 30-days of surgery due to respiratory failure after urgent zone 0 hybrid arch repair, yielding a 30-day/in-hospital mortality rate of 5% (0% elective, 33% non-elective). One patient with an aberrant left SAA and right descending thoracic aorta experienced a perioperative stroke, and no cases of paraplegia were observed (Table 10-1).

TABLE 10-1. 30-DAY/IN-HOSPITAL OUTCOMES

Variable	Total procedures (*N* = 20)	Hybrid/ Endovascular (*N* = 13)	Open (*N* = 7)	*P* Value
In-hospital death	0	0	0	
30-day/in-hospital death	1 (5%)	1 (7.7%)	0	> 0.99
Stroke (neurologic deficit lasting > 72 hours)	1 (5%)	1 (7.7%)	0	> 0.99
Permanent paraplegia/ paraparesis	0	0	0	

Data represented as number (percent). SCA = subclavian artery.

From Andersen et al. Reproduced with permission from the *Journal of Vascular Surgery*.[4]

SUBCLAVIAN ARTERY BYPASS GRAFT PATENCY, RE-INTERVENTIONS, AND SURVIVAL

Mean clinic follow-up at the time of original publication was 24 ± 21 months (median 18 months) with 21% (4 of 19) of patients lost to follow-up. During the follow-up interval, 16% (n = 3) of patients required re-intervention (Figure 10-11A). Two patients with native right SAAs required reintervention for RSCA bypass graft thrombosis. The third patient required aberrant RSCA ligation for type II endoleak 6 weeks after emergent acute type B dissection and aberrant right SAA repair. Primary subclavian artery bypass graft patency at 12 months was 100% for TEVAR-based repairs but 75% for open repairs owing to the two failed RSCA bypass grafts that required re-intervention (P=0.11, Figure 10-11B). Secondary patency was 100% as all subclavian artery bypass grafts were patent at most recent follow-up. Kaplan-Meier estimates of survival for the entire patient cohort were 95% and 73% at 1 and 3 years, respectively (P = 0.59, Figure 10-11C).

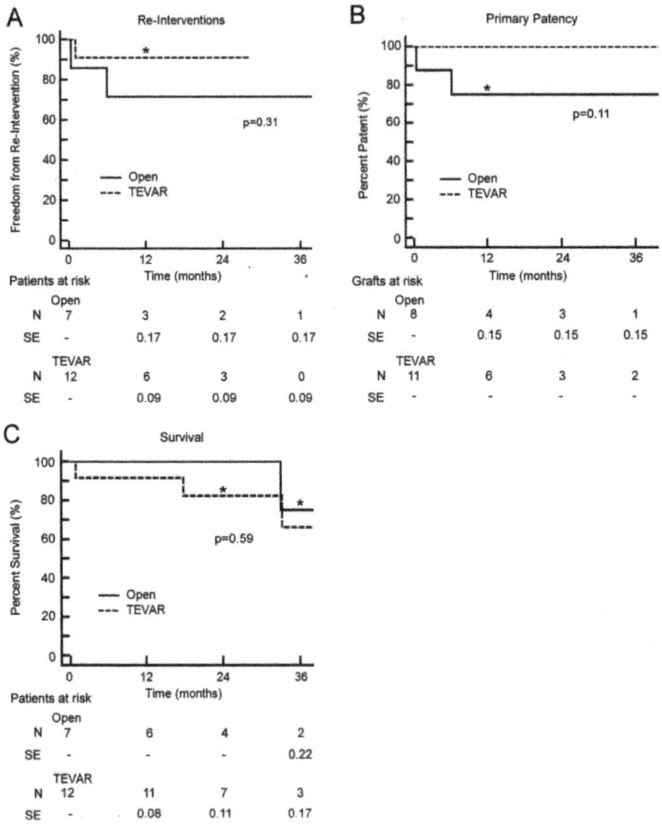

Figure 10-11. Kaplan-Meier estimates of (A) re-interventions, (B) primary subclavian artery bypass graft patency, and (C) survival stratified by operative approach. N = number at risk. SE = standard error. *denotes the time point at which standard error exceeds 10%. From Andersen et al. Reproduced with permission from the *Journal of Vascular Surgery*.[4]

CONCLUSION

SAAs are rare vascular lesions which require complex operative planning due to numerous anatomic and patient-specific considerations. Conventional open intrathoracic SAA repair requires sternotomy or thoracotomy for access and was associated with a mortality rate of 8% and a complication rate of 26% in a comprehensive meta-analysis.[3] Endovascular SAA repair has been shown to be associated with a lower rate of cardiopulmonary complications.[3] However, stent-grafting within the subclavian artery to exclude SAAs with covered stents has been associated with high rates of short-term thrombosis and failure (0–17%) due to compression, deformation, and fracture due to the rotationary forces experienced by the subclavian artery and the anatomic location under the clavicle.[3,8] Proximal SAA inflow exclusion by aortic endografting may therefore be a superior method of endovascular SAA treatment by avoiding the limitations of stent-graft placement within the subclavian artery. Our institutional results support this approach by demonstrating a 100% primary technical success rate, 100% primary subclavian artery bypass graft patency, and a 91% freedom from reintervention rate with TEVAR-based endovascular repair techniques. Modern TEVAR-based endovascular techniques therefore expand SAA repair options with excellent results and allow for less-invasive repair of SAAs as well as concomitant thoracic aortic pathology in many patients. The majority of SAAs, and nearly all aberrant SAAs, can be repaired using a TEVAR-based approach without the need for sternotomy or thoracotomy.

REFERENCES

1. Coselli JS, Crawford ES. Surgical treatment of aneurysms of the intrathoracic segment of the subclavian artery. *Chest.* 1987;91(5):704–8.
2. Austin EH, Wolfe WG. Aneurysm of aberrant subclavian artery with a review of the literature. *J Vasc Surg.* 1985;2(4):571–7.
3. Vierhout BP, Zeebregts CJ, van den Dungen JJ, Reijnen MM. Changing profiles of diagnostic and treatment options in subclavian artery aneurysms. *Eur J Vasc Endovasc Surg.* 2010;40(1):27–34.
4. Andersen ND, Barfield ME, Hanna JM, Shah AA, et al. Intrathoracic subclavian artery aneurysm repair in the thoracic endovascular aortic repair era. *J Vasc Surg.* 2013;57(4):915–25.
5. Lawrence PF, Gazak C, Bhirangi L, Jones B, et al. The epidemiology of surgically repaired aneurysms in the United States. *J Vasc Surg.* 1999;30(4):632–40.
6. Dent TL, Lindenauer SM, Ernst CB, Fry WJ. Multiple arteriosclerotic arterial aneurysms. *Arch Surg.* 1972;105(2):338–44.
7. Dougherty MJ, Calligaro KD, Savarese RP, DeLaurentis DA. Atherosclerotic aneurysm of the intrathoracic subclavian artery: A case report and review of the literature. *J Vasc Surg.* 1995;21(3):521–9.
8. Clagett GP. Upper Extremity Aneurysms. In: Rutherford RB, editor. *Vascular Surgery.* 6th ed. Philadelphia, PA: Elsevier Saunders; 2005. p. 1551–64.
9. Ota T, Okada K, Takanashi S, Yamamoto S, Okita Y. Surgical treatment for Kommerell's diverticulum. *J Thorac Cardiovasc Surg.* 2006;131(3):574–8.
10. Cina CS, Althani H, Pasenau J, Abouzahr L. Kommerell's diverticulum and right-sided aortic arch: A cohort study and review of the literature. *J Vasc Surg.* 2004;39(1):131–9.
11. Waterman AL, Feezor RJ, Lee WA, et al. Endovascular treatment of acute and chronic aortic pathology in patients with Marfan syndrome. *J Vasc Surg.* 2012;55(5):1234–40; discussion 40–1.

12. Lee TC, Andersen ND, Williams JB, Bhattacharya SD, et al. Results with a selective revascularization strategy for left subclavian artery coverage during thoracic endovascular aortic repair. *Ann Thorac Surg*. 2011;92(1):97–102; discussion-3.
13. Rajagopal K, Rogers JG, Lodge AJ, et al. Two-stage total cardioaortic replacement for end-stage heart and aortic disease in Marfan syndrome: Case report and review of the literature. *J Heart Lung Transplant*. 2009;28(9):958–63.
14. Hughes GC, Sulzer CF, McCann RL, Swaminathan M. Endovascular approaches to complex thoracic aortic disease. *Semin Cardiothorac Vasc Anesth*. 2008;12(4):298–319.
15. Hughes GC, Daneshmand MA, Balsara KR, et al. "Hybrid" repair of aneurysms of the transverse aortic arch: Midterm results. *Ann Thorac Surg*. 2009;88(6):1882–7; discussion 7–8.
16. Hughes GC. Aggressive aortic replacement for Loeys-Dietz syndrome. *Tex Heart Inst J*. 2011;38(6):663–6.
17. Ishimaru S. Endografting of the aortic arch. *J Endovasc Ther*. 2004;11 Suppl 2:II62–71.
18. Andersen ND, Williams JB, Hanna JM, et al. Results with an algorithmic approach to hybrid repair of the aortic arch. *J Vasc Surg*. 2013;57(3):655–67; discussion 66–7.

11

History of the Development of Endografts in the Americas

Juan C. Parodi, MD and Federico E. Parodi, MD

THE CONCEPTION OF THE IDEA AND THE FIRST STEPS

In 1976 I was a chief resident of vascular surgery at the Cleveland Clinic in Cleveland, Ohio. I acquired my previous training in general surgery at the University of Buenos Aires and the University of Illinois in Chicago.

The Division of Vascular Surgery at the Cleveland Clinic had a very busy practice; there were two staff members, Alfred Humphries and Edwin Beven, both excellent surgeons and teachers. Resection of abdominal aortic aneurysms (AAAs) was one of the most common operations performed in the division. The experience of the surgeons was remarkable, as was the pre- and post-operative care performed by the surgeons and physicians of vascular medicine (Jess Young and Ralph De Wolfe). In spite of the good care and treatment of the patients, complications were often seen, and mortality occurred with certain frequency.

One day in 1976, I told Al Humphries that I felt that we were being too aggressive with the old and often debilitated patients, and we needed to design a less traumatic way to repair the aneurysm.

In parallel with my surgical practice I was learning the Seldinger technique from an interventional radiologist who went to Cleveland from the Massachusetts General Hospital and very kindly acted as a mentor to me. One day, we were doing an AAA resection with Dr. Humphries, and I told him: "Most of the patients with aneurysms have big arteries, we could use the Seldinger technique, go retrograde to the aorta from the femoral artery, and deploy a thin but strong endograft covering a metal cage with barbs that would anchor and seal the aneurysm. My first drawings depicted two zig-zag rings of stainless steel, like those developed by Gianturco many years after, joined by two bars of metal welded to the rings, the Dacron was sutured to the metal.

I told Humphries, "I foresee a day in which patients will be walking to the operating room, will have the exclusion of the aneurysm under local anesthesia from the groin; we will put a band aid on the groin, and the patient will leave the operating room walking." Today several centers, including our own, do ambulatory surgery for some aneurysms. The procedure using closure devices was performed at the Cleveland Clinic in February of 2000. It was a live case transmitted to the Arizona Heart Center meeting in Phoenix in a celebration of the tenth anniversary of the first successful case of endoluminal exclusion of an abdominal aortic aneurysm in the world.

After finishing my training, I received offers from both Chicago and the Cleveland Clinic to continue working at these institutions, but my family preferred to go back to Buenos Aires.

In Buenos Aires I was doing experiments with stray dogs from the street, since I did not have support from industry or a university. I was using an aneurysmal graft to replace the abdominal aorta in dogs, and after a month I was excluding the aneurysm from the groin. I was welding the stainless steel rings by myself. My results were encouraging, but the quality of the "metal cage" and its integrity over time were not very good. As a model, I was using a graft in the shape of an aneurysm, I replaced the infra-renal aorta of dogs with it and after a few weeks implanted the "covered metal cage" from the femoral artery.

In 1988 I met Julio Palmaz during a meeting in Washington, DC. He was presenting his initial experience with his stent. I approached him, learned that he was also from Argentina, and we had a long conversation. I explained to him about my efforts from 1976 to 1988 and even about my failure to convince Toby Cosgrove (now CEO of the Cleveland Clinic) to explore the use of the covered metal cage to occlude the entry site of Type B aortic dissections. I asked him if I could use his stents to fix and seal the endograft. After hours of hesitation, he gave me a sample of his stents.

In Buenos Aires I visited an engineer, Carlos Sommer, who was producing missiles for export to Iran during its world with Iraq. He had the necessary high level of technology, and I persuaded him to produce a re-designed Palmaz stent with electro-erosion and electro-polishing using medical stainless steel produced in Sweden. He succeeded. The next step was to obtain a fabric graft. There was a company headed by a biochemist called Barone who produced for me a weft Dacron graft that was expandable at both ends according to my specifications. In that way we could use just one product for all sizes of aneurysm necks; the only variable was the size of the balloon, which was a valvuloplasty balloon produced in France by Bolt.

I performed 52 experiences with the new model, again with stray dogs, which I kept alive on the farm of a friend for 6 months. Results were remarkably good. I also introduced the aorto-uni-iliac device with occlusion using a plug of the contralateral iliac artery and a femoro-femoral bypass.

The First Case

The president of Argentina, who had learned that I was working on the project for many years, referred my first patient. The patient was a 74-year-old gentleman with back pain, an AAA, and severe COPD, which precluded him from having general anesthesia.

I had a long meeting with the patient and his family, explaining the procedure with precision and expressing our limitations in terms of knowing long-term results.

I remember showing them angiograms from before and after treatment and 6-month follow-up autopsies of the animals. They were very comfortable with the results, but their faces changed when I told them that the studies were from dogs, and the patient was going to be the first person in the world to have the procedure. They nevertheless accepted the terms and signed the informed consent form.

I constructed the device for him with extra-large Palmaz stents that I had redesigned to reach 30 mm in diameter. I sutured the graft to the stent and put two marks of gold at the end of the fabric. I used a 24-Fr Teflon sheath with a valve at the end, and I built a nose cone for the distal end with the end of the balloon partially inflated.

On September 7, 1990 I transferred the patient to the angio room, and under local anesthesia I exposed the right femoral artery. Julio Palmaz assisted me. I advanced a Wholey wire up to the descending aorta, and I used a pigtail to perform an angiogram. I gave 5000 U of heparin intravenously. I completed the arteriogram and advanced a super-stiff wire over the pigtail. Marks were made on the screen depicting the renal and iliac arteries. The 24-Fr Teflon sheath was placed in position over the wire and once the gold marks were positioned exactly under the renal arteries, the balloon was inflated for one minute.

With the same balloon, we distended the graft down to the distal gold mark. The final arteriogram was perfect. We saw no leaking, so we decided not to place the distal stent. The patient did well and was discharged the following day. An echogram showed good positioning of the graft and no leaks. It was encouraging that the patient reported to us that his back pain had subsided. That night after having dinner with Dr. Palmaz in a restaurant near the hospital, we went back to see our patients. That same day, I had performed an open replacement under general anesthesia. To our surprise, the endovascular case was having dinner while the first patient, who had had the open procedure, was still intubated. I told Julio, "If we can reproduce this procedure and the results are durable, it will be a major revolution in the way we treat aneurysms."

Later, we learned that Dr. Volodos in the Ukraine had tried to repair an AAA, but he had failed. The graft twisted and occluded the lumen, and he had to do an open conversion. Ours was, then, the first successful endovascular repair of AAA in history.

The first patient had an arteriogram one week later showing complete exclusion of the aneurysm: he came back, however, three months later with back pain. A CT scan showed a distal leak. We decided to place the second stent distally, after which the patient survived for 9 years, the aneurysm decreased in size, and no leakage was detected. The eventual cause of death was pancreatic cancer. Since this case, our approach has been to place two stents, and we have also introduced the aorto-uni-iliac endograft with occlusion of the contralateral iliac artery and a femoro-femoral bypass. Initially, we used detachable balloons produced by Bolt in France; later on we decided to use a Palmaz stent attached to a graft with a blind end.

The same week I operated on the first patient, a symposium of the "Spanish-Speaking Vascular Society" was held in Buenos Aires. I presented a video of the case and pictures of the device and patient. Gregorio Sicard was in the audience. He was very impressed and expressed his support for the procedure. He then invited me to be a visiting professor at Washington University in St Louis, where I became professor of surgery many years later. That was one of my most enriching experiences in academic surgery. Seventeen Nobel Prize recipients in medicine have been affiliated with Washington University. I continued to handle similar cases and published the initial experience in the *Annals of Vascular Surgery* in 1991.[1] The article had been previously rejected from the *Journal of Vascular Surgery*. After doing more than 50 cases, I then published my experience in the *Journal of Vascular Surgery*.

I received an invitation to present my experience in the Annual Meeting of the Society for Vascular Surgery. Craig Miller from Stanford was the other speaker during a breakfast session, and he gave me his assigned time as first speaker because, he said, most, if not all, of the people in the audience were there to listen to my talk. A great gesture from a great man.

Very soon we started to see complications, and we quickly realized the need to use the distal stent. The need to use the iliac arteries also became obvious.

Initially, I designed a bifurcated graft, which was deployed by attaching the contralateral limb to a guidewire after doing a crossover from the other side. Technically, it was successful but it also resulted in our first fatal complication. The patient was acidotic, had a base excess –21, mottled skin appeared in the lower extremities and abdomen. The complication was a massive micro-embolism caused by excessive instrumentation inside the aneurysm. The embolization included renal arteries and the superior mesenteric artery in addition to the pelvis and lower extremities. We abandoned attempts to perform bifurcations, and ended up inserting aorto-uni-iliac grafts, occluding the contralateral common iliac artery and performing a femoro-femoral bypass, but were unable to save the patient

We have had many visitors from all over the world and also have done live demonstrations in Nancy, France and Bronx, New York. The revolution was started and, as predicted in John Bergan's commentary to the first article, "Opposition will be mounted." And it was: the opposition was sometimes aggressive.

In spite of the opposition, I was sure that the procedure was reasonable and solid. Very soon other companies started producing endografts—Mintec and EVT and, later on, Aneurx.

By this time, we knew that nothing could stop the trend. One day I told John Manick from Boston and John Porter from Oregon: "If humankind was able to build the International Space Station, how could they not replace a vascular suture and affix a graft to the wall of the aorta with mechanical devices?"

I traveled a lot—France, Spain, and Sweden—but my favorite country has always been Italy. My family was originally from Genova (Parodi) and from Parma (D'Allasta), and I had good friends everywhere. The first city I visited as a professor was Verona, where I had been invited by Professor Vecchione, who is no longer with us. There, Drs. Adami and Scuro helped me to perform very successful surgeries. I went also to La Sapienza in Rome, to Milano with LuigiInglese and Tealdi, to Bologna with Stella, to Ravenna, Ferrara, Cerdegna, Palermo, and more. We had a wonderful time in Italy, and we motivated many people to begin using our techniques. We invited Tom Fogarty, who introduced the Aneurx device to Italy, to join us on a trip. Today, Italy is one of the leading countries in the world in terms of using endovascular treatments.

MISTAKES

During my life, I have made several mistakes, and among them was to include Drs. Palmaz and Barone in my patent, when in reality they were not involved as inventors. That caused me serious problems. The other big mistake was to include Johnson & Johnson in my project; they hindered the project and prevented the product I developed from reaching the market.

When J&J was ready to start trials in America, I was informed that they had decided to use a different device. The different device was one designed by Palmaz, who did not invite me to participate. His invention, which failed, was constructed with two covered Palmaz stents in parallel to make a bifurcated device. They tried the device, which failed, and my project was abandoned in spite of the success that I still have with it. Loyalty was not one of Palmaz's virtues, and J&J prevented the surgical community from acquiring a useful balloon-expandable endograft. In the past two years, St. George Medical (Freeport, Bahamas and Luminy, France) developed the Titan AAA, a bifurcated endograft with a proximal balloon-expandable stent. It is currently being marketed in Europe.

Barone refused to sign a contract or start a company with me, but he took the idea. He is still selling products in Argentina and making a great deal of money by promoting products based on my initial idea. My decisions as a businessman did not result in a great performance for my own bottom line.

While working with J&J, we learned about the work of Volodos in Ukraine. J&J sent a person to meet him. He never received the emissary, who went back to America saying that Volodos was not showing what he was doing and that Volodos had seen two consecutive catastrophes in his operating room. According to information this person collected, Volodos was opening aneurysms, placing the endograft inside, and then closing the aneurysm over it. I have no doubt that he was working on an idea similar to mine, but I was not able to meet him during my visits to Russia. I also learned that Russians had little idea about endografts, at least at the time of my visits. My intention was to establish a collaboration with him, but I couldn't make it happen. His work had had little, if any, impact on the international level.

Another big mistake I made occurred when I invented the endosutures. I was visiting Leon Hirsch at US Surgical Corporation, and I saw the Protract, a product used to apply spiral sutures to treat hernias laparoscopically. Immediately, I had an idea: "I can make this applicator flexible, with a low profile, and I will be able to apply endosutures to seal and fix endografts to prevent migrations and leaks." US Surgical assigned an engineer, Peter Ratcliff, who worked with me, and we filed patents. Tyco acquired US Surgical, and they decided to stop the project.

Alan Kaganof, a venture capitalist from Menlo Park, California came with Lee Bolduc to Buenos Aires, and they invited me to form a company. We were the three founders of APTUS. Alan had the idea of developing a complete endograft. I had recommended a different approach, but he did not pay any attention to my ideas. They excluded me from the company. I couldn't use my own product, and they diluted my participation in a similar way the founder of Facebook did with his initial collaborators. Now, the FDA has approved the endosuture (my product) alone, and I have no participation in the company. I write this to alert young investigators and to advise them not to be abused by businessmen as I was.

PRESENTATIONS

In the same week I operated on my first patient, at the meeting of the Spanish-Speaking Vascular Society, I presented a video of the operation.

I also presented my experience, by then supported by several additional cases, at a meeting including Frank Criado in Miami the following year. John Bergan, who was a faculty member of the meeting, became very excited and suggested that I publish the initial five cases, including one dissection, in the *Annals of Vascular Surgery* in 1991. The publication became very popular and opened the door to a new technology. Lazarus filed a patent in the 1980s, which developed with EVT and became the first FDA-approved device in America.

Frank Veith and Michael Marin invited me to do the first case in America with my primitive device; the case was successful and provided an injection of enthusiasm for all American interventionists. I continued to do cases at home in Buenos Aires, in America, and also in Europe and Israel. Most of the cases were successful and the patients remained in good condition for many years; recently, I received a CT scan from Ferrara of a case done 17 years ago with excellent results.

When I reached 50 cases with good follow-up, I presented my experience at the Society for Vascular Surgery, and I received multiple invitations to present and also to work in America and other countries. I have been a professor of surgery at Wake Forest, Wayne State, Washington University, University of Miami, and now I have an invitation from the University of Michigan. I have trained colleagues in South America, North America, Europe, Japan, China, Sweden, South Africa, and Israel.

DISSECTIONS, TRAUMA, AND OCCLUSIVE DISEASE

In 1979, I was unsuccessful in gaining the support of Toby Cosgrove for a project to treat type B dissections with a covered cage of metal to occlude the entry site.

In 1991 I treated the first dissection (abdominal) while successfully occluding the entry site. In 1995 I treated the first type A dissection on a patient with a contained rupture of the descending aorta using a covered Palmaz stent while stopping the heart with adenosine. The patient survived, and at 12 years post-surgery the aorta looked normal.

In 1997 I treated a patient with a complicated type B dissection (anuria and intestinal ischemia associated with limb ischemia). The patient was still alive in 2014.

In 1991 we treated a police officer with a subclavian A-V fistula after a gunshot wound. This was the first of hundreds of trauma cases treated endoluminally. In the illustration we show an aorto-cava fistula after a gunshot wound treated with a covered stent.

A general from the Pentagon brought his father who was 87 years old to have his aneurysm fixed under local anesthesia. He also observed one case of common carotid false aneurysm treated under local anesthesia using a covered Palmaz stent. Later on I was invited by the general, who was also a physician, to make a presentation for military surgeons at Walter Reed Hospital.

Occlusive disease

I thought that creating a barrier between the blood and the dilated artery after angioplasty could prevent hyperplasia. Dr. Michael Marin proved the concept in iliac arteries, but nobody paid attention until the Viabahn appeared. I had presented the concept of creating a barrier with polytetrafluoroethylene (PTFE) in the superficial femoral artery to prevent restenosis after angioplasty in Flagstaff, Arizona (W.L. Gore & Associates) in 1988; Jack Hoover had invited me. Later on, they developed the Viabahn.

FOGARTY

Tom Fogarty, a good friend, invited me to work for him in California. His company, Cardiovascular Concepts, was developing an endograft. I helped him, and that product ended up as the Aneurx product, which was very successful for many years.

WESLEY MOORE, TIM CHUTER, ROY GREENBERG

Drs. Moore and Chuter used the first FDA-approved devices in America and became pioneers in the field. Tim Chuter did the first fenestrated and branched grafts in America, but very soon Dr. Roy Greenberg appeared on the horizon and became the most experienced in the world with this new technology. He also introduced his own ideas for improvements in the products. Now surgeons at the Cleveland Clinic have performed more than 1000 cases of fenestrations with superb results. They also have one Parodi on their staff: my son Ezequiel.

ENDOGRAFTS IN AMERICA

More than 70% of aneurysms, Type B dissections, and transections are being treated with endografts in America. Mortality for aneurysms has dropped by half, and the survival benefit of endografts is proven. The incidence of ruptured aneurysms has dropped because more patients, who previously had been considered very high risk or inoperable, can now have the aneurysm treated. Covered stents (the concept I presented to Gore in Flagstaff in 1988) are widely used and produced by several companies.

Endoluminal treatment of aneurysms has established a new standard. Vascular surgery has evolved and has become a new specialty, almost completely different than it was 20 years ago. Volodos should be recognized as a pioneer, but his influence has been minimal in the endoluminal revolution.

Opening the operating room to everyone, showing our patients and images, presenting our successful cases as well as our failures, traveling all over the world to teach the technique, and collaborating with every single surgeon who wanted to learn the technique has made our group the trailblazers in the world for endografts.

REFERENCE

1. Parodi JC, Palmaz JC, Barone HD. Transfemoral intraluminal graft implantation for abdominal aortic aneurysms. *Ann Vasc Surg*. 1991;5:491–9.

12

Retrievable Inferior Vena Cava Filters: Advanced Techniques for Retrieval of Embedded Devices

Kush R. Desai, MD, Robert J. Lewandowski, MD, Robert K. Ryu, MD, and Robert L. Vogelzang, MD

Inferior vena cava (IVC) filters are utilized in patients with venous thromboembolic disease (VTE) in whom medical therapy has failed or is contraindicated, as well as for prophylaxis from VTE.[1] Two types of devices are used in clinical practice; retrievable/optional filters and permanent filters. Prospective studies have demonstrated that permanent IVC filters (pIVCF) decrease the risk of pulmonary embolism while increasing the risk of lower extremity deep venous thrombosis (DVT).[2, 3] Retrievable inferior vena cava filters (rIVCF) were developed to provide temporary protection from pulmonary embolism (PE) while minimizing the risk of filter related DVT.

Since their introduction, the placement of rIVCFs has increased dramatically, with a projected increase in the future.[4] Though designed to be removed when no longer indicated, the majority of filters are left in place permanently.[5, 6] Certainly, poor clinical follow up plays an important role in low retrieval rates; however, prolonged filter implantation has been associated with retrieval failure rates as high as 43%.[7] Furthermore, prolonged filter dwell time has been associated with complications including device fracture, migration, organ penetration by device components, and elevated risk of DVT.[8]

This chapter will explore the key clinical issues associated with rIVCFs. Specifically, it will briefly examine the differences between permanent and retrievable devices, the major obstacles to removal of rIVCFs, and the advanced techniques available to facilitate retrieval of embedded devices.

RETRIEVABLE IVC FILTERS AND PERMANENT IVC FILTERS ARE NOT EQUIVALENT DEVICES

Under 510(k) clearance, the US Food and Drug Administration (FDA) have approved all current commercially available rIVCFs for both retrievable and permanent indications. However, significant differences exist between pIVCFs and rIVCFs, largely due to the design constraints on rIVCFs; these devices must provide equivalent protection from PE while allowing removal when no longer indicated, presenting a significant challenge in engineering these devices.

Though studies have shown these devices provide excellent protection from pulmonary embolism,[9] numerous reports in the literature have shown rIVCFs are subject to device related complications, including fracture, migration/embolization,[10] and perforation/organ penetration,[11–14] relative to permanent devices. In a review of the FDA's own Manufacturer and User Facility Device Experience (MAUDE) database, Andreoli et al reported that nearly 87% of user reported adverse events were associated with rIVCFs, as opposed to approximately 13% associated with pIVCFs.[15] Another retrospective review found a complication rate of 9% in a series of 449 rIVCFs.[16] Furthermore, these complication rates appear to increase with dwell time; particularly fracture and embolization of filter components.[17–19] Devices that are in place for extended periods of time potentially encounter prolonged exposure to biomechanical rotational and torsional forces, which result in metal fatigue and eventually could result in compromised device structural integrity.[20, 21] Findings such as these prompted the FDA to issue a safety alert in 2010, advising all physicians responsible for patients with rIVCFs to have these devices removed as soon as they were no longer clinically necessary.[22]

IMPEDIMENTS TO REMOVAL OF RETRIEVABLE IVC FILTERS

The placement of rIVCFs is the province of multiple medical specialties, including interventional radiology, interventional cardiology, and vascular surgery. This significantly complicates monitoring of patients with these devices, and poor clinical follow up impedes retrieval of devices that are no longer indicated. Several studies have confirmed this theory, with reported retrieval rates as low as 8.5%.[23] The development of dedicated service lines for patients with these devices have positively impacted retrieval rates, with one study reporting an increase in retrieval rates from 29% to 60% after the establishment of a dedicated IVC filter service.[24]

Prior studies have identified prolonged rIVCF dwell time as a negative predictor for successful retrieval. In one study utilizing three different rIVCF devices in 200 patients, a dwell time of over 90 days was associated with retrieval failure.[25] A separate study utilizing a single device noted increased likelihood of failure at 6 months.[26] Findings from studies like these have led to the perception that prolonged dwell time rIVCFs should be left in situ due to the theoretical risk of vascular and perivascular injury during a retrieval procedure.[27] However, we have recently published a study demonstrating that filter removal can be performed regardless of filter dwell time with a failure rate of 3% or less when advanced endovascular techniques are employed. We found that there was a strong positive association with filter dwell time and the need for advanced filter techniques. Interestingly, despite the complex nature of some of these advanced retrieval procedures, our complication rates were low, and were not associated with filter dwell time.[28]

FILTER REMOVAL TECHNIQUES

Most rIVCF employ a somewhat conical design, including the Denali, G2X,/G2, Eclipse, Meridian (all Bard Peripheral Vascular Inc., Tempe, AZ), Celect, Gunther Tulip (both Cook Medical Inc., Bloomington, IN), ALN (ALN Implants Chirurgicaux, GHisonaccia, France), and Option/Option Elite (Argon Medical Devices, Plano, TX). These devices are designed to be retrieved via an internal jugular venous access. The OptEase (Cordis Corp., Miami Lakes, FL) is a non-conical polyhedron structure designed to be retrieved from a femoral venous access. A relative newcomer to the market, the Crux (Volcano Corp., San Diego, CA) has a helical design with hooks on both the caudal and cranial aspects of the filter, allowing retrieval from either jugular or femoral approach.

Standard Technique

Standard filter removal can be performed with a variety of devices; however, the basic underlying method is the same with the use of device to capture the filter (i.e. endovascular snare) and a sheath to coaxially collapse the filter and disengage filter elements from the caval wall. Most rIVCF manufacturers offer a retrieval kit; in our experience, these are rarely necessary to retrieve filters that are commercial available today.

Our approach to standard filter retrieval begins with a pigtail flush catheter, which is introduced over a wire caudal to the filter. Care is taken not to entangle the wire in the filter. After cavography is performed to assess for in situ filter thrombus, we place coaxial sheaths immediately cranial to the filter. We utilize a standard endovascular snare to capture the filter hook. Once captured, the filter is collapsed with the sheaths while gentle counter traction is applied via the snare.

Advanced Techniques in rIVCF Removal

Standard filter removal can fail for a variety of reasons, including filter tilt, encasement of the filter hook in the wall by a fibrin cap, incorporation of filter elements into the caval wall, significant extracaval perforation of filter elements, and filter fracture.

When filters are tilted significantly, standard straight sheaths and snare devices are often unable to capture the filter hook successfully. The use of curved inner sheath can add directionality and facilitate successful snaring of a hook that is significantly deviated from the central axis of the IVC (Figure 12-1). This technique is most useful when the filter hook is not embedded and no fibrin cap formation has taken place. In

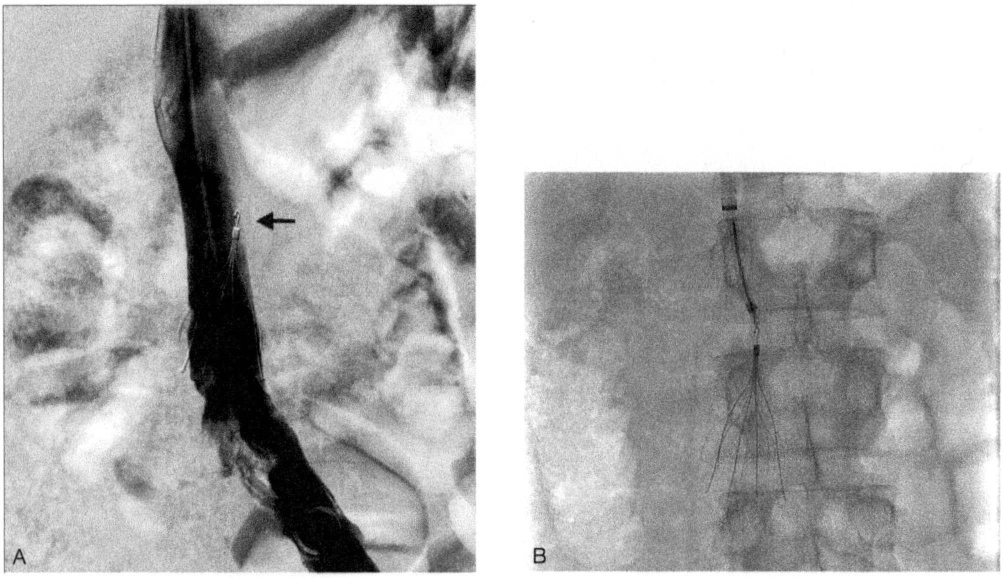

Figure 12-1. Curved sheath use for retrieval of tilted, nonembedded filters. (**A**) Filter hook is significantly tilted from the central axis of the cava (arrow). (**B**) Curved inner sheath provides greater directionality to enable successful snaring of the filter hook.

our practice, we utilize a Flexor sheath with Ansel 2 modification (Cook Medical Inc., Bloomington, IN).

Tip or hook embedded rIVCF present perhaps the most significant challenge to retrieval. Several techniques have been described as an approach to this problem, however we will highlight two that are most used in our practice, the loop snare and use of rigid endobronchial forceps.

The loop snare technique was originally described where a reverse curve catheter was guided through the filter struts, and a hydrophilic wire was advanced cranially.[27] The free end of the wire is then snared and externalized. This wire loop is then utilized to provide counter-traction while the sheath was coaxially collapsed over the filter (Figure 12-2). We do not perform this maneuver with regularity, primarily out of concern of causing fracture of filter elements while exerting counter-traction during coaxial collapse of the filter. Instead, we have developed a modified technique that targets the fibrin cap instead.[29] In our technique, we utilize a reverse curve catheter to engage the cap at the filter apex that is present in a large portion of these patients. A hydrophilic wire is then passed cranially and snared, forming a wire loop through the fibrin cap. The sheath is then advanced coaxially over the wire loop, either resulting in capture and collapse of the filter or disruption of the fibrin cap (Figure 12-3). If the latter occurs, a standard snare can be used to capture and retrieve the filter.

Rigid endobronchial forceps have been used to dissect fibrinous tissue from the filter apex and allow exposure and subsequent capture of the filter hook.[30] These forceps are usually malleable and can be shaped to provide the appropriate degree of curvature to reach a tilted, embedded filter apex. Once the fibrin encasing the apex has been

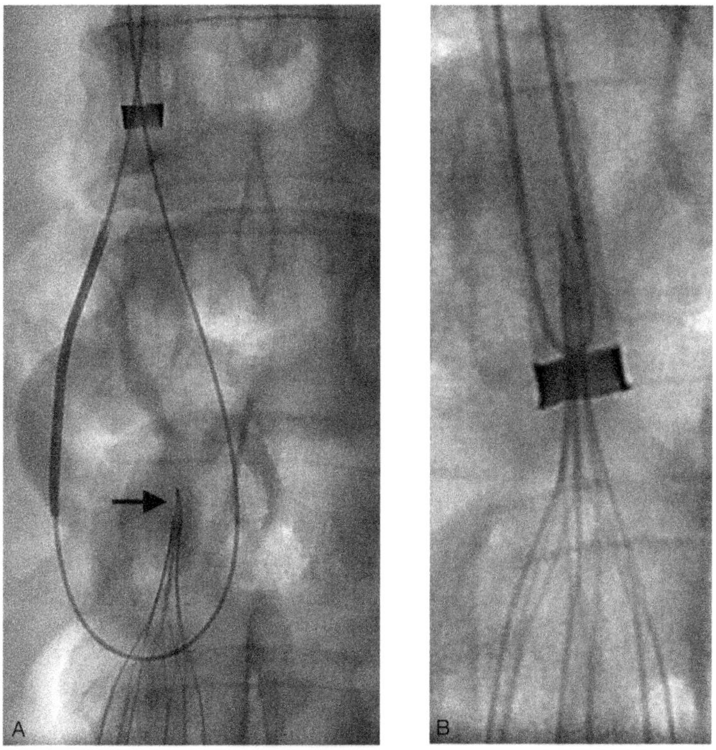

Figure 12-2. Loop wire through the filter. (**A**) Hydrophilic wire is looped through the filter struts with the aid of a reverse curve catheter. Note that the filter hook here has been fractured by prior filter retrieval attempt (arrow). (**B**) Utilizing tension on the looped wire, the sheath is coaxially advanced over the filter apex.

sufficiently removed, the filter hook can be captured with the forceps and the sheath can be advanced in a coaxial fashion to collapse and remove the filter (Figure 12-4). Care must be taken with forceps, however. Large curvatures of the forceps can cause caval distention and associated discomfort to the patient. Furthermore, tearing of the IVC wall can happen if the operator inadvertently grasps the caval wall instead of the fibrin tissue.

In some cases, a filter hook can be successfully captured, but the rIVCF cannot be collapse within the sheath, despite exertion of large forces. This occurs when there is incorporation of the filter struts into the wall. Laser extraction sheaths originally designed for pacemaker lead extraction have been successfully used to photothermally ablate fibrinous tissue encasing the filter struts into the caval wall, allowing filter removal without having to exert large and potentially hazardous forces during the retrieval procedure.[31] The CVX-300 Excimer laser system utilizes 12, 14, and 16 Fr, 50 cm sheaths which are introduced via a larger outer sheath. The laser is sequentially activated to ablate the encasing tissue and eventually allow filter collapse and removal (Figure 12-5). It is important to note that control of the filter apex/hook is required to successfully employ photothermal laser ablation; indeed it is common in our practice that other techniques need to be employed to free the filter apex prior to using the laser sheath.

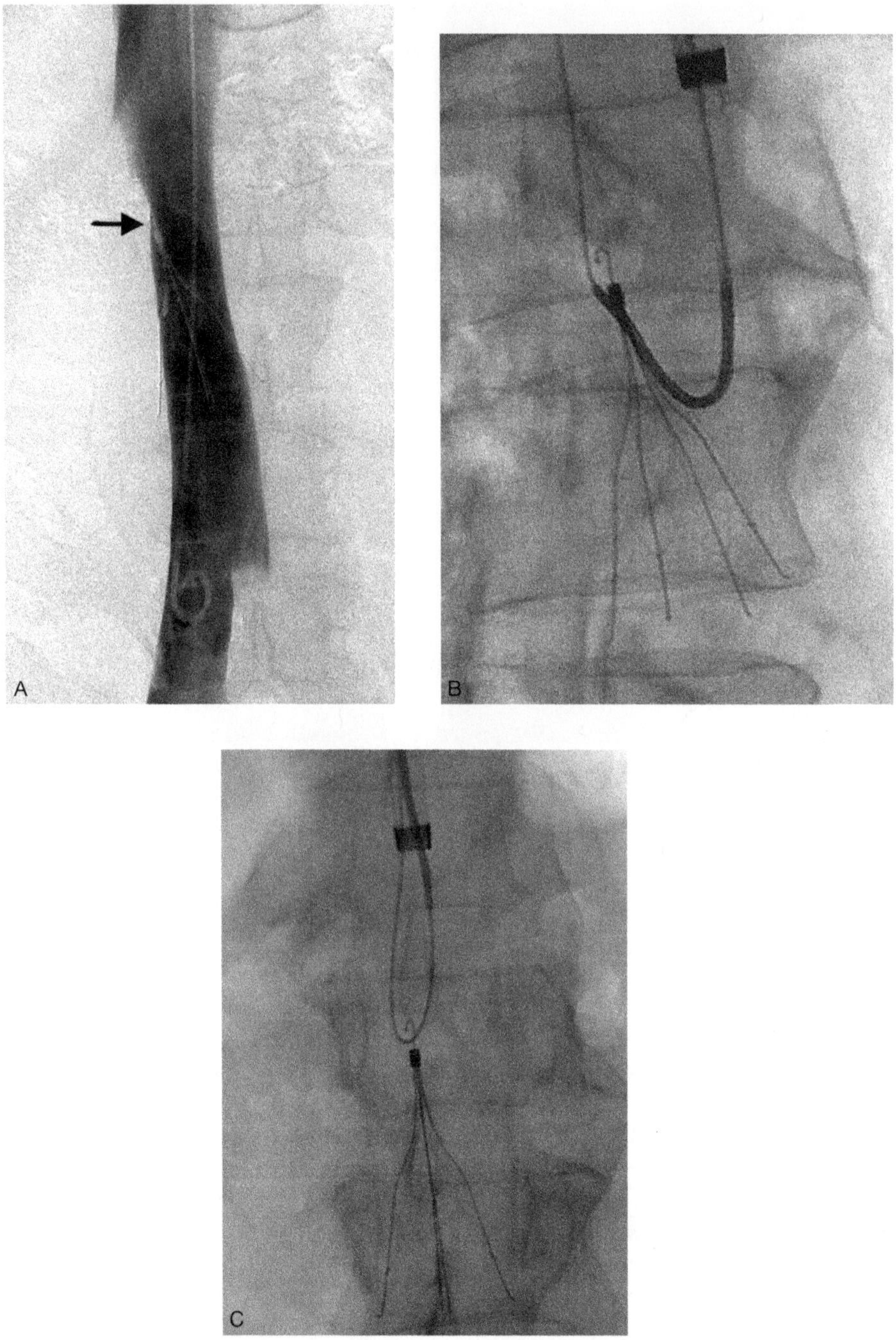

Figure 12-3. Loop wire capture of fibrin cap. (**A**) Digital subtraction cavogram demonstrates filter hook abutting the right lateral caval wall with suggestion of fibrin cap formation (arrow). Standard techniques failed to remove this device. (**B**) Reverse curve catheter utilized to engage fibrin cap. Hydrophilic wire is advanced cranially and captured with snare device. (**C**) Loop wire successfully engaged on fibrin cap. Note that no portion of the wire is through the filter struts.

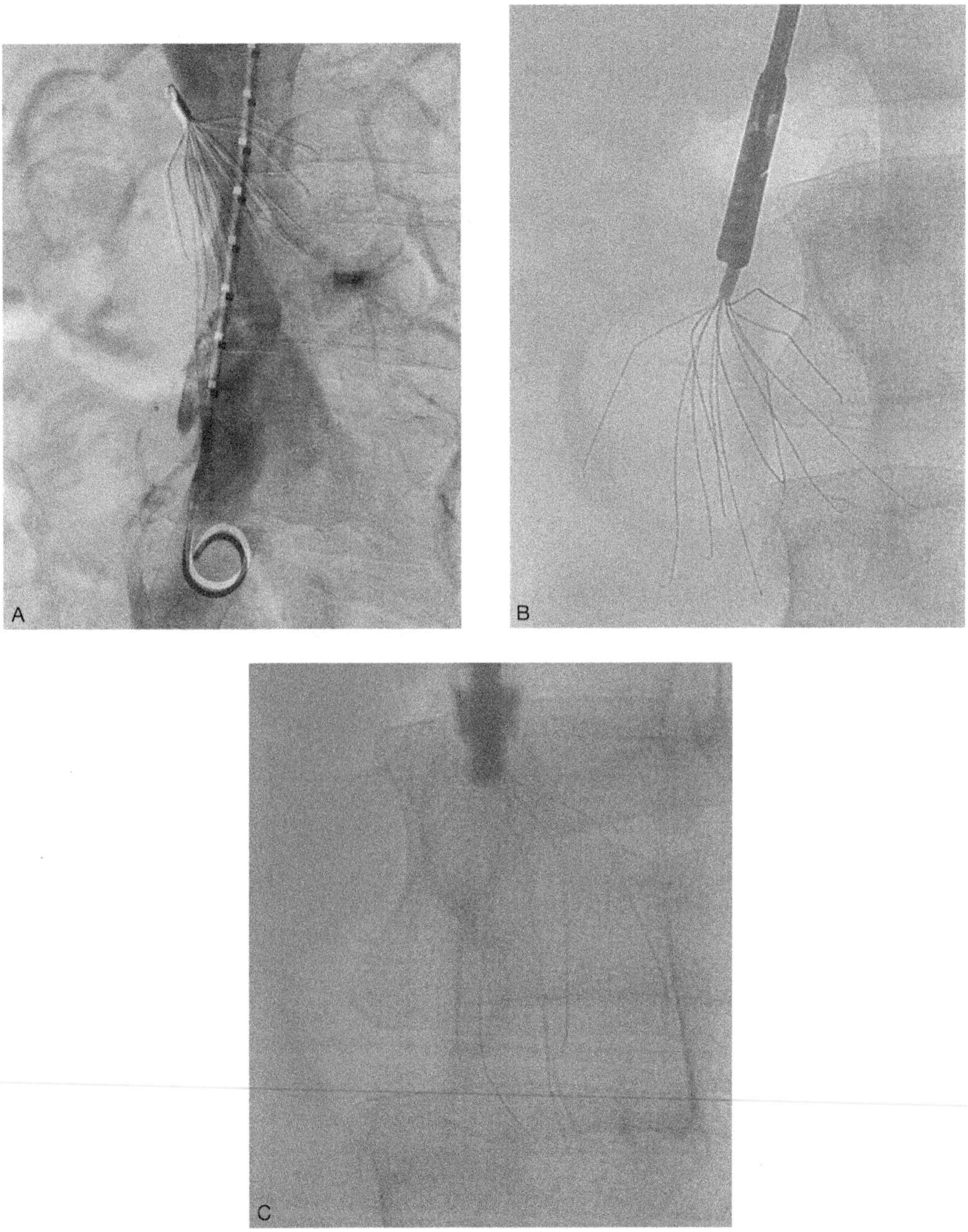

Figure 12-4. Endobronchial forceps in IVC filter retrieval. (**A**) Digital subtraction cavogram demonstrates embedded hook and multiple penetrated struts. (**B**) Rigid endobronchial forceps utilized to dissect fibrin off of hook and capture filter hook/apex. (**C**) Successfully captured filter can then be collapsed in sheath.

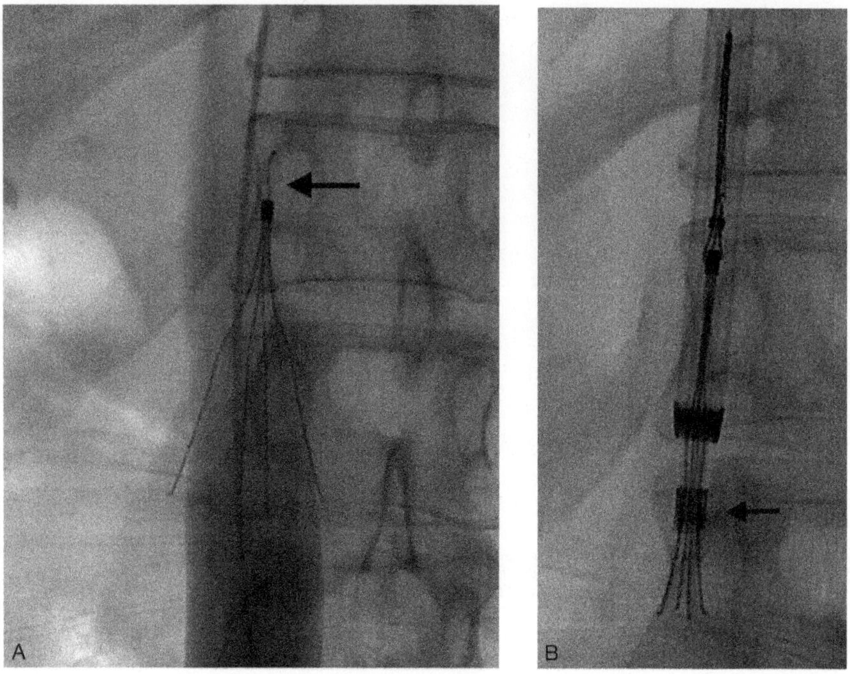

Figure 12-5. Photothermal laser ablation for embedded IVC filter struts. (**A**) Cavogram demonstrates lower portion of filter struts are penetrated. Note that the hook is straightened from prior filter retrieval attempt (arrow). (**B**) After snare capture of filter apex, the laser sheath (arrow) is sequentially activated to enable ablation of fibrinous scar tissue, thus enabling filter removal.

CONCLUSION

Retrievable inferior vena cava filters remain an important tool in providing temporary protection from PE in patients who cannot receive anticoagulation; increase in their use is to be expected with expanding prophylactic indications. With the continued growth in use of these devices, clinical follow up and surveillance of patients with these devices takes on heightened importance, particularly in light of device related complications, which appear to increase with prolonged filter dwell time. The development of advanced filter removal techniques fosters removal of the majority of devices regardless of their implantation time, and should be considered in all patients in which the rIVCF is no longer indicated.

REFERENCES

1. Duszak R, Jr., Parker L, Levin DC, Rao VM. Placement and removal of inferior vena cava filters: National trends in the medicare population. *JACR.* 2011;8(7):483–9.
2. Decousus H, Leizorovicz A, Parent F, et al. A clinical trial of vena caval filters in the prevention of pulmonary embolism in patients with proximal deep-vein thrombosis: Prevention du Risque d'Embolie Pulmonaire par Interruption Cave Study Group. *N Engl J Med.* 1998;338(7):409–15.

3. Group PS. Eight-year follow-up of patients with permanent vena cava filters in the prevention of pulmonary embolism: The PREPIC (Prevention du Risque d'Embolie Pulmonaire par Interruption Cave) randomized study. *Circulation.* 2005;112(3):416–22.
4. Smouse B, Johar A. Is market growth of vena cava filters justified? *Endovasc Today.* 2010;February 2010:74–7.
5. Helling TS, Kaswan S, Miller SL, Tretter JF. Practice patterns in the use of retrievable inferior vena cava filters in a trauma population: A single-center experience. *J Trauma.* 2009;67(6):1293–96.
6. Ray CE, Jr., Mitchell E, Zipser S, et al. Outcomes with retrievable inferior vena cava filters: A multicenter study. *JVIR.* 2006;17(10):1595–1604.
7. Marquess JS, Burke CT, Beecham AH, et al. Factors associated with failed retrieval of the Gunther Tulip inferior vena cava filter. *JVIR.* 2008;19(9):1321–7.
8. McLoney ED, Krishnasamy VP, Castle JC, et al. Complications of Celect, Gunther Tulip, and Greenfield inferior vena cava filters on CT follow-up: A single-institution experience. *JVIR.* 2013;24(11):1723–9.
9. Millward SF, Oliva VL, Bell SD, et al. Gunther Tulip retrievable vena cava filter: results from the Registry of the Canadian Interventional Radiology Association. *JVIR.* Sep 2001;12(9):1053–8.
10. Tam MD, Spain J, Lieber M, et al. Fracture and distant migration of the Bard Recovery filter: A retrospective review of 363 implantations for potentially life-threatening complications. *JVIR.* 2012;23(2):199–205 e191.
11. Durack JC, Westphalen AC, Kekulawela S, et al. Perforation of the IVC: Rule rather than exception after longer indwelling times for the Gunther Tulip and Celect retrievable filters. *Cardiovasc Intervent Radiol.* 2012;35(2):299–308.
12. Ford ME, Lippert JA, McGraw JK. Symptomatic filter penetration presenting as pancreatitis. *JVIR.* 2010;21(4):574–6.
13. Malgor RD, Labropoulos N. A systematic review of symptomatic duodenal perforation by inferior vena cava filters. *J Vasc Surg.* 2012;55(3):856–61 e853.
14. Putterman D, Niman D, Cohen G. Aortic pseudoaneurysm after penetration by a Simon nitinol inferior vena cava filter. *JVIR.* 2005;16(4):535–8.
15. Andreoli JM, Lewandowski RJ, Vogelzang RL, Ryu RK. Comparison of complication rates associated with permanent and retrievable inferior vena cava filters: a review of the MAUDE database. *JVIR.* 2014;25(8):1181–5.
16. Desai TR, Morcos OC, Lind BB, et al. Complications of indwelling retrievable versus permanent inferior vena cava filters. *J Vasc Surg. Venous and Lymphatic Disorders.* 2014;2(2):166–73.
17. Vijay K, Hughes JA, Burdette AS, et al. Fractured Bard Recovery, G2, and G2 express inferior vena cava filters: Incidence, clinical consequences, and outcomes of removal attempts. *JVIR.* 2012;23(2):188–94.
18. Nicholson W, Nicholson WJ, Tolerico P, et al. Prevalence of fracture and fragment embolization of Bard retrievable vena cava filters and clinical implications including cardiac perforation and tamponade. *Arch Intern Med.* 2010;170(20):1827–31.
19. Kuo WT, Robertson SW, Odegaard JI, Hofmann LV. Complex retrieval of fractured, embedded, and penetrating inferior vena cava filters: A prospective study with histologic and electron microscopic analysis. *JVIR.* 2013;24(5):622–30 e621; quiz 631.
20. Kuo WT, Robertson SW. Bard Denali inferior vena cava filter fracture and embolization resulting in cardiac tamponade: A device failure analysis. *JVIR.* 2015;26(1):111–5 e111.
21. Laborda A, Sierre S, Malve M, et al. Influence of breathing movements and Valsalva maneuver on vena caval dynamics. *World J Radiol.* 2014;6(10):833–9.
22. Administration USFaD. Removing Retrievable Inferior Vena Cava Filters: Initial Communication. http://www.fda.gov/MedicalDevices/Safety/AlertsandNotices/ucm221676.htm.

23. Sarosiek S, Crowther M, Sloan JM. Indications, complications, and management of inferior vena cava filters: The experience in 952 patients at an academic hospital with a level I trauma center. *JAMA Intern Med.* 2013;173(7):513–7.
24. Minocha J, Idakoji I, Riaz A, et al. Improving inferior vena cava filter retrieval rates: Impact of a dedicated inferior vena cava filter clinic. *JVIR.* 2010;21(12):1847–51.
25. Geisbusch P, Benenati JF, Pena CS, et al. Retrievable inferior vena cava filters: factors that affect retrieval success. *Cardiovasc Intervent Radiol.* 2012;35(5):1059–65.
26. Rosenthal D, Wellons ED, Hancock SM, Burkett AB. Retrievability of the Gunther Tulip vena cava filter after dwell times longer than 180 days in patients with multiple trauma. *J Endovas. Ther.* 2007;14(3):406–10.
27. Rubenstein L, Chun AK, Chew M, Binkert CA. Loop-snare technique for difficult inferior vena cava filter retrievals. *JVIR.* 2007;18(10):1315–8.
28. Desai KR, Lewandowski RJ, Salem R, et al. Retrieval of inferior vena cava filters with prolonged dwell time: A single-center experience in 648 retrieval procedures. *JAMA Intern Med.* 2015; doi: 10.1001/jamainternmed.2015.2561.
29. Esparaz AM, Ryu RK, Gupta R, et al. Fibrin cap disruption: An adjunctive technique for inferior vena cava filter retrieval. *JVIR.* 2012;23(9):1233–5.
30. Stavropoulos SW, Dixon RG, Burke CT, et al. Embedded inferior vena cava filter removal: Use of endobronchial forceps. *JVIR.* 2008;19(9):1297–301.
31. Kuo WT, Cupp JS. The excimer laser sheath technique for embedded inferior vena cava filter removal. *JVIR.* 2010;21(12):1896–9.

13

Mentorship and the Generational Divide in Surgery

Melina R. Kibbe, MD and Marco G. Patti, MD

Mentoring is usually the relationship between a senior individual (mentor) and a junior, less experienced individual (mentee), with the common purpose of developing the mentee's career. Successful mentorship requires shared goals, shared values, and mutual respect. In addition, this teacher–pupil relationship requires frequent, two-way communication, as well as a deep understanding of the many variables that can have an impact on this relationship. This chapter will describe in detail the importance of mentorship for junior faculty in a department of surgery in an academic medical center setting as well as the variables that can impact the mentor–mentee relationship. This chapter also describes how to establish and monitor a successful mentoring program in a department of surgery. Understanding the intricacies and who the key stakeholders are of a successful mentorship program is critical to any department of surgery as a successful mentorship program will result in the highest possible standards, improve quality, and allow for the recruitment and retention of faculty who will have high job satisfaction.

MENTORSHIP

A mentor is someone who imparts wisdom to and shares knowledge with a less experienced colleague. Traditionally, the mentorship relationship has been seen as both dyadic and hierarchical.[1] It is dyadic because it is a relationship between two people, the mentor and mentee, without the inclusion of other people. It is hierarchical because the mentor is usually several years older, and serves as a role model, teacher, advisor, and sponsor for the younger mentee.

In 1890, Dr. William Halsted became the first Chief of Surgery at John Hopkins Hospital and transformed surgical education by creating the residency program.[2] This was a major departure from the traditional European training in which the professor was the center of the attention. In Halsted's program the focus was on the trainee rather than on the teacher, and his model of "see one, do one, teach one" had the goal of giving increased amounts of responsibility to the resident that culminated with independence at the end of the training period.[3] Halsted also understood the importance of mentoring young surgeons with the goal of creating the teachers of the future. One mentor–mentee relationship that developed at John Hopkins Hospital during Halsted's tenure was between William Osler and Harvey Cushing. This wonderful model serves as an example of a classic dyadic mentorship that can last a lifetime.[4]

Even though changes in the training model occurred during the twentieth century (e.g., residents were allowed to live outside the hospital, they were provided with a stipend, etc.), the residency program created by William Halsted remained almost unchanged until the beginning of the twenty-first century. In 2003, the Accreditation Council for Graduate Medical Education established that residents could not engage in hospital activities more than 80 work hours per week in an effort to decrease mistakes caused by fatigue, improve the safety of patient care, and provide a more meaningful lifestyle for the trainees.[5] However, the change in work hours is just one—albeit very important—change that has occurred in the educational system, in the work force, and in society in general. For example, the increased level of supervision by the attending physician has also had a major impact in the development of independence. It is only with an understanding of these changes that any institution, particularly a department of surgery, can effectively develop a successful mentoring program to assist in the development of surgeons who enter the work force today and forge the leaders of tomorrow.

In addition to understanding the training paradigm shifts that have occurred, many other variables can have an important impact on the mentor-mentee relationship. To gain a deeper appreciation for these variables, a hypothetical example is provided of a mentor–mentee relationship between Dr. Taylor and Dr. Williams, both members of an academic department of surgery. Dr. Taylor was assigned by the department chair to mentor Dr. Williams when she joined the department as an assistant professor. During the past 12 months, it has become clear that the relationship is not working out. The chair decides to analyze the reasons behind this apparent failure. The factors that play an important role in the success or failure of such a relationship are discussed below.

GENERATIONAL IMPACT

Dr. Taylor is 64 years old, and Dr. Williams is 31 years old. That is a difference of 33 years, which makes Dr. Taylor a member of the baby boomer generation while Dr. Williams is part of Generation Y (i.e., the Millennials). This age gap is not unusual, because today the medical profession includes physicians who have trained over a 40-year span. Each generation has its own set of ideals, ethics, and culture; and each generation brings values that dramatically influence the way the world of surgery has been shaped.[6,7]

Baby Boomers (1944–1959)

Their parents had secure jobs and were optimistic about the future. They thought of themselves as a special generation, goal-oriented, hard-working, and driven to succeed. They valued work, power, and leadership. They believed in a hierarchical system. Their world was shaped by the Vietnam War.

Generation X (1960–1980)

Members of this generation were raised during a period of rapid social change. They experienced a significant shift in the family structure as often both parents worked and divorce was common. As compared to the Baby Boomers, they are a very heterogeneous generation (race, religion, and ethnicity). They had fast access to information through desktop technology. They are more self-reliant and independent, respecting talent more than academic rank and authority, and they appreciate the role of multiple mentors. They view education as something they need to endure in order to have a job that gives them financial security and the ability to enjoy leisure time. Work–life balance is a priority for this generation. Their world was shaped by the fall of the Berlin Wall.

Generation Y (1981–2000)

Their parents embraced family values, safety, and doing the right thing. The "Millennials" grew-up with computers, the internet, and a tremendous amount of easily obtainable information. They have a sense of entitlement, expect to express individual views without repercussions, and demand approachable and accessible mentors. They expect work–life balance, job flexibility, and will switch jobs more frequently than members of Generation X. Their world was shaped by the evolution of the AIDS epidemic.

Overall, generational changes have brought a different set of expectations, including more formalized education and training, and more stress on performance expectations, compensation, and quality of life. In our example above Dr. Taylor found it difficult to accept Dr. Williams' challenges to his own ideas and her frequent requests for earlier meetings as she wanted to leave in time to have dinner with her daughter. Faculty in general and mentors in particular have to acknowledge the characteristics of each generation, and accept them for what they are. It is important not to judge, particularly with one's own bias, the behavior of others and attribute right or wrong to their actions.

IMPACT OF GENDER

When Dr. Taylor trained in surgery almost all residents were men. Today the composition of the work force is completely different. In 2010, approximately 50% of all medical students were women.[8] Data show that even though women are more likely to pursue an academic career than men, they might also be more prone to leave academic medicine.[8] Lack of role models, frustration with research, inability to reach a satisfying work–life balance, and lack of effective mentoring have been identified as possible factors. In 1980, 9% of female faculty were at the rank of full professor. Thirty years later, that percentage has only increased to 12.5%.[9] Furthermore, in 2011, only six women served as the chair in a department of surgery among our 125 medical schools.[10] Thus, it appears that a glass ceiling for women in academic surgery is still present.

IMPACT OF RACE

Dr. Taylor is Caucasian and trained in a time when most residents were Caucasians of European descent. Dr. Williams is a member of an ethnic underrepresented minority. Today more ethnic underrepresented minorities have joined the work force even though they are still represented in dismal numbers among medical school faculty.[11,12] In the decade between 1990 and 2000, only 5% of the 1000 surgeons who completed a surgical training program were self-declared members of ethnic underrepresented minorities.[13] As a consequence, when starting an academic career underrepresented minorities will have very few role models and may feel isolated.[14]

IMPACT OF CULTURE

While Dr. Taylor graduated from medical school in a leading American institution, Dr. Williams is a foreign medical graduate. She trained abroad, and then successfully passed all the required examinations in order to have her medical degree recognized so that she could apply to a residency program in the United States. Because of the shortage of American-born applicants to general surgery programs, the number of foreign medical graduates will increase over time. It is, therefore, important to understand and respect the cultural differences that exist and that might affect career development. For some foreign-born surgeons, a process of assimilation into the American culture eventually occurs with complete acceptance of new values. For others, it is only a process of acculturation whereby the individual adapts to the cultural context in which he or she lives but preserves the values and ethics of the country of origin.

IMPACT OF SPECIALIZATION

After completion of his residency, Dr. Taylor's practice was that of a general surgeon, taking care of patients with a variety of different diseases, from breast to colon cancer, and from cholecystitis to peptic ulcer disease. He continues to take emergency room calls and feels that he can take care of any problem that he is presented with; he does not embrace the concept of subspecialization. He finds it difficult to accept the fact that Dr. Williams completed a fellowship in colorectal surgery, and she only takes care of patients with inflammatory bowel disease or colorectal cancer, mostly using a laparoscopic approach. While she makes herself available to all her patients, she prefers not to participate in the general call pool as she does not feel she can provide the same level of service that Dr. Taylor can. She has no problem referring patients with diseases outside of this narrow scope to her colleagues who have similarly embraced the concept of subspecialization.

THE MENTOR'S MENTOR

Dr. Taylor's mentor belonged to the Silent Generation (1925–1942), who are usually described as unimaginative, cautious, but able to adapt easily. It was a classic dyadic type of mentorship, almost filial in nature, based on absolute faith and trust on the part of the mentee. It was a Halstedian type of apprenticeship that focused mostly on the clinical aspects of surgery. He respected, admired, and appreciated his mentor. In fact, he rarely challenged him. Sometimes he finds that Dr. Williams' remarks fall short of recognizing the effort, energy, and time that he puts into her career development. On the other hand, Dr. Williams wants to be a surgeon scientist with a translational research component in addition to a solid clinical practice. She has slowly come to the realization that while Dr. Taylor is an excellent clinician, she needs separate mentors for her research, to navigate the academic world, and to reach a manageable work–life balance. In her department there is no formalized, structured, or supervised mentoring program. Neither the mentor nor the mentee fill out evaluation forms. At best, once a year the Vice Chair for Academic Affairs meets with the faculty for 20 minutes to ask how things are going, with minimal to no follow-up.

NEED FOR WORK–LIFE BALANCE

This is probably the most frustrating aspect of Dr. Williams' relationship with her mentor. Dr. Taylor's wife is a stay-at-home mom who took care of their three children and the household and never worked. This home environment allowed Dr. Taylor to spend long hours in the hospital without firm family commitments. Often his children were in bed by the time he got home and he ate a late dinner alone. In retrospect, he wishes he had spent more time with his family and missed fewer important events in their lives. He admits that he was never able to find a way to do that. Dr. Williams' husband is a lawyer, and they have two children. When asked, she admits that finding a balance between her career and her family is the most important priority to her. They want to be real parents for their children, making sure they get proper exposure to a solid educational environment, music, sports, languages, and different cultures.

Overall, it is clear that the only thing that Dr. Taylor and Dr. Williams have in common is that they are both surgeons. They are part of a mentor–mentee relationship that is doomed to failure. While Dr. Williams is aware of the problems, she realizes that there is no easy way out. The Chairman of the Department of Surgery, a baby boomer himself, does not understand the value of establishing a formal and structured mentorship program, and the Vice Chair for Academic Affairs is just going through the motions meeting with the faculty once every 12 months.

Although this is a hypothetical mentor–mentee relationship, it is unfortunately quite common in many academic institutions. This relationship illustrates the challenges and obstacles present in establishing a mentorship program. It demonstrates the lack of a formal statement of the mentee's ambitions and goals as an academic surgeon and the lack of the mentor's expertise to provide useful mentoring. A successful mentoring relationship must have mutual interests and meet the needs and expectations of each. The following section describes key elements that must be present in order to establish a successful mentorship program.

ESTABLISHING A MENTORSHIP PROGRAM WITHIN A DEPARTMENT OF SURGERY

Mentorship has been recognized as a key element of a successful career as it has a very important influence on career guidance, research productivity, and personal development. Furthermore, as academic institutions have become parts of larger healthcare systems, including community hospitals, mentorship programs have to take into consideration the mentorship needs of the surgeons who practice in these hospitals and who, for the most part, do not have academic aspirations. Key participants of an effective mentorship program include: (1) the mentor; (2) the mentee; (3) the department; and (4) the institution.

The Mentor

Mentors are usually midcareer or senior faculty, at the rank of associate professor or professor. They are considered successful in their careers and ready to guide younger faculty. Mentors can be described according to the following different categories:

- ***The parent.*** The parent mentor serves as a role model. The parent mentor is trustworthy, open, honest, and committed to the mentee's best interest. He/she has connections, power, and resources. In today's academic environment, the parent mentor most likely was part of a classic dyadic mentor–mentee relationship when he/she was younger.
- ***The godfather.*** He/she gives very clear directions. The godfather mentor is powerful and well connected. He/she caters to the mentee's needs, but it can be at a cost. Since the godfather's interests come first, it may difficult for the mentee to establish independence.
- ***The big brother/sister.*** This mentor is a helpful person of the same age or slightly older than the mentee. This relationship is also known as peer mentoring. The big brother/sister is a trusted person who the mentee can turn to for advice. This person may not have the best answers, however, and may not have resources or power, and might experience the same struggles as the mentee.
- ***The patron.*** The patron mentor is a distant supporter from whom the mentee can seek advice, or with whom the mentee can even share projects. The patron mentor is successful and well-connected, and is willing to help and receive little, or nothing, in return.

Mentors are often persons who have the desire to leave a legacy that gives an additional meaning to their professional and personal life. They acknowledge the benefits of this activity in terms of personal satisfaction, pride in developing the next generation, greater research productivity, increased professional recognition when working with well-performing mentees, and improved technical expertise.[15] However, mentoring can be jeopardized by several elements:

1. increased demands in terms of clinical and research productivity, and administrative tasks;
2. lack of recognition of the mentoring activity at an academic level;
3. lack of incentive; and
4. lack of mentoring skills.[16,17]

These elements should be considered and acknowledged when developing a mentoring program.

HOW TO IDENTIFY AND DEVELOP MENTORS WITHIN THE DEPARTMENT

The mentors should have demonstrated knowledge, a successful track record, and interest in the mentee's area of academic pursuit (i.e., basic/translational research, outcomes/health services research, education research, global surgery, etc.). They must be patient, honest, supportive, accessible, and have good communication skills. Strauss and colleagues from St. Michael's Hospital in Ontario and the University of California San Francisco completed interviews with 54 faculty members and identified characteristics of successful and failed mentoring relationships (Table 13-1).[18] An effective mentor should help with career guidance such as navigating the political environment of the institution,

TABLE 13-1. CHARACTERISTICS OF SUCCESSFUL AND UNSUCCESSFUL MENTORING RELATIONSHIPS[18]

Characteristics of Mentoring Relationships	
Successful Relationships	**Unsuccessful Relationships**
Reciprocity (i.e., two-way street)	Poor communication
Mutual respect	Lack of commitment
Clear expectations	Personality differences
Personal connection (i.e., chemistry with one another)	Perceived (or real) competition
Shared values	Conflict of interest (i.e., competing agendas)
	Lack of experience on the part of the mentor

networking, and creating opportunities. Most mentees especially appreciated it when their mentors did not try to solve their problems but rather helped them to find a solution.

While some individuals, particularly those who had good mentors themselves, are ready to serve this role, others need formal training. Positive mentoring behaviors are common, but not universally innate, and when absent must be taught like any other skill. The department leaders should define a list of mentor qualifications. Formal training programs for mentors should be established for faculty members who do not have the minimum qualifications or who need additional skills.[17] This goal can be achieved by providing books on mentoring or through workshops and seminars.[19] At Northwestern University, our department held a "Mentoring the Mentor" workshop for all faculty. Faculty was subdivided into small groups by rank, and skilled mentor educators from the medical school served as facilitators. Every level of mentor benefited from this program. Mentors should have proper academic recognition for their mentoring. For instance, their mentorship activity should be part of the annual review process and be considered during the evaluation for promotion and tenure. Finally, proper financial incentives should be established, such as merit awards or as part of the compensation plan.

The Mentee

The role of the mentee in a successful mentoring relationship is as important as the role of the mentor. Mentees must have a clear understanding of their needs and goals before entering such a relationship. As stressed by Zerzan and colleagues in their guide for mentees, there are five main domains in which mentees usually need guidance.[20]

- ***Research.*** Identifying a valuable project, developing methods, finding collaborators, drafting manuscripts, and writing grant applications.
- ***Professional development.*** Establishing clear goals, choosing jobs, negotiating, and creating an effective network system.
- ***Academic guidance.*** Understanding the culture of the department and the institution, and navigating the treacherous waters of academic life.[21]
- ***Skill development.*** Managing time, resources, and clinical skills.
- ***Personal.*** In today's academic world, one of the most challenging aspects of the mentoring relationship is providing guidance on establishing balance between the professional and personal life.

In addition to the five domains above, there are concepts that mentees must clearly understand. First, it is difficult to find a mentor who is an expert in all of these areas. It is recommended to choose more than one mentor. For instance, Dr. Williams might be best served by having an overall academic career mentor, a research mentor, and a clinical mentor. For women, it might be easier to seek guidance from another woman, particularly for work–life balance issues. For minorities, it might be helpful to have a mentor with similar background and ethnic origin.[12] Second, mentorship is a two-way street. The mentee cannot always be on the receiving side, but must be willing to help the mentor when needed. Third, it is important for the mentee to assume an active role, taking responsibility and ownership of the relationship. Mentees must make their goals clear, communicate in a straightforward way, and address potential conflicts. This is defined as "managing up" in the business world, and it makes the role of a mentor much easier and the relationship more satisfying.[22] A tool that is extremely helpful is the Mentee Self-Evaluation Form (Figure 13-1). This document should be completed by the mentee prior to each semi-annual meeting with the mentor, and should serve as a template or point of discussion during the mentee–mentor meetings.

The Department

The Chair and department leaders must recognize the importance of a formal and structured mentorship program. They cannot wait passively for junior and senior faculty to form relationships. The Department must assume an active role.[18] The Department must recognize the many benefits that can result from an effective program such as high morale, high job satisfaction, better quality and safety, improved retention, and the ability to recruit promising faculty.

Kashiwagi and colleagues searched the MEDLINE EMBASE and Scopus databases for articles that described mentoring programs.[19] Although no programs reported long-term results, they identified several components that served a role in establishing a successful mentoring program:

- ***Planning committees***. Several programs were overseen by a team or a committee. Their responsibilities included program design, identifying mentors, assessing the pairing of mentors with mentees, monitoring the mentor–mentee relationship, and intervening when necessary. In order to assess the relationship, it is essential that mentors and mentees fill out annual or semi-annual evaluation forms (Figures 13-2 and 13-3) that document their satisfaction with the relationship and with the established goals. These forms should be regularly reviewed by an external group such as this, along with the department chair, in order to identify areas of conflict or areas that need work. Intervention is needed when a clear conflict has been identified and needs resolution. Objective measures of mentee progress should include manuscripts, grants, committee memberships (departmental, hospital, medical school, or university), membership in professional societies, leadership positions, promotions, and retention rates. Individual data from–mentee pairs should be included in forms. These forms will also provide subjective data regarding the program. Periodic review of the mentorship program—using these forms as objective data for a starting point—should occur and lead to a process of continued improvement of the mentorship program.

MENTEE SELF-EVALUATION FORM

Mentee Name:____________________________ Date:____________________

Division:________________________________ Rank:____________________

Mentor Name:____________________________

Describe your academic interests:

List major accomplishments over the past 6–12 months:

List institutional committees you currently serve on (i.e., departmental, hospital, med school, university:

List societies you currently belong to:

State 3 short-term goals (i.e., 1 year goals):

1)

2)

3)

State your long-term goal(s)

State 3 areas where you feel a mentor could help you most:

1)

2)

3)

Indicate how the Department of Surgery can help your professional career development:

Indicate any roadblocks you have encountered with your career development that you would like to discuss with your mentor:

Figure 13-1. Example of a Mentee Self-Evaluation Form

EVALUATION OF THE MENTEE BY THE MENTOR

Mentor Name:______________________________

Mentee Name:______________________________ Date:____________________

Mentee Division:______________________________ Mentee Rank:______________

1. How often are you meeting with your mentee?
   a. Is this frequent enough?
2. Did you discuss the mentee's short-term career goals?
3. Did you discuss the mentee's long-term career goals?
4. Did you discuss the promotion and tenure process with the mentee?
5. Did you discuss the mentees academic interests?
6. Did you discuss committee assignments?
   a. Are these assignments appropriate?
   b. Are there committees the mentee should serve on that would benefit his/her career?
7. Did you discuss society involvement?
   a. Are there societies the mentee should belong to?
8. Did you ask the mentee if there were any roadblocks or challenges he/she perceived or encountered that might impact his/her career development?
9. Are there collaborators the mentee needs?
10. What additional topics did you discuss with the mentee?
11. Indicate 3 goals you and the mentee discussed that will be addressed at the next visit:
    a. 1)
    b. 2)
    c. 3)
12. Is there additional training or education the mentee requires or desires?
13. Indicate areas needing improvement that you discussed with your mentee.
14. Is additional support required from the Division/Department/Institution to support the mentee?
15. Do you feel the mentee has benefited from your mentorship?
16. Have you benefited from your mentorship relationship?
17. Are you satisfied with your mentee's progress?
18. Are you satisfied with the departmental mentoring program?
    a. If not, how can the department help?

Figure 13-2. Example of a Mentee Evaluation Form.

EVALUATION OF THE MENTOR BY THE MENTEE

Mentor Name:____________________________

Mentee Name:____________________________ Date:____________________

Mentee Division:____________________________ Mentee Rank:________________

1. How often are you meeting with your mentor?
   a. Is this frequent enough?
2. Did you discuss your short-term career goals with your mentor?
3. Did you discuss your long-term career goals with your mentor?
4. Did you discuss the promotion and tenure process with your mentor?
5. Did you discuss your academic interests with your mentor?
6. Did you discuss committee assignments with your mentor?
   a. Are your assignments appropriate?
   b. Are there additional committees you would like/not like to serve on?
7. Did you discuss society involvement with your mentor?
   a. Are there societies you do not currently belong to, but would like to?
8. Did you discuss any roadblocks or challenges you have encountered that might impact your career development?
9. Are there collaborators you would like to work with?
10. What additional topics did you discuss with your mentor?
11. Indicate 3 goals you and your mentor discussed that will be addressed at the next visit:
    a. 1)
    b. 2)
    c. 3)
12. Is there additional training or education you require or desire?
13. Indicate areas needing improvement that you discussed with your mentor?
14. Is additional support required from the Division/Department/Institution to support your academic career?
15. Do you feel your mentor is satisfied with your progress?
16. Have you benefited from the relationship with your mentor?
17. Are you satisfied with your mentor?
18. Are you satisfied with the departmental mentoring program?
    a. If not, how can the department help?

Figure 13-3. Example of a Mentor Evaluation Form.

- *Pairing of mentors and mentees.* Often the mentees choose their mentors, a process defined as informal mentoring. This is favored in general by mentees and avoids mentors choosing whomever they consider to be the best mentees with the highest potential for success. If the mentee cannot identify a mentor, however, the department chair should provide a list of potential mentors to the mentee or assign a mentor. This is known as formal mentoring and is more often doomed to failure when little time is invested in properly identifying a mentor most suitable to the mentee.
- *Contracts.* Departments that have a more developed mentora–mentee program use contracts. At the initiation of the mentor–mentee relationship, the mentee and mentor read and sign a Mentee Contract (Figure 13-4) and Mentor Contract (Figure 13-5). This simple document, a copy of which is kept in the department's administrative offices for the chair to monitor, guarantees that both parties in the relationship understand the expectations established in the beginning of the relationship. The contract can also be used during faculty evaluation and as a means of starting discussions when issues arise between the mentor and the mentee. They can also be used by the mentors as evidence of engagement in an important activity of the department.
- *Mentoring activities.* A good mentor–mentee relationship will have frequent contact and a myriad of activities and good exchange of information between the mentor and the mentee. These activities go beyond the regular annual and semi-annual meetings established between the mentor and mentee. This includes attending certain events together, such as lectures, seminars, and courses. The mentor may also attend national or international meetings with the mentee and introduce the mentee to other faculty, broadening the mentee's network.
- *A formal curriculum for mentees.* A variety of courses exist that mentees can attend to further their career development. This includes: career development courses, such as the ones offered by the Association for Academic Surgery (AAS) or the Association of American Medical Colleges (AAMC); courses on how to be a better educator, like the Surgeons as Educators Course developed by the American College of Surgeons (ACS); or specific courses based on research needs, such as obtaining advanced degrees, peer-review manuscript writing, grant writing courses, and so forth.
- *Funding/recognition of mentoring efforts.* It is important for the mentor to receive recognition of his/her efforts, thereby incentivizing the mentor. This could be in the form of awards from the department or medical school, or recognition of the effort as part of a compensation plan. Mentoring efforts should also be recognized during annual reviews and upon consideration for promotion and tenure. It is the chair's role to make certain that faculty realize that mentoring is highly valued by the department, school, and institution.

DeCastro and colleagues surveyed 1,708 clinician-researchers between 2010 and 2011 who received National Institutes of Health (NIH) K08 and K23 career development awards between 2006 and 2009.[23] Even though the study had limitations, such as the self-reporting nature of data collection and the fact that the participants had already shown the ability to secure NIH funding, it clearly identified mentoring aspects that were significantly and positively associated with career satisfaction. These factors included the amount of time spent with the mentor, mentor behavior, mentor prestige, collegiality of the mentor–mentee relationship, and extent of mentorship in various roles. The authors concluded that to address the issue of faculty attrition, academic departments should consider implementing a formal mentoring program that includes mentor training.

MENTEE CONTRACT

Name of Mentee: ______________________________

Name of Mentor: ______________________________

Specialty: ______________________________

Rank: ______________________________

As the Mentee, I agree to:

- be committed to a career in academic surgery
- be committed to the mission of the Department of Surgery
- develop a career development plan with input from my mentor(s)
- spend regular time committed to academic pursuits (i.e., teaching, research, etc.)
- ensure that procedures are followed according to policy and ethical guidelines (i.e.,experimental, analytical, human-subject, animal, etc.)
- be intellectually committed to the research project and overall career development
- be a collaborative researcher
- share learned insights with the mentor(s) and other collaborators and investigators
- attend all official mentor-mentee meetings.official mentor-mentee meetings.
- complete the mentee self-evaluation form before each semi-annual mentor-menteemeeting
- be accessible, communicate clearly, and answer emails promptly
- promptly advise the mentor of any issues (intellectual, practical, or personal) that may affect my work
- be mindful of all project deadlines

In addition, I agree to:

- commit 100% effort to my career development
- meet with my mentor on a regular basis

______________________________ ______________________________

Signature Print Name

__/__/____ Date

Figure 13-4. Example of a Mentee Contract.

MENTOR CONTRACT

Name of Mentor:______________________________

MentorSpecialty:______________________________

Name of Mentee:______________________________

Mentee Specialty:______________________________

As the Mentor, I agree to:

- commit time to and be available for the mentor-mentee relationship
- ensure that the mentee understands the specific criteria by which he/she will be evaluated for promotion and tenure
- help the mentee create their career development plan and annually review and revise the plan accordingly
- assist the mentee in understanding institutional policies and procedures, especially in regard to programmatic development, grant applications, educational commitments, and other activities that may be unfamiliar for young faculty
- offer advice and guidance, and when necessary, intervention with administration, faculty, or trainees on behalf of the mentee
- introduction of the mentee to key faculty collaborators and staff
- timely and accurate feedback
- respect and nurture the ideas of the mentee, independent of the mentor's interests
- prioritize the mentee's research interest above that of the mentor's interests
- help the mentee to solve problems and not solve them directly
- be familiar with, and sensitive to, issues of faculty diversity and be able to relate to the special needs and concerns of women and minorities
- help ensure that the mentee is fully integrated within the academic infrastructure of the institution, including identification of relevant conferences, seminars, and meetings
- provide supervision and critical review of the mentee's early work, including manuscripts, grant applications, presentations, etc.

In addition, I agree to:

- commit a minimum of 5% effort to this mentor-mentee relationship
- attend the Department of Surgery Mentoring Workshop
- attend the mentee's presentations at department and national meetings, as time permits, and provide critical feedback.

______________________________ ______________________________

Signature Print Name

__/__/____ Date

Figure 13-5. Example of a Mentor Contract.

A key element of any mentoring program is close supervision of the existing mentor–mentee relationships. By definition, such relationships reflect an imbalance of power, and supervision is needed to ensure that the mentor does not exploit the relationship. Departments must establish policies and procedures for reviewing the mentor–mentee relationship on an annual basis to detect potential areas of conflict or a failing mentor–mentee relationship. If either of these situations arises, procedures should be in place for resolving potential conflicts, including processes for assessing alleged violations. On the part of the mentor, failure is often expressed as the mentee not performing according to the initial plan or lacking respect for the mentor or for his or her time. On the part of the mentee, failure is often expressed as the mentor not giving the mentee proper credit for their work. For example, the mentor taking ownership of research, grants, and/or intellectual property such as publications and patents; the mentor asking the mentee to focus on the mentor's research; or the mentor not allowing the mentee to explore their own ideas independently from the mentor's research.[17] This is why it is very important that evaluations are independently filled out annually or semi-annually by both the mentor and mentee and the relationship analyzed every 6 months by an independent third party. If the relationship is deemed failed, an exit strategy such as a "no fault divorce" should be implemented.[24]

The Institution

An effective mentoring program cannot be established by the chair in a department of surgery without the open and transparent approval and support of the institution. The medical school and hospital benefit substantially from the existence of a mentoring program:

- ***Economic gain.*** Successful research programs bring federal and nonfederal support to a medical school. These dollar amounts are made publically available. The facilities and administrative costs (aka indirect costs) associated with some research grants helps to support the infrastructure of the medical school.
- ***Recruitment and retention.*** A department with a solid mentoring program would likely have more faculty successful with their research endeavors, leading to more research dollars and larger research programs. This in turn raises the profile of the department, and hence the medical school and allows for the recruitment and retention of faculty, a key ingredient for the success of the hospital, medical school, and department.
- ***Programmatic development.*** A strong track record of success from the faculty in a department allows the institution to plan and invest in the development of future programs deemed important to the mission and goals of the department. This could represent clinical programs or research such as basic science research, translational research, outcomes and health services research, or educational research.
- ***Ranking.*** All of the above improve the national reputation of the department and institution, creating a cycle by which new hires have the background and potential to be the leaders of the future.

The institution can help by providing economic support for the program and by acknowledging the work of the department in general and the mentors in particular (i.e., promotion and tenure, compensation plan, etc.). The goal of such programs is bigger than the individuals who participate, as it guarantees continuity by forging the leaders of the future.

CONCLUSION

Mentorship is an important aspect of any academic department of surgery. Establishing a formal mentoring program can have far-reaching implications that include quality, program development, job satisfaction, research funding, and faculty recruitment and retention. However, establishment of a program is not enough. Annual or semi-annual review of the mentor–mentee relationships by an independent third party is critical to the success of the program and can provide meaningful metrics about the impact the program has on the department and the medical school. Successful development and implementation of a mentoring program will impact the overall quality of an academic department of surgery.

REFERENCES

1. Barondess JA. President's address: a brief history of mentoring. *Trans Am Clin Climatol Assoc.* 1995;106:1–24.
2. Kotsis SV, Chung KC. Application of the "see one, do one, teach one" concept in surgical training. *Plast Reconstr Surg.* 2013;131:1194–1201.
3. Cameron JL. William Stewart Halsted: our surgical heritage. *Ann Surg.* 1997;255:445–58.
4. Duffy TP. The Osler-Cushing Covenant. *Perspect Biol Med.* 2005; 48(4):592–602.
5. ACGME program requirements for graduate medical education in general surgery. 2008. Available at: www.acgme.org/acgmeweb/Portals/0/PDFs/archive/409_psychosomatic_PRs_RC.pdf. Accessed August 9, 2012.
6. Jonhson SA, Romanello ML. Generational Diversity: Teaching and learning approaches. *Nurse Educ.* 2005; 30(5):212–6.
7. Johnston S. See one, do one, teach one: developing professionalism across the generations. *Clin Orthop Relat Res.* 2006; 449:186–92.
8. Levine RB, Lin F, Kern DE, Wright SM, Carrese J, et al. Stories from early-career women physicians who have left academic medicine: a qualitative study at a single institution. *Acad Med.* 2011; 86(6):752–8.
9. Varkey P, Jatoi A, Williams A, et al. The positive impact of a facilitated peer mentoring program on academic skills of women faculty. *BMC Med Educ.* 2012 Mar 23;12:14.
10. Zhuge Y, Kaufman J, Simeone DM, et al. Is there still a glass ceiling for women in academic surgery? *Ann Surg.* 2011;253(4):637–43.
11. Johnson JC, Williams B, Jayadevappa R. Mentoring program for minority faculty at the University of Pennsylvania School of Medicine. *Acad Med.* 1999; 74(4):376–9.
12. Kosoko-Lasaki O, Sonnino RE, Voytko ML. Mentoring for women and underrepresented minority faculty and students: Experience at two institutions of higher education. *J Natl Med Assoc.* 2006;98(9):1449–59.
13. Newman LA, Pollock RE, Johnson-Thompson MC. Increasing the pool of academically oriented African-American medical and surgical oncologists. CANCER Supplement. 2003;97(1):329–34.
14. Singletary SE. Mentoring surgeons for the 21st century. *Ann Surg Oncol.* 2005; 12(11):848–60.
15. Coates WC. Being a mentor: What's in it for me? *Acad Emerg Med.* 2012; 19:92–97.
16. Straus SE. Chatur F, Taylor M. Issues in the mentor-mentee relationship in academic medicine: A qualitative study. *Acad Med.* 2009; 84(1):135–9.
17. Keyser DJ, Lakoski JM, Lara-Cinisomo S, et al. Advancing institutional efforts to support research mentorship: A conceptual framework and self-assessment tool. *Acad Med.* 2008; 83(3):217–25.

18. Straus SE, Johnson MO, Marquez VC, Feldman MD. Characteristics of successful and failed mentoring relationships: A qualitative study across two academic health centers. *Acad Med.* 2013; 88(1):82–9.
19. Kashiwagi DT, Varkey P, Cook DA. Mentoring programs for physicians in academic medicine: A systematic review. *Acad Med.* 2013; 88(7):1029–37.
20. Zerzan JT, Hess R, Schur E, et al. Making the most of mentors: A guide for mentees. *Acad Med.* 2009; 84(1):140–4.
21. Simone JV. Understanding academic medical centers: Simone's maxims. *Clin Cancer Res.* 1999; 5:2281–5.
22. Drucker PF. Managing oneself. Harvard Business Review.1999; 77(2):64–74.23.
23. DeCastro R, Griffith KA, Ubel PA, Stewart A, Jagsi R. Mentoring and the career satisfaction of male and female academic medical faculty. *Acad Med.* 2014; 89(2):1–11.
24. Sanfey H, Hollands C, Gantt NL. Strategies for building an effective mentoring relationship. *Am J Surg.* 2013; 206:714–8.

14

Are Vascular Surgeons Unique?

Victor J. Davila, MD and Samuel R. Money, MD, MBA

Charles Darwin is known as the father of evolution. His voyages to the Galapagos Islands had a lasting influence on his theory of natural selection. In particular, his observation of varied species of finches, all of which are native to the Galapagos Islands and not found anywhere else in the world, shaped his ideas on the topic. Darwin noticed in his travels to the Galapagos Islands that each individual island has a unique ecosystem, and each island also curiously has a particular and very distinct type of finch that inhabits it. Each type of finch has adapted in isolation to be particularly well suited to survival on its own island. Inspired by this unique phenomenon, Darwin wrote in his text *On the Origin of Species*: "It is not the strongest of the species that survive, nor the most intelligent, but the one most responsive to change." These finches, in isolation, are not special in any obvious way. Darwin noted that the "feathers, coloration, general structure, and tone of voice bear a remarkable resemblance to their mainland counterparts." However, when taken together, these finches are fascinatingly unique as each type of Galapagos finch has a highly adapted beak, specifically designed to thrive in its own island ecosystem. This adaptation is the reason why these finches have survived for centuries in a rather harsh environment and what makes them special, especially to Darwin who first observed this evolution in action.[1]

HOW ARE VASCULAR SURGEONS *NOT* DIFFERENT?

Like the Galapagos finches, vascular surgeons do not seem to be particularly special in any way. In fact, vascular surgeons are no different than general surgeons, orthopedic surgeons, otolaryngologists, neurosurgeons, interventional radiologists, or interventional cardiologists in many ways. Vascular surgeons operate in the abdomen as do general surgeons. Vascular surgeons operate on extremities, just like orthopedic surgeons, hand surgeons, and plastic surgeons. Vascular surgeons operate in the neck, so do neurosurgeons and otolaryngologists. Vascular surgeons perform endovascular procedures along with interventional cardiologists and radiologists. The procedures that vascular surgeons are qualified to perform are not what set them apart. With so much overlap and subspecialization in the many fields of medicine, there will always be another specialty looking to perform the same type of procedure. For this reason, vascular surgeons are not able to merely state that they are blood vessel experts and expect patients to flock to them over any other specialty. However, what has made vascular surgeons so unique from other surgical specialties, has been their repeated ability, like Darwin's finches, to adapt over time.

HOW ARE VASCULAR SURGEONS DIFFERENT?

Technology

Disruptive innovation is an idea, technology, or process which changes the market and solves problems better than the status quo.[2] Vascular surgery has seen several waves of disruptive innovation over the last several decades. Endovascular aneurysm repair and percutaneous peripheral interventions are the prime examples. The landscape of vascular surgery has evolved significantly, from large incisions to puncture sites and from bypasses to balloons. In general, vascular surgeons have learned to embrace these technical advances in procedural intervention, and this ability to adapt—to embrace technology and changing times—is what sets vascular surgery apart from our general surgery and cardiothoracic surgery counterparts.

Disruptive innovation occurs in all industries. iTunes, Amazon, and digital photography have revolutionized the music industry, consumer product marketplace, and photography industry respectively. The healthcare industry is no different and vascular surgery has seen a wave of disruptive innovation wash over and change the landscape of how vascular pathology is treated. Endovascular aneurysm repair and peripheral interventions have become staple procedures in the vascular surgeon's armamentarium.

Other medical specialties have not adopted disruptive innovation in a timely manner. When endoscopy was belittled as a "lesser" procedure by general surgeons, the gastroenterologists seized the opportunity and worked hard to become experts at endoscopy; today, almost all colonoscopies and upper endoscopies are referred to them versus general surgeons. Further, even what is considered a staple general surgery procedure, the cholecystectomy, is now able to be performed endoscopically. In a similar fashion, when percutaneous coronary intervention began, the cardiothoracic surgeons criticized it as trivial and inferior to coronary bypass. Now, a majority of patient with coronary artery disease are treated by cardiologists who have no idea how to perform a sternotomy. As these examples tend to illustrate, both general surgery and cardiothoracic surgery professions were generally slow to adapt to change, and, as a consequence, are often even today embroiled in "turf" battles with medical (non-surgical) subspecialties. The collective general surgery and cardiothoracic surgery experience stand in stark contrast to vascular surgery. Whereas other surgical specialties have struggled over time, vascular surgery has been routinely recognized for its ability to embrace disruptive technology like endovascular aneurysm repair and percutaneous peripheral interventions.

Broader Toolkit

Vascular surgeons are also unique in the multitude of approaches they have available to solve simple and complex problems. General surgeons may be able to bypass a stenosis or occluded artery, and interventional radiologists may be able to angioplasty or stent the same stenosis. Vascular surgeons can however do both, and therefore decide which procedure is best depending on the individual patient. Vascular surgeons are able to choose the right tool from all of the available tools, which gives them the ability to treat the patient in a more holistic way, and the patients reaps the benefits for having a more customized approach to their situation. Vascular surgeons fundamentally have more options than other specialties when deciding what intervention, if any, to perform. While this wealth of alternatives may seem overwhelming especially to young vascular surgeons, the options allow a vascular surgeon to be mechanically focused on delivering the best patient care in each and every situation.

Clinic/Continuity of Care

Like quality of care that comes as a result of possessing a broad toolkit, vascular surgeons are also known for their continuity of care. Vascular surgeons are not always called upon to immediately perform a procedure. We have a highly toned expertise in decision making which takes years to develop. Our evaluation is called upon by other specialties when they are unsure of the next step in treatment whether it is open surgery, endovascular therapy, or conservative management. Interventional radiologists are called upon typically to perform procedures only, and, in many instances, meet the patient for the first time when they are prepped and draped on the interventional radiology procedure table. Vascular surgeons are known for thorough evaluation, preoperative planning, choosing the right procedure, and following the patients progress if they need future intervention—and their care typically follows from the first point of patient contact all the way through to problem resolution and long-term follow up. Unlike other surgical or procedure-driven specialties, a patient who visits a vascular surgeon's office may need further intervention, and vascular surgery is one of the few surgical specialties known for its continuity of care with the patient. The fact that these patients are generally some of the sickest in the health care population encourages this continuity of care. Vascular surgery patients are complicated and need a physician who understands their specific needs and situation to be able to help them make the most informed decision when planning medical intervention. The vascular surgeon should be the first person at the bedside when needed to discuss these frequently complicated matters. For these reasons, vascular surgeons are unique in their ability, when called upon, to deliver true continuity of patient care.

Importance of Realistic Expectations and Accepting Failure

In general and broadly speaking, surgeons are known for being very meticulous and not accepting of failure. Gallbladders, thyroids, breast masses, and intestines are removed every day, and these patients typically never need additional intervention. Unlike other surgical specialties, however, vascular surgeons do not always have the luxury of talking with their patients about fixing their vascular problems, but rather temporizing them. The patient populations that a vascular surgeon typically treats are older, higher risk, and have multiple comorbidities. The types of problems that vascular surgeons are called upon to treat often involve preserving limbs and lives. The reality of a vascular surgery practice is that blood flow can be restored, but re-stenosis frequently occurs, and grafts can fail. When patients are consented for peripheral interventions, they are told the failure rates in terms of years or months until another balloon needs to be inflated, or graft revised. Vascular surgeons routinely manage sicker and sicker patients as the general population ages, and they are increasingly dealing with complication rates that are statistically higher than other specialties. Vascular surgeons are more accepting of failure, knowing that not every problem can be fixed—which is unique to vascular surgery and very important when it comes to patient care. Setting realistic expectations with patients and allowing patients to choose their most desired treatment modality is an area where vascular surgery excels.

"Many Different Finches"

The Galapagos finches each found a particular way to adapt and thrive in their environment; similarly, vascular surgeons have also found many different ways to adapt the knowledge and skills gained during training to a particular medical system. Solo practice physicians, group practice physicians, academic surgeons, mentors in training programs, surgeons known for a particular skill set of open or endovascular surgery have all found their own niche, albeit in different ways. The most important skill is not what we know, but how we adapt to our environment in a way that allows us to create the best patient experience. In the United States there are approximately 3,500 board-certified vascular surgeons, and no two vascular surgeons have identical practices. Furthermore, the specific doctors, procedures, and patients are not what make vascular surgery unique. Vascular surgeons have learned how to evolve our practice of treating vascular pathology to the disease process and use all of the available tools at our disposal. Simply put, like Darwin's finches, what has made vascular surgeons unique from other surgical specialties has been our ability to successfully adapt over time, and, in doing so, deliver best in class patient care.

FUTURE CHALLENGES

As technology and treatment modalities evolve, so must the vascular surgeon. We must not simply accept the current state of technology and be satisfied with our accomplishments. We must be able to create or accept new technology as it becomes available. This constant thirst for being able to do better will ensure that we continue to be at the cutting edge of vascular treatment.

Another change that is occurring in the medical system is a mentality of shift work. Current training programs mandate a shift work style of medical education. The 80-hour work week has sometimes mandated the shift to night float systems and 12-hour work days. Previous generations of surgeons were trained under the paradigm of always being available for the patient, every day, all day.[3] Younger physicians have shifted priorities to enable more personal time without the constant need for pagers and hospital visits. This shift from a surgeon–patient relationship to a shift work mentality will be challenging to manage and may cause the relationship between a vascular surgeon and the patients to deteriorate. This is something that we must be acutely aware of as this transition becomes more apparent.

In addition to a shift work paradigm, vascular surgeons are increasingly becoming part of hospital systems or other multispecialty groups. With this change, the patient relationship is also threatened. It no longer matters who is performing the procedure, interventional radiology, interventional cardiology, general surgery, or vascular surgery. We must continue to be eager to take care of our patients and not see any procedure as too diminutive as to not warrant our attention. Central lines, dialysis access problems, thrombolysis; none of these problems are sexy, but they are under the auspices of vascular surgery, and we must make sure to not lose our basic foundation as other specialties try to pick up vascular expertise. We should always be the first ones called on to deal with vascular problems, but we must encourage this in our medical colleagues and accept all consults with care and respect for the patient, the condition, and the referring physician.

Dr. Frank Veith spoke of Darwin and the theory of natural selection in his presidential address to the Society for Vascular Surgery in 1996. He stated almost 20 years ago that "vascular surgeons must acquire endovascular skills. . . . If we do not, the need for our services will decrease, we will gradually be replaced, and our numbers diminish, heading towards eventual extinction."[4] Vascular surgeons have evolved their practices and have established their position as experts in open surgery and endovascular procedures. This competitive pressure was also met head on with change in vascular surgery training programs, both the 5+2 and 0+5 models, to allow more exposure and more emphasis on endovascular skill acquisition.

Vascular surgeons must be finches and continue to evolve with the changing landscape of treatment of vascular pathology.

REFERENCES

1. Darwin CR. *On the Origin of Species.* Vol. XI. The Harvard Classics. New York: P.F. Collier & Son, 1909–14; Bartleby.com, 2001.
2. Bower JL, Christensen CM. Disruptive technologies: Catching the wave. *Harvard Business Review,* January–February 1995.
3. Hutter MM, Kellogg KC, Ferguson CM, et al. The impact of the 80-hour resident workweek on surgical residents and attending surgeons. *Ann Surg.* 2006;243(6):864–75.
4. Veith FJ. Presidential address: Charles Darwin and vascular surgery. *J Vasc Surg.* 1997;25:8–18.

15

Interpreting Randomized Controlled Trials of Vascular Treatments: Why They Can Be Misleading*

Frank J. Veith, MD

Good randomized controlled trials (RCTs) published in leading peer-reviewed journals are considered the best possible basis for determining good medical practice. However, such trials have several limitations. These include flaws and weaknesses in the design and the timeliness of RCTs. Progress in a treatment method or control arm may invalidate a trial. So too can defects in patient selection, physician competence, randomization, applicability, endpoints, and the population being studied. Idiosyncratic flaws can also invalidate a RCT. Another problem with RCTs is the possibility that author error or bias will render the conclusions of the article reporting the trial misleading. This can occur even when the report is published in a leading journal. This plus further misinterpretation (spinning) of the trial results or conclusions by others can make the effect of the trial misleading with an unintended detrimental result on medical practice. The problem can be compounded when Guidelines are based on such errors or bias-based conclusions. All physicians should recognize these value-limiting processes so that RCTs can be evaluated adequately and fairly. In that way they can be used along with good physician judgment to optimize the care delivered to individual patients and to society at large.

Randomized controlled trials (RCTs) are considered part of level 1 evidence or the "Holy Grail" of medical evidence.[1] Such trials, especially when published in leading journals, are deemed by many the best possible basis for determining medical practice. In vascular disease, leading journals include the *New England Journal of Medicine, The Lancet*, the *Journal of Vascular Surgery, Circulation*, the *European Journal of Vascular & Endovascular Surgery*, the *Journal of Endovascular Therapy*, the *Journal of Vascular and Interventional Radiology* and several others. Articles in these journals form the scientific

* Portions of this chapter are reproduced from an article in the *Journal of Vascular Surgery*,[22] and other portions are reproduced from an article in *Vascular*[20]; used with permission from Elsevier and Sage Publications.

basis for what vascular surgeons and other vascular specialists do in the management of patients with noncardiac vascular disease. It is assumed that these journals are peer-reviewed and edited with objectivity and that their content is unbiased and reflects the truth or near to the truth. So when RCTs are published in these leading journals, they have an enormous impact on the standards of medical practice for physicians and surgeons dealing with vascular disease patients.

This chapter will show why this is not always the case and how RCTs, even when reported in leading journals, can be misleading by two mechanisms. The first is by timeliness or design flaws in the RCTs. The second is by misinterpretation of even well-designed, valid RCTS so that they are rendered misleading. This can occur when the conclusion expressed in the article reporting the RCT is inconsistent with the trial's data because of error or bias in interpreting the trial's results. It can also occur when others interpret the results of a trial in an erroneous or biased fashion. An additional purpose of this chapter is to show how guidelines based on flawed or misinterpreted RCTs can also be misleading and harmful to good patient care.

PERSPECTIVE ON RCTs AND LEVEL 1 EVIDENCE

Legitimate disagreement exists about the need for and the value of level 1 evidence to support various aspects of medical practice. Some believe practice should always be based on the support of Level 1 evidence and good RCTs. Because of the flaws and weaknesses in RCTs and because they are hard to do, however, others believe that such Level 1 evidence support is rarely needed. Both these viewpoints have some merit. Although good, valid RCTs can be an excellent basis for determining medical practice, their possible flaws and weaknesses must be always recognized and considered. RCTs and Level 1 evidence are not always absolute, inviolate or timeless. Appropriate evidence-based information or guidelines may not always be available, applicable, or correct. Accordingly physician judgment must be exercised in the application of RCTs to clinical decisions in various circumstances and will always be required for the optimal practice of medicine.

FLAWS AND WEAKNESSES OF RCTs

These occur in two groups, which are shown in Table 15-1 with examples of the flaws and weaknesses of RCTs cited.

Timeliness Flaws (Table 15-1, Items 1 and 2)

In the simplest terms, RCTs usually compare a new treatment against an old treatment or a new treatment against no treatment. In each instance the treatment under evaluation is compared against a control arm (old treatment or no treatment). If in a RCT the new treatment is proven to be ineffective, and then the technology, patient selection or operator skills for the new treatment improve in a major way, the original RCT becomes obsolete or invalid on the basis of timeliness (Table 15-1, Item 1). An example would be the Endarterectomy Versus Angioplasty in Patients with Symptomatic Severe Carotid Stenosis (EVA-3S) trial in which carotid stenting (CAS) proved to

TABLE 15-1. FLAWS AND WEAKNESSES OF RCTS THAT RENDER THEM LESS APPLICABLE OR INVALID[22]

No.	Flaws and weaknesses	Examples
1	Treatment under evaluation Technology or patient selection improves	CAS vs CEA RCTs (EVA-3S[2] and others)
2	Progress in control Treatment	Asymptomatic CS CEA+BMT vs BMT RCTS (ACAS[3], ACST[4])
3	Poor or unrepresentative patient selection	CAS vs CEA (SAPPHIRE[5,6])
4	Inadequate experience or competence of operators	CAS vs CEA – CAS operators (EVA-3S[2], ICSS[7]) CEA operators (SAPPHIRE[5])
5	Imperfect randomization	(SAPPHIRE[5]—see text)
6	Non-applicability to reality	CAS vs CEA (CREST[8]—see text)
7	Ideosyncratic flaws – delay in application of treatment	EVAR vs no treatment in unfit patients (EVAR 2[11])
8	Imperfect population randomized	CAS vs CEA – asymptomatic patients included—power decreased (CREST[8])
9	Inappropriate primary endpoints	CAS vs CEA – MI included (SAPPHIRE[5], CREST[8])

be less safe and have worse outcomes than carotid endarterectomy (CEA).[2] With improvements in CAS technology, patient selection, and operator experience and skill, the conclusions of this trial may no longer be valid.

On the other hand, if there is a valid RCT proving a given treatment effective against a control arm and there is improvement in the latter, the conclusions of the trial become obsolete and no longer valid. Examples would be trials comparing CEA and best medical therapy (BMT) against a control group receiving BMT alone, like the Asymptomatic Carotid Atherosclerosis Study (ACAS) or Asymptomatic Carotid Surgery Trial (ACST).[3,4] Since BMT for stroke prevention has improved dramatically since patients were entered into these trials (up to 2003), the demonstration that CEA plus BMT is better than current BMT alone is no longer valid (Table 15-1, Item 2).

DESIGN FLAWS (TABLE 15-1, ITEMS 3–9)

Inappropriate patient selection for randomization can invalidate the conclusion of a RCT. An example of this flaw was in the Stenting and Angioplasty with Protection in Patients at High Risk for Endarterectomy (SAPPHIRE) trial comparing CAS versus CEA in high-risk patients with carotid stenosis (CS).[5] Patients were selected for randomization because they were high risk for CEA but not necessarily for CAS, thus biasing the study against the open surgical procedure.[6] SAPPHIRE had the additional flaw of including 71% asymptomatic patients and yet having unacceptably high 30-day stroke and death rates (~6%).[6]

The competence and experience of the operators performing the treatment under evaluation can be suboptimal. If this is true, the conclusions of the RCT can be invalid or at least open to question. Some have made the case that such experience and competence issues have impaired the validity of the EVA-3S and International Carotid Stenting Study (ICSS) trials that compare the outcomes of CAS and CEA in symptomatic carotid stenosis patients.[2,7] Whether or not these issues invalidated these trials remains controversial.

Adequacy of patient randomization is another issue that can weaken or invalidate the conclusions of RCTs. SAPPHIRE is one example, since many more patients were excluded from randomization and treated by CAS than were randomized to the CAS arm.

If the operators who perform the procedure under evaluation in a RCT are so experienced and skillful that they are not representative of the vascular specialists performing the procedure in the population at large, then the results of the trial cannot apply to the general population of patients who are treated by less skilled operators. In the Carotid Revascularization Endarterectomy vs. Stenting Trial (CREST) trial, those performing CAS were only vetted to enter patients after they were shown to have a high level of experience and skill.[8] Thus the CAS results in CREST may not be representative of those generally performing the procedure in the "real world." This possibility is supported by the higher adverse event rates with CAS in population-based studies than in CREST.[8,9,10]

Some RCTs are weakened or invalidated by idiosyncratic flaws that are specific to that trial. One example of this flaw existed in the EVAR 2 trial in which endovascular abdominal aortic aneurysm repair (EVAR) was compared to no treatment in patients deemed unfit for open repair. A major flaw in this trial was the lengthy delay after randomization to EVAR (average 57 days) until the procedure was performed.[11] During that delay, nine of the patients died from aneurysm rupture before having the scheduled EVAR. The trial showed no difference in mortality between the two groups. The conclusion reached was that EVAR offered no benefit in these unfit aneurysm patients.[11] If the nine patients who died from rupture before their scheduled EVAR was performed had been treated more promptly, the trial's results and conclusions would likely have been very different.

Some otherwise excellent and valid RCTs are negatively impacted by inclusion of inappropriate patients in the randomization process. One example of this was in the CREST trial, which included both symptomatic and asymptomatic patients (see below).[8] Many believe that symptomatic and asymptomatic CS are somewhat different disease processes with different plaque characteristics, embolic potential, and stroke potential. Because of the inclusion of the asymptomatic patients, the statistical power of the findings in CREST was reduced and the value of the study was weakened.

Finally, the choice of inappropriate endpoints for determining safety and efficacy of the treatment under evaluation may weaken some otherwise good RCTs. Inclusion of myocardial infarction (MI) as part of a composite adverse event rate endpoint in CAS versus CEA trials (SAPPHIRE and CREST) is an example.[5,8] Although the case may be made for or against this inclusion, whether or not MIs are equivalent to strokes remains controversial, especially since the primary purpose of both CAS and CEA is to prevent death and disability from strokes. All of these flaws and weaknesses can reduce the value of a RCT or invalidate it completely. They must be considered in using and applying RCTs to clinical situations.

BIASED OR ERRONEOUS CONCLUSIONS AND INTERPRETATIONS OF RCTs

There is an even more insidious problem with some RCTs. This is the impact of bias in the interpretation of trial results that unfairly alter the conclusions reached in the article reporting the trial. These biased or erroneous conclusions can appear directly in articles describing RCTs with some of the flaws and weaknesses already discussed. Even more importantly, such biased and misleading conclusions can be reached in reports of otherwise flawless studies published in the foremost journals. Because of the high regard in which these exemplary RCTs are held, such misleading conclusions may have an important detrimental influence on medical practice.

This problem can be further enhanced by a second, usually bias-related mechanism, namely the way RCTs and their conclusions can be misinterpreted or "spun" by others to support their special interests. Such misinterpretation can even find their way into guideline documents produced by respected professional societies.

To exemplify these issues this chapter will present a detailed analysis of the CREST trial and a more superficial overview in tabular form of several other highly respected RCTs that have been reported in leading peer-reviewed and widely read journals.

CREST

The *CREST trial* was designed to compare CAS and CEA in symptomatic patients with CS.[8] CREST has been regarded as a well-designed and well-conducted RCT. Some have claimed that its results changed everything in the field, and it has been spun beyond that. In this regard CREST formed the basis for an important part of the so-called American Heart Association (AHA) Guideline on Management of Patients with Extracranial Carotid and Vertebral Artery Disease, which were also approved by 13 other organizations.[12] These Guidelines reached the conclusion that *"CAS is indicated as an alternative to CEA for symptomatic patients at average or low risk of complications associated with endovascular intervention..."*

The facts and data in CREST may not justify its conclusions, and more importantly, the way CREST is being interpreted in the AHA Guideline and spun by others may not be reasonable and valid. CREST was conceived in 1997, funded by the NIH in 1999 and randomized and analyzed 2502 patients from 2000–2008. It was originally designed to compare CAS and CEA for the treatment of moderate and high grade CS in recently symptomatic (6 months) patients. Allegedly, because adequate numbers of patients could not be recruited, asymptomatic patients were included in 2005. The 4-year results in 1262 CAS-treated patients and 1240 CEA-treated patients were reported in June 2010.[8]

The primary endpoint was a composite of death, stroke, and MI. This endpoint was reached by 4 years in 7.2% of the CAS patients and 6.8% of the CEA patients

(p = .51). The conclusions reached in the NEJM report was that the risk of CAS and CEA "did not differ significantly" in patients with symptomatic and asymptomatic CS. Because of this conclusion the CREST trial was spun to demonstrate the equivalence of CAS and CEA in both symptomatic and asymptomatic CS patients. In addition the AHA Guideline implies that this is the case.

Are these conclusions justified? To make that judgment one must examine in greater detail the data from CREST and its flaws (some already mentioned), remembering that the purpose of CEA and CAS is to prevent strokes, disability and death from CS. Table 15-2 shows some of the data details from CREST. There were substantially more deaths and strokes in the CAS-treated patients than those treated by CEA. Only when MIs were included were the adverse events similar in the two groups.

Other flaws existed in CREST (some already mentioned). Adding asymptomatic CS patients to the study diluted its power and prevented significance from being reached in some of the adverse events shown in Table 15-2.

The composite endpoint weakened the trial. MIs are not the equivalent of strokes. This is borne out by the greater degree of disability after a stroke than after an MI that has been observed in many studies including CREST. Moreover, even after a minor stroke with full motor and sensory recovery, patients often have evidence of brain damage with loss of memory, intelligence, and altered affect. Although it has been pointed out that even minor MIs are associated with decreased life expectancy and this was observed in CREST, the same is true after minor strokes, and this was documented in CREST.[13] Although further subgroup analyses from CREST have been enlightening and although everyone is entitled to their bias, the detailed CREST data in Table 15-2 seem to speak for themselves.

There is another potential flaw in CREST. The CAS-treated patients received more intensive antiplatelet therapy during and after their procedure than did the CEA patients. This may have contributed to the decreased incidence of MIs in the CAS group.

So what is the value of CREST and how should it be used? It clearly shows that both CAS and CEA can be performed with low morbidity and mortality rates. CREST, like most RCTs, however, has its flaws, which must be considered in any interpretation of its results. Moreover, CREST should be considered with other RCTs comparing CAS versus CEA in symptomatic CS patients, particularly the most recent European trial, ICSS, the results of which were published at the same time as those of CREST.[7,8] Although ICSS may also have its flaws, it showed that CAS was associated with a higher stroke rate and more diffusion weighted magnetic resonance imaging cerebral defects than CEA.

TABLE 15-2. DATA DETAILS FROM CREST[8,22]

Adverse events	No. CAS-treated patients (total = 1262)	No. CEA-treated patients (total = 1240)	*p* value
Deaths	9	4	0.18
Total Strokes	52	29	0.01
Major Strokes (Ipsilateral)	11	4	0.09
Minor Strokes (Ipsilateral)	37	17	0.01
Minor MIs	14	28	0.03

In both ICSS and CREST, however, the CAS procedures did not reflect the current state of the art. Accordingly, it is likely that with better stents (membrane or mesh covered), better embolic protection (reversal or cessation of flow), cervical access to avoid aortic arch problems, better patient selection and better operator skills, the results of CAS will be better than they were in these two most recent good trials; however, this must be shown by appropriate future RCTs.

With regard to asymptomatic patients, CREST does not add much since it did not include a BMT arm. A trial that does include a BMT arm (like CREST 2) is sorely needed. Until then and until we can have better methods to identify asymptomatic CS patients at high risk of having a stroke, it is likely that many, if not most, such patients should be treated by BMT and undergo no invasive intervention, but this remains highly controversial.

What about the AHA Guidelines and its conclusion, largely based on CREST, that "CAS is an alternative to CEA" in symptomatic average- and low-risk patients. A Webster's dictionary definition of *alternative* is "choice between two things."[15] This implies equivalence. In view of the considerations about CREST and its data details in Table 15-2, it would seem that the AHA Guidelines' conclusion that CAS is an alternative to CEA is not yet justified except when there are clear contraindications to CEA in a symptomatic patient requiring invasive treatment. High or long lesions or infected, scarred, or immobile necks represent examples of such contraindications.

OTHER MISLEADING RCTs

What about some other vascular RCTs published in leading journals and how they may be misleading? Some of these, their stated conclusions, more appropriate conclusions, and their date and site of publication are summarized in Table 15-3. The most misleading of these trials was SAPPHIRE, a deeply flawed trial, which was published twice in the *NEJM*, and spun widely at medical meetings and in the lay press to spell the death knell of CEA.[5,6,14]

IMPROVE TRIAL

The IMPROVE trial compares the value of open repair and endovascular aneurysm repair (EVAR) for the treatment of ruptured abdominal aortic aneurysms (RAAAs). Although some believe EVAR, if it can be done, is the best treatment for RAAAs, others claim the superior results for EVAR in this setting are due to favorable patient selection for EVAR. So the best treatment for RAAAs remains controversial. The IMPROVE trial was a large, multicenter trial conducted in 29 UK centers and one Canadian center designed to settle this controversy. Of 1265 clinically diagnosed RAAA patients considered, 615 were randomized to either an Endovascular Strategy Group or an Open Repair Group.[18] Randomization was carried out before CT scans were obtained. Mortality at 30 days for the 316 patients randomized to the Endovascular Strategy Group was 35%, whereas it was 37% for the 297 patients

TABLE 15-3. OTHER RCTS THAT REACHED MISLEADING CONCLUSIONS

RCT	Publication site	Year	Trial conclusion	Flaws	Appropriate conclusion
ACAS ACST	*JAMA* *Lancet*	1995[3] 2010[4]	CEA decreased stroke risk (SR) more than BMT; CEA for ACS[a] reduces 10 year SR from 2% to 1% per year	Obsolete BMT; decreasing SR with ACS	Need RCT in ACS of CAS & CEA vs BMT; Need way to identify high SR patients; BMT best for most ACS patients
SAPPHIRE	*NEJM* *NEJM*	2004[5] 2008[14]	No significant difference in outcome of CAS & CEA at 30 days, 1, or 3 years	71% asymptomatic CAS patients; ~6% 30-day death & stroke rate	High-risk ACS patients should be treated with BMT not by CAS or CEA
EVAR II	*Lancet*	2005[11]	In unfit patients EVAR did not improve survival over no intervention	½ of deaths (9) in EVAR arm due to rupture before treatment; average delay = 57 days	Timely EVAR justified in some unfit patients (see text)
EVAR I	*NEJM*	2010[17]	EVAR and open repair had equivalent long-term mortality with increased graft complications, need for reinterventions and cost		EVAR prolonged patient survival longer than open repair
IMPROVE	*BMJ*	2014[18] 2015[21]	EVAR strategy for RAAAs not decr mortality	>½ pts randomized to endov strat had open repair	EVAR has lower mortality than open repair if EVAR can be done

[a] ACS = Asymptomatic carotid stenosis.

randomized to the Open Repair Group. On the strength of these findings, the conclusion of the main paper describing the early mortality in the IMPROVE trial read in part:

"A strategy of endovascular repair was not associated with significant reduction in 30-day mortality."[18] This was widely quoted on the internet and in a *Vascular News* headline as: "NO DIFFERENCE BETWEEN ENDOVASC & OPEN REPAIR."[19]

To appreciate why these conclusions are misleading, it is necessary to examine the detailed results of the IMPROVE trial, which are shown in Table 15-4.[18,20] Such an examination reveals that of the 316 patients randomized to an Endovascular Strategy, only 154 or less than one-half were actually treated by EVAR. In these 154 patients, 30-day mortality was only 27%, whereas in the 112 patients in this group actually treated by open repair it was 38%. Of the 297 patients randomized to Open Repair, 36 were actually treated by EVAR, with a 30-day mortality of 22%, and 220 were actually treated by open repair with a 30-day mortality of 37%. When the two groups were combined, the 30-day mortality of the patients actually treated by EVAR was 25%, whereas it was 38% for those patients actually treated by open repair, a highly significant difference ($p < .002$).[20]

TABLE 15-4. DETAILED 30-DAY MORTALITY DATA FROM THE IMPROVE TRIAL[18,20]

316 patients randomized to endovascular strategy[a]			
Treatment	**Number of patients treated**	**Number of deaths in 30 days**	**30-day mortality (%)**
EVAR	150	38 } 42	25.3 } 27.3
EVAR Attempted Converted to open repair	4	4	100
Open repair	112	43	38.4
No Repair	17	16	94.1

[a] Eight patients had a symptomatic unruptured AAA but were included in this treatment analysis; 33 patients had another non-aneurysmal diagnosis and were not included in this treatment analysis.

297 patients randomized to open repair[b]			
Treatment	**Number of patients treated**	**Number of deaths in 30 days**	**30-day mortality (%)**
EVAR	36	8	22.2
Open repair	220	81	36.8
No repair	19	19	100

[b] Fourteen patients had a symptomatic unruptured AAA but were included in this treatment analysis; 22 patients had another non-aneurysmal diagnosis and were not included in this treatment analysis.

Actual treatment results in the two randomized groups combined			
Treatment	**Number of patients treated**	**Number of deaths in 30 days**	**30-day mortality (%)**
EVAR	186	46	24.7
Open repair	336	128	38.1

Although IMPROVE was a well-conducted trial that produced and will continue to produce some valuable information, its main finding regarding the similarity of 30-day and 1-year[21] mortality was rendered misleading by the primary flaw in the trial that more than half of the patients randomized to the Endovascular Strategy Group actually underwent open repair. This produced an intention-to-treat analysis that was totally misleading. A better conclusion to this part of the IMPROVE trial would have been: "EVAR produces a lower treatment mortality than open repair for RAAAs, if EVAR can be performed."[20]

CONCLUSIONS

All these RCTs show that unjustified conclusions can sometimes be reached in leading peer-reviewed journals.[22] This occurs because of flaws in the RCTs, unrecognized author bias, or both. More importantly, these unjustified conclusions and the trials on which they are based can be further misinterpreted or spun to reach even more erroneous or unjustified conclusions. Presumably, much of this spinning results from the bias or biases that all of us in medicine have. By being aware of the influence of bias along with the possible flaws that RCTs can have, we should be able to interpret and use RCTs fairly and optimally for the care of patients.

REFERENCES

1. Sackett DL, Rosenberg WM: The need for evidence-based medicine. *J R Soc Med.* 1995;88(11):620–4.
2. Mas JL, Chatellier G, Beyssen B, et al. Endarterectomy versus stenting in patients with symptomatic severe carotid stenosis. *N Engl J Med.* 2006;355:1660–71.
3. Endarterectomy for asymptomatic carotid artery stenosis. Executive Committee for the Asymptomatic Carotid Atherosclerosis Study. *JAMA.* 1995;273:1421–8.
4. Halliday A, Harrison M, Hayter E, et al. Asymptomatic Carotid Surgery Trial (ACST) Collaborative Group. 10-year stroke prevention after successful carotid endarterectomy for asymptomatic patients (ACST-1): a multicentre randomised trial. *Lancet.* 2010;376:1074–84.
5. Yadav JS, Wholey MH, Kuntz RE, et al. Protected carotid-artery stenting versus endarterectomy in high-risk patients. *N Engl J Med.* 2004;351:1493–501.
6. Naylor AR, Golledge J: High risk plaque, high risk patient or high risk procedure? *Eur J Vasc Endovasc Surg.* 2006;32(5):557–60.
7. International Carotid Stenting Study Investigators, Ederle J, Dobson J, Featherstone RL, et al. Carotid artery stenting compared with endarterectomy in patients with symptomatic carotid stenosis (International Carotid Stenting Study): an interim analysis of a randomised controlled trial. *Lancet.* 2010;375:985–97.
8. Brott TG, Hobson RW 2nd, Howard G, et al. CREST Investigators. Stenting versus endarterectomy for treatment of carotid-artery stenosis. *N Engl J Med.* 2010;363:11–23.
9. Sidawy AN, Zwolak RM, White RA, et al. Risk-adjusted 30-day outcomes of carotid stenting and endarterectomy: results from the SVS Vascular Registry. *J Vasc Surg.* 2009; 49(1):71–9.
10. Giles KA, Hamdan AD, Pomposelli FB, Wyers MC, Schermerhorn ML. Stroke and death rates after carotid endarterectomy and carotid artery stenting with and without high risk criteria. *J Vasc Surg.* 2010;52:1497–1504.
11. EVAR trial participants. Endovascular aneurysm repair and outcome in patients unfit for open repair of abdominal aortic aneurysm (EVAR trial 2): randomised controlled trial. *Lancet.* 2005;365(9478):2187–92.
12. Brott TG, Halperin JL, Abbara S, et al. 2011 ASA/ACCF/AHA/AANN/AANS/ACR/ASNR/CNS/SAIP/SCAI/SIR/SNIS/SVM/SVS Guideline on the Management of Patients With Extracranial Carotid and Vertebral Artery Disease A Report of the American College of Cardiology Foundation/American Heart Association Task Force on Practice Guidelines, and the American Stroke Association, American Association of Neuroscience Nurses, American Association of Neurological Surgeons, American College of Radiology, American Society of Neuroradiology, Congress of Neurological Surgeons, Society of Atherosclerosis Imaging and Prevention, Society for Cardiovascular Angiography and Interventions, Society of Interventional Radiology, Society of NeuroInterventional Surgery, Society for Vascular Medicine, and Society for Vascular Surgery Developed in Collaboration with the American Academy of Neurology and Society of Cardiovascular Computed Tomography. *J Am Coll Cardiol.* 2011;57(8):1002–44.
13. Blackshear JL, Cutlip DE, Roubin GS, et al. Myocardial Infarction After Carotid Stenting and Endarterectomy:Results From the Carotid Revascularization Endarterectomy Versus Stenting Trial. *Circulation.* 2011: Published online DOI: 10.1161 CIRCULATIONAHA. 110.008250
14. Gurm HS, Yadav JS, Fayad P, et al. SAPPHIRE Investigators. Long-term results of carotid stenting versus endarterectomy in high-risk patients. *N Engl J Med.* 2008;358:1572–9.

15. Webster's New World College Dictionary. Available at: http://www.yourdictionary.com/alternative. Last accessed on 8/2/2015.
16. Paraskevas KI, Veith FJ, Riles TS, Moore WS: Is carotid artery stenting a fair alternative to carotid endarterectomy for symptomatic carotid artery stenosis? A commentary on the AHA/ASA guidelines. *J Vasc Surg*. 2012;55:585–7.
17. United Kingdom EVAR Trial Investigators. Greenhalgh RM, Brown LC, Powell JT, et al. Endovascular versus open repair of abdominal aortic aneurysm. *N Eng J Med.* 2010;362(20):1863–71.
18. IMPROVE trial Investigtors, Powell JT, Sweeting MJ, Thompson MM, et al. Endovascular or open repair strategy for ruptured abdominal aortic aneurysm: 30 day outcomes from IMPROVE randomised trial. *BMJ*. 2014;348:f7661.
19. IMPROVE Trial 30-Day Results: No difference between endovascular and open repair for ruptured aneurysms. *Vascular News*. 2014;61:1–2.
20. Veith FJ, Rockman CB. The recent randomized trials of EVAR versus open repair for ruptured abdominal aortic aneurysms are misleading. *Vascular*. 2015;23:217–9.
21. Grieve R, Gomes M, Sweeting MJ, et al. Endovascular strategy or open repair for ruptured abdominal aortic aneurysm: one-year outcomes from the IMPROVE randomized trial. *Eur Heart J*. 2015 Apr 7. pii: ehv125. [Epub ahead of print].
22. Veith FJ: How can good randomized controlled trials in leading journals be so misinterpreted? *J Vasc Surg*. 2013;57(2 Suppl):3S–7S.

16

Preoperative Planning for Hemodialysis Access

Godfrey Parkerson, MD and Karl A. Illig, MD

Too many surgeons view construction of arteriovenous access (AV access) as a chore, often delegated to junior partners, faculty, or residents. As such, when approached in such a manner, results can be poor. The modern approach to AV access planning emphasizes careful preoperative evaluation including, critically, ultrasonic vein mapping to plan the access choice that has the greatest chance of working in the short-term, while keeping in mind the long-term potential sequence of events to keep the patient as healthy as possible.

It is best to consider access choices as a series of preferences, although certain conditions MUST be met. A general algorithm is presented in Table 16-1, but the following is a useful guide in determining the choice of access:

Absolute requirements:

- Adequate arterial inflow to provide at least 500cc/min flow, and
- Unobstructed venous outflow to the right atrium

General preferences, in rough order of significance (note that exceptions to each exist):

- Establishing AV access is better than relying on a catheter in the long-term
- An autologous fistula is better than a prosthetic graft
- The nondominant arm is preferable to the dominant arm
- Start distally and work proximally

HISTORY AND RISK FACTORS

Patients being considered for AV access are seen for a thorough history and physical exam. Several components of the patient's medical and surgical situation can have a large impact on pre-operative planning and post-operative expectations. With the multiple comorbidities and hospitalizations common in the patient with end-stage renal disease (ESRD), it is important that surgeons investigate each patient's medical history to optimize success of the operation.[1]

TABLE 16-1. GENERAL ALGORITHM FOR AV ACCESS DECISION-MAKING

Mandatory for either side to be used:

- Adequate arterial inflow (absence of significant stenosis, ideally arterial size greater than 2–3 mm at the wrist (undefined higher) with minimal calcification at site(s) of anastomosis)
- Unobstructed venous outflow (or realistic endovascular or surgical options to achieve it); ideally no pacemaker or AICD in place

Next steps, in rough order of preference (although the order may vary according to patient factors):

- Cephalic vein at wrist and centrally >3 mm? Use better arm if so; if equally good, use nondominant arm. RADIOCEPHALIC AVF
- Cephalic vein at upper arm and centrally >3 mm? Use better arm if so; if equally good, use non-dominant arm. BRACHIOCEPHALIC AVF
- No usable cephalic vein?
  - Patient acceptable risk, reasonable life expectancy?
    - » Basilic vein >3 mm? Use better arm if so; if equally good, use non-dominant arm.
      - If >4 mm, ONE STAGE TRANSPOSED BRACHIOBASILIC FISTULA
      - If <4 mm, TWO STAGE BRACHIOBASILIC FISTULA
  - Patient poor risk, unusually poor life expectancy, or tenuous catheter dependence:
    - » Consider AVG (ACUSEAL if immediate access of benefit)
- All steps above: If vein borderline consider AVG

If cephalic and basilic veins are not usable in either arm, or if patient has unusual risk or unusually limited life expectancy:

- AVG – forearm to brachial veins, upper arm (we prefer axillary-based loop)

If arterial inflow is adequate, but veins are obstructed and cannot easily be decompressed and reconstructed:

- HeRO

If arterial inflow and venous outflow adequate only on opposite sides:

- Chest wall/necklace AVG

If venous outflow stenotic ONLY at costoclavicular junction:

- Consider anterior thoracic outlet decompression with plasty/stent, AVF or AVG as above

If central veins stenotic but catheter in place:

- HeRO/ACCUSEAL combination

If SVC is occluded:

- Leg AVF (preferred) or AVG
- Exotic recanalization

End Stage Renal Disease

It's obvious that patients being evaluated for AV access will have Chronic Kidney Disease (CKD), but the degree and duration of their renal disease is an important factor when evaluating a patient for AV access creation. According to KDOQI guidelines, ideally patients should have AVF placed at least 6 months prior to anticipated hemodialysis (HD) therapy, and 3–6 weeks earlier if an AV graft is to be placed. These guidelines are set to allow for use of the permanent AV access at the start of HD therapy, thus avoiding the need for catheter-based access and associated complications. Placement of AV access before progression to HD therapy also allows for fistula maturation in a healthier environment not subjected to the oxidative stress associated with uremia and dialysis. Lower failure-to-mature rates and increased patency rates have been shown in AV access placed before commencing dialysis versus those placed afterward.[2] While the intervals set by the KDOQI guidelines are usually enough time for maturation and wound-healing, they may not be appropriate for all patients. A retrospective cohort study of 150 patients with late-stage CKD and preemptive AVF creation found that only 49% of the patients were actually receiving HD at mean follow-up of 10 months. Of the patients on HD therapy, 65% were using their AVF while 35% were not because of failure to create a working fistula. In the patients not on HD, 55% had their fistula abandoned either due to death, transplant, HD refusal, or AVF failure.[3] Although preemptive AVF creation is advantageous if catheter placement can be avoided, not all patients will benefit as about half of such patients never received HD (at 10 month follow up). The timing of AVF creation is a decision that should be made with awareness of multiple patient-related factors that may affect incidence of HD therapy and success/maturation of the access. Discourse between the surgeon, the nephrologist, and the patient can help refine the decision and timing for AV access creation to optimize success and avoid unnecessary surgery.

Diabetes Mellitus

The prevalence of diabetes is high among the CKD patient population. Patients with diabetes have been shown to have lower AVF patency compared to non-diabetic patients and centers have reported increased use of prosthetic grafts in diabetic patients.[1] The poor patency rates reported are presumably due to increased vessel calcification and decreased vessel compliance predominantly with regard to the arterial supply. Certain preoperative strategies can help to reduce these deleterious effects and achieve satisfactory maturation and patency rates. In their comprehensive review, Smith et al. found that the use of careful preoperative vessel imaging contributed to similar primary AVF outcomes in diabetic versus nondiabetic patients.[1] Although diabetic patients may require more proximal access than nondiabetic patients, studies have yielded primary access survival rates comparable to that of nondiabetic patients.[4] One important risk in diabetic patient is the increased incidence of ischemic complications after AV access creation. Although rare, ischemic monomelic neuropathy is a complication occurring exclusively in diabetic patients. It occurs almost exclusively with AV access created above the brachial artery bifurcation. In addition, steal occurs more commonly in patients with diabetes, particularly those with small and calcified forearm vessels.

History of Steal

In patients with a history of prior hemodialysis access, prior complications are thought to predict subsequent events in the contralateral arm. Patients with a history of ischemic steal syndrome on one side are at increased risk for steal with future fistula and graft creation on the other. Surgeons should be particularly cautious in patients who require access creation on their dominant extremity as untreated ischemic complications can have catastrophic effects on patient quality of life. Experience has revealed several strategies to reduce the probability of steal. These strategies include limiting arteriotomy to 0.4–0.7mm in length and the use of more proximal arteriotomy sites.

Age and Life Expectancy

According to the United States Renal Data System (USRDS), the adjusted incidence rate of the ESRD in the U.S. population from 2000 to 2011 has grown by 7.1% in the population aged 75 years and older. Data from meta-analyses have shown that radiocephalic AVFs have reduced patency and increased primary failure rates in elderly patients,[5] and as such a lower threshold to create a brachiocephalic fistula may be warranted. Research has varied regarding the effect of specific access options on quality of life in the elderly population, but patterns in certain cohorts have been identified. Particularly in patients aged >80y who are female and/or had prior hemodialysis access, brachiocephalic fistulas have been shown to provide improved patency and quality of life over radiocephalic fistulas.[6] Consideration of primary AV grafts may be appropriate in elderly patients with comorbidities that predict no long-term life expectancy. Starting with a graft would avoid the complications associated with catheter-based access while awaiting fistula maturation and would provide the patient with a functional access for the remaining months of their lives.

Obesity

Obese patients (defined as those with BMI > 30) can present a challenge for AV access creation. Superficial veins are often difficult to visualize on physical exam, and these patients frequently require duplex ultrasound for evaluation of venous circulation. With the use of duplex vein mapping, obese patients have the same frequency of suitable venous anatomy as non-obese patients.[1] In a study comparing 1486 patients with BMI >30 and those <30, BMI was not found to be a predictor of AVF revision or failure. On the other hand, patients with BMI >35 had increased risk of failure to mature.[7] Historically, many surgeons have avoided creation of AV fistulas in obese patients preferring graft-based AV access options, the argument being that veins in obese patients often require increased operative time and/or multiple operations to superficialize the venous outflow. This is particularly true for super-obese patients and autogenous access requiring venous transposition such as brachial-basilic and brachial-brachial fistulas. When performing these procedures in obese patients, we generally plan for longer operative times and often opt for general over regional anesthesia. We have found substantial success with autogenous access creation even in obese patients and have actually tended to steer away from prosthetic access if possible due to an observed increased incidence of re-intervention. We do discuss superficialization at initial evaluation with the patient.

Hypotension

Diastolic hypotension (defined as diastolic pressure <60mmHg) has been associated with decreased 12-month survival of AVFs even after exclusion of patients with early fistula failure.[1] The same trend holds true for both AVF and AV grafts in pre-dialysis patients with diastolic hypotension.[1] As such early attempts at more proximal access locations may be warranted in patients with diastolic hypotension to avoid thrombosis and necessary return to the OR for revision or creation of subsequent access. Hypotensive patients may also have decreased baseline Doppler signals at the wrist, which surgeons must be aware of when evaluating Doppler signals for steal syndrome after completion of the AV anastomosis.

ARTERIAL AND VENOUS EXAM

Traditionally, Allen's test has been performed (or at least recommended) as an integral part of the physical exam. Most high-volume access centers and surgeons, however, have failed to find any prognostic benefit with this maneuver, especially in the age of widespread availability of duplex ultrasound. What is probably more important than patency of the Palmer arch is patency of the radio and/or owner arteries. If both of these are patent, but the arch is occluded, in fact, this may be protective of steal after radiocephalic fistula creation. If duplex examination shows that both form vessels are not patent, consideration may be strong to start higher.

Examination is useful for assessing venous patency in patients without much subcutaneous body fat, but can be very misleading in the obese. A visible antecubital cephalic vein predicts upper arm cephalic patency, but, again, ultrasound is critical to ensure that everything is wide open. A palpable radial pulse suggests adequate inflow, but if any question arises, hemodynamic assessment should be undertaken. Finally, attention should obviously be paid to evidence of venous outflow obstruction, including scars suggestive of prior catheter placement, dilated chest wall and shoulder veins, and, obviously, a swollen arm or pacemaker in place.

IMAGING

Duplex Ultrasound

The modern cornerstone of presurgical evaluation is now thorough duplex ultrasound (DUS) examination of the arteries and veins ("vein mapping"). Randomized controlled trials have shown 10–20% increased success of AVF creation with DUS over physical examination in radiocephalic fistula creation.[1] The KDOQI guidelines now recommend preoperative duplex ultrasound for all patients undergoing evaluation for AV access creation. Multiple studies have shown an increase in the rate of autogenous access creation with the use of preoperative DUS, but the effect on maturation and functional patency rates remains uncertain.

Factors obtainable using DUS that have been shown to affect early patency include arterial diameter, venous diameter, and presence of anatomic anomalies. Small arterial diameters <1.5–3.0 mm are associated with increased rates of nonmaturation, but agreement on minimum diameters has not been established.[8] For radiocephalic fistulas (RCF) at the wrist, radial artery diameters >2 mm were shown to have significantly higher success rate than radial artery diameters <2 mm (59% vs. 40%).[1] Criteria for minimum venous diameter range greatly, typically judged to be from 2.0 to 4.0 mm. Success rates for cephalic vein diameters <2 mm are significantly less than those with diameter >2 mm (29% vs. 71%).[1]

Venography

Duplex ultrasound has become the preferred imaging modality for most surgeons prior to AV access creation, but the sensitivity and specificity of DUS still falls short of digital subtraction angiography (DSA). DSA provides direct visualization of the selected veins, especially those that make up the central venous circulation. Reports have shown sensitivities less than 80% for DUS compared to DSA in detection of central venous stenoses.[8] While venous waveforms may help suggest the presence of central stenosis or occlusion, DUS has a limited ability to precisely locate these abnormalities. Adequate assessment of central venous circulation is especially important for patients with history of central venous catheterization (in whom the prevalence of central venous stenosis or obstruction can be as high as 40%).[8] The use of iodinated contrast in patients who are not yet on dialysis is the obvious drawback. For patients with eGFR <30 mL/min/1.73 m^2, the risk of contrast induced AKI is 30–40%, with a 2–8% risk of precipitating the need for dialysis, and in patients with diabetes and eGFR < 60 mL/min/1.73 m^2 the incidence of contrast-induced AKI has been reported as high as 50%.[9] We do not routinely obtain venography, but save this for people with relatively high suspicion of venous outflow abnormalities (visible dilated veins, pacemaker in place, any degree of arm swelling, or a history of subclavian or multiple jugular central venous catheters). If venography is obtained, it's important to use superficial tourniquets, both to dilate the superficial veins peripheral to the tourniquets and also to better visualize the deep veins.

ARTERIAL FACTORS

Arterial diameter and degree of atherosclerosis measured on DUS have significant effects on patency of AV fistulas. While arterial diameter has not been shown to affect patency at more proximal sites, radial artery diameters of less than 2 mm have been correlated with decreased fistula success rates at the wrist. Additionally, the degree of atherosclerosis has been correlated with increased rates of thrombosis and inability to support dialysis at 1 year post-fistula creation.[1] Awareness of anatomic variants such as a high radial take-off may help surgeons avoid potential ischemic complications in patients with poor collateral ulnar circulation, and/or choose the best vessel for inflow. In our vascular lab, every evaluation for hemodialysis access includes bilateral brachial pressures (with optional forearm and finger pressures if any question exists as to perfusion), duplex evaluation of brachial, radial, and ulnar artery sizes, documentation of the presence or absence of atherosclerosis and calcification, and documentation of anatomic abnormalities or anomalies.

VENOUS FACTORS

Diameter has served as the primary venous trait assessed in the planning stages of AV access for decades, even before the widespread availability of duplex ultrasound. As discussed above, the cut-off for a minimum vein diameter for successful creation of other AV access configurations has not been agreed upon. A recent single center retrospective review of patients who had undergone brachiocephalic and brachiobasilic AVF demonstrated that minimum vein diameter of <2.7mm was associated with significantly increased failure rates (> 33%) and decreased long-term patency compared to those a minimum diameter of ≥3.3 mm. Models adjusting for age, diabetes, gender, and preoperative dialysis status found that increased minimum vein diameter alone was associated with decreased risk of failure to mature and increased long term patency in brachiocephalic and brachiobasilic fistulas.[10] In our lab the venous evaluation for hemodialysis access includes direct duplex imaging of the axillosubclavian veins for patency, venous diameter of cephalic vein measured from its origin to its termination noting evidence of phlebosclerosis and anatomic abnormalities, and venous diameter of the basilic vein measured from its origin to its insertion into the deep system noting evidence of phlebosclerosis and anatomic abnormalities (the length of the true basilic vein is noted, but we use the entire basilic and brachial/axillary venous complex dissected high into the axilla for routine brachiobasilic transposed AV fistulas, so this is not critical). Patients with previous failed access may also have assessment of the brachial veins for possible brachial–brachial AVF. Although the ideal cut-off for minimum vein diameter has yet to be established, utilization of imaging still allows surgeons stratify the venous outflow options for each individual patient and plan the access configuration that has the greatest chance of success.

ANESTHESIA

Before making the incision, every patient undergoing AV access creation must be evaluated for appropriate anesthesia. The choice of anesthesia has traditionally been a joint decision between surgeon and anesthesiologist based on the given patient's tolerance of general anesthesia and endotracheal intubation. Regional anesthesia (brachial plexus block) produces significant vasodilatation, which may improve maturation and short term patency rates. Malinzak and Gan have documented that regional anesthesia improved vasodilation in cephalic and basilic veins as well as increased AVF blood flow in the immediate post-operative period compared to general and local anesthesia.[11] This advantage of regional anesthesia has led us to steer away from local anesthesia and utilize regional anesthesia (brachial plexus block) whenever patients can tolerate it. In our experience, the most common factors limiting the utilization of regional anesthesia have been patient anxiety and inability to lie still or lie flat, and our practice of dissecting well into the axilla to eliminate a tethered "swing point" in patients requiring transposed brachiobasilic fistula creation. Although no prospective randomized trials have been completed, the collection of evidence suggests that regional anesthesia may be preferred in any patient willing to have their surgery performed while awake.

PUTTING IT ALL TOGETHER: CHOICE OF ACCESS

The optimal location or configuration of initial autogenous fistula creation remains a hotly debated and intensely researched subject in the field of hemodialysis access, and one that is surprisingly difficult to construct an algorithm for. The KDOQI guidelines attempt to standardize the selection of initial autogenous AV access, ranking forearm/wrist radiocephalic fistulas as the first preferred configuration for AV access followed by elbow brachiocephalic and finally transposed brachiobasilic fistulas. While the evidence presented in the KDOQI guidelines provides adequate support for these recommendations, it fails to take into account several of the factors that we have discussed so far. In addition, "value judgments" such as utilization of a good cephalic vein vs. arm dominance, forearm grafts vs. transposed fistulas, the value of staging certain fistulas, and so on are not addressed.

Radiocephalic Fistula

The radiocephalic fistula (RCF) has traditionally been the first option for permanent AV access. The KDOQI guidelines recommend a wrist radiocephalic fistula (Cimino) as the preferred option for primary AV access creation, and many surgeons feel confident attempting RCF in patients who meet the minimum vein diameter of ≥2 mm (although many would use 3.0 mm as a better predictor of success). The main benefits of RCF's lie in the simplicity of the operation (low risk) and excellent patency rates after maturation. A major problem encountered with RCFs is, however, their poor initial maturation rates. Diabetic and elderly patients are two groups in which RCF creation should be approached with caution. Patients with diabetes have been shown to have lower maturation rates of RCF's (30%) compared to brachiocephalic and brachiobasilic fistulas (73%, 100%) with cumulative patency rates as much as 45% lower as compared to upper arm fistulas.[12] A recent meta-analysis of RCFs fistulas in elderly patients has likewise documented decreased 12 and 24 months patency rates as compared to upper arm AV access.[5] Additionally, a factor that surgeons sometimes fail to consider is patient preference and cosmetic concerns. Some patients, particularly the young, may be highly concerned about appearance and the ability to conceal their access sites. For these patients, more proximal configurations should be considered to allow the fistula or graft to be hidden under the sleeve.

Brachiocephalic Fistula

According to the KDOQI, the preferred site for primary autogenous access if a RCF is not possible is the brachiocephalic fistula (BCF) at the elbow. This fistula offers the advantages of a single short incision for creation as well as good maturation (66–75%) and patency rates. The main drawback in creation of BCF over RCF is the increased incidence of ischemic symptoms and median nerve injury. Although BCFs have increased risk with regard to RCFs, thc risk remains low. In comparison to other brachial artery based access configurations, the creation of a BCF requires less time and dissection and offers equal if not superior patency. While there is no consensus agreement on anatomic criteria for BCFs, we use 3 mm as the minimum vein diameter to consider creation of a BCF.

Transposed Brachiobasilic Fistulas

The last choice of AV access configuration addressed by the KDOQI guidelines is the transposed brachiobasilic fistula (TBBF). If creation of an RCF or BCF is not likely to succeed, this is the next option. The main disadvantage of TBBF creation lies in the obligation to widely expose the basilic (and usually brachial/axillary) vein to allow for transposition. As general anesthesia is more commonly required, the patient's medical comorbidities and physical exam findings can have significant effects on the success and ease of TBBF creation. Obese patients may require more time for exposure, transposition, and superficialization around/through large amounts of adipose tissue. The incision required for TBBF is larger, and wound complications are thus greater. The larger dissection also results in increased time required to complete the operation (although the operation is easily performed in less than 90 min). To address some of these concerns, some have advocated that the procedure be done in two stages, saving transposition (i.e., most of the morbidity) for only those who achieve initial patency. This approach may be useful for obese patients or patients with marginal anatomy to hopefully allow for vein dilation and lengthening to ease maturation and transposition, but preliminary results have not shown overwhelming benefit. Two recent meta-analyses have shown no differences in terms of overall maturation rate or post-operative complications in one- versus two-stage TBBF.[13,14] Although TBBF is traditionally not attempted unless options for RCF or BCF have been precluded, the performance of TBBF in terms of patency is excellent, and perhaps the best-performing fistula of all. Koksoy et al. randomized patients with prior failed distal access to receive either BCF or TBBF. All patients had minimum vein diameter of >3 mm. Their study showed no statistically significant difference in primary or secondary patency at 42 months between BCF and TBBF.[15] The largest series reporting outcomes of TBBFs shows maturation rates of almost 90%.[16] Patient-specific risk factors mentioned previously should be considered and may be the deciding factor in patients with marginal cephalic vein and suitable basilic vein. While more distal access options may offer shorter and less demanding operations, the TBBF remains an excellent access option that should be considered when anatomy is suitable.

Transposed Brachial-Brachial Fistula

In patients with absolutely no suitable superficial vein, many will proceed to nonautogenous upper extremity access using prosthetic graft. Although not traditionally thought of as a first line autogenous access option, a brachial artery to brachial vein fistula (transposed in one stage or two) can serve as an excellent autogenous access option. Data have suggested that brachial-brachial fistulas have equal patency to TBBF and improved primary patency and functional patency compared to prosthetic upper arm AV access.[17,18] The decision for staged versus unstaged brachial-brachial access creation depends on patient-specific factors (overlying tissue depth, vein length) and surgeon preference, but the brachial vein is more often highly branched and inherent to the artery, and we thus prefer a staged approach in virtually all circumstances.

Prosthetic Upper Extremity AV Access

When autogenous AV access in the upper extremity has been exhausted or is unavailable, the only upper extremity option for most patients is a non-autologous upper extremity AV graft (AVG). Although it is axiomatic that long-term function is less when compared with autologous access, there are some clear advantages to prosthetic access. Standard PTFE-based AVG's can be cannulated within 3-6 weeks of creation, and with varying degrees of success several previous graphs and the new trilayer prosthetic (ACUSEAL; Gore, Inc; Flagstaff Arizona) can be cannulated within 24 hours. Because "maturation" is nearly certain, an AVG serves as a good first option for patients with limited life expectancy, fast-approaching dialysis needs, or unusually urgent need for catheter removal. Rosas and Fieldman conducted a cost-utility analysis evaluating autogenous vs prosthetic access and found a difference of only 0.13 QALY's. They also found that cost-effectiveness of the fistula first strategy was significant only when fistula maturation rate was >36%.[19] The configuration of upper extremity AVGs is largely based on patient preference and physician experience. Patients who are not concerned about the appearance of their access site may receive forearm straight or loop grafts. Those who prefer a more discrete AV access usually receive curved or loop brachial artery based grafts. Finally, grafts derived from bovine, ovine, porcine, and cultured human cell sources are all available or will soon be; although no clear evidence of benefit exists, the possibilities are encouraging that we will have better options in the near future.

CHALLENGES AND SOLUTIONS

Central Vein Stenosis

Early access failure is often due to venous outflow stenosis. While the vein itself can be stenotic, this is usually identifiable by preoperative imaging and easily corrected. By contrast, stenosis or occlusion of the more central veins has been reported to be present in up to 40% of patients with history of central venous catheterization,[8] and in our experience seems to be surprisingly prevalent even in those without. Patients with symptomatic CVS in the setting of a functioning AV access typically present with prolonged post-cannulation bleeding, arm swelling, failed maturation, or even access thrombosis. When access sites opposite to the side of stenosis are not available, surgeons are forced address the central vein stenosis directly in order to create upper extremity AV access. The KDOQI recommends percutaneous transluminal venoplasty with or without stenting as the first line treatment for central venous stenosis, but results of this therapy have been disappointing as a whole. Treatment of asymptomatic CVS should be avoided as studies have shown that it results in faster progression of CVS.[20] For stenosis occurring at the costoclavicular junction (CCJ) the cause is often due extrinsic bony compression which is less amenable to PTA and stenting alone. These cases should be considered dialysis-associated venous thoracic outlet syndrome. The treatment of venous thoracic outlet syndrome generally requires bony decompression in the form of first rib resection.[21] In patients with symptomatic CCJ stenosis recognized after AV access creation, several small studies have found satisfactory rates of access salvage after first rib resection.[22,23] In patients with confirmed symptomatic CCJ stenosis and history of failed AV Access, we have found success performing first rib resection with simultaneous new AV access creation to relieve symptoms of CVS. Despite the available treatments for CVS, some patients still fail to achieve functional upper extremity AV access by standard autogenous or prosthetic configurations. For these patients, surgeons should be prepared to offer more complex AV access options.

HeRO Grafts

The Hemodialysis Reliable Outflow (HeRO) graft (Cryolife Inc., Kennesaw, GA) has become an increasingly popular option for catheter-dependent patients with central venous occlusion or stenosis preventing upper extremity AV access. The driving force behind the graft's approval and use has been the 69% lower incidence of infection shown in HeRO grafts compared to tunneled dialysis catheters.[24] The patency and infection rate of the HeRO graft compared to alternate lower extremity AVG has been similar, but with more interventions (2.21/year) required to maintain HeRO patency.[25] Preoperatively, surgeons should measure each patient's ability and willingness to undergo interventions to maintain patency after implantation. Patients with poor follow up and those with a history of steal may be better candidates for alternate AV access options in the trunk or lower extremities.

Lower Extremity AV Access

Conventionally patients seeking permanent dialysis access without upper extremity options have received lower extremity AV access. The typical lower extremity autogenous access involves transposition of the femoral vein to the lateral thigh with anastomosis to the distal SFA. Prosthetic lower extremity access arrangements vary greatly. Surgeons have typically avoided lower extremity AV access in obese patients as they tend to require several interventions often for infection post-operatively. The greatest drawback of lower extremity prosthetic AV access is the increased infection rate compared to upper extremity. Antiniou et al. performed an extensive review of the literature regarding lower extremity prosthetic and autogenous AV access and divided patients into three groups based on configuration: autogenous, prosthetic upper thigh, and prosthetic mid-thigh. As expected, infection rates were significantly greater at 18.39% for prosthetic thigh access. The data also revealed a greatly increased primary patency of autogenous fistula (83%) over upper (48%) and mid-thigh (43%) prosthetic. Rates of secondary patency were significantly greater for autogenous as well. While autogenous access provided greater patency, the rate of steal syndrome resulting in limb ischemia with autogenous access was three times greater at 20.7% compared to prosthetic access. Ischemic complications were particularly high in elderly diabetic patients with a long history of ESRD.[26] For this subset of patients, avoidance of lower extremity access creation is likely the best strategy. While lower extremity access may provide durable access options for some patients, physicians must be able to weigh the benefits with impact of potential complications on each patient's current state of health.

Chest Wall or Truncal AV Access

As medical technology has expanded and guidelines set in place, the longevity of patients with ESRD has increased. This has challenged surgeons to provide vascular access for patients in whom upper extremity access has been exhausted. One example for patients with patent central venous circulation is the prosthetic axilloaxillary loop access. In a prospective cohort study, Kendall et al placed prosthetic axilloaxillary loop grafts in both non-obese and obese patients seen as high risk for thigh AV access. They achieved 59% secondary patency at 1 year overall with no infections in the non-obese cohort.[27] The axilloaxillary loop graft serves as a viable alternative for patients with open central venous circulation in whom lower extremity AV access for whatever reason (amputation, history of lower extremity steal, severe PAD, etc.) cannot be attempted. Several other prosthetic complex access configurations have been studied in small numbers, but strong data supporting when and how to employ them has been lacking. Ultimately, the decision to embark on more complex AV access options is a joint decision between the physician and patient with the appropriate strategy determined by the patient's history, imaging, and physical exam.

AN ALGORITHM FOR PLANNING ACCESS

Multiple algorithms have been published to address optimization of the success of AV-access patient populations. Although the validity of these algorithms have not all been verified by reproduction in separate studies, each algorithm incorporates important facets that should be considered when planning AV access. In their scoring system to predict autogenous AV access maturation Lok et al. used age > 65yo, white race, presence of peripheral vascular disease, and presence of coronary artery disease to assign points 445 patients who had their first fistula creation for HD access. They found a correlation between scores and rates of successful maturation in their patient series.[28] It is important to note that the scoring system fails to identify a significant number of the previously discussed risk factors which may confound their results. Table 16-1 presents the general algorithm used in our practice encompassing the major factors discussed above.

SUMMARY

The exact choice of access is not currently definable: too many variables exist. In general, autologous access is preferred over prosthetic, which in turn is preferred over catheter use, but exceptions exist. Additionally, distal access is preferred over proximal access, and superficial veins over deep, but veins and arteries don't always cooperate. What is probably certain is that preoperative examination of the arterial inflow, venous conduit, and venous outflow using duplex ultrasound is critically important, and that the decision should be made by an experienced access surgeon in conjunction with the patient. Finally, the "access whisperer" will think several steps ahead. This is not a one-time surgical event, but a relationship between the physician and the patient. There must be a plan B, a plan C, and so on, if one is to keep these patients alive.

REFERENCES

1. Smith GE, Gohil R, Chetter IC. Factors affecting the patency of arteriovenous fistulas for dialysis access. *J Vasc Surg.* 2012;55:849–55.
2. Kalantarinia K, Campbell A, Mourad S, et al. Timing of hemodialysis Vascular access placement determines access outcomes. *Am J Kidney Dis.* 2010;55:B67.
3. Kimball TA, Barz K, Dimond KR, et al. Efficiency of the kidney disease outcomes quality initiative guidelines for preemptive vascular access in an academic setting. *J Vasc Surg.* 2011;54(3):760–6.
4. Konner K, Hulbert-Shearon TE, Roys EC, Port FK. Tailoring the initial vascular access for dialysis patients. *Kidney Int.* 2002;62:329–38.
5. Lazarides MK, Georgiadis GS, Antoniou GA, Staramos DN. A meta-analysis of dialysis access outcome in elderly patients. *J Vasc Surg.* 2007:45:420–6.
6. Weale AR, Bevir P, Neary, et al. Radiocephalic and brachiocephalic arteriovenous fistula outcomes in the elderly. *J Vasc Surg.* 2008;47:144–50.
7. Chan MR, Young HN, Becker YT, Yevzlin AS. Obesity as a predictor of vascular access outcomes: Analysis of the USRDS DMMS Wave II study. *Semin Dial.* 2008;21:274–9.
8. Planken RN, Tordoir JHM, Duijm LEM, et al. Current techniques for assessment of upper extremity vasculature prior to hemodialysis vascular access creation. *Eur Radiol.* 2007;17:3001–11.
9. Goldfarb S, McCullough PA, McDermott J, Gay SB. Contrast-induced acute kidney injury: Specialty-specific protocols for interventional radiology, diagnostic computed tomography radiology, and interventional radiology. *Mayo Clin Proc.* 2009;84(2):170–9.
10. Dageforde LA, Harms KA, Feurer ID, Shaffer D. Increased minimum vein diameter on preoperative mapping with duplex ultrasound is associated with arteriovenous fistula maturation and secondary patency. *J Vasc Surg.* 2015;71:170–6.
11. Malinzak EB, Gan TJ. Regional anesthesia for vascular access surgery. *Anesth Analg.* 2009;109(3):976–80.

12. Hakaim AG, Nalbandian M, Scott T. Superior maturation and patency of primary brachiocephalic and transposed basilic vein arteriovenous fistulae in patients with diabetes. *J Vasc Surg.* 1998;27(1):154–7.
13. Cooper J, Power AH, DeRose G, et al. Similar failure and patency rates when comparing one- and two-stage basilic vein transposition. *J Vasc Surg.* 2015;61(3):809–16.
14. Wooster M, Dansey K, Gabbard W, Illig KA. One- versus two-stage brachiobasilic arteriovenous fistulae: A meta-analysis. *Ann Vasc Surg.* 2015; in press.
15. Koksoy C, Demirci RK, Balci D, et al. Brachiobasilic versus brachiocephalic arteriovenous fistula: A prospective randomized study. *J Vasc Surg.* 2009:171–7.
16. Glass C, Porter J, Singh M, et al. A large scale study of the upper arm basilic transposition for hemodialysis. *Ann Vasc Surg.* 2010;24(1):85–91.
17. Casey K, Tonnessen BH, Mannava K, et al. Brachial versus basilic vein dialysis fistulas: A comparison of maturation and patency rates. *J Vasc Surg.* 2008;47:402–6.
18. Greenberg JI, May S, Suliman A, Angle N. The brachial artery-brachial vein fistula: expanding the possibilities for autogenous fistulae. *J Vasc Surg.* 2008;48:1245–50.
19. Rosas SE and Fieldman HI. Synthetic vascular hemodialysis access vs native arteriovenous fistula: A cost-utility analysis. *Ann Surg.* 2012;255(1):181–6.
20. Renaud CJ, Francois M, Nony A, et al. Comparative outcomes of treated symptomatic versus non-treated asymptomatic high grade central stenosis in the outflow of predominantly dialysis fistulas. *Nephrol Dial Transplant.* 2012;27:1631–8.
21. Illig KA. Management of central vein stenoses and occlusions: the critical importance of the costoclavicular junction. *Semin Vasc Surg.* 2011;24(2): 113–8.
22. Glass C, Dugan M, Gillespie D, et al. Costoclavicular venous decompression in patients with threatened arteriovenous hemodialysis access. *Ann Vasc Surg.* 2011;25(5):640–5.
23. Illig KA, Gabbard W, Calero A, et al. Aggressive costoclavicular junction decompression in patients with failing AV access. *Ann Vasc Surg.* 2015;29(4):698–703.
24. Katzman HE, McLafferty RB, Ross JR, et al. Initial experience and outcome of a new hemodialysis access device for catheter-dependent patients. *J Vasc Surg.* 2009;50:600–7.
25. Steerman SN, Wagner J, Higgins JA, et al. Outcomes comparison of HeRO and lower extremity arteriovenous grafts in patients with long-standing renal failure. *J Vasc Surg.* 2013; 57:776–83.
26. Antiniou GA, Lazarides MK, Georgiadis GS, et al. Lower-extremity Arteriovenous Access for Haemodialysis: A systematic Review. *Eur J Vasc Endovasc Surg.* 2009;38:365–72.
27. Kendall TW, Cull DL, Carsten CG, et al. The role of prosthetic axilloaxillary loop access as a tertiary arteriovenous access procedure. *J Vasc Surg.* 2008;48:389–93.
28. Lok CE, Allon M, Moist L, et al. Risk equation determining unsuccessful cannulation events and failure to maturation in arteriovenous fistulas (REDUCE FTM I). *J Am Soc Nephrol.* 2006;17(11):3204–12.

17

Basilic Vein Transposition for Hemodialysis: A Review

Marc H. Glickman, MD

The basilic vein transposition was first described by Dagher[1] in 1976 and since then several modifications and changes have been described. The basilic vein lies deep in the upper arm and several different techniques have been described to superficialize this vein for puncture for dialysis. In 2001 this procedure became more common and became part of the KDOQI guidelines in recommendation for access in patients to maintain" the fistula first" concept. After failure of either a radial cephalic fistula or brachial cephalic fistula, the guidelines recommend placement of a brachial basilica vein transposition for hemoaccess. There are several techniques that have been described to obtain satisfactory results with this method of access creation. These include placing the fistula in two stages rather than one stage. There are also techniques also described in elevation of the vein as opposed to transposition that recent data appears to show improvement in outcomes. These various techniques will be discussed in this review article. New concepts also to improve outcomes with this procedure will also be part of the discussion as well.

ONE-STAGE VERSUS TWO-STAGE TECHNIQUE

There have been multiple reports and articles concerning the advantages and disadvantages of performing the basilic vein operation for dialysis access. This includes the presence of a long upper arm incision, which can be fraught with complications such as wound breakdown and infection, poor maturation and often-lengthy times to cannulation due to creation of edema from the transposition portion of the procedure. There have been numerous articles demonstrating the advantages or disadvantages of this procedure over using prosthetic grafts. However, concurrence in the literature demonstrates a lower incidence of infection and the need for fewer interventions over its superiority to prosthetic grafts for access. A disadvantage noted in the literature is its higher rate of nonmaturation, running up to 38% in the literature.

There may be several reasons for this high nonmaturation rate. The major reason could be technical as a smaller, friable vein may be more difficult to handle and thereby resulting in torque of the vessel. This torque can result in stenosis and early graft failure and could be the result of such a high rate of fistula nonmaturation. Another reason, described by Anaya-Ayala et al.[2] could be related to anatomical variation of the basilic vein. They describe three variations of the anatomy of the basilic vein. Only 66% of all patients have "normal" anatomy, which is described as the basilic vein entering one of two paired brachial veins close to the axilla. 17% of patients have a type 2 anatomy which describes the basilica vein entering one of the paired brachial veins low in the arm. The last type, three, was seen in 17% of patients where the basilic vein enters a single brachial vein low in the arm. This last type of anatomy could have a confounding influence on fistula maturation and complications including venous hypertension. Their findings suggest that 34% of all patients have abnormal anatomy of the basilic vein and this reason alone could account for the reason for a high nonmaturation rate of this fistula.

The basilic vein fistula can be formed in either a one-stage or a two-stage method. The theoretical concept of a two-stage procedure was to allow for the basilic vein to mature and with a larger vein, the hopes would be that this could reduce technical complications and result in improved outcomes. The one-stage method offers benefits of one procedure and can result in a shorter duration for access cannulation. Also patients are more satisfied with one procedure rather than with two procedures. As stated, the advantage of the two-stage, theoretically, is technical with the ease of mobilizing a larger, thicker and arterialized vein. To date, however, there is no clear-cut report demonstrating the superiority of one method over the other. The purpose of this report is to summarize present data on the comparison of one-stage vs. two-stage basilic vein transposition

Agarwal et al.[3] reported a retrospective study of 144 patients at one center. Forty-two percent had a one-stage procedure, and 58% had a two-stage procedure. There was no direct reason why one group underwent one-stage vs. two-stage except for surgeon preference. Results demonstrated that 90% of one-stage procedures matured compared to 75% of two-stage ($P = 0.92$). Mean time to initiation of cannulation was similar in the two groups, 142 days for one-stage and 146 days for two-stage. Secondary patency rates were similar between the two groups ($P = 0.12$) (Table 17-1) Their conclusion from this report demonstrated that basilic vein transposition in two stages confers only a modest reduction in maturation rates and secondary patency and should only be used considered if a prosthetic conduit is being considered due to a small basilic vein.

Kakkos et al.[4] reported on a retrospective study of 173 patients, 76 patients receiving a one-stage and 98 patients receiving a two-stage procedure. Failure to mature was equivalent in groups, 15% for one-stage and 18% for two-stage. Time to fistula access was decreased for the one-stage at 68 days vs. 132 days for the two-stage ($P < 0.001$). However, there was a significantly lower complication rate for the two-stage procedure including reduction in wound hematomas, venous hypertension when compared to the one stage procedure ($P < 0.001$). This study demonstrated that a two-stage procedure produced a functioning access with less morbidity but at a cost of longer time to cannulation.

In a more recent study, Kakkos[5] reported on a randomized, prospective controlled trial comparing primary and staged basilic vein transposition. In this study, 16 patients

TABLE 17-1. STUDIES COMPARING PATENCY OF A ONE-STAGE VERSUS A TWO-STAGE PROCEDURE FOR FORMING A BASILICA VEIN FISTULA

Agarwal	1 year: Secondary patency	2 year	3 year	4 year	
One stage	86%	75%	69%	57%	
Two stage	76%	71%	49%	25%	
Vrakas	1 year: assisted primary patency	2 year: assisted primary patency	1 year secondary patency	2 year: Secondary patency	
One Stage	77%	57%	79%	57%	
Two Stage	95% $P = 0.017$	77% $P = 0.026$	95% $P = 0.026$	77% $P = 0.026$	
Syed	1 year primary patency	2 year primary patency	3 year primary patency	1 year secondary patency	2 year secondary patency
One stage	82%	81%	51%	91%	80%
Two Stage	67%	27%	18%	81%	61%
Reynolds	Primary Functional Patency—1 year	Primary Functional patency—2 years	Secondary functional patency—1 year	Secondary functional patency—2 years	
One stage	61% p = .047	34%	80% p = .015	41%	
Two Stage	88%	88%	94%	94%	

who had basilic veins greater than 2.5 mm were randomized with primary placement of the fistula ($N = 9$) and staged ($N = 7$). This small study was concluded early due to the significant maturation difference between the two groups. The primary procedure had a maturation rate of 33% (3/9) while the staged procedures had a maturation rate of 100% (7/7, $P = .011$, Fisher's exact test). Their conclusion noted higher maturation rates with staged procedures and this reflected in improved secondary patency rates due to a higher number of patients that matured.

Vrakas et al.[6] in 2013 reported on a retrospective study looking at 149 patients. Again these patients were not randomized and underwent their procedure due to surgeon preference. Sixty-five patients underwent a one-stage procedure, and 84 patients underwent a two- stage procedure. Primary failure was similar in both groups. Results are in Table 17-1.

They did not see any difference in complication rates between the two procedures. Their conclusion from this study demonstrated improved functional patency rates with a two-stage procedure over a one-stage both at the one-year and two-year time frames.

Syed et al.[7] reported a retrospective review of 106 patients: 29 patients who underwent a one-stage procedure, and 77 patients who underwent a two-stage procedure. Primary failure was found to be similar in both groups. Primary patency and secondary patency rates are demonstrated in Table 17-1. Their conclusion was that the one-stage procedures provided better patency rates but at the primary and secondary rates for all years.

Reynolds et al.[8] in 2011 presented 90 patients in a retrospective review of basilic vein transpositions. Sixty patients underwent the one-stage procedure, whereas 30 patients underwent the two-stage procedure. The primary procedure was performed by different surgeons than the two-stage procedure. Also, the second part of the two- stage procedure was more of an elevation rather than a transposition. They demonstrated no difference in early failures between the two groups. However, primary patency and secondary patency as well as functional patency were improved with the two-stage procedure (Table 17-1).

Lastly, Glickman et al.[9] presented their data for a comparison of one-stage vs. two-stage procedures for basilic vein transposition. This again was a retrospective study of 316 patients, 270 patients who underwent one-stage and 46 patients who underwent a two-stage procedure. The one-stage group had an 83% maturation rate and the two-stage group had an 89% maturation rate. The one-stage group had a 7.4% complication rate and the two-stage had a 2.27% complication rate ($P = 0.075$). One year primary patency rate for one-stage was 33% and two-stage was 45% ($P = 0.01$). Secondary patency rates at one year was 63.9% for one-stage and 73.9% for two-stage ($P = 0.26$): 0.98 procedures per year were required to maintain patency in one-stage patients, whereas 0.63 procedures per year were required to maintain patency in two-stage patients ($P = 0.08$). They concluded from this study, that a two-stage procedure provided statistically improved primary patency and trended in improvement in secondary patency, reduced interventions to maintain patency and fewer complications post operatively.

ELEVATION AND NEW FRONTIERS

Dagher1 described the basilic vein techniques with one long incision and the vein being rerouted laterally through a subdermal tunnel. Another method that is used to utilize the basilic vein is an elevation method, where after the anastomosis is performed, the vein is elevated within the incision by closing the subcutaneous fascia beneath the skin and over the vein. Another potential method for elevation is also to perform a lipectomy in the same area of the vein.

Korkut et al.[10] reported a series of 350 cases over a 4-year period that used the elevation technique. Mean time to first puncture was 52 days. They describe a primary patency rate of 92%, 78%, 64%, and 54% at 1, 2, 3, and 4 years, respectively. Secondary patency rates were 93%, 81%, 66% and 56% at 1, 2, 3, 4 years. This technique suggests that reducing the angle of the basilic vein/axillary area can reduce intimal hyperplasia.

Effat et al.[11] performed a randomized prospective study comparing the elevation technique with standard basilic vein transposition. The study was performed from October 2010 to December 2011. One hundred and four patients were randomized within this study. Although there was no statistical difference in patency rates, the patients who underwent elevation technique had improved primary and secondary patency rates at 1 and 2 years over the standard transposition technique. The elevation technique did require a slightly longer time to cannulation than the standard operation.

A new device approved by the FDA, the Venous Window Guide or V wing, may offer another alternative to the transposed portion of the basilic vein procedure or elevation technique. This device is composed of a single piece of titanium allowing for repeated access of the AVF through a single puncture site, similar to a buttonhole technique. This device would be implanted and sewn to the mature basilic vein and placed subcutaneously in the vein's natural bed. Although this device was not used in this fashion in the majority of the original trial, several cases in the trial were used in this fashion.[12] Using this device would allow the vein to lie in its natural bed, reduce any torque and allow earlier use of the basilic vein for cannulation.

The NEAT clinical study in Canada is providing exciting potential for use in basilic vein access creation. The trial utilizes the EVERLINQ catheters and system to create a percutaneous fistula in the forearm region. Small bursts of radiofrequency energy are used to connect the artery to the vein to create a small fistula in the forearm area. This creation may allow for a "percutaneous "first stage and create a large basilic vein for either an elevation, transposition or V wing procedure. Although the data is not complete as of this writing, the potential seems significant to the author.

CONCLUSION

Defined data on whether to perform a one-stage over a two-stage procedure is not apparent, although Kakkos' small but significant prospective data adds some clarity to the debate. Technical advantages of a two-stage procedure are apparent to the surgeon, using a larger thicker vein can create a better conduit to perform and create the functional fistula. Patient satisfaction needs to be considered as well as many ESRD patients get "surgical fatigue" and often do not show up for the second procedure or delay it significantly. The new endovascular approach to fistula creation may result in not only creating improved patient satisfaction but also improve both long-term and short-term results.

REFERENCES

1. Dagher F, Gelber R, Ramose E, Sadler J. The use of the basilic vein and brachial artery as an A-V fistula for long term hemodialysis. *J Surg Res.* 1976;20:373–6.
2. Anaya-Ayala JE, Younes HK, Kaiser CL, et al. Prevalence of variant brachial-basilic vein anatomy and implications for vascular access planning. *J Vasc Surg.* 2011;53:3,720–3.
3. Agarwal A, Mantell M, Cohen R. Outcomes of single-stage compared to two-stage basilic vein transposition fistulae. *Semin Dial.* 2014;27(3):298–302. doi:10.1111/sdi.12170, 2013.
4. Kakkos S, Haddad GK, Weaver RK. Basilic vein transposition: What is the optimal technique? *Eur J Vasc Endovasc Surg.* 2010;39(5):612–9.
5. Kakkos S, Tsolakis I, Papadoulas S, et al. Randomized controlled trial comparing primary and staged basilic vein transposition. *Front Surg.* 2015; 2:14. doi: 10.3389/fsurg.2015.00014
6. Vrakas G, Defigueiredo F, Turner S. A comparison of the outcomes of the one-stage and two-stage brachiobasilic arteriovenous fistula. *J Vasc Surg.* 2013;58:5: 1300–4.
7. Syed F, Smolock C, Duan C. Comparison of outcomes of one-stage basilic vein transpositions and two-stage basilic vein transposition. *Ann Vasc Surg.* 2012; 26(6):852–7.
8. Reynolds T, Zayed M, Kim K, et al. A comparison between one-and two-stage brachiobasilic arteriovenous fistulas. *J Vasc Surg.* 2011;53(6):1632–9.
9. Chen B, Glickman M. Basilic vein transposition. *VASA* 2010, Las Vegas.
10. Korkut AK, Kosem M. Superficialization of the basilica vein technique in brachiobasilic arteriovenous fistula: Surgical experience with 350 cases during 4 years. *Ann Vasc Surg.* 2010;24(6):762–7.
11. Effat M. Staging of brachiobasilic arteriovenous fistulae, Does it worth Effort? VSE9–EVC9, May 29– June 1, 2013, Hurghada Egypt.
12. Hill AA, Vasudeven T, Young NP, et al. Use of an implantable needle guide to access difficult or impossible to cannulate arteriovenous fistulae using the buttonhole technique. *JVA.* 2013;14(2):164–9.

18

Dialysis Vascular Access and Transvenous Cardiac Devices

Haimanot Wasse, MD, MPH and Dirk Hentschel, MD

Cardiac implantable electronic devices (CIED) are implanted for the treatment of cardiac rhythm disturbances and include pacemakers (PMs) and implantable cardioverter-defibrillators (ICDs). Their placement in U.S. chronic kidney disease (CKD) and end-stage renal disease (ESRD) patients has increased over time, and it is estimated that 10% of U.S. hemodialysis patients have a CIED.[1]

CKD and ESRD patients commonly experience cardiac rhythm disorders in which a pacemaker is indicated. Further, while an ICD significantly improves survival in CKD and ESRD patients with underlying ischemic heart disease, cardiomyopathy and congestive heart failure who experience ventricular tachycardia or fibrillation (secondary prevention), the survival benefit is not as significant as that attributed to ICD placement in the general population.[2] Specifically, a meta-analysis found a nearly three-fold higher mortality in ESRD patients with ICD than non-ESRD patient with ICD.[3] ICD placement for primary prevention shows survival benefit in patients with CKD-3a and b; however, overall mortality in CKD-4 patients is such that no survival benefit after ICD placement is observed.[4] This may reflect higher mortality of the device placement procedure and subsequent clinical events such as infection or device exchange and competing mortality from comorbid conditions. Alternatively, benefits of ICD placement may be attenuated by noncardiovertable rhythms such as bradycardia and asystole.

CIED AND CENTRAL VENOUS STENOSIS

CIED-related central venous stenosis can occur in non-ESRD and ESRD patients, and stenosis can develop from the venotomy site to any portion of the vessel wall that is in contact with the CIED leads and extend to the superior vena cava.[5] Among a series of non-ESRD patients evaluated six months following transvenous pacemaker placement,

64% were noted to have developed central venous stenosis, however only 2.6% were clinically symptomatic.[6] The presence of an ipsilateral upper extremity arteriovenous access, however, can significantly increase venous return by adding 1000–2000 mL/min mean blood flow, unmasking clinically significant stenosis with venous hypertension manifesting as arm swelling and development of collateral veins. While arm swelling is not universal after ipsilateral CIED and dialysis access placement, the majority of published case studies and case series report the onset of complications due to venous hypertension within 6 months of concurrent access and device presence.

CIED AND VASCULAR ACCESS PATENCY

Reports from limited case series have examined whether the presence of a CIED influences arteriovenous (AV) access patency. In one report, the outcomes of AV access creation were compared between patients with ipsilateral (n = 19) versus contralateral (N = 17) CIED placement.[7] Patients with ipsilateral CIED placement experienced a primary AV access failure rate of 78.9% versus 35.3% in patients with contralateral placement (P = 0.02).[7]

CENTRAL VEIN STENOSIS AFTER CIED LEAD PLACEMENT

Implantation of cardiac devices is associated with stenosis and occlusion of the central veins, ranging from between 3.6 and 33% for occlusion and between 10 and 65% for stenosis.[8–10] In 7–14% of patients, there are pre-existing stenoses of the central veins.[8,9] It is unclear if this is due to cannulation of the veins at a prior point in time or truly a natural occurrence. Lead entry through the subclavian or cutdown to the cephalic vein does not appear to make a difference,[9,11–14] neither does left versus right-sided insertion.[13,14] However, clinical symptoms occur only in a minority of patients with documented central venous stenosis (1-5%). Symptomatic cases can be treated with angioplasty and stent placement,[15–23] but long-term success is not well documented. In the largest retrospective study, 50% of stenoses had recurred after 26 months.[15] While these reports describe placement of stents across the central venous stenosis with CRMD leads in place, more recently lead extraction prior to angioplasty and stent placement with subsequent insertion of new CRMD leads has been performed.[24,25] Recent expert consensus guidelines of the Heart Rhythm society recommend lead extraction prior to stent placement to avoid lead entrapment complications and future lead extractions.[26] There is concern that bacteremia is more common in dialysis patients necessitating lead removal more frequently, such that lead entrapment would pose a great difficulty. The only available retrospective study addressing the question of increased complication rates for CRMDs in ESRD patients documents a higher rate of device related complications such as lead dislodgement and elevated defibrillator thresholds, hematoma formation at the insertion site, and a non-significant trend to higher incidence of pocket infections[27]; in total, major complications were reported in 29% of dialysis patients compared to 5% in non-ESRD patients. On the other hand, presence of renal failure (OR = 1.76) and older age (OR = 1.63 per 20 years) are risk factors for in-hospital mortality in patients admitted with CRMD infections.[28]

Available data on central vein stenosis in dialysis patients with autogenous AV or prosthetic accesses and ipsilateral cardiac device leads is limited. One retrospective center analysis of 495 transvenous pacemaker insertions identified 14 patients with ipsilateral dialysis accesses.[29] Ten of these 14 patients (71%) had clinical symptoms; eight of these had a total occlusion of the subclavian vein and required ligation of the dialysis access. The four asymptomatic patients died from unrelated causes within 6 months after implantation of the cardiac device. Tourret and colleagues report a case of symptomatic subclavian vein stenosis immediately after creation of an autogenous AV access 21 months after an ipsilateral pacemaker was inserted.[30] In this case, the access had to be ligated to control symptoms. Ten other cases from the literature are reviewed in this report, with time of symptoms after AVF creation ranging from immediately to two years. In total of six AVFs were abandoned due to symptoms,[31–34] three underwent angioplasty, but eventually had to be ligated,[35] and one underwent angioplasty and placement of a stent and remained patent 8 months after the intervention.[36] Ultimately, ipsilateral dialysis accesses and CRMDs should be avoided.

CIED-INSERTION SITES: IMPLICATIONS AND OUTCOMES

1) Subclavian Vein

Since the 1980s, it has been known that subclavian vein catheters are associated with subclavian vein stenosis and thrombosis.[37] Schillinger established that three weeks after removal of a Shaldon hemodialysis catheter, stenoses were present in 42% of patients who had a subclavian vein catheter, but only in 10% who had internal jugular vein catheters.[38] A report on the natural history of subclavian vein stenoses in dialysis patients finds a stenosis in just over 50% of patients at the time of removal of subclavian vein catheters. Some of these stenoses improve, but after 3–6 months, 28% of subclavian veins had stenosis severity of greater than 30%.[39] Insertion of tunneled hemodialysis catheters into the subclavian veins should be considered a measure of last resort as ipsilateral long-term access options can be severely jeopardized.

We recommend avoiding insertion of CIEDs leads via subclavian veins ipsilateral to an existing or planned hemodialysis access. Contralateral insertion may be acceptable if life expectancy of the patient in question is limited. However, in young and middle-aged patients, alternative CIED lead insertion sites should be explored.

2) Cephalic Vein

The cephalic vein has been used for CIED lead insertion for many decades. It is typically ligated distally, thereby complicating ipsilateral forearm accesses and excluding an upper arm autologous brachial-cephalic access. When evaluated, the incidence of central venous stenosis is not different for cephalic vein versus subclavian vein insertion. Ipsilateral cephalic vein insertion of CIED leads to an existing or planned hemodialysis access is contraindicated. Contralateral insertion requires careful weighing of life expectancy and need for new vascular access.

3) Femoral Vein

Traditional indications for CIED lead placement using a femoral approach include use in children, occluded thoracic central veins, anomalies in the central thoracic veins, and the presence of a very thin anterior chest wall such that it cannot accommodate a device pocket.[40,41] The femoral route has also been demonstrated as successful in children where endovascular lead placement is often not possible due to small subclavian vein size.[42] Advantages of the femoral approach as compared to an open thoracic approach for epicardial lead placement are lower morbidity from anesthesia and surgery, as well as cost. Weinstein et al. reported on 100 consecutive cases of temporary pacing via the femoral route and found minimal complications.[43] The largest series of permanent femoral pacing systems in adults was published by Ellestad and French.[44] They described the ease of 95 pacemaker implantations via the femoral/iliac route. Atrial lead displacement was the major complication occurring in 21%. Mathur et al reported the next largest series in 27 adult patients.[41] No thromboses or lead fractures were observed but atrial lead displacement occurred in 20% in this series. The authors reported that during the last 4 years of the study, no atrial lead displacements occurred and this was attributed to increased operator experience. Two pacemaker pocket pre-erosions required the pulse generators to be repositioned. A more recent study by Garcia Guerrero et al described their experience with the transfemoral approach for 12 permanent pacemaker systems.[45] Their lead displacement rate was 0%. Furthermore, they described a modification of previous techniques in which the pocket is in the anterior thigh rather than the lower abdomen.

Clinical success with the transfemoral route appears to be supported in the literature in-spite of limited numbers. The reported disadvantages of femoral lead placement include a slightly higher risk of lead detachment and thromboembolism. Rates of such complications in earlier reports of the femoral approach have seemingly abated with more modern active fixation leads, lower device pocket location (thigh and pelvis versus abdominal), and increasing operator experience. While the ability to measure such risks is skewed given that the two largest series of the femoral approach in adults are 95 and 27 patients, we feel that known risks do not outweigh the benefits of preserving the central venous circuit of CKD patients. Therefore, we recommend adding the CKD/dialysis patient to the list of indications for this approach based on the current literature.

4) Internal Jugular Veins

The internal and external jugular veins are established as insertion sites of choice for tunneled hemodialysis catheters (KDOQI Vascular Access Guidelines 2006).[46] The catheter is tunneled in a gentle curve to avoid kinking as the catheter traverses the clavicle. Transvenous pacing using the internal jugular vein was described first with ligation of the vein,[47] and then without.[48] Brodman and Furman reported on 90 patients, 5% of the total population, in whom cephalic and external jugular vein lead insertion was not possible.[49] The internal jugular vein was ligated, in apparent follow-up, and for up to 7 years they did not report out-of-the-ordinary complications. Lead fracture rates of cephalic, external and internal jugular veins in 2226 patients with a total of 2563 leads (total of 100 lead fractures) were reported by Alt et al in 1987.[50] While fracture rates were higher for internal jugular vein insertion than for cephalic or external jugular vein, these particular rates are not annualized, nor are they differentiated by type of lead. The study spans the years 1965 to 1980, and includes three different types of lead wire (Elema, singlefilar and multifilar coil), with different length of follow-up. Since this report, there has not been a large study including the internal jugular vein as lead insertion sites.

5) Epicardial Leads

Given the risk of development of central venous stenosis from transvenous CIED lead insertion, it is useful to consider alternate routes when indicated. The central veins can be avoided completely with surgical placement of an epicardial left ventricular lead CIED, as the leads traverse through the subcutaneous tissue. Data among pediatric populations show similar complication and survival rates between endocardial versus epicardial lead placement.[51–53] Recent data from a large series of 216 adult non-ESRD patients undergoing epicardial lead CIED placement with 5-year follow-up demonstrated a decrease in epicardial LV pacing threshold during the initial 6 months following implantation, that then stabilized, and a cumulative incidence of device infection of 9.6% compared with 3%–4% reported in patients with transvenous leads.[54] The authors attribute this to a more complicated patient population that previously underwent device replacements and upgrades, risk factors for infection. De novo epicardial lead CIEDs had an infection rate of 1.6 per 100 CIED-years versus 4.7 per 100 CIED-years among patients receiving a replacement device.

Overall, epicardial systems could be considered an alternate option for patients with advanced CKD or ESRD, particularly those with limited venous access options, but require surgical expertise as placement requires a thoractomy.

6) Subcutaneous Devices

Subcutaneous ICDs have a single lead for sensing and defibrillation and are tunneled subcutaneously without the need for imaging at the time of implantation, offering an advantage over surgically placed epicardial leads that require a cardiothoracic surgeon. They are primarily used in young patients to treat ventricular fibrillation and avoid transvenous lead placement, but lack pacing capability and are not indicated for ventricular tachycardia.[55] Although long-term subcutaneous lead survival has not yet been documented, no primary lead failures have been reported to date.[55] When compared with transvenous CIEDs, subcutaneous ICDs offer several advantages, including relative ease of extraction. To date, data is limited in the ESRD patient population, however, a series of 27 dialysis patients demonstrates that subcutaneous ICDs can be successfully placed in long-term dialysis patients with an AV access, are not associated with excess risk of implant related complications or inappropriate shocks,[56] and offer the advantage of minimization of the risk of central venous stenosis and the potential for reduced risk of infection.

MANAGEMENT OF CIED–ASSOCIATED CENTRAL VENOUS STENOSIS

Percutaneous balloon angioplasty (PTA) without stent placement is considered the standard treatment for symptomatic central vein stenosis with reported primary patency rates of up to 50% and secondary patency up to 86% at 12 months.[57] The concern with repeated PTA is long-term CIED lead stability, yet to date, there is no evidence that PTA has a negative impact on lead function.[57] In the setting of failed PTA, reports describe use of stent insertion,[58] however because this results in CIED lead entrapment, significant difficulty in patient management can arise when the leads require removal, such as in the case of sepsis or endocarditis. In accordance, the Heart Rhythm Society expert consensus on transvenous lead extraction recommends CIED lead removal prior to stent deployment at sites of CIED-lead associated stenosis.[26]

CIED AND CKD PATIENT PROGRESSING TOWARDS ESRD

In planning for hemodialysis access in the late-stage CKD patient, the primary goal is preventing central venous stenosis. To this end, the American Society of Diagnostic and Interventional Nephrology published recommendations in 2012 related to CIED placement in CKD and ESRD patients, partly summarized in Figure 18-1.[57] For patients preparing to initiate dialysis in whom a CIED is recommended, it is suggested that the cardiologist, nephrologist, and primary physician review the risks and benefits of CIED therapy, anticipated vascular access requirements, dialysis modality and prognosis. From there, thorough vessel mapping is warranted via Doppler ultrasound or venography in advance of CIED placement, and CIED leads should be placed contralateral to the side of anticipated dialysis access. Among patients with an existing CIED, new AV access should be placed contralateral to the CIED. It is recommended that epicardial leads be considered in patients requiring a new CIED, or CIED lead replacement in order to avoid central venous stenosis.

In the setting of CIED-related central stenosis, PTA without stent placement is the preferred treatment and stent-entrapment of CIED leads should be avoided. Given the high risk of catheter-related blood stream infection, concurrent CIED and central venous catheter use should be avoided. Finally, it is recommended that wearable cardioverter defibrillators should be considered for patients at risk of sudden cardiac death, particularly in the setting of an infection preventing immediate CIED placement or in those transitioning from central venous catheter to use of an arteriovenous access.

CIED-RELATED INFECTION IN END-STAGE RENAL DISEASE PATIENTS

The severity of renal dysfunction is associated with an increased risk of CIED infection.[59] The number of ESRD patients hospitalized for CIED-related infection has increased over the past decade and is most recently estimated at 300.3 versus 6.1 hospitalizations per 100,000 persons compared with nondialysis groups, respectively.[60] Moreover, ESRD patients experience twofold greater in-hospital mortality following CIED infection-related hospitalization.[60]

Surgical Management of CIED-Related Infection

In a recent retrospective analysis of patients admitted to Mayo Clinic between 1991-2008, 415 patients were identified as having CIED infection, defined as the presence of presence of a pocket infection or bacteremia.[61] Of the 415 patients, 17 (4%) were hemodialysis patients; of these, 53% had a concurrent tunneled dialysis catheter in place. All HD patients presented with positive blood cultures, while pocket infections were more likely in non-HD patients. Further, HD patients were more likely to be diagnosed with CIED-infective endocarditis compared to those in the non-HD group (41% vs. 21%, respectively). The two leading pathogens were coagulase-negative staphlococci (29%) and methicillin-resistant staphylococcus aureus (29%).

The primary surgical approach to CIED infection in the HD patients was CIED removal (82%) and the success of device removal was similar between HD and

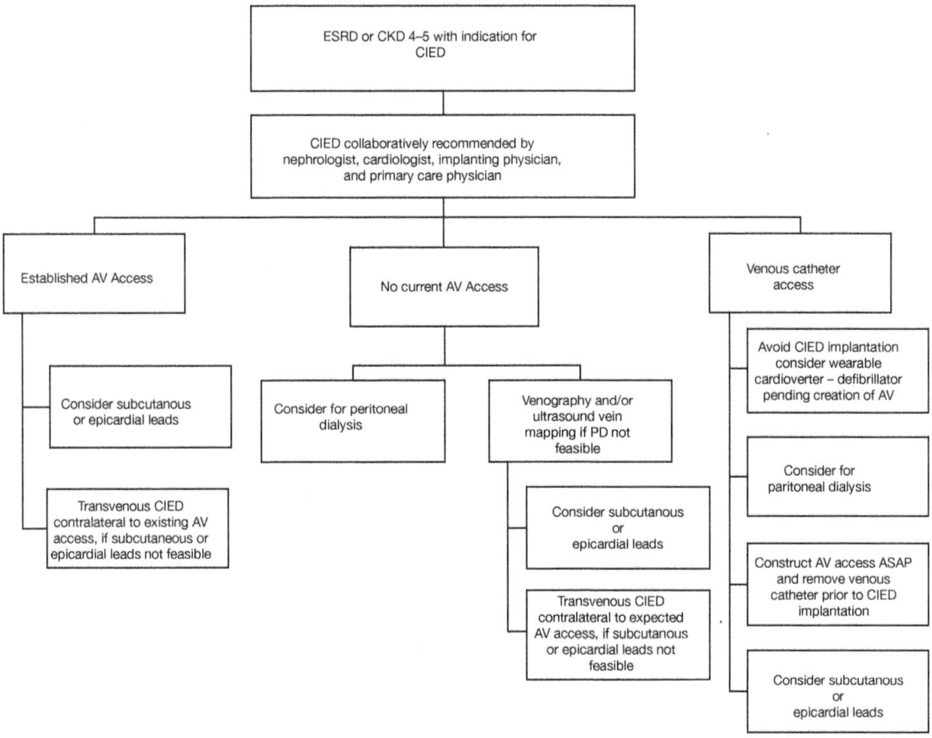

Figure 18-1. CIED Implantation in CKD stage 4–5 and ESRD patients. Modified from Figure 4 in Saad TF, Hentschel DM, Koplan B, et al.[57]

non-HD patients. By day 90 following diagnosis, 76% of HD patients survived vs. 92% non-HD patients, and by study end (average 2.2-year follow-up), 59% of HD patients died vs. 32% of non-HD patients, suggesting that mortality remains elevated in HD patients despite CIED-device removal.

CONCLUSIONS

CIED-associated central venous stenosis is best prevented through the careful selection of sites for transvenous CIED leads and ipsilateral placement to an existing or future AV access. This is best accomplished through close communication between the patient, nephrologist, cardiologist, interventionalist and access surgeon. CIED-related central stenosis may be avoided through surgical placement of subcutaneous or epicardial leads.

REFERENCES

1. Charytan DM, Patrick AR, Liu J, et al. Trends in the use and outcomes of implantable cardioverter-defibrillators in patients undergoing dialysis in the United States. *Am J Kidney Dis. The official journal of the National Kidney Foundation.* Sep 2011;58(3):409–17.

2. Herzog CA, Li S, Weinhandl ED, Strief JW, Collins AJ, Gilbertson DT. Survival of dialysis patients after cardiac arrest and the impact of implantable cardioverter defibrillators. *Kidney Int.* Aug 2005;68(2):818–25.
3. Sakhuja R, Keebler M, Lai TS, et al. Meta-analysis of mortality in dialysis patients with an implantable cardioverter defibrillator. *Am J Cardiol.* Mar 1 2009;103(5):735–41.
4. Nakhoul GN, Schold JD, Arrigain S, et al. Implantable cardioverter-defibrillators in patients with CKD: A propensity-matched mortality analysis. *Clinical journal of the American Society of Nephrology : CJASN.* Jul 7 2015;10(7):1119–27.
5. Asif A, Carrillo R, Garisto JD, et al. Epicardial cardiac rhythm devices for dialysis patients: Minimizing the risk of infection and preserving central veins. *Semin Dial.* Jan-Feb 2012;25(1):88–94.
6. da Costa SSD, Neto AS, Costa R, Caldas JG, Martinelli M. Incidence and risk factors of upper extremity deep vein lesions after permanent transvenous pacemaker implant: A 6-month follow-up prospective study. *Pace.* Sep 2002;25(9):1301–6.
7. Tan CS, Jie C, Joe J, et al. The impact of transvenous cardiac devices on vascular access patency in hemodialysis patients. *Semin Dial.* Nov-Dec 2013;26(6):728–32.
8. Oginosawa Y, Abe H, Nakashima Y. The incidence and risk factors for venous obstruction after implantation of transvenous pacing leads. *Pacing Clin Electrophysiol.* Nov 2002;25(11):1605–11.
9. Korkeila P, Nyman K, Ylitalo A, et al. Venous obstruction after pacemaker implantation. *Pacing Clin Electrophysiol.* Feb 2007;30(2):199–206.
10. Goto Y, Abe T, Sekine S, Sakurada T. Long-term thrombosis after transvenous permanent pacemaker implantation. *Pacing Clin Electrophysiol.* Jun 1998;21(6):1192–5.
11. Lickfett L, Bitzen A, Arepally A, et al. Incidence of venous obstruction following insertion of an implantable cardioverter defibrillator. A study of systematic contrast venography on patients presenting for their first elective ICD generator replacement. *Europace.* Jan 2004;6(1):25–31.
12. Sticherling C, Chough SP, Baker RL, et al. Prevalence of central venous occlusion in patients with chronic defibrillator leads. *Am Heart J.* May 2001;141(5):813–6.
13. Zuber M, Huber P, Fricker U, Buser P, Jager K. Assessment of the subclavian vein in patients with transvenous pacemaker leads. *Pacing Clin Electrophysiol.* Dec 1998;21(12):2621–30.
14. Haghjoo M, Nikoo MH, Fazelifar AF, Alizadeh A, Emkanjoo Z, Sadr-Ameli MA. Predictors of venous obstruction following pacemaker or implantable cardioverter-defibrillator implantation: A contrast venographic study on 100 patients admitted for generator change, lead revision, or device upgrade. *Europace.* May 2007;9(5):328–32.
15. Kalman PG, Lindsay TF, Clarke K, Sniderman KW, Vanderburgh L. Management of upper extremity central venous obstruction using interventional radiology. *Ann Vasc Surg.* May 1998;12(3):202–6.
16. Qanadli SD, El Hajjam M, Mignon F, et al. Subacute and chronic benign superior vena cava obstructions: Endovascular treatment with self-expanding metallic stents. *AJR Am J Roentgenol.* Jul 1999;173(1):159–64.
17. Slonim SM, Semba CP, Sze DY, Dake MD. Placement of SVC stents over pacemaker wires for the treatment of SVC syndrome. *J Vasc Interv Radiol.* Feb 2000;11(2 Pt 1):215-s9.
18. Grace AA, Sutters M, Schofield PM. Balloon dilatation of pacemaker induced stenosis of the superior vena cava. *Br Heart J.* Apr 1991;65(4):225–6.
19. Teo N, Sabharwal T, Rowland E, Curry P, Adam A. Treatment of superior vena cava obstruction secondary to pacemaker wires with balloon venoplasty and insertion of metallic stents. *Eur Heart J.* Sep 2002;23(18):1465–70.
20. Gilard M, Perennes A, Mansourati J, et al. Stent implantation for the treatment of superior vena cava syndrome related to pacemaker leads. *Europace.* Apr 2002;4(2):155–8.
21. Lanciego C, Rodriguez M, Rodriguez A, Carbonell MA, Garcia LG. Permanent pacemaker-induced superior vena cava syndrome: successful treatment by endovascular stent. *Cardiovasc Intervent Radiol.* Nov-Dec 2003;26(6):576–9.

22. Park HW, Kim W, Cho JG, Kang JC. Multiple pacing lead-induced superior vena cava syndrome: Successful treatment by balloon angioplasty. *J Cardiovasc Electrophysiol.* Feb 2005;16(2):221–3.
23. Lam YY, Chan JY. An unusual case of non-malignant superior vena cava obstruction. *Hong Kong Med J.* Jun 2006;12(3):232–4.
24. Chan AW, Bhatt DL, Wilkoff BL, et al. Percutaneous treatment for pacemaker-associated superior vena cava syndrome. *Pacing Clin Electrophysiol.* Nov 2002;25(11):1628–33.
25. Bolad I, Karanam S, Mathew D, John R, Piemonte T, Martin D. Percutaneous treatment of superior vena cava obstruction following transvenous device implantation. *Catheter Cardiovasc Interv.* May 2005;65(1):54–9.
26. Wilkoff BL, Love CJ, Byrd CL, et al. Transvenous lead extraction: Heart Rhythm Society expert consensus on facilities, training, indications, and patient management: This document was endorsed by the American Heart Association (AHA). *Heart Rhythm.* Jul 2009;6(7):1085–104.
27. Dasgupta A, Montalvo J, Medendorp S, et al. Increased complication rates of cardiac rhythm management devices in ESRD patients. *Am J Kid Dis.* 2007;49(5):656–63.
28. Voigt A, Shalaby A, Saba S. Rising rates of cardiac rhythm management device infections in the United States: 1996 through 2003. *J Am Coll Cardiol.* Aug 1 2006;48(3):590–1.
29. Teruya TH, Abou-Zamzam AM, Jr., Limm W, Wong L. Symptomatic subclavian vein stenosis and occlusion in hemodialysis patients with transvenous pacemakers. *Ann Vasc Surg.* Sep 2003;17(5):526–9.
30. Tourret J, Cluzel P, Tostivint I, Barrou B, Deray G, Bagnis CI. Central venous stenosis as a complication of ipsilateral haemodialysis fistula and pacemaker. *Nephrol Dial Transplant.* May 2005;20(5):997–1001.
31. Stone WJ, Wall MN, Powers TA. Massive upper extremity edema with arteriovenous fistula for hemodialysis. A complication of previous pacemaker insertion. *Nephron.* 1982;31(2):184–6.
32. Korzets A, Chagnac A, Ori Y, Katz M, Zevin D. Subclavian vein stenosis, permanent cardiac pacemakers and the haemodialysed patient. *Nephron.* 1991;58(1):103–5.
33. Deighan CJ, McLaughlin KJ, Simpson K, Jones JM. Unsuspected subclavian vein stenosis resulting from a permanent pacing wire. *Nephrol Dial Transplant.* Nov 1996;11(11):2333–4.
34. Cavatorta F, Campisi S, Zollo A. Subclavian vein stenosis: A potentially serious complication in chronic hemodialysis patients with permanent cardiac pacemakers. *Int J Artif Organs.* Jun 1997;20(6):316–8.
35. Chuang CL, Tarng DC, Yang WC, Huang TP. An occult cause of arteriovenous access failure: Central vein stenosis from permanent pacemaker wire. Report of three cases and review of the literature. *Am J Nephrol.* Sep-Oct 2001;21(5):406–9.
36. Konner K, Vorwerk D. Permanent pacemaker wires causing subclavian vein stenosis in presence of AV fistula—Is it ever wrong to try angioplasty and stenting? *Nephrol Dial Transplant.* Aug 1997;12(8):1735–8.
37. Bozzetti F, Scarpa D, Terno G, et al. Subclavian venous thrombosis due to indwelling catheters: A prospective study on 52 patients. *JPEN. J Parenter Enteral Nutr.* Nov-Dec 1983;7(6):560–2.
38. Schillinger F, Schillinger D, Montagnac R, Milcent T. Post catheterisation vein stenosis in haemodialysis: Comparative angiographic study of 50 subclavian and 50 internal jugular accesses. *Nephrol Dial Transplant.* 1991;6(10):722–4.
39. Hernandez D, Diaz F, Rufino M, et al. Subclavian vascular access stenosis in dialysis patients: Natural history and risk factors. *J Am Soc Nephrol.* Aug 1998;9(8):1507–10.
40. Barakat K, Hill J, Kelly P. Permanent transfemoral pacemaker implantation is the technique of choice for patients in whom the superior vena cava is inaccessible. *Pacing Clin Electrophysiol.* Apr 2000;23(4 Pt 1):446–9.
41. Mathur G, Stables RH, Heaven D, Ingram A, Sutton R. Permanent pacemaker implantation via the femoral vein: An alternative in cases with contraindications to the pectoral approach. *Europace.* Jan 2001;3(1):56–9.

42. Costa R, Filho MM, Tamaki WT, et al. Transfemoral pediatric permanent pacing: Long-term results. *Pacing Clin Electrophysiol.* Jan 2003;26(1 Pt 2):487–91.
43. Weinstein J, Gnoj J, Mazzara JT, Ayres SM, Grace WJ. Temporary transvenous pacing via the percutaneous femoral vein approach. A prospective study of 100 cases. *Am Heart J.* May 1973;85(5):695–705.
44. Ellestad MH, French J. Iliac vein approach to permanent pacemaker implantation. *Pacing Clin Electrophysiol.* Jul 1989;12(7 Pt 1):1030–3.
45. Garcia Guerrero JJ, De La Concha Castaneda JF, Fernandez Mora G, et al. Permanent transfemoral pacemaker: A single-center series performed with an easier and safer surgical technique. *Pacing Clin Electrophysiol.* Jul 2005;28(7):675–9.
46. National Kidney Foundation. KDOQI Clinical Practice Guidelines and Clinical Practice Recommendations for 2006 Updates: Hemodialysis adequacy, peritoneal dialysis adequacy and vascular access. *Am J Kid Dis.* 2006;48: S1–S322.
47. Leininger BJ, Neville WE. Use of the internal jugular vein for implantations of permanent transvenous pacemakers. Experiences with 22 patients. *Ann Thorac Surg.* Jan 1968;5(1):61–5.
48. Rao G, Zikria EA. Technique of insertion of pacing electrode through the internal jugular vein. *J Cardiovasc Surg (Torino).* May-Jun 1973;14(3):294.
49. Brodman R, Furman S. Pacemaker implantation through the internal jugular vein. *Ann Thorac Surg.* Jan 1980;29(1):63–5.
50. Alt E, Volker R, Blomer H. Lead fracture in pacemaker patients. *Thorac Cardiovasc Surg.* Apr 1987;35(2):101–4.
51. Cecchin F, Frangini PA, Brown DW, et al. Cardiac resynchronization therapy (and multisite pacing) in pediatrics and congenital heart disease: Five years experience in a single institution. *J Cardiovasc Electr.* Jan 2009;20(1):58–65.
52. Dodge-Khatami A, Johnsrude CL, Backer CL, et al. A comparison of steroid-eluting epicardial versus transvenous pacing leads in children. *J Card Surg.* Sep-Oct 2000;15(5):323–9.
53. Beaufort-Krol GC, Mulder H, Nagelkerke D, Waterbolk TW, Bink-Boelkens MT. Comparison of longevity, pacing, and sensing characteristics of steroid-eluting epicardial versus conventional endocardial pacing leads in children. *J Thorac Cardiovasc Surg.* Mar 1999;117(3):523–8.
54. Buiten MS, van der Heijden AC, Klautz RJ, Schalij MJ, van Erven L. Epicardial leads in adult cardiac resynchronization therapy recipients: A study on lead performance, durability, and safety. *Heart Rhythm.* Mar 2015;12(3):533–9.
55. Lewis GF, Gold MR. Clinical experience with subcutaneous implantable cardioverter-defibrillators. *Nature Rev Cardiol.* Jul 2015;12(7):398–405.
56. El-Chami MF, Levy M, Kelli HM, et al. Outcome of Subcutaneous Implantable Cardioverter Defibrillator Implantation in Patients with End-Stage Renal Disease on Dialysis. *J Cardiovasc Electrophysiol.* 2015;26(8):900–4.
57. Saad TF, Hentschel DM, Koplan B, et al. Cardiovascular implantable electronic device leads in CKD and ESRD patients: Review and recommendations for practice. *Semin Dial.* Jan-Feb 2013;26(1):114–23.
58. Saad TF, Myers GR, Cicone J. Central vein stenosis or occlusion associated with cardiac rhythm management device leads in hemodialysis patients with ipsilateral arteriovenous access: a retrospective study of treatment using stents or stent-grafts. *J Vasc Access.* 2010 Oct-Dec;11(4):293–302.
59. Tompkins C, McLean R, Cheng A, et al. End-stage renal disease predicts complications in pacemaker and ICD implants. *J Cardiovasc Electrophysiol.* Oct 2011;22(10):1099–104.
60. Opelami O, Sakhuja A, Liu X, et al. Outcomes of infected cardiovascular implantable devices in dialysis patients. *Am J Nephrol.* 2014;40(3):280–7.
61. Hickson LJ, Gooden JY, Le KY, et al. Clinical presentation and outcomes of cardiovascular implantable electronic device infections in hemodialysis patients. *Am J Kid Dis.* Jul 2014;64(1):104–10.

19

Management of Infected AV Grafts

Samir K. Shah, MD and C. Keith Ozaki, MD

In 2010, there were approximately 384,000 patients with end-stage renal disease on hemodialysis in the United States.[1] The prevalence of renal failure and its attendant costs—$23.6 b in Medicare costs in 2010—has led to a focus on renal replacement strategies and outcomes generally in the renal failure population.[1] Hemodialysis stands as the most common renal replacement therapy. Despite the manifold advantages of autogenous reconstructions for hemodialysis access, including improved patency, decreased infection rates, and lower medical costs, arteriovenous grafts (AVGs) remain a common form of hemodialysis access.

INCIDENCE, RISK FACTORS, AND PREVENTION

Of the numerous complications that can affect AVGs perhaps the most important is infection. Indeed, infection affects 3.5 to 17% of prosthetic AVGs and is the second most common cause of access loss.[2–4]

AVG infection is most common in the first year after surgery: Minga[5] reported that 59% of infections occurred within one year of surgery while Ryan[2] reported that 86% were apparent within six months. In the latter report, 75% of infections occurring within a month were located at an incision while 78% of those presenting later than a month occurred in the body of graft, remote from any incisions. These observations prompted the authors to speculate that infections in the immediate postoperative period may reflect contamination at the time of surgery while later infections represent inoculation during graft access.

Factors associated with AVG infection include hypoalbuminemia,[5,6] number of surgical revisions,[7] lower extremity grafts,[3] diabetes,[6] limited ambulatory ability,[8] frequent hospitalization,[8] graft age,[8] patient age,[6] and poor hygiene.[7] Not all of these variables have been consistently associated with infection; for example, Minga has found that diabetes and lower extremity grafts are not associated with infection.[5]

Generic measures employed to prevent perioperative surgical site infections should also be applied to AVG surgery. Examples include maintenance of sterile technique, perioperative antibiotic use, avoiding contact between prosthetic material and skin surfaces, intraoperative normothermia, and optimization of diabetes to avoid hyperglycemia. Special mention should be made of vancomycin prophylaxis, which was shown by Zibari and colleagues in a randomized trial to reduce AVG graft infection compared to no antibiotics.[9] Aseptic technique at dialysis centers is also critical: 47% of AVG infections in one trial occurred in the body of the graft, suggesting infection during access.[2]

BACTERIOLOGY

Gram-positive pathogens are involved in an overwhelming majority of AVG infections. Specifically, *Staphylococcus aureus* is the most common cultured pathogen, accounting for 60% of infections, followed by *Staphylococcus epidermidis* (15%–22%). Gram-negative bacteria cause a minority of infections.[2,5] Intraoperative cultures are not uniformly positive, likely because of the effect of pre-culture antibiotic administration and the difficulty of culturing some organisms such as *Staphylococcus epidermidis*.

DIAGNOSIS

AVG infection most often presents with local signs. In a series of 57 PTFE infections from the Cleveland Clinic, all patients had at least one local sign, most commonly induration, while 28% had no systemic signs whatsoever.[10] In Ryan's series of 51 infected grafts, the most common presentation (occurring in 45%) was exposed graft or a sinus tract (Figure 19-1).[2] Alternative local presentations include purulent drainage, erythema, pseudoaneurysm, and hemorrhage (Figures 19-2 and 19-3). Hemorrhage can be controlled by direct pressure over the inflow and outflow of the conduit. If there is difficulty then a blood pressure cuff is temporarily placed on the affected limb proximal to the graft, and inflated to a pressure greater than the patient's systolic pressure. Patients may additionally present with remote manifestations (e.g. septic emboli, generalized sepsis) with or without local signs.

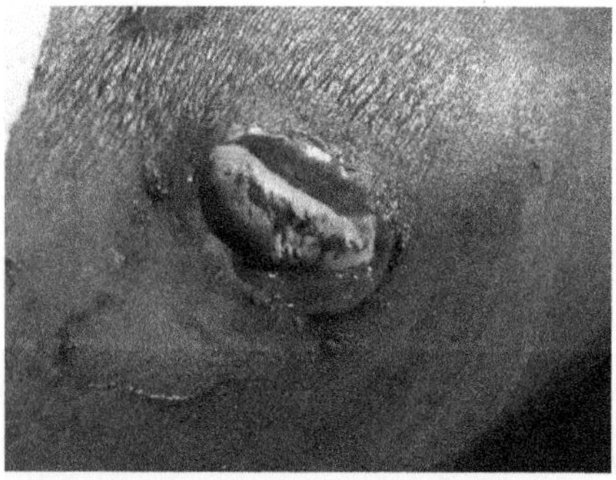

Figure 19-1. Exposed PTFE AVG with evidence of repeated cannulation. Image provided courtesy of Dirk Hentschel, MD.

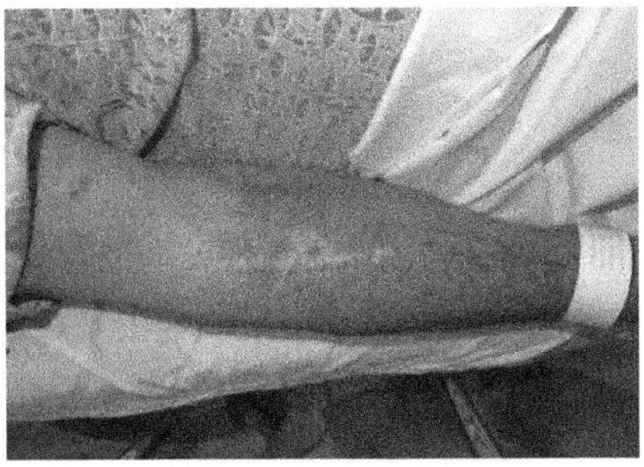

Figure 19-2. Erythema associated with a thrombosed AVG superinfected by repeated cannulation attempts. Extensive perigraft purulence was found during excision. Image provided courtesy of Dirk Hentschel, MD.

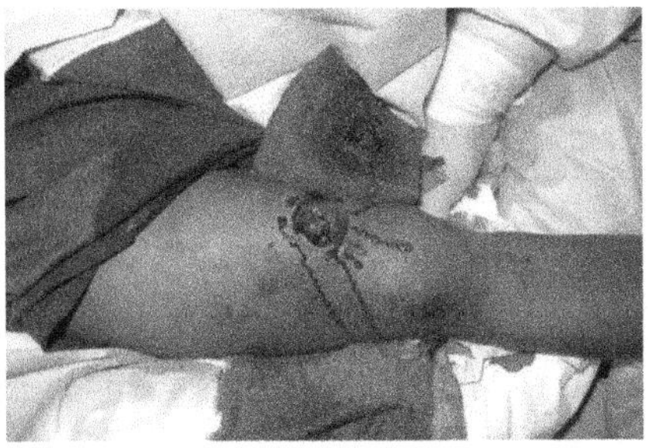

Figure 19-3. AVG infection presenting with focal hemorrhage. Image provided courtesy of Dirk Hentschel, MD.

Ultrasound is a useful adjunct to physical examination to gauge the extent of infection, particularly gross involvement of the anastomoses, which will impact management (see below). Ultrasound can also help identify vein for autogenous reconstruction or patching, and to clarify arterial anatomy.

In cases of suspected infection without clear localizing signs, groups have described the use of PET[11] and indium-111-labeled leukocyte scintigraphy[12] to clarify the status of the graft. Palestro reported a series of 30 indium scintigrams on patients with suspected PTFE AVG infections.[12] Of these 15 occurred in patients ultimately shown by intraoperative exam to have infection, all of who had scintigraphy consistent with infection. Only one patient with a thrombosed AVG had a false positive study. An added advantage of nuclear imaging was the ability to identify infections remote from the graft, which occurred in two patients in Palestro's report.

MANAGEMENT AND OUTCOMES

Prosthetic AVG infection generally mandates surgical excision. Strategies fall into three major categories: total, subtotal, and partial graft excision. Total excision consists of complete removal of prosthetic material and is indicated for extensive infection along the length of the graft, anastomotic involvement, or presentation with severe sepsis or shock. After debridement and irrigation of infected tissues, the wounds are left completely or partially open for drainage. Total graft excision has the advantage of removing all potentially infected prosthetic material and thereby theoretically minimizing recurrent infection. Disadvantages include the sacrifice of existing dialysis access and the corollary need for a temporary dialysis catheter and dissection through previously operated fields. Some arteriotomies may be amenable to primary closure while others will require vein patching. The venous outflow is closed primarily.

Subtotal graft excision implies removal of the entire graft save for a portion at the arterial anastomosis. Any open wounds are excluded by way of occlusive barriers from the field, and the clean arterial portion of the graft is exposed, divided, oversewn, then the outflow pushed into the soft tissue tunnel and sealed over. This clean wound is then closed, and again a barrier dressing applied. Finally, the infected portion of the conduit is explored and the inflow limb is pulled into the field through the now contaminated incisions. Subtotal graft excision has a profile of advantages and disadvantages similar to total graft excision except that the prosthetic cuff may be oversewn to close the arteriotomy. However, prosthetic cuff infection is a possible source of recurrent infection, and Schild reported that this was the cause in 17% of 132 procedures to address graft infection.[4] His group consequently argues against subtotal graft excision.

Partial graft excision involves segmental excision with bypass around the infected field to restore AVG continuity. As above, the infected field is initially excluded and dissection performed on uninfected, well-incorporated graft proximally and distally. Conduit is then tunneled around the infected field. Incisions are closed and covered before excising the infected graft segment. It is employed by some groups for focal AVG infection with no anastomotic involvement or systemic sepsis. This option preserves the AVG for hemodialysis and avoids extensive anastomotic re-operative dissection, but at the risk of incomplete removal of infected material.

Outcomes after partial graft excision have been mixed. Ryan reported a 74% success rate albeit at a short median follow up of 8 months.[2] Schutte and Schwab in series of 17 and 91 patients had salvage rates of 70% and 91%, respectively.[13,14] Nevertheless, relative to total excision, partial graft excision has been associated with more infectious complications and need for additional surgical procedures.[10,13] Thirty-day mortality is similar.[10] Schutte's report had a statistically insignificant trend toward more hemorrhage and systemic sepsis in patients undergoing partial graft excision compared to total excision[13]; Ryan reported no life-threatening hemorrhages or infections from attempts at graft salvage.[2]

Reconstruction of the arterial system (via autogenous patch or interposition vein graft) is the standard practice when grafts are removed from an artery. Brachial artery ligation is usually unnecessary but may be performed safely if there is concern about the integrity of the arteriotomy closure in an infected field. Schanzer reports on 21 patients with AVF graft infection with brachial anastomotic involvement where the brachial arteriotomy was oversewn followed by routine ligation distal to the profunda brachii artery.[15] Normal hand perfusion was assessed clinically preoperatively and again postoperatively at 6 months—there were no cases of hemorrhage or hand ischemia.

While creation of new access at an alternative site may be deferred until resolution of sepsis, some groups have reported success with immediate cryopreserved vein reconstruction. Matsuura and colleagues reported a series of 43 PTFE AVG infections treated with total graft excision and immediate cryopreserved femoral vein reconstruction.[16] Thirty-two of these preserved femoral veins were placed in tunnels parallel to the excision site while the remaining 11 patients had *in situ* reconstruction because of adjacent thrombosed AVGs and the lack of alternative tunneling sites. All were accessed within 14 days. Postoperative infection was rare: one patient with *Candida albicans* infection constitutes the sole case of the series, presenting with wound dehiscence and hemorrhage on postoperative day 94. Primary and secondary patencies at one year were 42% and 68%. However, this strategy can be expensive and care must be taken to avoid use in renal transplantation candidates because of the risk of allosensitization that may preclude transplantation.

Irrespective of the surgical strategy adjunctive antibiotic administration is an essential component of the treatment. Empiric antibiotics to cover methicillin-resistant *S. aureus* and Gram-negative bacilli are initially appropriate. Cultures should be used when available to tailor therapy. Antibiotic therapy durations in the literature range from two to six weeks after surgery.

In summary, with the rising incidence of the metabolic syndrome and aging population it is likely that prosthetic AVG infections will remain a morbid problem for patients and an expensive challenge for providers. Management strategies tailored to individual patient circumstances offer reasonable clinical outcomes in these patients.

REFERENCES

1. Malas MB, Canner JK, Hicks CW, et al. Trends in incident hemodialysis access and mortality. *JAMA Surg.* 2015;150(5):441–8. doi:10.1001/jamasurg.2014.3484.
2. Ryan SV, Calligaro KD, Scharff J, Dougherty MJ. Management of infected prosthetic dialysis arteriovenous grafts. *J Vasc Surg.* 2004;39(1):73–8. doi:10.1016/j.jvs.2003.07.002.
3. Akoh JA, Patel N. Infection of hemodialysis arteriovenous grafts. *J Vasc Access.* 2010;11(2):155–8.
4. Schild AF, Perez E, Gillaspie E, et al. Arteriovenous fistulae vs. arteriovenous grafts: A retrospective review of 1,700 consecutive vascular access cases. *J Vasc Access.* 2008;9(4):231–5.
5. Minga TE, Flanagan KH, Allon M. Clinical consequences of infected arteriovenous grafts in hemodialysis patients. *Am J Kidney Dis.* 2001;38(5):975–8. doi:10.1053/ajkd.2001.28583.
6. Powe NR, Jaar B, Furth SL, et al. Septicemia in dialysis patients: Incidence, risk factors, and prognosis. *Kidney Int.* 1999;55(3):1081–90. doi:10.1046/j.1523-1755.1999.0550031081.x.
7. Nassar GM, Ayus JC. Infectious complications of the hemodialysis access. *Kidney Int.* 2001;60(1):1–13. doi:10.1046/j.1523-1755.2001.00765.x.
8. Anderson JE, Chang AS, Anstadt MP. Polytetrafluoroethylene hemoaccess site infections. *ASAIO J Am Soc Artif Intern Organs. 1992.* 2000;46(6):S18–S21.
9. Zibari GB, Gadallah MF, Landreneau M, et al. Preoperative vancomycin prophylaxis decreases incidence of postoperative hemodialysis vascular access infections. *Am J Kidney Dis.* 1997;30(3):343–8.
10. Tabbara MR, O'Hara PJ, Hertzer NR, et al. Surgical management of infected PTFE hemodialysis grafts: Analysis of a 15-year experience. *Ann Vasc Surg.* 1995;9(4):378–84. doi:10.1007/BF02139410.
11. Carlos MG, Juliana R, Matilde N, et al. Hidden clotted vascular access infection diagnosed by fluorodeoxyglucose positron emission tomography. *Nephrol Carlton Vic.* 2008;13(3):264–5. doi:10.1111/j.1440-1797.2007.00837.x.
12. Palestro CJ, Vega A, Kim CK, et al. Indium-111-labeled leukocyte scintigraphy in hemodialysis access-site infection. *J Nucl Med Off.* 1990;31(3):319–24.
13. Schutte WP, Helmer SD, Salazar L, Smith JL. Surgical treatment of infected prosthetic dialysis arteriovenous grafts: Total versus partial graft excision. *Am J Surg.* 2007;193(3):385–8; discussion 388. doi:10.1016/j.amjsurg.2006.09.028.

14. Schwab DP, Taylor SM, Cull DL, et al. Isolated arteriovenous dialysis access graft segment infection: The results of segmental bypass and partial graft excision. *Ann Vasc Surg.* 2000;14(1):63–6.
15. Schanzer A, Ciaranello AL, Schanzer H. Brachial artery ligation with total graft excision is a safe and effective approach to prosthetic arteriovenous graft infections. *J Vasc Surg.* 2008;48(3):655–8. doi:10.1016/j.jvs.2008.04.030.
16. Matsuura JH, Rosenthal D, Wellons ED, et al. Hemodialysis graft infections treated with cryopreserved femoral vein. *Cardiovasc Surg.* 2002;10(6):561–5.

20

Bioengineered Vascular Access Grafts

Ehsan Benrashid, MD, David N. Ranney, MD, and Jeffrey H. Lawson MD, PhD

Patients with end-stage renal disease (ESRD), of which the most common form of renal replacement therapy (RRT) is hemodialysis (HD), account for a large proportion of healthcare expenditures. Unfortunately, because of the restricted availability of kidneys for transplantation, many patients spend years on the transplant waiting list, or are simply ineligible for renal transplantation due to advanced age or other exclusion criteria. In the meanwhile, many ESRD patients are maintained on HD, with well-established guidelines stating that, provided adequate anatomy, initial vascular access should be through upper extremity arteriovenous fistula (AVF).[1] This landmark surgical technique, as first described by Drs. Brescia, Cimino, and Appel, revolutionized the care of patients with ESRD.[2] Along with the development of the first true access method/"device" several years prior—the Scribner shunt[3]—these two medico surgical advances were directly responsible for the establishment and rapid advances in the fields of nephrology and vascular access. However, owing to limitations in individual anatomy, prior access procedures, and a host of other factors, placement of AVF is not always a realistic option for patients with ESRD. Hence, other strategies and materials for vascular access have been developed in the past 50 years, such as the tunneled dialysis catheter or arteriovenous graft (AVG).

Unfortunately, these "alternative" or "non-preferential" vascular access options are not without complications—such as thrombosis, central venous stenosis, poor patency when compared to AVF, and infection. As such, numerous attempts have been made, especially in the case of AVG, to create less thrombotic blood-contacting surfaces and materials more resistant to infection. With the advent of the field of bioengineering, along with the rapid development of tissue engineering techniques, alternative *biologic* graft materials to the more conventional *synthetic* polytetrafluoroethylene (PTFE) and expanded PTFE (ePTFE) have been developed. Additionally, it is becoming apparent that these bioprosthetic devices are emerging as potential options for readily available "off the shelf" access.[4] Given the rapidly growing interest in bioengineered vascular grafts (BEVGs) for HD access—with potential extension to other cardiovascular indications—and our institutional experience as one of the first groups in the United States to implant these devices for dialysis access in patients, we set as our objective for this chapter to describe the historical context, development, and potential clinical application of BEVGs.

HISTORICAL CONTEXT OF BEVGs

The historical context and setting for BEVG development and use in the modern era is important to understand, as many prior attempts at creation of vascular conduits concerned the utilization and creation of heterografts or allografts through various modification techniques of pre-existing, or "native," artery or vein. As such, our aim for this section is to briefly discuss the initial tissue engineering attempts for vascular tissue of heterologous origin—or what is oftentimes termed as a "bioprosthetic vascular conduit."[5]

Heterograft Dialysis Access Conduit Development and Utilization

The initial creation of a truly bioengineered blood vessel can be considered as that described by Rosenberg et al. in the 1960s,[6] with enzymatic degradation of what was assumed to be antigenic components ("muscle and elastica") in bovine carotid artery grafts. In their initial experience, implantation of these devices as thoracic or thoraco-abdominal aortic replacement in canine models yielded acceptable patency results, with further microscopic examination showing almost complete lining of the graft with a native intimal layer and a relative paucity of inflammatory infiltrate in the vessel layers.[6] Shortly thereafter, enzymatically-treated bovine carotid artery became commercially available for use as vascular conduit as the Artegraft® (Artegraft, North Brunswick, NJ). Importantly, it should be noted that this bioprosthetic device was available several years before the first widely accepted synthetic vascular conduits, in the form of PTFE and ePTFE, were available off the shelf. However, several studies demonstrating limitations of the Artegraft® device, in particular its susceptibility to thrombosis and aneurysm or pseudoaneurysm formation at HD cannulation sites,[7–10] along with the eventual widespread acceptance of improved PTFE-based grafts, resulted in their decreased use.

Many subsequently postulated that aneurysmal degradation of the first iteration of the Artegraft® was largely a result of the proteolytic breakdown process in the manufacturing of these grafts. As a result of these initial studies with bovine heterografts, further interest was spurred in developing a biologic alternative to PTFE and ePTFE. For instance, additional bioprosthetic bovine collagen-based prostheses were developed in the form of the Solcograft-P® (Solco Basle Ltd., Birsfelden-Basle, Switzerland), which demonstrated adequate short-term patency, but had an astonishingly high rate of aneurysm formation over one study period and was hence abandoned.[11] More recent improvements in the manufacturing process have resulted in the most recent iteration of the Artegraft®, which by at least one study appears to be a suitable alternative for dialysis access in patients who are otherwise poor AVF candidates.[5]

Continued modifications to the manufacturing process subsequently yielded the BioPolyMeric® (BPM) graft (St. Jude Medical, Inc., Saint Paul, MN), which was a glutaraldehyde-tanned bovine carotid artery graft initially developed for infrainguinal reconstruction.[12] Reports of the utilization of this device, which was taken off the market prior to this initial publication, are however limited in regard to dialysis access applications, although patency rates when used in infrainguinal reconstruction were comparable to PTFE. A final device adjunct in the realm of bovine heterograft development, a glutaraldehyde-tanned bovine mesenteric vein graft, ProCol® (Hancock Jaffe Laboratories, Inc., Irvine CA), has been shown to demonstrate acceptable patency results in "high risk" or anatomically unfavorable (for AVF) dialysis access patients.[13,14] The authors should note that interestingly enough, given an extremely poor patency rate over the short-term, this product was deemed unacceptable for use in additional vascular surgical applications—such as infrainguinal reconstruction[15]—although ProCol® remains available as a readily available HD access conduit at this date.

ALLOGRAFT DIALYSIS ACCESS CONDUIT DEVELOPMENT AND UTILIZATION

The first true attempts at creation and widespread marketing of a readily available human-based, or allogenic, bioprosthetic graft device was through the efforts of Dardik et al., who described the use of human umbilical veins (derived from umbilical cords) treated with glutaraldehyde.[16] In this study the authors describe the creation of the graft from the chemical and structural modification of it utilizing a polyester fiber mesh, to its implantation as upper and lower extremity AVG conduit in a primate model (baboon). Notably, the authors determined that functionality was maintained in 7/9 upper extremity AVG over a four-month period, with no incidence or propensity toward aneurysm despite weekly needle punctures. Subsequent studies utilizing this so-called, but now defunct, Dardik Biograft® (Meadox Laboratories, Oakland, NJ) as vascular prosthesis in humans demonstrated comparable patency to autogenous saphenous vein in lower extremity arterial reconstruction, with apparently fewer overall infectious complications.[17,18] Notably, access-specific studies utilizing the Dardik Biograft® demonstrated a complication rate (as defined by infection, thrombosis, aneurysm, or steal) of approximately 50%, with the overwhelming majority of these complications due to thrombosis of the bioprosthetic graft.[19] Reinforcing the aforementioned work of Rubio and Farrell demonstrating a particular propensity for graft thrombosis,[19] *in vitro* studies of the Dardik Biograft® demonstrated that the graft, over the short-term (mimicking the peri-implantation period) had a particularly increased propensity toward thrombogenicity as measured by platelet aggregation studies.[20]

An additional readily available human-derived bioprosthetic dialysis access conduit is available in the form of cryopreserved femoral or saphenous vein, in its most recent iteration the CryoVein® (CryoLife, Inc., Kennesaw, GA). Initial studies demonstrated comparable patency of these devices to PTFE in dialysis access, although their placement was associated with a particular propensity for pseudoaneurysm formation, as in the initial Artegraft® studies.[21,22] The very first iteration of this bioprosthetic conduit, the Synergraft® (CryoLife, Inc., Kennesaw, GA), was not, however, supported for HD access applications relative to PTFE (in patients without suitable anatomy for upper extremity AVF). This was due to the fact that the Synergraft® demonstrated, again, a higher propensity for aneurysm formation and an almost two-times higher rate of access failure—30% failure in Synergraft® vs. 15% in PTFE.[23] Additionally, 65% of cryopreserved femoral vein grafts were found to have a major complication in one study, with a concomitant poor primary patency of 28% over 17 months in patients at high risk for access site infection.[24] Several of the very first studies with this first iteration of a readily available human bioprosthetic graft were terminated due to CryoLife's FDA-mandated recall of several vascular prostheses. It should be noted that the Synergraft®, is currently commercially available for cardiac surgical applications, and owing to CryoLife's decellularization process, purports a paucity of induction of the immune response, making it beneficial for patients with potential future requirements for transplantation. As will be discussed, this lack of induction of the immune response is a vital component in the design and implantation of BEVG, as many patients are candidates for renal transplantation.

SELECTION CRITERIA FOR BEVG

As can be demonstrated, BEVGs appear to be best served in patient populations in which the patient does not want to or cannot be subjected to the morbidity of an additional procedure (i.e., concomitant femoral or saphenous vein harvesting), or in patients that have already exhausted this option (i.e., prior saphenous vein harvest). As described above, for the indications of dialysis access, BEVGs appear to be most useful in patients with unsuitable anatomy for AVF, prior failed AVG prostheses, or in access site infection or risk of infection. Prior to the description of the development and utilization of BEVGs, it should be noted that these devices are to be considered clinically feasible only if they meet the following criteria.[4,25,26]

- Maintain a low incidence of infectious complications.
- Do not generate an antigenic response.
- Remain patent to a degree that rivals autogenous tissue as conduit.
- Withstand degradation, but are porous enough to allow for cellular migration and seeding.
- Maintain adequate suture strength and are easily suturable.
- Have the ability to remodel.
- Are responsive to physiologic stimuli.
- Have an anti-thrombotic blood-contacting interface.
- Are durable.
- Are cost-effective.
- Are readily available.

EMERGENCE AND CLINICAL USE OF BEVG

Aside from the aforementioned bioprosthetic devices, true tissue- or bio-engineered vascular grafts were initially brought into the foray by the pioneering work of Weinberg and Bell in 1986,[27] who described the creation of an *in vitro,* multilayered collagen tube from animal collagen and bovine endothelial and smooth muscle cells (SMCs), utilizing a Dacron structural scaffold upon which these cellular constituents were seeded. Subsequently, a completely de-novo human cell–based "vascular tube" was created by L'Heureux et al. in 1993, with omission of any synthetic scaffold incorporated into the graft itself—as the graft was cultured *in vitro* around a glass mandrel.[28] Unfortunately, both of these devices were plagued by poor mechanical strength and were susceptible to degeneration, and due largely to these concerns, clinical trials were not performed.[27,28]

Given the limitations in the strength and durability of these initial BEVG, a series of strategies to modify the structural characteristics have been done in the years since. These modification processes have targeted the timeframe over which the graft is degraded, as well as the strength characteristics of the bio-scaffold material itself, which is utilized as the structural framework from which the hollow vascular tube graft is created. Briefly, examples have included modification of the BEVG culture medium or thickness of the scaffold to stiffen the graft itself, or attempts to line the device with chemical moieties that stimulate extracellular matrix (ECM) production and deposition.[29–32]

Despite modifications to the manufacturing process of BEVG, the idea that the endogenous vascular remodeling process must remain intact has always remained at the forefront of the creation of these vessels. This is of utmost importance as the structural scaffold upon which many of these grafts are created, which are composed of materials that must be degraded over time, such as polyglycolic acid or polyglycerol sebacate, must allow endogenous ECM remodeling to take place for graft incorporation. Other techniques to manipulate the environment under which the graft is synthesized include creating the graft under pulsatile conditions (a "biomimetic" approach – designed to simulate neovessel formation),[33] or utilization of the body as a "bioreactor." In this latter technique, hollow synthetic tubular scaffolds were implanted into body cavities (i.e., peritoneal or pleural cavities) and subsequently seeded *in vivo* with what was later determined to be myofibroblasts, collagen, and mesothelium.[34,35] In essence, this eliminated both a large proportion of the *in vitro* process of BEVG synthesis and, theoretically, any potential future antigenicity should the device be implanted in the organism that served as the initial "bioreactor." Criticisms of the "bioreactor" approach centered over the length of time required for BEVG creation with this technique and potential for antigenicity when used as an allotransplanted, as opposed to the aforementioned autotransplanted graft, and have not been extended to human subjects to this date.

Additional work by the group of Dahl et al. in which BEVG were decellularized after their initial creation set the stage for potential "off-the-shelf" availability of these devices for use in many vascular applications.[36] In principle, the decellularization process allows for what essentially is a hollow ECM-component tube to be stored and subsequently either: 1) seeded with the patient's own endothelium as derived from a small superficial venous biopsy; or 2) implanted into subjects at a later date, with the thought that the remodeling process will result in a structure that eventually forms a three-layered blood vessel. Notably these grafts, despite the detergents utilized in the decellularization process, did not appear to be more susceptible to mechanical stress or aneurysmal degeneration in animal models, unlike prior bioprosthetic iterations.[36] Finally, additional pioneering work in the field of tissue engineering by L'Heureux and colleagues yielded the technique of "sheet-based tissue engineering," in which fibroblasts cultured in conditions promoting ECM deposition form a flat sheet, which can be layered or rolled into a cylindrical tube resembling a blood vessel.[37] Importantly, this technique avoided the utilization of any synthetic compounds (which would need to be subject to degradation) in the formation of the neovessel.

Given the excitement over the potential for these conduits to remodel and function as native vascular tissue, the group of Shinoka et al. performed what can be considered the first reported human implantation of BEVGs, in the form of a pulmonary arterial conduit into a child with single ventricle physiology and pulmonary atresia after a prior failed repair.[38] This was largely based on this group's series of experiments in which they showed the feasibility of congenital cardiac application of these devices by demonstrating both patency and durability of BEVGs when utilized as conduit in pulmonary arterial replacement in an ovine model.[39] It should be noted that the initial BEVG implanted in a human was synthesized much in the same manner as this group's ovine model, instead using the child's autogenous vein constituents as the source of cells subsequently seeded onto a biodegradable scaffold.[38] Utilizing similar BEVG manufacturing techniques, these authors have remarkably gone on to complete implantation of their BEVGs in a cohort of 42 patients, with mid-term results demonstrating acceptable patency and a relatively low rate of reintervention, with no graft loss at this mid-term time point.[40] It should be noted that any BEVG produced as described by this study must be done so in a proactive fashion, as they are seeded with autologous bone marrow constituents, and hence were not necessarily readily available for implantation.

A final technical modification to the synthesis process of BEVGs is in electrospinning, in which application of an electric field guides the formation of polymers around structures that can be crafted to resemble vascular tubes.[41] Recent modifications to the electrospinning process have resulted in the co-spinning of collagen and elastin fibers to the create a three-layered vessel—with an intact and separate intimal, medial, and adventitial layer—more closely mimicking the three-layered nature of blood vessels and hence conferring structural stability to the TEVG.[42] Despite their promise and ease of synthesis, electrospun BEVG have yet to be implanted in clinical trials.

Subsequently, interest in the realm of BEVG application as a conduit was stimulated in the vascular access device market. In part, this is due to the fact that: 1) currently available synthetic graft materials (i.e., PTFE, Dacron, Teflon) are poor options for conduit given poor patency relative to AVF and a higher incidence of infectious complications; and 2) if the BEVG should fail in its dialysis application, most patients with ESRD can be dialyzed through, at a minimum, an indwelling central venous catheter (amongst the other modalities available). This is in opposition to utilization of BEVGs as a conduit in infrainguinal bypass procedures, where the morbidity of graft loss due to thrombosis or other factors may necessitate amputation.

As such, the first application of BEVG technology was reported in the first iteration of the Cytograft® (Cytograft Tissue Engineering, Inc., Novato, CA).[43] This device, which was made utilizing autologous fibroblasts and endothelial cells from each respective patient, was implanted in 10 subjects whom had a history of failed dialysis access. Despite primary patency comparable to conventional synthetic materials over the short term (78% at 1 month, 60% at six months), with 9/10 grafts reported as being successfully cannulated following implantation, 2/9 of these grafts underwent early structural failure, with several device failures and complications thought secondary to the graft eliciting the endogenous immune response.[44] A subsequent foray into the dialysis access market by Cytograft was via the Lifeline® graft, which was created in a more proactive fashion than the Cytograft®, by isolating autologous endothelial cells and fibroblasts from a respective patient and forming the BEVG several months prior to implantation (stored at –80°C).[45] In doing so, Cytograft performed the initial attempts at producing a personalized, "off-the-shelf" conduit for HD access, which could be stored and subsequently implanted at a later time. Later work utilizing the Lifeline® graft, this time with non-self donor cells to construct an "allogenic graft," demonstrated eventual graft failure in 2/3 patients, with the last additional patient succumbing to sepsis prior to determination of any short-term patency results.[46] Despite these poor results, one insight gleaned by the authors of this study was that these allogenic BEVG did not induce a systemic immune response, through examination of human leukocyte antigen (HLA) sensitization, panel reactive antibody values, or cross-reactivity tests.[46] This remains vital to these devices being of potential use in the long-term, as induction of any immune response from antigen present on substrates utilized during graft synthesis or HLA sensitization—both from non-self BEVG constituent donors—could render future renal transplantation at risk.

Further clinical work was then performed through development of the Humacyte Acellular Vessel (HAV; Humacyte, Inc., RTP, NC), which utilizes aortic vascular smooth muscle cells to seed a biodegradable synthetic scaffold, which is then decellularized prior to implantation (hence removing antigenic cells), producing a final acellular graft which can in theory be stored for some time—again, bringing to light the importance of "off the shelf access."[47] In initial animal models, utilization of the HAV as an AVG in baboons, or as conduit for coronary or peripheral bypass in canines, resulted in the majority of conduits patent at 1, 3, and 6 months for the AVG model, and at 1 week, 1 month, and 1 year in the arterial bypass model.[47] Current studies with the HAV are being performed for both HD access and arterial reconstruction indications, with 60 grafts currently implanted in six centers worldwide for HD access, and 20 lower extremity arterial bypass grafts implanted in one center in Europe.[48] Follow-up is ongoing, but a significant number of these grafts implanted for both indications have been functioning for over two years (unpublished data, JHL).

A final clinical application of BEVG, which although extraneous to the realm of dialysis access, we would be remiss to mention was recently described in the work of Olausson et al.[49] These authors describe their utilization of decellularized donor iliac vein subsequently seeded with host stem cells to relieve extrahepatic portal venous obstruction in a child (through interposition grafting), in order to avoid transplantation and lifelong immunosuppression, with an adequate result.

LIMITATIONS, CHALLENGES, AND FUTURE DIRECTIONS OF BEVG

As mentioned, there are several limitations and challenges for BEVG that must be considered, especially when utilized in the realm of HD access. Chief among these is the lack of antigenicity of the compounds and cells utilized in synthesis of both the bio-scaffold and graft itself, as stimulation of the immune response would raise concern for rejection in any subsequent solid organ transplantation. As mentioned in the text, preliminary studies have demonstrated a lack of the immune response to grafts created from allogenic donors,[46] although mid- and long-term immune response data for both the HAV and the Lifeline® graft are incumbent on ongoing clinical trials. Additionally, as previous authors have demonstrated dramatically increased costs with bioprosthetic grafts (five to 10 times greater than that for PTFE),[24] questions remain given the potential cost for BEVG. This cost conundrum is magnified when one considers that, at baseline, each patient on HD has been shown to account for approximately $80,000 in Medicare funds alone on an annual basis,[50] although more durable access may result in average decreased costs over time.

Additional concerns remain over the durability of the graft in terms of dialysis access, and whether the endogenous remodeling process will be so robust as to cause aneurysmal degeneration of chronically needled segment of the BEVGs utilized for HD, as prior bioprosthetic graft devices have been shown prone to. Finally, one must take into account the fact that the time to creation of these BEVGs is of utmost importance, hence our highlighting of the concepts of "ready availability" and "off-the-shelf access." Studies have demonstrated that grafts such as the HAV, which can be synthesized from cadaveric donor tissue and are eventually decellularized and stored as an essentially hollow ECM tube are designed to be readily available.[47] Admittedly, aside perhaps from the acutely infected dialysis access, the ready availability of BEVG may not drastically impact the HD patient in need of access, as there remain backup modalities and access choices for RRT, however unfavorable they are. However, with the possibility that extension of BEVGs to other clinical applications such as coronary or peripheral arterial bypass is on the horizon given these pending clinical trials, the underlying urgency regarding availability and timeliness of conduit creation is further magnified.

A final but separate note must be made about a rapidly evolving field, that of three-dimensional (3D) printing of neovessels in which the printing of materials in a repetitive fashion cumulatively forms a complex object with 3D geometry.[51] Theoretically, this process can result in the formation of not only hollow vascular tubes, but also both solid and hollow organs, such as the kidney and bowel, respectively. Several groups have demonstrated *in vitro* formation of BEVGs through 3D printing,[52–54] with some utilizing endothelial cells as the precursor "bio ink." It must be mentioned, again, that similar to the other modalities as mentioned above, these techniques have yet to be validated in clinical trials. It should be noted, however, that 3D bioprinting shows some promise in the fact that it can produce vessels in a relatively rapid and customized fashion, and thus subsequently overcomes some of the aforementioned time limitations of BEVGs synthesized via "more conventional" methodology.

CONCLUSION

Vascular access technology has experienced several seminal events in its history, dating as far back as the 1950s, which have dramatically altered the course of the fields of both vascular surgery and nephrology. The recent development of BEVG, along with more modernized approaches to the synthesis and creation of these devices reflects a tremendous volume of work done by basic scientists, bioengineers, and clinicians alike. In part, this represents a reaction to the inadequacy of synthetic and bioprosthetic vascular conduits for patients with difficult access or that are not necessarily suitable for autogenous AVF, or who have expended other access options. As described, BEVGs have the capability to dramatically impact the realm of dialysis access, oncologic vascular reconstructive, and coronary or peripheral arterial bypass procedures, amongst other indications, if they display physiologic responses to endogenous vasoactive compounds, remain anti-thrombotic, resistant to infection, durable, easy to handle, and above all, are readily available. Indeed, the current utilization of dialysis access technology initially developed almost half a century ago may seem archaic when compared to other treatment alternatives afforded to vascular surgery patients by modern technical advances, such as in the case of the ever-evolving endovascular approaches to the treatment of peripheral arterial and aortic pathology. Ongoing clinical trials will allow us to determine if these BEVGs meet the minimum requisite criteria as a viable dialysis conduit for the difficult vascular access patient.

REFERENCES

1. National Kidney Foundation. K/DOQI clinical practice guidelines for chronic kidney disease: evaluation, classification, and stratification. *Am J Kidney Dis.* 2002;39:S1–266.
2. Brescia MJ CJ, Appel K, Hurwich BJ. Chronic hemodialysis using venipuncture and a surgically created arteriovenous fistula. *N Engl J Med.* 1966;275:1089–92.
3. Scribner BH CJ, Buri R, Quinton W. The technique of continuous hemodialysis. *Trans Am Soc Artif Intern Organs.* 1960;10–11:88–103.
4. Manson RJ, Unger JM, Ali A, Gage SM, Lawson JH. Tissue-engineered vascular grafts: autologous off-the-shelf vascular access? *Semin Nephrol.* 2012;32:582–91.
5. Harlander-Locke M, Jimenez JC, Lawrence PF, et al. Bovine carotid artery (Artegraft) as a hemodialysis access conduit in patients who are poor candidates for native arteriovenous fistulae. *Vasc Endovasc Surg.* 2014;48:497–502.
6. Rosenberg N, Henderson J, Lord GH, Bothwell JW. An Arterial Prosthesis of Heterologous Vascular Origin. *JAMA.* 1964;187:741–3.
7. Merickel JH, Anderson RC, Knutson R, Lipschultz ML, Hitchcock CR. Bovine carotid artery shunts in vascular access surgery. Complications in the chronic hemodialysis patient. *Arch Surg.* 1974;109:245–50.
8. Chinitz JL, Tokoyama T, Bower R, Swartz C. Self-sealing prosthesis for arteriovenous fistula in man. *Trans Am Soc Artif Intern Organs.* 1972;18:452–7.
9. Rosenberg N, Thompson JE, Keshishian JM, VanderWerf BA. The modified bovine arterial graft. *Arch Surg.* 1976;111:222–6.
10. Hertzer NR, Beven EG. Venous access using the bovine carotid heterograft: Techniques, results, and complications in 75 patients. *Arch Surg.* 1978;113:696–700.
11. Schroder A, Imig H, Peiper U, Neidel J, Petereit A. Results of a bovine collagen vascular graft (Solcograft-P) in infra-inguinal positions. *Eur J Vasc Surg.* 1988;2:315–21.
12. Holdsworth RJ, Naidu S, Gervaz P, McCollum PT. Glutaraldehyde-tanned bovine carotid artery graft for infrainguinal vascular reconstruction: 5-year follow-up. *Eur J Vasc Endovasc Surg.* 1997;14:208–11.
13. Widmer MK, Aregger F, Stauffer E, et al. Intermediate outcome and risk factor assessment of bovine vascular heterografts used as AV-fistulas for hemodialysis access. *Eur J Vasc Endovasc Surg.* 2004;27:660–5.
14. Katzman HE, Glickman MH, Schild AF, Fujitani RM, Lawson JH. Multicenter evaluation of the bovine mesenteric vein bioprostheses for hemodialysis access in patients with an earlier failed prosthetic graft. *J Am Coll Surg.* 2005;201:223–30.
15. Kovalic AJ, Beattie DK, Davies AH. Outcome of ProCol, a bovine mesenteric vein graft, in infrainguinal reconstruction. *Eur J Vasc Endovasc Surg.* 2002;24:533–4.
16. Dardik H, Ibrahim IM, Dardik I. Arteriovenous fistulas constructed with modified human umbilical cord vein graft. *Arch Surg.* 1976;111:60–2.
17. Dardik H, Ibrahim IM, Baier R, Sprayregen S, Levy M, Dardik, II. Human umbilical cord. A new source for vascular prosthesis. *JAMA.* 1976;236:2859–62.
18. Hirsch SA, Jarrett F. The use of stabilized human umbilical vein for femoropopliteal bypass. Experience with 133 operations with 5-year follow-up. *Ann Surg.* 1984;200:147–52.
19. Rubio PA, Farrell EM. Modified human umbilical vein graft arteriovenous fistulae as a source of angioaccess in maintenance hemodialysis. *Cardiovasc Dis.* 1980;7:51–7.

20. Goldman M, Gunson B, Hawker RJ, McCollum CN. Human umbilical vein and polytetrafluorethylene arterial grafts compared in an artificial circulation. *Br J Surg*. 1983;70:4–6.
21. Madden RL, Lipkowitz GS, Browne BJ, Kurbanov A. Experience with cryopreserved cadaveric femoral vein allografts used for hemodialysis access. *Ann Vasc Surg*. 2004;18:453–8.
22. Matsuura JH, Johansen KH, Rosenthal D, Clark MD, Clarke KA, Kirby LB. Cryopreserved femoral vein grafts for difficult hemodialysis access. *Ann Vasc Surg*. 2000;14:50–5.
23. Madden RL, Lipkowitz GS, Browne BJ, Kurbanov A. A comparison of cryopreserved vein allografts and prosthetic grafts for hemodialysis access. *Ann Vasc Surg*. 2005;19:686–91.
24. Bolton WD, Cull DL, Taylor SM, et al. The use of cryopreserved femoral vein grafts for hemodialysis access in patients at high risk for infection: A word of caution. *J Vasc Surg*. 2002;36:464–8.
25. Sell SA, McClure MJ, Garg K, Wolfe PS, Bowlin GL. Electrospinning of collagen/biopolymers for regenerative medicine and cardiovascular tissue engineering. *Adv Drug Deliv Rev*. 2009;61:1007–19.
26. Thomas AC, Campbell GR, Campbell JH. Advances in vascular tissue engineering. *Cardiovasc Pathol*. 2003;12:271–6.
27. Weinberg CB, Bell E. A blood vessel model constructed from collagen and cultured vascular cells. *Science* 1986;231:397–400.
28. L'Heureux NS, Germain LS, Labbe RS, Auger FA. In vitro construction of a human blood vessel from cultured vascular cells: A morphologic study. *J Vasc Surg*. 1993;17:499–509.
29. Girton T, Oegema T, Grassl E, Isenberg B, Tranquillo R. Mechanisms of stiffening and strengthening in media-equivalents fabricated using glycation. *J Biomech Eng*. 2000;122:216–23.
30. Girton T, Oegema T, Tranquillo RT. Exploiting glycation to stiffen and strengthen tissue equivalents for tissue engineering. *J Biomed Mater Res*. 1999;46:87–92.
31. L'Heureux N, Paquet S, Labbe R, Germain L, Auger F. A completely biological tissue-engineered human blood vessel. *FASEB J*. 1998;12:47–56.
32. Walles T, Herden T, Haverich A, Mertsching H. Influence of scaffold thickness and scaffold composition on bioartificial graft survival. *Biomaterials*. 2003;24:1233–39.
33. Niklason LE, Gao J, Abbott W, et al. Functional arteries grown in vitro. *Science*. 1999;284:489–93.
34. Campbell J, Efendy J, Campbell G. Novel vascular graft grown within recipient's own peritoneal cavity. *Circ Res*. 1999;85:1173–8.
35. Chue WL, Campbell GR, Caplice N, et al. Dog peritoneal and pleural cavities as bioreactors to grow autologous vascular grafts. *J Vasc Surg*. 2004;39:859–67.
36. Dahl SL, Koh J, Prabhakar V, Niklason LE. Decellularized native and engineered arterial scaffolds for transplantation. *Cell Transplant*. 2003;12:659–66.
37. L'Heureux N, Dusserre N, Konig G, et al. Human tissue-engineered blood vessels for adult arterial revascularization. *Nat Med*. 2006;12:361–5.
38. Shin'oka T, Imai Y, Ikada Y. Transplantation of a tissue-engineered pulmonary artery. *N Engl J Med*. 2001;344:532–3.
39. Shinoka T, Shum-Tim D, Ma P, et al. Creation of viable pulmonary artery autografts through tissue engineering. *J Thorac Cardiovasc Surg*. 1998;115:536–46.
40. Shin'oka T, Matsumura G, Hibino N, et al. Midterm clinical result of tissue-engineered vascular autografts seeded with autologous bone marrow cells. *J Thorac Cardiovasc Surg*. 2005;129:1330–8.
41. Matthews JA, Wnek GE, Simpson DG, Bowlin GL. Electrospinning of collagen nanofibers. *Biomacromolecules*. 2002;3:232–8.
42. Boland ED, Matthews JA, Pawlowski KJ, Simpson DG, Wnek GE, Bowlin GL. Electrospinning collagen and elastin: preliminary vascular tissue engineering. *Front Biosci*. 2004;9:1422–32.
43. L'Heureux N, McAllister TN, de la Fuente LM. Tissue-engineered blood vessel for adult arterial revascularization. *N Engl J Med*. 2007;357:1451–3.

44. McAllister T, Maruszewski M, Garrido S, et al. Effectiveness of haemodialysis access with an autologous tissue-engineered vascular graft: A multicentre cohort study. *Lancet.* 2009;373:1440–46.
45. Wystrychowski W, Cierpka L, Zagalski K, et al. Case study: First implantation of a frozen, devitalized tissue-engineered vascular graft for urgent hemodialysis access. *J Vasc Access.* 2011;12:67–70.
46. Wystrychowski W, McAllister TN, Zagalski K, Dusserre N, Cierpka L, L'Heureux N. First human use of an allogeneic tissue-engineered vascular graft for hemodialysis access. *J Vasc Surg.* 2014;60:1353–7.
47. Dahl S, Kypson A, Lawson J, et al. Readily available tissue-engineered vascular grafts. *Sci Transl Med.* 2011;3:68ra9.
48. Benrashid E, McCoy CC, Youngwirth LM, et al. Tissue Engineered Vascular Grafts: Origins, Development, and Current Strategies for Clinical Application. *Methods.* 2015. http://dx.doi.org/10.1016/j.ymeth.2015.07.014 [Epub ahead of print]
49. Olausson M, Patil PB, Kuna VK, et al. Transplantation of an allogeneic vein bioengineered with autologous stem cells: A proof-of-concept study. *Lancet.* 2012;380:230–7.
50. USRDS. Atlas of chronic kidney diesase and end-stage renal disease in the United States. United States Renal Data System (2013). Available from htttp://www.usrds.org/atlas.aspx. Accessed 31 July 2015.
51. Murphy SV, Atala A. 3D bioprinting of tissues and organs. *Nat Biotechnol.*2014;32:773–85.
52. Cui X, Boland T. Human microvasculature fabrication using thermal inkjet printing technology. *Biomaterials.* 2009;30:6221–7.
53. Lee VK, Kim DY, Ngo H, et al. Creating perfused functional vascular channels using 3D bioprinting technology. *Biomaterials.* 2014;35:8092–102.
54. Zhao L, Lee VK, Yoo SS, Dai G, Intes X. The integration of 3-D cell printing and mesoscopic fluorescence molecular tomography of vascular constructs within thick hydrogel scaffolds. *Biomaterials.* 2012;33:5325–32.

21

Endovenous Ablation of the Saphenous Vein for Prevention and Healing of Venous Ulcers

Randolph Todd C. Jones, MD and Mark A. Adelman, MD

Venous lower extremity ulcers (VLUs) represent the most severe clinical manifestation of chronic venous insufficiency. Proper identification of patients with or at risk of developing a venous leg ulcer is paramount. To this end the SVS and AVF clinical practice guidelines for the management of venous leg ulcers proposed the following definition: A venous ulcer is an open skin lesion of the leg or foot that occurs in an area affected by venous hypertension.[1] Several other definitions exist in the international literature; for example, the Scottish and French healthcare system guidelines are more specific; both stipulate that the wound must remain unhealed for one month (or four weeks) and be pathophysiologically due to venous hypertension.[2-3] The American Venous Forum consensus statement defines a VLU as a "full thickness defect of the skin, most frequently in the ankle region, that fails to heal spontaneously and is sustained by CVD."[4]

The diagnosis of a VLU must be differentiated from other causes of lower extremity ulcers (i.e., vasculitis, peripheral arterial disease etc.), to that end these authors prefer a more specific definition of: a full thickness defect of the skin that occurs below the knee in an area affected directly by chronic venous insufficiency (confirmed by duplex ultrasonography, plethysmography, or another accepted venous imaging modality), which fails to heal spontaneously for at least 4 weeks, and is not due to another underlying pathophysiologic process (e.g., peripheral arterial disease).

The majority of clinical issues arising from chronic venous insufficiency are, by nature, quality of life issues. That being said, the presence of a VLU can cause significant morbidity to any patient, let alone one that has multiple co-morbid factors (such as super infection of the ulcer bed in the setting of diabetes or peripheral arterial disease). VLUs can also have significant psycho-social and economic effects, with many patients reportedly being embarrassed about the appearance of their legs, and the significant stress associated with managing a chronically open wound on a day to day basis. In the United States alone, more than 6 million patients are affected with VLUs, at a cost of over $2.5 billion annually.[5]

WORK-UP

Patients presenting with venous leg ulceration need work-up for both venous and arterial insufficiency. The etiologies of VLU are numerous, and it is imperative that the presence of arterial insufficiency be evaluated before proceeding with any ulcer therapy. All patients should receive a thorough history and physical, including documentation of the presence and quality of lower extremity pulses (femoral, popliteal, dosal pedis, and posterior tibial), as well as an ankle-brachial index (and pulse volume recordings where necessary). Moreover, less common but more morbid and potentially life-threatening etiologies need to be considered or excluded from the differential diagnosis (e.g., malignancy, vasculitis, necrotizing soft tissue infections).

As with all disease processes, a detailed understanding of the involved anatomy is essential to proper diagnosis and treatment. The venous system is one of, if not the most complex and anatomically variable components of the human body. Understanding or memorizing every single anatomic variant of the venous system is not necessary; however the use of standardized nomenclature when describing the individual anatomic variants of each patient is necessary. To this end these authors recommend all practitioners use and understand the International Consensus Committee on Venous Anatomical Terminology.[6]

We also recommend the use of the CEAP (Clinical class, Etiology, Anatomy, and Pathophysiology) classification system, VCSS (Venous Clinical Severity Score), and a venous disease specific quality of life assessment for each patient.[1] Both CEAP and VCSS (shown in Table 21-1) represent imperative standardized clinical documentation for the diagnosis and proper management of chronic venous insufficiency, particularly in patients with VLUs. They allow for a common language and documentation system which can be used and understood between multiple different practitioners regarding the exact etiology and severity of a patient's venous disease.

Recently quality of life (QOL) questionnaires have also begun to be added to the repertoire of practitioners as a way to judge the baseline impact of a patient's venous disease on their day to day life, as well as a way to track their progress over the course of their treatment. These Authors, and many other practitioners, believe QOL assessment to be the most important clinical indicator of the severity of an individual patient's disease, and will judge the effectiveness, or failure, of treatment based on the improvement (or lack thereof) of a QOL questionnaire score. There are many different commercially available, and validated QOL questionnaires on the market (e.g., CIVIQ, AVVQ). Given that the vast majority of chronic venous insufficiency is at its nature, a quality of life issue, these authors consider the inclusion of a QOL assessment for each patient paramount to the proper management and quality control of applied treatments.

All patients with a venous leg ulcer should undergo diagnostic and anatomical evaluation using duplex ultrasonography by an experienced ultrasonographer trained in the evaluation of both the deep and superficial venous systems. Duplex ultrasonography is widely available, has a high degree of diagnostic accuracy, is of low cost, and is now considered to be the gold standard for the diagnosis of peripheral venous insufficiency.

TABLE 21-1. VCSS

	None: 0	Mild: 1	Moderate: 2	Severe: 3
Pain or other discomfort (ie, aching, heaviness, fatigue, soreness, burning) Presumes venous origin		Occasional pain or other discomfort (ie, not restricting regular daily activities)	Daily pain or other discomfort (ie, interfering with but not preventing regular daily activities)	Daily pain or discomfort (ie, limits most regular daily activities)
Varicose veins		Few: scattered	Confined to calf or thigh	Involves calf and thigh
Venous edema		Limited to foot and ankle area	Extends above ankle but below knee	Extends to knee and above
Skin pigmentation	None or focal	Limited to perimalleolar area	Diffuse over lower third of calf	Wider distribution above lower third of calf
Induration	Limited to perimalleolar area	Limited to perimalleolar area	Diffuse over lower third of calf	Wider distribution above lower third of calf
Active ulcer number	**0**	**1**	**2**	**3 or more**
Active ulcer duration (longest active)		<3 mo	>3 mo but <1 y	Not healed for >1 y
Active ulcer size (largest active)		Diameter <2 cm	Diameter 2–6 cm	Diameter >6 cm
Use of compression therapy	Not used	**1** Intermittent use of stockings	**2** Wears stockings most days	**3** Full compliance: stockings

Using duplex ultrasonography a practitioner can document the specific anatomy of the patient with a suspected VLU, as well as the location of specific refluxing veins (superficial, deep, or perforating veins). It is important to document the specifics relating to the location, diameter, degree of reflux, and any connection to tributaries associated with or contributing to any associated advanced skin changes (hyperpigmentation, lipodermatosclerosis, or atrophie blanche) or the ulcer bed. For the purposes of this chapter, we will focus on the important elements specific to great and small saphenous reflux and their anatomic variants. The presence of reflux in the deep (both peripheral, and central), or perforating, venous systems and its management, is extremely important; but it is beyond the scope of this chapter and will be discussed in detail elsewhere in the text. However, if central venous obstruction (iliocaval) is clinically suspected, these authors believe that it should be appropriately evaluated (either by MRV, CTV, or directly by IVUS or venography) and the need for intervention via open venous reconstruction, or endovascular methods considered before proceeding with any superficial venous reflux treatment.

Clinical documentation of the exact location, diameter (in at least 2 dimensions), depth, and the presence (or absence) of exudates, infection or surrounding inflammation is also paramount to the management of any VLU, and is important for the tracking of clinical progress and healing.

The duration of a non-healing ulcer is very important in determining treatment options. In many cases lower extremity ulcers may have been present for several months, and even years. The patient may have had no prior treatment for their ulcer(s), or the ulcer may have been refractory to medical and/or surgical therapies. In either case it is necessary to rule out both infection, and malignancy, as either of these can be the precipitating factor in non-healing VLUs. In the presence of significant pain and surrounding erythema, one must consider the possibility of infection; which may be present even in the absence of a purulent exudate or a surrounding cellulitis. Cultures should be taken only in this scenario. A painless ulcer, that has been refractory to conservative medical or surgical therapy, may be of malignant etiology. Biopsy of any suspicious lower extremity ulcer should be considered.[7]

ENDOVENOUS SURGICAL APPROACH

Prior to the treatment of perforating veins, superficial truncal valvular insufficiency should be addressed. There are several efficient endovenous methodologies that can be used to interrupt incompetent saphenous veins; each technique has its individual advantages and disadvantages. Proper technique selection is essential to clinical success.

Previously described endovenous techniques include ultrasound guided chemical, mechanicochemical, laser, and radiofrequency ablation. Common steps to all four techniques includes the use of duplex ultrasound, to gain needle access to the saphenous vein in question (Figure 21-1), or a communicating tributary in close proximity; after which the chosen ablative device or chemical is introduced into the vein via a catheter, or directly through the needle access.

Specific consideration should be given to the anatomic relation of the ulcer to the refluxing saphenous vein in question. Generally, great saphenous reflux causes its maximal effect and is related to VLUs in the area of the medial ankle and leg (i.e., near its anatomic origin), while reflux of the small saphenous vein may be the related to ulcers on the lateral ankle (again, near its anatomic origin). This being said, refluxing and dilated tributaries of any vein can travel in the subcutaneous tissues in nearly any direction to exert their effect and contribute to ulcer development. The authors again emphasize the importance of proper and detailed duplex ultrasonography and examination in determining the exact source of venous hypertension related to a healed or active ulcer bed.

Several studies have documented the efficacy of endovenous ablative techniques to aid in the healing of VLUs. However, no studies exist that show a superiority of surgical techniques over medical therapy alone (i.e., conservative measures combined with local wound care and compression). In 2013 the Cochrane Database published a review after attempting to determine the effects of superficial endovenous ablation on the healing and prevention of recurrence in patients with active or healed venous ulcers. They were unable to identify any randomized controlled trials which met their inclusion criteria at that time on the effects of endovenous ablation of the superficial veins on ulcer healing, recurrence or quality of life; and cited a need for adequately powered, high quality randomized controlled trials comparing endovenous thermal ablation with compression therapy.[8] In 2014 the Society for Vascular Surgery conducted a review and

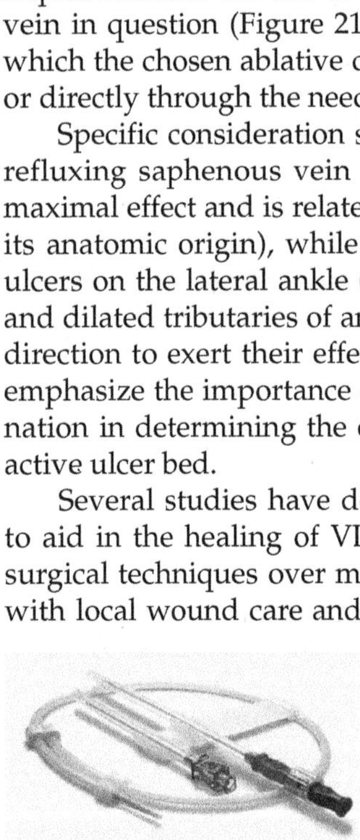

Figure 21-1. An 0.018″ microintroducer set, which includes a 21-G needle, 0.018″ guidewire, and a 4-Fr introducer sheath, just one of many available access kits.

meta-analysis of surgical interventions versus conservative therapy for VLUs; which also found that current evidence did not support the superiority of endovascular interventions compared with compression alone.[9] There does exist evidence the surgical therapy increases the interval to recurrence of VLUs or decreases the recurrence rate of VLUs altogether.[10,11]

There is a paucity of high quality randomized controlled trials demonstrating evidence regarding the efficacy of endovenous ablative techniques in the primary prevention of ulcer formation and the healing of VLUs versus compression alone. Despite this, most clinicians feel that the endovenous ablative techniques in patients at risk for formation of VLUs (those patients with C4b disease), or with active VLUs, does have clinical value to prevent the formation of ulcers and assist in healing of active VLUs. The current SVS and AVF clinical practice guidelines recommend endovenous ablation of incompetent superficial axial veins in addition to standard compressive therapy to:

1. Improve ulcer healing (grade 2C recommendation)
2. Prevent formation of ulcers in patients at risk (C4b disease) with superficial axial incompetence directed at the bed of the affected skin (grade 2C recommendation)
3. Decrease VLU recurrence rates in both patients with C5 (grade 1C recommendation) and C6 disease (grade 1B recommendation)[1]

Endovenous Thermal Ablation

Endovenous thermal ablation with either radiofrequency ablation or endovenous laser ablation of the saphenous veins is a well-documented and described procedure with a high degree of efficacy. Both techniques are relatively equivalent in efficacy and safety,[12,13] and these authors suggest that the individual practitioners choose whichever thermal ablative devices they are most familiar with.

It should be noted that access to the most peripheral portions of the saphenous veins is precluded with the use of thermal ablative techniques. The saphenous nerve comes in close proximity to the great saphenous vein 10–15 cm below the knee, and as such is at risk for thermal injury in the lower leg if using laser or radiofrequency ablation. The sural nerve begins to approximate the small saphenous vein just below the heads of the gastrocnemius muscle and is also susceptible to thermal injury when ablating below this location. In a subset of patients who have undergone endothermal ablation of the small and/or great saphenous veins, there will continue to be reflux peripheral to the lowest point of ablation post-procedurally. These authors would advocate that practitioners consider the use of endo-chemical or pharmacomechanical ablative techniques to treat vein segments in these areas in patients who are at high risk of ulcer development, recurrence, or persistent non-healing of a VLU. This approach mitigates the possibility of compounding a VLU with concomitant saphenous or sural neuropathy secondary to thermal injury of the nerve at these locations.

Endochemical and Pharmaco-mechanical Ablation

Ultrasound guided chemical ablation can be needle or catheter directed. The initial steps are essentially the same; however, catheter directed sclerotherapy involves the use of a guidewire and the modified Seldinger technique to introduce it into the

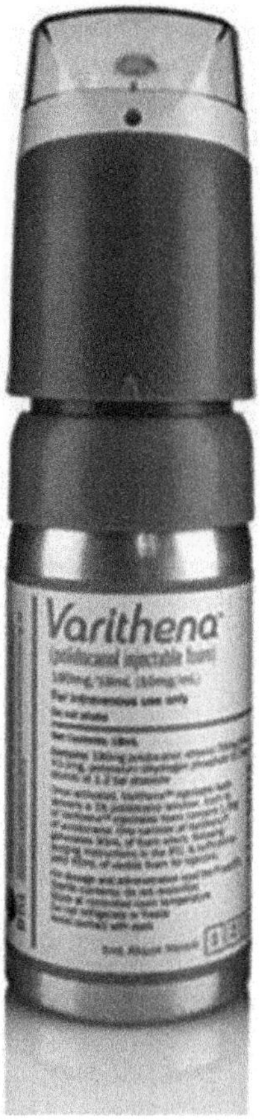

Figure 21-2. Varithena Canister.

saphenous vein, and/or it's communicating tributaries. Currently approved sclerosants are sodium tetradecyl sulfate (Sotradecol), and polidocanol (Asclera). The use of a proprietary foam sclerosant (Varithena®) for ablation of the saphenous vein has recently been approved by the FDA (BTG, Philadelphia, Pennsylvania, see Figure 21-2); however injection of physician-made foam has been well documented in the literature, but represents off-label use of either polidocanol or sodium tetradecyl sulfate. If a foamed sclerosant is used, the patient should be placed in trendelenburg position during the injection process, and proximal pressure should be applied to minimize the amount of foam that enters the central venous system. Although the rate of treatment failure is higher with the use of a sclerosant versus endothermal ablative techniques,[14] it has the distinct advantage of being easily repeatable, with success rates approaching that of endothermal techniques with repetition.

ClariVein® (Figure 21-3) is the only commercially available and FDA approved device for pharmaco-mechanical ablation of the saphenous veins. It consists of a long wire with an angled tip which rotates causing mechanical agitation of the endothelium via a motorized mechanism located within the handle of the device. It also allows for simultaneous injection of liquid sclerosant from the tip of the catheter as it is withdrawn from the vein. There is no need for the use of tumescent anesthesia with this device, and the risk of thermal

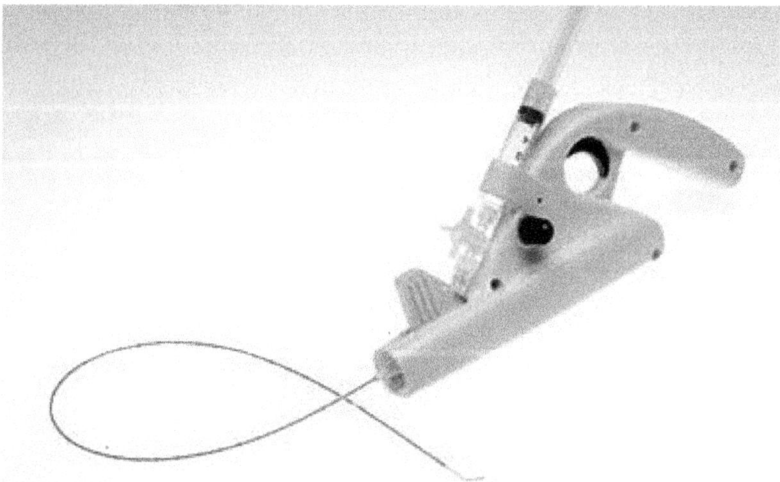

Figure 21-3. ClariVein device.

damage to nerves or the overlying skin is obviated. It has been reported to have a clinical success rate of up to 96% at two years.[15]

Intraoperative Considerations for the Use of Sclerosants

When using endochemical ablation techniques (foamed or liquid) the interventionalists should ensure that needle or catheter access is within the desired saphenous vein. Through the needle, blood should be aspirated, and should be of obvious venous source. If there is any question about location of the needle or catheter, it should be withdrawn, and access should be reattempted. Finally, the interventionalists should use ultrasound while injecting a foam sclerosant to monitor central progression of the foam towards the deep venous system.

POST-OPERATIVE CARE

Postoperatively we place all patients into 30–40 mmHg compression stockings. In addition to the compression garment, we also ask our patients to ambulate for several minutes in the office before leaving.

Patients should be seen for routine follow up at 1 week, and duplex ultrasound at 1 month to assess for efficacy of the closure. These authors recommend against routine duplex within the 1st post-operative week, as it has been suggested that it has little effect on outcomes.[16] In patients with healed ulcers, or C4b disease, routine follow up at 3 months should be performed with duplex ultrasound to check the efficacy of the closure; although a lesser time interval would be reasonable if the clinician had reason to be more concerned about recurrent or active ulceration.

CONCLUSION

There is a distinct absence of high quality randomized controlled trials demonstrating the superiority of endovenous ablative techniques in the primary prevention of and healing of venous leg ulcers over compression alone. However, evidence exists that endovenous surgical interventions are at least equivalent to the best medical therapy in the promoting the healing of VLUs. Moreover, despite the lack of compelling data, it seems to make pathophysiologic sense that interruption of chronic superficial venous insufficiency that has been shown to be anatomically related to sites of active VLUs or sites at risk of development of a VLU (areas of C4b disease) should improve VLU healing rates, and decrease the risk of VLU formation in at risk patients. Given this, these authors will continue to advocate for the use of endovenous ablative techniques in combination with the best medical therapy to aid in the prevention, healing, or recurrence of venous leg ulcers. If truncal venous ablation is unsuccessful in the healing of ulceration, intensive interrogation of perforating veins using duplex ultrasound should be performed. If a perforating vein measuring 3.5 mm in diameter with greater than 0.5 seconds of valvular reflux time perfuses the ulcer bed, perforator ablation or interruption should be considered.

SUGGESTED READINGS

1. *Management of venous leg ulcers: Clinical practice guidelines of the Society for Vascular Surgery and the American Venous Forum.*© 2014 AVF and SVS.
2. *Handbook of Venous Disorders,* 3rd edition. Peter Glviczki, 2009. Guidelines of the American Venous Forum.

REFERENCES

1. O'Donnell T, Passman A, Marston W, et al. Management of venous leg ulcers: Clinical practice guidelines of the Society for Vascular Surgery and the American Venous Forum. *J Vasc Surg*. 2014;60(2):3S–59S
2. Scottish Intercollegiate Guidelines Network—update of SIGN 26. The care of patients with chronic (venous) leg ulcers. August 2012. Available at: http://www.sign.ac.uk/pdf/sign120.pdf. Accessed June 6, 2015.
3. Haute Autorité de Santé (HAS). Clinical practice guidelines. Managing venous leg ulcers excluding dressings. June 2006. Available at: http://www.has-sante.fr. Accessed June 6, 2015.
4. Gloviczki P. Handbook of Venous Disorders, 3rd edition. 2009. *Guidelines of the American Venous Forum*. London, UK: Hodder Arnold.
5. Simka M, Majewski E. The social and economic burden of venous leg ulcers: Focus on the role of micronized purified flavonoid fraction adjuvant therapy. *Am J Clin Dermatol.* 2003;4:573–81.
6. Caggiati A, Bergan J.J, Gloviczki P, et al. Nomenclature of the veins of the lower limbs: An international interdisciplinary consensus statement. *J Vasc Surg*. 2002;36:416–22.
7. Senet P, Combemale P, Debure C, et al. Malignancy and chronic leg ulcers: The value of systematic wound biopsies: a prospective, multicenter, cross-sectional study. *Arch Dematol.* 2012;148(6):704–8.
8. Samuel N, Carradice D, Wallace T, et al. Endovenous thermal ablation for healing venous ulcers and preventing recurrence. *Cochrane Database Syst Rev*. 2013;10:CD009494.
9. Mauck KF, Asi N, Undavalli C, et al. Systematic review and meta-analysis of surgical interventions versus conservative therapy from venous ulcers. *J Vasc Surg*. 2014;60:60S–72S.
10. Van Gent WB, Hop WC, Van Praag MC, et al. Conservative versus surgical treatment of venous leg ulcers: A prospective, randomized, multicenter trial. *J Vasc Surg*. 2006;44:563–71.
11. Gohel MS, Barwell JR, Taylor M, et al. Long-term results of compression therapy alone versus compression plus surgery in chronic venous ulceration (ESCHAR): randomised controlled trial. *BMJ*. 2007;335:83.
12. Theivacuma NS, Darwood R, Gough MJ. Neovascularization and recurrence 2 years after treatment for sapheno-femoral and great saphenous reflux: A comparison of surgery and endovenous laser. *Eur J Vasc Endovasc Surg*. 2009;38:203–7.
13. Rasmussen L, Lawaetz M, Bjoern L, et al. Randomized trial comparing endovenous laser ablation and stripping of the great saphenous vein with duplex outcome after 5 years. *J Vasc Surg*. 2013;58:421–6.
14. O'Hare JL, Earnshaw JJ. Randomised clinical trial of foam sclerotherapy for patients with a venous leg ulcer. *Eur J Vasc Endovasc Surg*. 2010;39:495–9.
15. Witte ME, Reijnen MM, de Vries JP, et al. Mechanicochemical endovenous occlusion of varicose veins using the ClariVein device. *Surg Technol*. 2015;25:219–25.
16. Jones RTC, Kabnick LS. Perioperative duplex ultrasound following endothermal ablation of the saphenous vein: Is it worthless? *J Invasive Cardiol*. 2014;26(10):548–50.

22

May–Thurner Syndrome: Practical Approach to Diagnosis and Treatment

Johnathon Rollo, MD and Brian G. DeRubertis, MD

HISTORY

May–Thurner Syndrome (MTS) has been recognized as a clinically significant entity for nearly 60 years. The presence of intraluminal webs in the iliac veins was first described by McMurrich in a 1908 autopsy series.[1] He discovered the lesions in 33 of 107 unselected autopsy specimens, and suggested it as a pathologic condition contributing to vein thrombosis. In the seminal 1957 paper by May and Thurner,[2] the syndrome explains Virchow's observation in 1851 that iliofemoral DVT was five times more likely to occur on the left leg than the right. They described an anatomical variant in which the left common iliac vein produced "venous spurs" in response to chronic overlying pulsation from the right common iliac artery.[3] In 1967 Crockett observed that 65% of patients with iliofemoral deep venous thrombosis (DVT) had evidence of left common iliac vein (LCIV) compression on venography, and the left leg was affected in 83% of unilateral cases.[4] In early 20th century autopsy series, 20%–30% of randomly selected patients had evidence of LCIV compression and venous adhesions without DVT. In addition, he noted multiple anatomical variations that accounted for compression of LCIV, vena cava, left external iliac vein and right common iliac venous compression. This gave further evidence that LCIV compression was a contributing etiologic factor for symptomatic unilateral venous swelling, claudication and iliofemoral DVT.[4]

Treatment of chronic venous claudication and post phlebitic syndrome throughout most of the twentieth century consisted of morbid and invasive surgical venous bypass. Only with modern cross-sectional imaging technology and the advent of routine venous angiography did the true prevalence of MTS become apparent, and intravascular treatment options develop. In the early 1990s, the use of catheter directed thrombolysis and venography for the treatment of iliofemoral DVT frequently identified compression of the LCIV and these procedures offered the ability to treat the underlying conditions with iliocaval stenting. In 1991 the first series of central venous stenting for chronic obstruction was reported.[5] With the development of advanced endovascular technology, iliac vein stenting for chronic total occlusion (CTO) and symptomatic May–Thurner syndrome has become standard practice, largely replacing the relatively morbid open surgical venous reconstructions. Debate persists as to the role of imaging in diagnosis of MTS and indications for stenting symptomatic lesions.

PREVALENCE

Chronic venous disease (CVD) is a very common, costly malady particularly in western countries. The spectrum of disease affects more than 30 million people in the USA alone. Over 500,000 patients in this country suffer from nonhealing venous ulceration.[6] MTS is increasingly recognized as a major contributing factor in lower extremity venous pathologies including iliofemoral DVT, post-phlebitic syndrome, chronic venous insufficiency (CVI). The true incidence rate of MTS is unknown and perhaps ranges from 20% to 30% according to the autopsy studies in the early twentieth century. The incidence of LCIV compression in iliofemoral DVT is likely under-reported as the majority of patients do not undergo lysis, venography, or axial imaging. When patients with left iliofemoral DVT do undergo more extensive imaging than duplex ultrasound alone, LCIV stenosis is discovered with a high frequency, in contradistinction to traditional teaching which had ascribed MTS as the underlying etiology of iliofemoral DVT in the minority of cases.[7] In recent a large series of 1000 patients with CVD of all CEAP classifications who underwent intravascular ultrasound (IVUS) imaging, nonthrombotic compression of the CIV was noted in 53% of cases, and post-thrombotic stenosis in 40%. Stenting of iliac vein stenosis produced symptomatic relief in 75% of these patients.[8]

CVI was previously thought to be a result of vein reflux and for two centuries treatment has been directed at the saphenous vein. However, new imaging technologies, including IVUS and more prevalent venous angiography, have pointed toward compression of the iliac vein as a major contributing factor in patients thought to suffer from superficial axial vein reflux alone. In 2010, Raju et al. reported a series of 470 patients with CVI who underwent iliac vein stenting for non-thrombotic iliac vein lesions without concomitant treatment of superficial axial vein reflux. With iliac stenting alone, the ulcer healing rate was 54% in C6 limbs, complete symptom resolution occurred in 36%, and partial symptom relief was attained in 55%.[9] However, the clinical significance of MTS in CVD continues to be a matter of some debate, as approximately 50% of the general population has some degree of LCIV compression on IVUS and axial imaging.

PATHOPHYSIOLOGY

In classic MTS, the left common iliac vein is compressed against the fifth lumbar vertebral body by the right common iliac artery as the artery crosses in front of the vein. (Figure 22-1). Additional anatomic variants produce compression of the IVC, right common iliac vein and left external iliac vein by the right common iliac artery or left hypogastric artery. In LCIV compression by the right common iliac artery, the point of

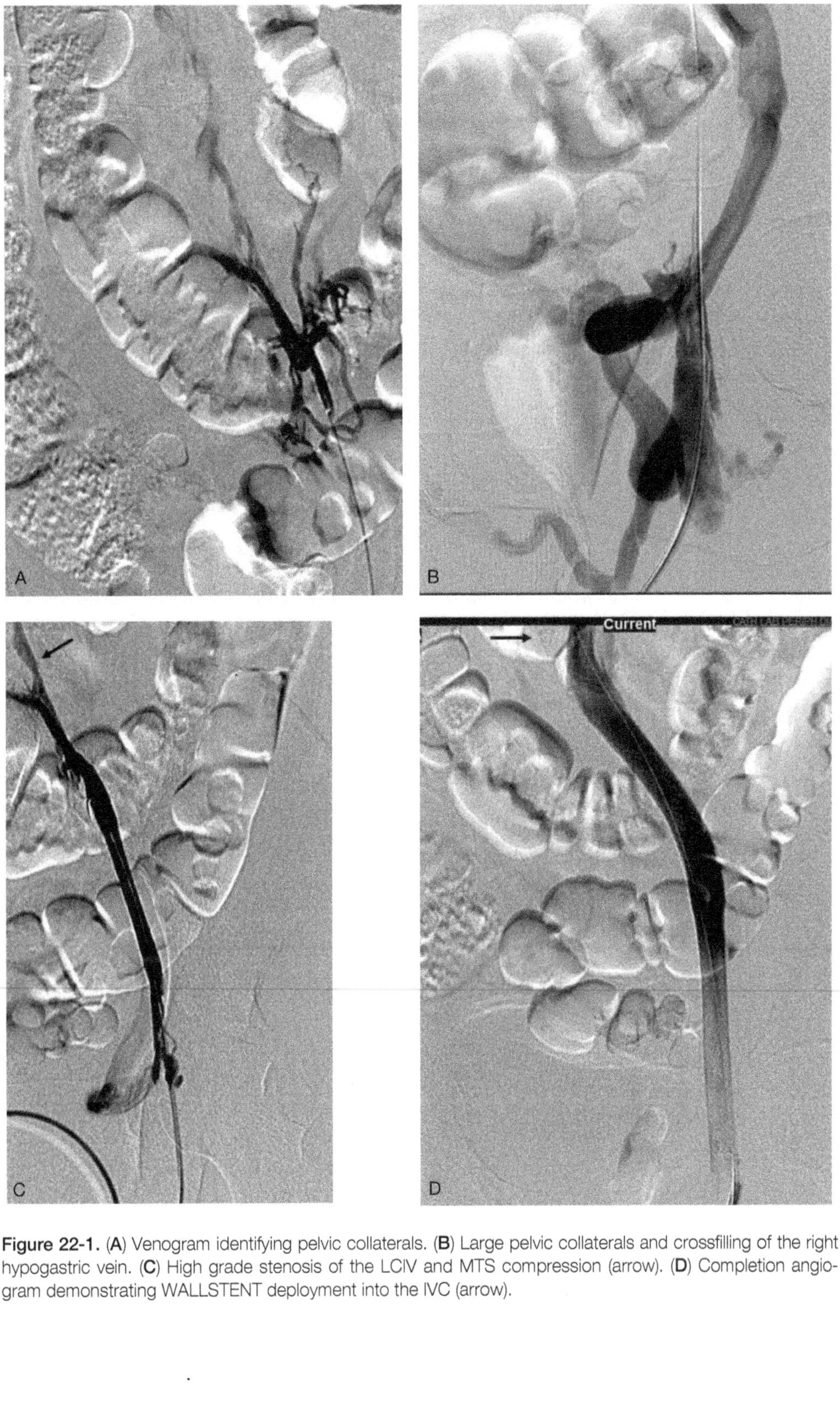

Figure 22-1. (**A**) Venogram identifying pelvic collaterals. (**B**) Large pelvic collaterals and crossfilling of the right hypogastric vein. (**C**) High grade stenosis of the LCIV and MTS compression (arrow). (**D**) Completion angiogram demonstrating WALLSTENT deployment into the IVC (arrow).

maximal compression can vary, sometimes affecting solely the LCIV but other times leading to significant compression of the caval confluence, and therefore stenting of this compression generally requires extension of the central portion of the stent significantly into the vena cava. In addition to classic LCIV compression, related venous compression syndromes can include compression of the left external iliac vein by the left hypogastric artery as it crosses over the vein into the pelvis. Similarly, the right hypogastric artery can sometimes lead to pathologic venous compression of the right external iliac vein by the same mechanism.

In addition to the obvious venous flow abnormalities caused by significant compression of these structures, the chronic compression can lead to structural changes within the vein. Chronic pulsation of the artery is thought to cause elastin and collagen deposition intraluminally, and intimal fibrosis therefore results, leading to formation of venous spurs and webs. These pathologic changes can ultimately result in development of unilateral chronic leg swelling and ultimately contributes to venous thrombosis. External compression of the iliac vein is therefore a ubiquitous finding but not the only contributing factor.

Previously thought to be primarily a disease of women and isolated to the left leg, more recent study has found that venous compression syndromes occur commonly in both men and women, and can involve the right leg by one of the mechanisms described above. In one study of asymptomatic individuals, the venous compression lesions were found as frequently in men, but women were found to have higher degrees of stenosis. In a large modern series of symptomatic patients with MTS without reflux, the female: male ratio was 4.7:1, Left: right 3:1 and mean age 51 years.[10] Therefore, venous compression syndromes should be considered in patients of all ages, regardless of sex or lesion laterality, and the utility of axial imaging or contrast venography should be discussed with any patient with iliofemoral DVT.

The pathogenic role of compressive lesions in the iliac veins has come under question with the findings that 20%–50% of the general population has these lesions at baseline. What makes these lesions symptomatic in some and silent in others is not well understood. Multiple large series have demonstrated significant clinical benefit in correcting these lesions with negligible morbidity. MTS may be thought of as a "permissive" condition that predisposes a person to thrombosis when a "second hit" occurs, such as initiation of oral contraceptives, prolonged immobility, malignancy or hypercoagulable state. The presence of intraluminal webs and external compression could increase the leg morbidity from conditions such as new distal DVT, heart failure, saphenous vein valvular incompetence, cellulitis, lymphedema, or fluid shifts. While asymptomatic or minimally symptomatic individuals require no screening for or treatment of venous compression syndromes, recognition of the role that venous compression syndromes can play in any patient with leg swelling or iliofemoral DVT should not be neglected.

CLINICAL PRESENTATION

MTS can present in the acute phase as a new iliofemoral DVT, or be discovered in work-up for CVD. Acute DVT presents with sudden onset of leg pain, swelling and edema, but can also be asymptomatic. While massive iliofemoral DVT can produce phlegmasia cerulea dolens, resulting from venous hypertension obstructing arterial inflow, this condition is luckily quite uncommon. Most patients with iliofemoral DVT present with acute onset of mild to moderate leg pain or discomfort, accompanied by swelling and edema. The standard of care for the diagnosis of lower extremity DVT is duplex ultrasonography because of its high degree of sensitivity and specificity, and many patients are diagnosed with this modality and started on anticoagulation alone without further imaging or interventional treatment.

CVD presents as a more indolent course. Patients have a range of clinical findings from telangectasia and varicose veins, edema, pigmentation and lipodermatosclerosis to venous ulcers. These typically localize to a "gaiter" distribution above the medial malleolus. The clinical, etiologic, anatomic and pathologic (CEAP) classification system defines the spectrum of CVD ranging from 0 with no visible disease to 6 with non-healing venous ulcers. The contribution of MTS to this disease process was previously thought to be minimal, but a paradigm shift has occurred with modern imaging and endovascular therapeutic options leading to heightened awareness of proximal venous obstruction.

DIAGNOSIS

As routine history, physical exam and standard imaging for CVD or acute DVT will not reveal MTS pathology, all patients with unilateral leg swelling and/or unilateral DVT should be considered for additional diagnostic imaging and interventional treatment, depending on the age of the patient, his or her functional capacity and other comorbidities. Since up to 50% of healthy patients have some evidence of compression of the iliac veins on axial imaging, screening for MTS is impractical, but this does not mean that the potential contribution of venous compression syndromes should be disregarded in those patients who develop leg swelling or DVT.

While axial imaging with CT or MRV can be highly sensitive for detecting venous compression syndromes, the static nature of these imaging modalities does not allow for assessment of the physiologic impact of the compression. The authors therefore favor the use of contrast venography, which can identify aberrations in normal of venous flow patterns, and IVUS, which can precisely pinpoint the degree and location of maximal compression. Venography in the AP view alone will demonstrate flattening and widening of the LCIV in MTS, but will fail to demonstrate actual narrowing of the vein in the majority of cases. While venography in the left anterior oblique and cranial caudal view can more accurately demonstrate this narrowing, the best technique for assessment of the degree of stenosis is IVUS, which can be used to assess both diameters and cross-sectional area. Despite the difficulties with demonstrating the venous narrowing on contrast venography, this imaging modality is invaluable in terms of identifying venous flow pattern derangements and collateralization, which is a sign of physiologically relevant chronic venous obstruction. On venographic assessment, it is important to note the degree of retroperitoneal collateralization and contralateral cross-filling to the right iliac venous system through hypogastric collaterals. In addition, contrast stagnation within the left iliac venous system represents a pathologic stenosis, and simultaneous contrast injections in both femoral veins can show asymmetry between the flow patterns in both iliac veins. Venographic and IVUS assessment of potential MTS patients typically requires only local anesthesia and can be accomplished with minimal risk on an outpatient basis.

TREATMENT

The treatment of MTS was previously in the realm of open surgical bypass procedures which carried high morbidity and mortality. Currently the treatment of choice is venography and IVUS guided endovascular stent placement. There is limited role for angioplasty alone as the venous system is highly compliant and recoil is certain.

The treatment of MTS must be preceded by a thorough history, physical, consideration of hypercoagulable states and appropriate diagnostic imaging. Since some degree of LCIV compression is present in many asymptomatic individuals, those that receive benefit from stent placement are patients with physiologically relevant compression and significant life limiting symptoms. Consideration of treating patients with mild leg swelling should be preceded by a trial period of compression stocking use. Compression stockings alone may eliminate the need for any procedure. Those that fail compression stocking use have undergone duplex ultrasound for DVT and venous insufficiency and continue to have life limiting symptoms should be referred for venography and IVUS imaging. In the setting of post thrombotic syndrome, repeat duplex imaging is essential to determine the extent of prior DVT and post-thrombotic venous luminal scarring, both of which can affect the decision regarding the location of the access site.

While diagnostic imaging is typically done under local anesthesia, we generally perform iliac vein stenting under conscious sedation because of the associated back pain that often accompanies stent implantation. Access depends on several factors, including whether the patient's presenting symptom is an acute DVT or nonthrombotic leg swelling. For patients with non-thrombotic leg swelling, an antegrade common femoral vein (CFV) puncture is appropriate, while those with a prior (or chronic) DVT that may have significant scarring of the CFV generally require puncture of the femoral vein in the proximal thigh in order to allow for extension of the stent more peripherally across the inguinal ligament if needed. Alternatively, the prone approach with popliteal venous access may be used, and this is typically the preferred access route for patients with acute iliofemoral DVT that will require lysis before stenting the MTS compression. Following initial access, patients with acute iliofemoral DVT are treated with lysis or pharmacomechanical thrombectomy, and once all acute thrombus has been treated the underlying venous compression syndrome is addressed.

Treatment of the venous compression syndrome begins with contrast venography, in which contrast stagnation, contralateral cross-filling to the right iliac venous circulation, and/or significant retroperitoneal collateralization suggests a physiologically significant stenosis is present. (Figure 22-1) On IVUS, the finding of a >50% stenosis with or without intravascular webs indicates a lesion that may benefit from stenting, particularly coupled with the above venography findings.

Additionally, IVUS is employed to determine the precise point of maximal compression and to guide size and location of stent placement. We typically use self-expanding stainless steel stents (WALLSTENT, Boston Scientific, Marlborough, MA), which are used to cover the area of maximal compression and any associated post-thrombotic scarring. Centrally, the stent must extend *into* the IVC for a distance of 1–2 cm, and peripherally to normal healthy vein, including the infrainguinal segment if necessary (Figure 22-1).

Stent diameter is based on IVUS measurement (utilizing the transverse diameter of the compressed vein as well as the proximal vein segment as a guide for stent selection). Large diameter stents should be used to achieve normal vein diameter (14–22 mm) in the common iliac and erring on the side of oversizing 10%–20%, with the most common stent diameters being 16–18 mm. Undersizing should be avoided as it can lead to stent migration. In addition, adequate stent overlap of at least 2 cm should be achieved without any skip areas. All diseased areas should be treated. At the completion of stent placement, repeat venogram and IVUS imaging should be performed to evaluate luminal gain and assess stent apposition to the vein wall. Post stent balloon angioplasty is performed to smooth out the stent wall and oppose overlying stent segments. Our group takes IVUS measurements to compare pre- and post-stenting cross-sectional area and diameter changes.

Chronic total occlusions can present a technical challenge, but even daunting initial venograms can prove to be straight-forward cases. The use of hydrophilic wires, angled support catheters, and long 5–6F sheaths are typically all that is needed for crossing long occlusions. Wire perforation of the vein in the occluded segment is generally without consequence, and can be withdrawn and advanced to a more appropriate intraluminal course. Once crossing into IVC is confirmed by IVUS or venography, the occluded segment is sequentially dilated up to diameters of 14–18 mm, and then stent implantation follows as described above.

Complications from the procedure are rare, and the most common issue perioperatively is back pain which can be managed by oral analgesics and muscle relaxants. Early stent thrombosis can occur, and when it does it generally results from inadequate lesion coverage, as it is important to adequately treat all flow limiting lesions. Puncture site hematomas are infrequent, but because many of these patients are on full anticoagulation and antiplatelet therapy they can occur.

Anticoagulation with heparin is performed intra-procedurally, with activated clotting times (ACT) of 250–300 achieved before stent implantation. Post-operatively, aspirin 81 mg daily and clopidigrel 75 mg daily is used for all stented patients for a period of three months, at which point we favor single antiplatelet therapy with aspirin alone. In patients with a history of hypercoagulable state or those treated with lysis for acute DVT before correction of the MTS lesions, appropriate systemic anticoagulation is continued according to national guidelines.

Post-intervention, patients are imaged with duplex US to confirm patency of the iliac venous system within 2 weeks. Their symptoms are re-assessed and most patients note significant clinical improvement shortly following the procedure. Repeat duplex ultrasound is performed at a 3-month follow-up appointment, then at yearly intervals thereafter.

OUTCOMES

Multiple large series of iliac vein stenting for MTS have been reported with excellent long-term outcomes. Overall, primary patency is higher in patients who present with nonthrombotic MTS (leg swelling) than in patients who present with MTS in association with DVT. An early series of 39 patients published series by O'Sullivan et al. in 2000 reported 87% technical success rate and 79% one year stent primary patency.[11] Of note, those patients that did not require pre-op thrombolysis had 100% primary patency and complete resolution of symptoms at 1 year. In other large series of 395 patients with combined obstruction and reflux, 3-year patency of limbs stented for primary MTS without thrombosis was 100%. In post-thrombotic patients, this rate dropped to 82%. In all comers, complete relief from pain (78%), swelling (36%) and healed ulcers (86%) was achieved at 3 years. Data from these retrospective studies was carried out to 5 years with satisfactory long-term results with 74% of patients having partial pain and swelling relief and 58% long-term ulcer healing rates. This is achieved with minimal morbidity and no mortality from these procedures.[5]

In our early recent series of 22 patients with MTS with or without thrombosis, 100% technical success was achieved. 94% of patients achieved symptom relief and 83% reduced their CEAP score. We achieved a reduction of pain and swelling by 80% and venous claudication by 100%. Primary patency in this group was 87.5% and secondary patency was 100%.[12]

CONCLUSIONS

May–Thurner syndrome is an important contributor to the development of chronic venous disease, acute iliofemoral DVT and post-thrombotic syndrome. This entity first described in 1908 has new relevance with the advent of axial imaging, angiography and endovascular surgery. With current technology, MTS can be diagnosed and treated in the outpatient setting with minimal risk. With proper patient selection based on clinical history, physiologically relevant venogram findings, and IVUS imaging, iliac venous compression can now be treated with endovascular stenting with an expectation of excellent long-term results. This disease process should be considered in all patients presenting with acute iliofemoral DVT or unilateral chronic venous disease.

REFERENCES

1. McMurrich JP. The occurrence of congenital adhesions in the common iliac veins and their relation to thrombosis of the femoral and iliac veins. *Am J M Sc.* 1908;135:342–6.
2. May R, Thurner J. The cause of the predominately sinistral occurrence of thrombosis of the pelvic veins. *Angiology.* 1957;8:419–27.
3. Negus D, Fletcher EW, Cockett FB, Thomas ML. Compression and band formation at the mouth of the left common iliac vein. *Br J Surg.* 1968;55:369–74.
4. Cockett FB, Thomas ML, Negus D. Iliac vein compression—its relation to iliofemoral thrombosis and the post-thrombotic syndrome. *Br Med J.* 1967; 2: 14–9.
5. Elson, JD, Becker, GJ. Vena caval and central venous stenoses: management with Palmaz balloon-expandable intraluminal stents. *J Vasc Intervent Radiol.* 1991 2(2), 215–23.
6. Wakefield TW, Dalsing MC. Venous Disease. In: Mulholland M, Lillemoe K, eds. *Greenfield's Surgery*, 5th ed. Philadelphia: Lippencott Williams and Williams; 2011. pp. 1785–6.
7. Patel, NH, Stookey, KR. Endovascular management of acute extensive iliofemoral deep venous thrombosis caused by May–Thurner syndrome. *J Vasc Intervent Radiol.* 2000;11(10):1297–302.
8. Raju S, Neglen P. High prevalence of non-thrombotic iliac vein lesions in chronic venous disease: a permissive role in pathogenicity. *J Vasc Surg.* 2006;44(1):136–43; discussion 144. PubMed PMID: 16828437.
9. Raju, S, Darcey, R. Unexpected major role for venous stenting in deep reflux disease. *J Vasc Surg.* 2010; 51(2):401–8; discussion 408.
10. Birn J, Vedantham S. May–Thurner syndrome and other obstructive iliac vein lesions: Meaning, myth, and mystery *Vasc Med.* 2015; 20:74–83, December 10, 2014.
11. O'Sullivan, G J, Semba, C P. Endovascular management of iliac vein compression (May–Thurner) syndrome. *J Vasc Intervent Radiol.* 2000;11(7): 823–36.
12. DeRubertis BG, Alktaifi A, Jimenez JC, et al. Endovascular management of nonmalignant iliocaval venous lesions. *Ann Vasc Surg.* 2013 Jul;27(5):577–86.

23

Diagnosis and Treatment of Pelvic Congestion Syndrome

Richard Pin, MD and David L. Gillespie, MD

Chronic pelvic pain, described as lower abdominal or pelvic discomfort lasting greater than 6 months, affects upwards of 10 million women in the United States and accounts for 10% to 15% of outpatient gynecologic visits.[1] Despite thorough evaluation, the etiology of chronic pelvic pain remains undiagnosed in a large proportion of these women. Over the past several years as scientific evidence has grown, pelvic congestion syndrome (PCS) has been considered a potential cause of chronic pelvic pain when more prevalent causes, such as endometriosis or pelvic adhesions, have been excluded. Pelvic congestion was first described by Richet in 1857 as a "tubo-ovarian varicocele" and later characterized by Taylor in 1949 as a clinical entity with congestion and hyperemia of the female reproductive system. PCS results from venous reflux of ovarian, gluteal, or periuterine veins. Associated clinical symptoms include dysmenorrhea, dyspareunia, and dysuria. Frequently perineal and vulvar varices are present. Patients typically present in the third to fifth decades of life and multiparity and family history are considered risk factors.

ANATOMIC CONSIDERATIONS

The veins of the pelvis drain into either the internal iliac veins or the ovarian veins. The internal iliac veins have parietal and visceral tributaries. The parietal tributaries include the superior and inferior gluteal, sciatic, sacral, ascending lumbar, and obturator veins. The visceral veins include the uterine and vesicovaginal plexus. Valves are infrequently found on the internal iliac vein or its tributaries, only present approximately 10% of the time.[2] The internal iliac vein joins the external iliac vein to form the common iliac vein that drains into the inferior vena cava (IVC). The ovarian veins provide drainage to the parametrium, cervix, mesosalpinx, and pampiniform plexus, which is the vast network of small veins that drain the ovaries (Figure 23-1). Typically,

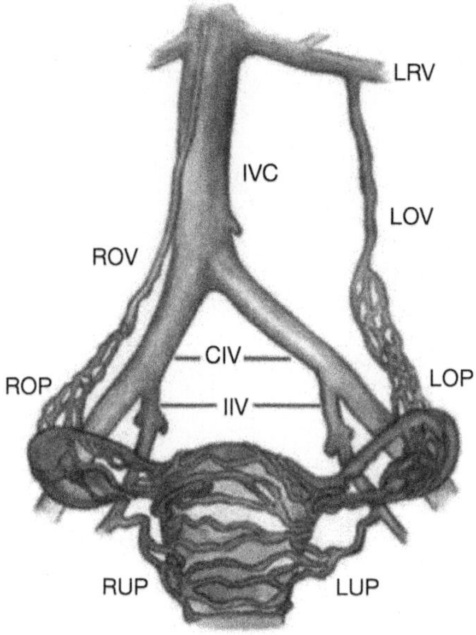

Figure 23-1. The ovarian veins provide drainage to the parametrium, cervix, mesosalpinx, and pampiniform plexus, which is the vast network of small veins that drain the ovaries.

the left ovarian vein drain into the left renal vein and the right ovarian vein drains into the IVC. In 10% of women however, the right ovarian vein drains into the right renal vein instead of the IVC. In contrast to the iliac veins, valves are present in the ovarian veins 80 to 90% of the time.[3] A normal ovarian vein measures less than 5mm in diameter. It is not uncommon though for reflux to occur in the ovarian veins and for the ovarian veins to enlarge without causing chronic pelvic pain or associated pelvic symptoms.[4] PCS is therefore a clinical diagnosis that is supported, but not defined, by anatomic or functional imaging criteria.

PATHOPHYSIOLOGY

Valvular reflux in the ovarian vein is considered to be the root cause of PCS.[5] During pregnancy, hormonal changes induce uterine growth and dilatation of ovarian and uterine veins, increasing vein capacity by 60%. This stress in turn can lead to valvular reflux and a higher rate of PCS in multiparous women. Obstruction of ovarian vein outflow can also produce reflux. A well-described phenomenon of left renal vein compression between the aorta and superior mesenteric artery, also known as nutcracker syndrome, leads to increased venous pressure in the left ovarian vein with subsequent valvular incompetence (Figure 23-2).[3] A pressure gradient develops in the left renal vein compared to the inferior vena cava, and in the non-compensated form can be measured during catheterization. Less common causes of reflux include a malpositioned, retroverted uterus with ovarian vein kinking, and May–Thurner syndrome with compression of the left common iliac vein between

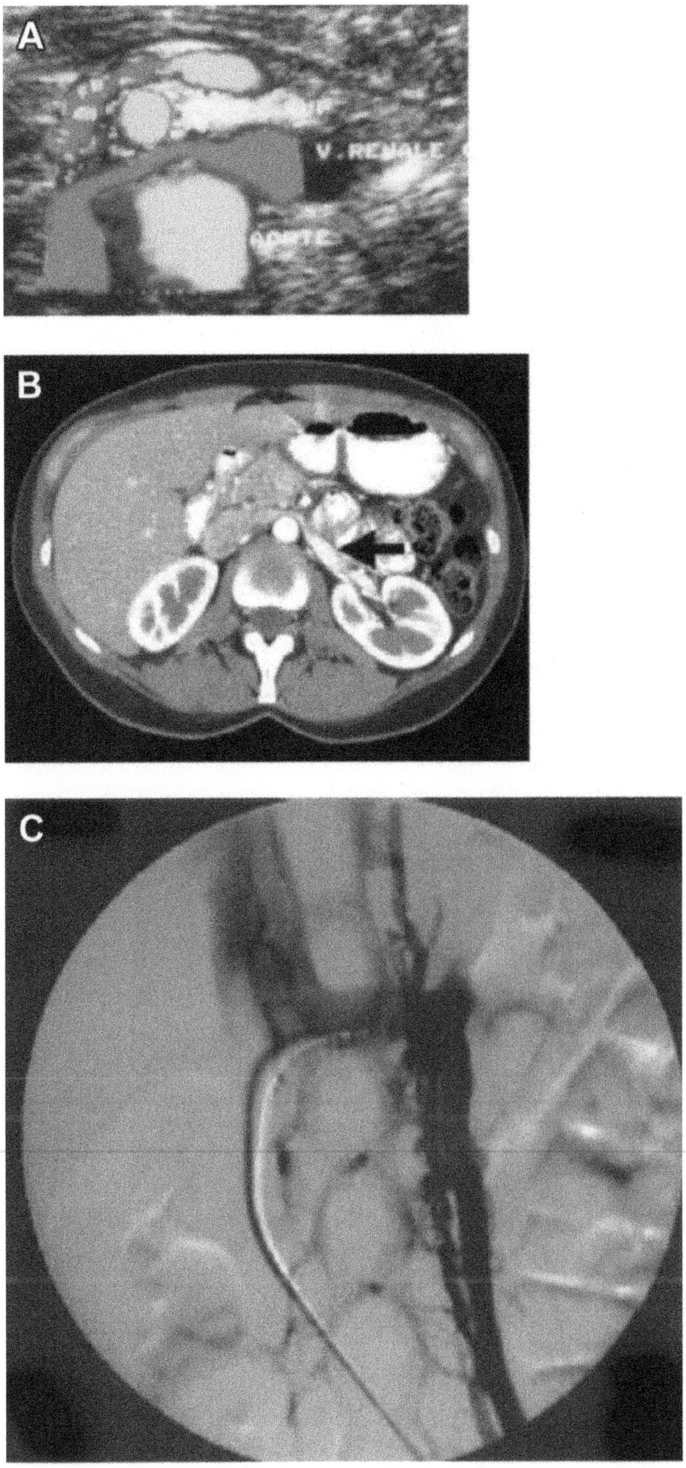

Figure 23-2. A well-described phenomenon of left renal vein compression between the aorta and superior mesenteric artery, also known as nutcracker syndrome, leads to increased venous pressure in the left ovarian vein with subsequent valvular incompetence.

the aorta and the spine resulting in increased pressure within the internal iliac vein and its tributaries. Regardless of the pathophysiology, the ovarian vein reflux leads to pelvic varicosities, cross-pelvic venous collaterals, and painful pelvic venous congestion.

PRESENTATION

Patients with PCS often present with chronic dull lower abdominal pain associated with dysuria and bladder irritability. Symptoms worsen towards the end of the day particularly with long periods of standing, and during the premenstrual period.[6] It is not uncommon for women to have pain during and after intercourse, non-specific gastrointestinal symptoms, and generalized lethargy and depression. Physical exam reveals vulvar and lower extremity varicosities, cervical motion tenderness, and point tenderness over the ovaries.[7] Hemorrhoids and buttock varicosities may be present as well. Patients with chronic pelvic pain are usually worked up for more common etiologies such as endometriosis, fibroids, and pelvic inflammatory disease before PCS is considered. As other causes of chronic pelvic pain are excluded, non-invasive imaging modalities can support the diagnosis of PCS.

DIAGNOSTIC STUDIES

Pelvic ultrasound can determine the diameter of the ovarian veins, antegrade or retrograde flow in the ovarian veins, and dilated tortuous arcuate veins in the myometrium. Ovarian veins are considered varicosed when their diameter is greater than 6mm. Ultrasound sensitivity for detection of dilatation in the left ovarian vein approaches 100%, and 67% in the right ovarian vein.[8] Imaging should be performed with the patient standing and with valsalva maneuvers to improve sensitivity. Stenosis or obstruction in the iliac veins, vena cava, and left renal vein can also be assessed with ultrasound. In cases where pelvic ultrasound is not diagnostic, magnetic resonance venography (MRV) or computed tomography venography (CTV) can provide a higher sensitivity for lower pelvic varices and can also provide more discerning information as to other pelvic structures that could be causing extrinsic compression. These modalities are limited however by their static nature and inability to provide directional blood flow information, and they are performed with the patient supine, which can underestimate the degree of pelvic collaterals and ovarian vein size. More recent advances in time-resolved MRV (TR-MRV) can determine antegrade or retrograde flow in the ovarian veins based on time-lapsed images for 1 to 3 minutes after contrast injection, and is likely the most accurate non-invasive test for pelvic venous reflux.[9] CTV and MRV may not be good modalities for follow-up studies after intervention as coils may cause significant scatter artifact.

The gold standard for diagnosis of pelvic reflux and PCS is venography. It is reserved for patients whose non-invasive testing has been equivocal or when percutaneous intervention is being contemplated. Approach through the femoral vein is common, although basilic and jugular vein approaches are also used. Bilateral internal iliac veins and ovarian veins should be selectively catheterized and evaluated in reverse Trendelenberg and with valsalva maneuvers.

TREATMENT

Various treatment options exist for PCS. Pharmacologic therapy consists of medications to suppress ovarian function or cause vasoconstriction of dilated veins. Medroxyprogesterone acetate (MPA) and the GnRH analogue goserelin have been used with modest effect.[10] Both essentially cause a chemical ovarian ligation and estrogen replacement therapy is frequently required. In addition, the results are transient with diminishing clinical response over time.

Psychotherapy is many times co-administered with pharmacotherapy to improve long-term effects as there is a close relationship between psychological and somatic factors in chronic pelvic pain arising from PCS.[11] Side effects of MPA and goserelin are frequent and consist of bloating, weight gain, night sweats, vaginal dryness, mood changes, and decreased fertility. With these prominent side effects and limited efficacy, medical therapy is not considered optimal for the long-term treatment of PCS.

Percutaneous endovascular intervention is considered first line treatment of PCS due to ovarian and pelvic vein incompetence.[6] Right femoral vein or jugular vein access is the most common approach. A sheath is brought into the vena cava and the left renal and left ovarian veins are catheterized, as well as the right ovarian vein. A Cobra 2 catheter usually makes for efficient left renal vein catheterization and a Simmons 2 catheter works well for engaging the right renal vein. Bilateral internal iliac veins are also catheterized and evaluated. Venograms are performed with the patient in reverse Trendelenberg and with Valsalva maneuvers. Incompetent ovarian veins demonstrate reflux of contrast and dilatation (Figure 23-3). In addition, cross-pelvic collaterals and thigh and vulvar varicosities may also be demonstrated. Treatment for ovarian vein reflux can then be performed with embolization techniques. Thrombogenic coils or plugs may be used to occlude the ovarian vein or hypogastric veins.[12] In addition, thrombogenic particles or sclerosants can be delivered more distally into hypogastic vein branches.[13] The decision to treat one or both ovarian veins is determined by the anatomy of the pelvic reflux. Certainly, if venous reflux is demonstrated in bilateral ovarian veins and symptoms are severe, both ovarian veins should be occluded. However, if reflux is clearly limited to one ovarian vein, or if symptoms seem unilateral and the ipsilateral ovarian vein is dilated, then only one ovarian vein may need to be embolized. Clinical judgment and experience should guide the physician in these circumstances. Potential complications of embolization include coil or plug migration into the pulmonary system.[14] This risk is higher in larger caliber veins (>12mm). To mitigate this complication, coil diameters should be oversized 30% greater than the diameter of the vein. Other potential complications include venous perforation and venous access site hematoma.

Surgical treatment for PCS can provide symptomatic relief in acceptable surgical candidates who fail endovascular therapy. Open extraperitoneal resection of the ovarian vein can be accomplished through an abdominal or flank incision with good relief of chronic pelvic pain and low morbidity.[15] Likewise laparoscopic transperitoneal ovarian vein resection has been described, but experience has been anecdotal, and

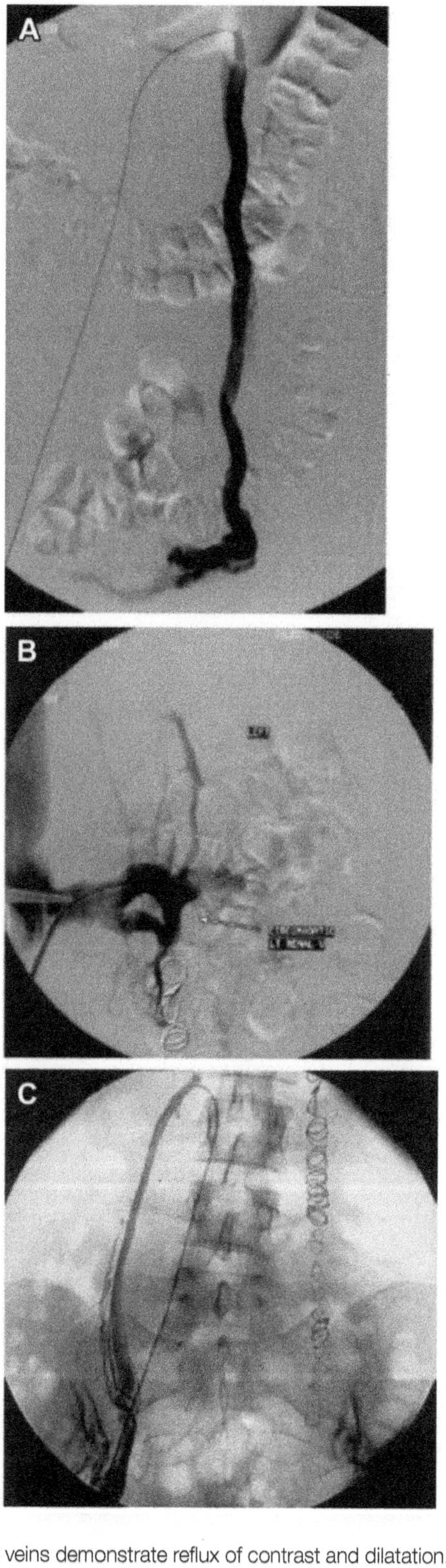

Figure 23-3. Incompetent ovarian veins demonstrate reflux of contrast and dilatation.

insufflation of the peritoneal cavity itself effaces and compresses venous structures underestimating the size of varices.[16]

VENOUS OBSTRUCTION

There are two obstructive causes of PCS: nutcracker syndrome and May–Thurner syndrome. Nutcracker syndrome occurs when the left renal vein is compressed as it crosses between the aorta and superior mesenteric artery. Many times a "bird's beak" type appearance will be visualized in the renal vein, and a ratio of diameter between the dilated and stenotic portion of the vein is 5 to 1 or greater.[17] Diagnosis with pressure gradients across the area of stenosis often is unreliable as the syndrome can be compensated or non-compensated. The normal gradient between the IVC and left renal vein is less than 1 mmHg and in those with non-compensated renal vein hypertension it is greater than 3 mmHg.[3] In those patients with renal vein hypertension, the pressure gradient may be an effective tool to measure the adequacy of treatment, which from a percutaneous standpoint would involve stenting the left renal vein. This option is quite feasible in any patient who can undergo venogram as it is usually performed percutaneously at the time of angiographic diagnosis. The main complication of left renal vein stenting is migration of the stent into the right atrium.[18] To limit this occurrence, the stent should be oversized 20% and stent length should be optimized so that there is an adequate length of contact between the external stent wall and the left renal vein endothelium. Open surgical options also exist and include transposition of the renal vein,[19] transposition of the superior mesenteric artery,[20] or ovarian vein to inferior mesenteric vein bypass.[21] These procedures are usually limited to patients who have failed percutaneous stenting, or young healthy patients with severe symptoms who wish a durable surgical result. When the left renal vein crosses posterior to the aorta and compression occurs between the aorta and vertebra (posterior nutcracker syndrome), open surgical transposition of the left renal vein, as opposed to percutaneous stenting, may be a preferred initial treatment option in healthy patients. In patients with PCS related to May–Thurner syndrome, the left common iliac vein is compressed between the right common iliac artery anteriorly and vertebra posteriorly. Such extrinsic compression may not be well visualized with two dimensional contrast-based imaging. Instead, using intravascular ultrasound (IVUS) in this situation provides cross-sectional detail allowing for visualization of venous stenosis in a different plane. IVUS can then be used to guide treatment of May–Thurner syndrome with iliocaval stenting.[22]

CONCLUSION

Although it accounts for as many as 30% of outpatient gynecologic visits for chronic pelvic pain, PCS is a frequently underdiagnosed etiology. Many times it is a diagnosis of exclusion after other etiologies such as endometriosis or fibroids have been excluded. Corresponding symptoms include dyspareunia, dysuria, and vulvar varicosities. Diagnosis involves transvaginal or transabdominal ultrasound to assess for dilated and refluxing ovarian and pelvic veins. Other imaging modalities include

CTV and MRV. Formal venogram is the gold standard and percutaneous intervention can be performed at the same setting. Percutaneous options include embolization of refluxing ovarian or hypogastric veins as well as stenting of the left renal vein in the context of nutcracker syndrome, and stenting of the left common iliac vein in the setting of May–Thurner syndrome. Significant reduction in chronic pelvic pain can be achieved in 70%–85% of patient with a percutaneous approach. Open surgery is typically reserved for patients who fail endovenous therapy and for those who are an acceptable surgical risk.

REFERENCES

1. Ignacio EA, Dua R, Sarin S, et al. Pelvic congestion syndrome: diagnosis and treatment. *Semin Intervent Radiol.* 2008;25:361–8.
2. Ahlberg NE, Bartley O, Chidekel N. Right and left gonadal veins. An anatomical and statistical study. *Acta Radiol Diagn (Stockh).* 1966;4:593–601.
3. Kurklinsky AK, Rooke TW. Nutcracker phenomenon and nutcracker syndrome. *Mayo Clin Proc.* 2010;85:552–9.
4. Rozenblit AM, Ricci ZJ, Tuvia J, Amis ES, Jr. Incompetent and dilated ovarian veins: a common CT finding in asymptomatic parous women. *AJR Am J Roentgenol.* 2001;176:119–22.
5. Scultetus AH, Villavicencio JL, Gillespie DL, et al. The pelvic venous syndromes: analysis of our experience with 57 patients. *J Vasc Surg.* 2002;36:881–8.
6. O'Brien MT, Gillespie DL. Diagnosis and treatment of the pelvic congestion syndrome. *J Vasc Surg.* 2014; 5:96–106.
7. Beard RW, Kennedy RG, Gangar KF, et al. Bilateral oophorectomy and hysterectomy in the treatment of intractable pelvic pain associated with pelvic congestion. *Br J Obstet Gynaecol.* 1991 98(10):988–92.
8. Malgor RD, Labropoulos N. Diagnosis of venous disease with duplex ultrasound. *Phlebology.* 2013;28:158–61.
9. Yang DM, Kim HC, Nam DH, et al. Time-resolved MR angiography for detecting and grading ovarian venous reflux: comparison with conventional venography. *Br J Radiol.* 2012;85:e117–e122.
10. Farquhar CM, Rogers V, Franks S, et al. A randomized controlled trial of medroxyprogesterone acetate and psychotherapy for the treatment of pelvic congestion. *Br J Obstet Gynaecol.* 1989;96:1153–62.
11. Champaneria R, Daniels JP, Raza A, et al. Psychological therapies for chronic pelvic pain: systematic review of randomized controlled trials. *Acta Obstet Gynecol Scand.* 2012;91:281–6.
12. Meneses L, Fava M, Diaz P, et al. Embolization of incompetent pelvic veins for the treatment of recurrent varicose veins in lower limbs and pelvic congestion syndrome. *Cardiovasc Intervent Radiol.* 2013;36:128–32.
13. Sichlau MJ, Yao JS, Vogelzang RL. Transcatheter embolotherapy for the treatment of pelvic congestion syndrome. *Obstet Gynecol.* 1994;83:892–6.
14. Yamasaki W, Kakizawa H, Ishikawa M, et al. Migration to the pulmonary artery of nine metallic coils placed in the internal iliac vein for treatment of giant rectal varices. *Acta Radiol Short Rep.* 2012;1(6).
15. Rundqvist E, Sandholm LE, Larsson G. Treatment of pelvic varicosities causing lower abdominal pain with extraperitoneal resection of the left ovarian vein. *Ann Chir Gynaecol.* 1984;73:339–41.
16. Gargiulo T, Mais V, Brokaj L, et al. Bilateral laparoscopic transperitoneal ligation of ovarian veins for treatment of pelvic congestion syndrome. *J Am Assoc Gynecol Laparosc.* 2003;10:501–4.

17. Kim KW, Cho JY, Kim SH, et al. Diagnostic value of computed tomographic findings of nutcracker syndrome: correlation with renal venography and renocaval pressure gradients. *Eur J Radiol.* 2011;80:648–54.
18. Liu Y, Sun Y, Wu XJ, et al. Endovascular stent placement for the treatment of nutcracker syndrome. *Int Urol Nephrol.* 2012;44:1097–100.
19. Salehipour M, Khezri A, Rasekhi A, Zand F. Left renal vein transposition for treatment of the nutcracker syndrome. *Arch Iran Med.* 2006;9:161–2.
20. Thompson PN, Darling RC 3rd, Chang BB, et al. A case of nutcracker syndrome: treatment by mesoaortic transposition. *J Vasc Surg.* 1992;16:663–5.
21. Xu D, Gao Y, Chen J, et al. Laparoscopic inferior mesenteric–gonadal vein bypass for the treatment of nutcracker syndrome. *J Vasc Surg.* 2013;57:1429–31.
22. Xzabia CA, Clark AL, Doyle AJ, et al. The incidence of contralateral iliac venous thrombosis after stenting across the iliocaval confluence in patients with acute or chronic venous outflow obstruction. *J Vasc Surg.* 2014;3:253–9.

24

Nutcracker Syndrome: Current Trends in Diagnosis and Treatment

John V. White, MD, Connie Ryjewski, APN, Jennifer Grant, MD, and Lewis B. Schwartz, MD

As Chairman of the Department of Anatomy at the University of Toronto from 1930 to 1965, Dr. John Charles Grant performed countless anatomical dissections, had specimens collected for illustration, and from these created Grant's Atlas of Anatomy. Among his seminal observations was compression of the left renal vein between the superior mesenteric artery (SMA) and the abdominal aorta. His initial report, published in 1937, was the first description of the anatomic relationship of these three structures.[1] It was not, however, until 1950 that the physiologic significance of left renal vein compression between the SMA and aorta was noted by El Sadr and Mina as they evaluated the surgical treatment of varicocoele.[2] Despite these early efforts, Nutcracker Syndrome has remained somewhat enigmatic, with little additional evidence to identify those with the Syndrome and indications for treatment.

Nutcracker phenomenon is defined as the presence of compression of the left renal vein between the superior mesenteric artery and the abdominal aorta as seen on axial imaging studies in the absence of symptoms. This form of **anterior compression** is a common finding on CT scan and has been noted in more than 20% of patients without associated symptoms[3] (Figure 24-1A,B). **Posterior compression** in which a retroaortic left renal vein is compressed between the aorta and the vertebral bodies or in which a circumaortic left renal vein is compressed are less common anatomic abnormalities that may cause Nutcracker phenomenon (Figures 24-2A,B and 24-3). Nutcracker Syndrome is the constellation of symptoms generated by restriction of venous outflow through the left renal vein and its manifestations are similar in all forms of compression. Although the prevalence has not been clearly defined, the syndrome is far less common than the phenomenon of renal vein compression. The anatomic relationship between the superior mesenteric artery, the left renal vein, and the aorta is likely present at birth. The factors that cause conversion

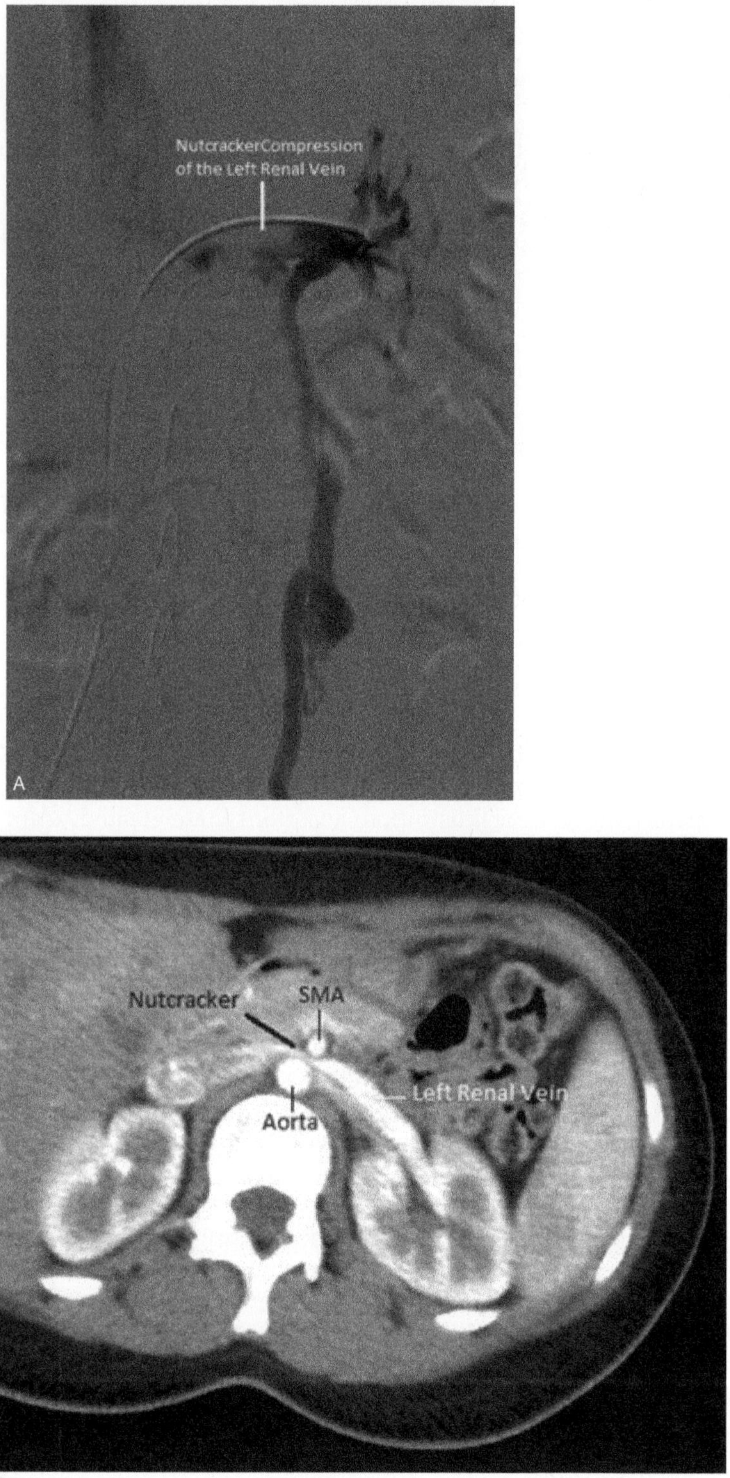

Figure 24-1. Anterior compression of the left renal vein. (A) Venographic appearance of compression. (B) CT confirmation of compression.

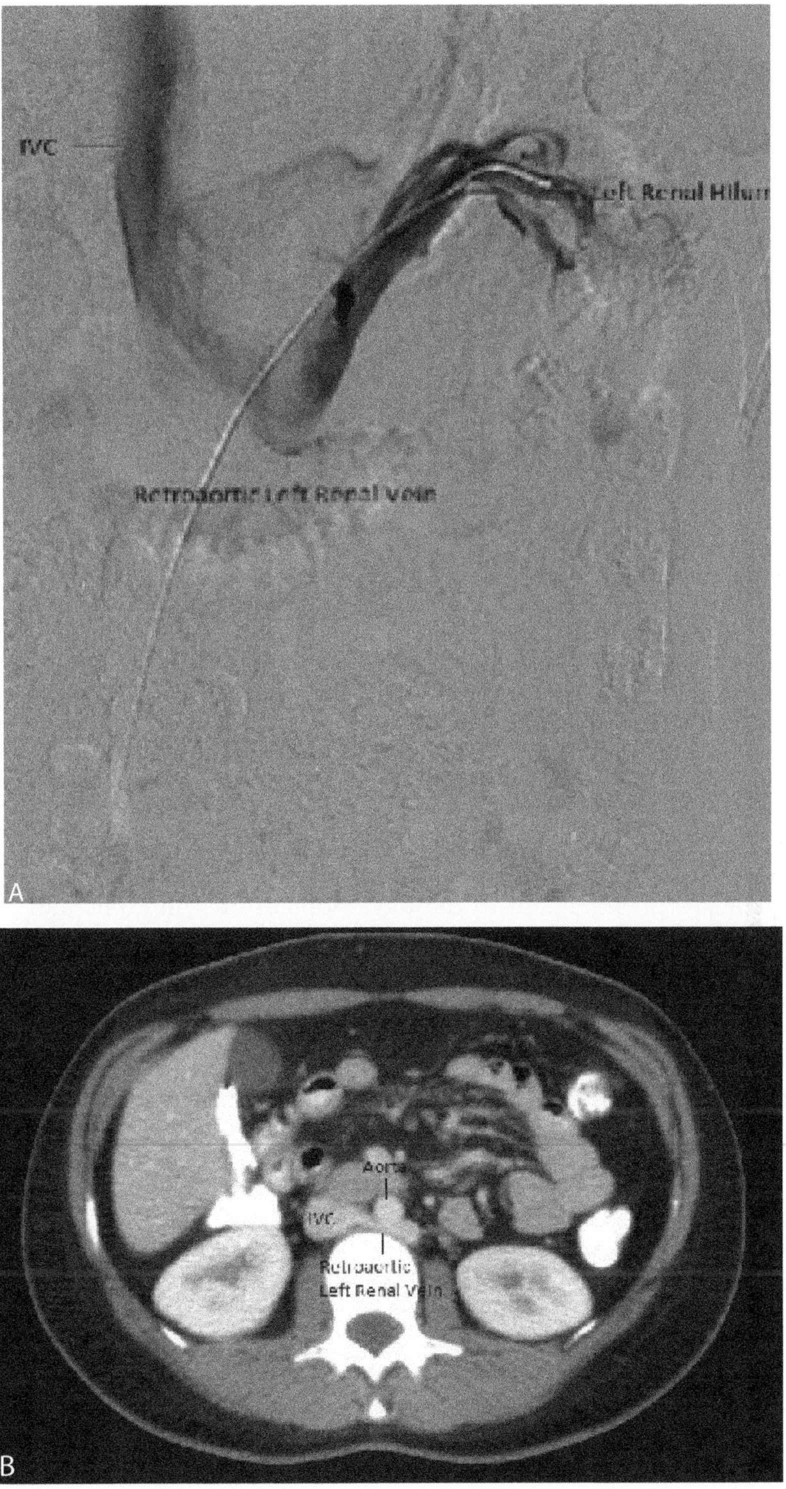

Figure 24-2. Posterior Compression of a retroaortic left renal vein. (A) Venographic appearance of a retroaortic renal vein. (B) CT confirmation of a retroaortic left renal vein with compression by the aorta.

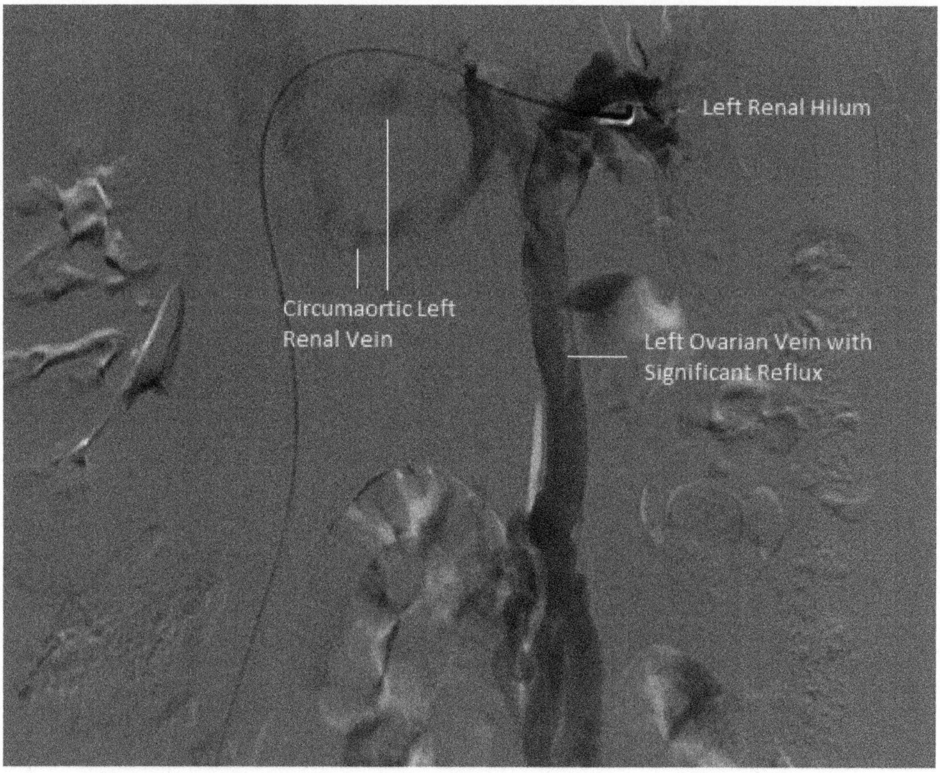

Figure 24-3. Compression of a circumaortic left renal vein.

from Nutcracker phenomenon to the development of symptoms and Nutcracker Syndrome have not yet been identified.

PATHOPHYSIOLOGY AND SYMPTOMS

The symptoms of Nutcracker Syndrome stem from both the compression of the left renal vein and the adaptive response to this compression. The normal course of the left renal vein as it extends from the renal hilum to the inferior vena cava is to pass anteriorly over the abdominal aorta at a level that is 0.5–2 cm distal to the origin of the superior mesenteric artery. The SMA usually originates at an angle of 45° or greater from the aorta. As the artery continues distally, it creates a space for the left renal vein that is often cushioned with a fat pad anteriorly (Figure 24-4A). This protected environment permits the rapid movement of venous blood from the kidney to the inferior vena cava. Left renal vein drainage usually requires less than a 1 mm Hg gradient to move blood swiftly from the left renal hilum into the IVC.[4] Indeed, renal parenchymal function is based upon a high flow, low pressure venous system that is capable of processing more than 10–20% of the cardiac output at any given time.

The anatomic changes that must occur to cause left renal vein compression are unclear but several have been identified. Origination of the superior mesenteric artery

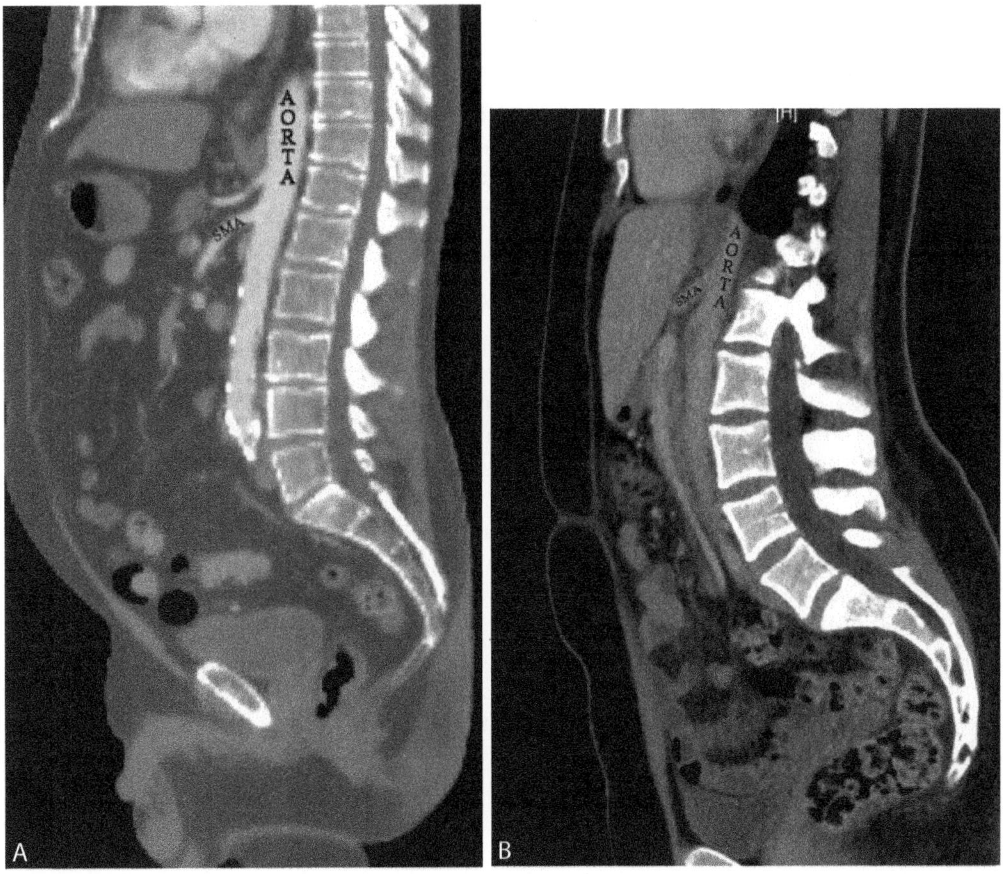

Figure 24-4. CT anatomy of the mesoaortic angle. (A) Normally, the superior mesenteric artery separates from the aorta at an angle of 45° or greater, leaving a space for the left renal vein. (B) In the setting of a very narrow angle of less than 20° compression of the left renal vein may occur.

at an acute angle from the aorta can cause this vessel to press the left renal vein against the aorta thereby obstructing venous flow (Figure 24-4B). It has also been suggested that a high left renal vein may abut the superior mesenteric artery at its origin causing compression. Finally, ptosis of the left kidney stretching the left renal vein over the aorta may also cause venous compression and inhibition of venous return from the left kidney. Compression may worsen when the patient is upright because of the downward pull on the superior mesenteric artery by the intestines, decreasing the space between this vessel and the aorta. The severity of the compression and the degree of luminal reduction of the left renal vein needed to cause symptoms have not, as yet, been quantified. It is also unclear as to whether such compression of the left renal vein is constant or intermittent.

Inhibition of venous outflow from the left renal vein will cause a rise in intraparenchymal venous pressures leading rupture of the small venules adjacent to the tubules causing focal edema and hematuria.[5] The parenchymal edema is likely the cause left flank pain often reported as an intermittent of constant aching discomfort. The hematuria is usually intermittent and may be micro or macroscopic. These are the two most common presenting symptoms of Nutcracker Syndrome.

The adaptive response to venous compression is often the source of secondary symptoms of Nutcracker Syndrome. The chronic elevation in left renal venous pressure initiates the development of alternate routes of venous outflow. The alternate pathways arise from the tributaries of the left renal vein, including the suprarenal vein comprised of the inferior phrenic and the adrenal veins, the lumbar vein which connects to the ascending lumbar and hemiazygous veins, and the gonadal vein. These tributaries are generally significantly smaller in diameter than the left renal vein but are capable of enlarging to carry renal venous outflow. Of these, the left gonadal vein is the most common alternate venous drainage pathway. As the vein diameter increases in response to rising left renal venous pressures, the single valve is rendered incompetent and reflux is initiated. In males this reflux generally presents as a varicocoele within the first 2 decades of life. Beyond the childhood years, there seems to be a preponderance of women who manifest Nutcracker Syndrome. With incompetence of the ovarian vein valve, flow is directed from the left renal vein to the pelvis. As reflux through the ovarian vein increases, blood is forced into the left peri-ovarian pampiniform plexus and perimetrial veins. These veins may become quite engorged causing women to experience a shift in discomfort from the left flank to the left pelvis due to pelvic venous congestion.[6] The symptoms of pelvic congestion syndrome, including constant aching in the left lower quadrant of the abdomen in the area of the left ovary, worsening menstrual discomfort, menorrhagia, and dyspareunia, have all been reported in association with Nutcracker Syndrome. As a greater proportion of the left renal venous outflow is diverted through the left ovarian vein into the pelvis, lower abdominal symptoms increase in both severity and duration.

Finally, although reflux into left renal venous tributaries may be the source of additional discomfort, it may also be the reason that left renal vein thrombosis is rare in Nutcracker Syndrome. This fact distinguishes it from the two other major venous compression syndromes, Thoracic Outlet and May-Thurner Syndromes, both of which have limited venous outflow from the compressed segment and have a recognized risk of major venous thrombosis.

DIAGNOSIS

The major challenge to the timely diagnosis of Nutcracker Syndrome is clinical suspicion. The subtlety and often nonspecific nature of the symptoms, such as left flank pain and microscopic hematuria, frequently delay consideration of this clinical problem. Patients with a history of left flank pain, intermittent hematuria, and the development of pelvic pain should undergo renal evaluation and evaluation for extrinsic compression of the left renal vein by pancreatic masses, aneurysms, para-aortic lymphadenopathy or other retroperitoneal mass lesions. If a cause of patient symptoms is not determined, then evaluation for Nutcracker Syndrome should be considered. Once the diagnosis is suspected, there are few standards by which confirmatory can be interpreted.

A combination of axial and physiologic imaging studies is preferred to establish the diagnosis of Nutcracker Syndrome. Ultrasound has been recommended as an initial imaging study to evaluate the left renal vein. Color duplex imaging, preferably performed on the fasting patient, should include both the left renal vein and its major tributaries. Performance of the study with the patient in the upright position may serve to exaggerate findings of left renal vein diameter and peak systolic velocity measurements medial and lateral to the point of compression. Peak systolic velocity ratios within the left renal vein medial and lateral to the point of superior mesenteric artery compression are most commonly recommended but there is little agreement on the threshold levels. A PSV ratio of greater than 4.7 in children has been reported as having a sensitivity of 100% and a specificity of 90%.[7] Using a threshold PSV ratio in the adult of greater than 4 is associated with a sensitivity of 69%–90% and a specificity of 89%–100%.[8] Unfortunately, most of these studies involve only small numbers of patients, usually children with hematuria, preventing their broad applicability to adult women. There are also several factors that limit the precise performance of the test, including patient habitus, bowel gas, and renal abnormalities, thereby reducing the value of this modality for the diagnosis of Nutcracker Syndrome in the adult.

Contrast enhanced CT or MRI axial imaging provides a clear assessment of the left renal vein and its relationship to the superior mesenteric artery and the aorta (Figures 24-1B and 24-4A,B). The axial images permit the direct evaluation of the left renal vein as it crosses over the aorta. In patients in whom there is complete obstruction of the left renal vein under the superior mesenteric artery, the diagnosis is easily made.[9] However, there are no specific standards for establishing the presence of a hemodynamically significant narrowing of the left renal vein.[10] Some authors have reported that calculation of the aortomesenteric angle is of value in determining clinically relevant compression of the vein, with most symptomatic patients having an angle less than 30°.[9,10] While a severely acute angle is consistent with compression of the left renal vein, it is not sufficient to establish the diagnosis. Magnetic resonance imaging offers the same degree of information and the same interpretive challenges.

Contrast venography remains one of the most useful tests for confirming the presence and clinical significance of nutcracker phenomenon. It can determine the pathways of venous outflow from the left kidney and restriction of venous flow in the area of the superior mesenteric artery. Many authors suggest that a pressure gradient of 3 mm Hg or more between the renal vein lateral to the superior mesenteric artery and the inferior vena cava at the level of the renal vein is diagnostic. While this does indicate some compromise of venous flow through the left renal vein, this value can be misleading.[11]

It is our preference, in all patients in whom Nutcracker Syndrome is suspected, to obtain a CT scan of the abdomen with intravenous contrast only to assess the configuration of the left renal vein and the aortomesenteric angle. If findings suggest severe compression of the left renal vein, we subsequently obtain contrast venography of the renal veins, the inferior vena cava, and the iliac venous system bilaterally to fully evaluate the flow patterns of the major veins of the abdomen and pelvis. We believe that Nutcracker phenomenon represents a venous flow disorder and establish the diagnosis on the basis of the pattern of venous outflow from the left kidney. Venous flow should be directed from smaller veins to larger veins in the cephalad direction. We perform venography with the patient in 20° reverse Trendelenburg position with low pressure hand injections of contrast into the various target vessels. Therefore, if on low pressure injection of contrast into the left renal vein, flow carries it into the suprarenal vein, the ovarian vein, and/or the lumbar vein, then there is likely a hemodynamically significant restriction of renal venous outflow caused by the superior mesenteric artery. While gradients may be helpful in the early stages of Nutcracker phenomenon, the pressure within the hilar portion of the left renal vein may decrease to near normal levels as flow into the ovarian vein and other collateral veins increases. If a patient has symptoms consistent with Nutcracker Syndrome, has significant compression of the left renal vein on CT scan associated with a narrow aortomesenteric angle, and venographic evidence of a left renal venous flow disorder with a majority of venous drainage from the left kidney directed into venous collaterals, then intervention is considered.

TREATMENT

While there is little consistency regarding the indication for treatment of those with Nutcracker Syndrome, our goal for intervention is improvement in quality of life through resolution of left flank and/or pelvic pain. Therefore, a treatment program that eliminates these major presenting symptoms should be developed for each patient. In many cases, improvement in left renal vein drainage alone may not reduce or eliminate pelvic pain due to reflux through a large incompetent left ovarian vein. In such patients, both may need to be treated. Numerous treatments have been developed to accomplish these goals. Endovascular approaches with left renal vein stenting and/or coiling of the left ovarian vein have been used successfully in addition to minimally invasive and open surgical procedures developed to improve left renal vein drainage and reduce reflux into the pelvis (Table 24-1). While each may be effective, each of these therapies requires careful patient selection.

The most common surgical approach currently employed is open left renal vein transposition.[12] This procedure improves left renal vein drainage by slightly altering the course of the left renal vein so that it enters the inferior vena cava 2–3 cm more distally (Figure 24-5A,B). While the procedure has been performed using advanced minimally invasive techniques, it is most often performed through a midline incision.[13] The procedure requires isolation and mobilization of the left

TABLE 24-1 TREATMENT OPTIONS FOR NUTCRACKER SYNDROME

Surgical Options

- Transposition of the left renal vein
- Patch venoplasty of the left renal vein
- Left renocaval bypass with saphenous vein
- Transposition of the left gonadal vein to the IVC
- Inferior mesenteric vein – gonadal vein bypass
- Splenorenal bypass
- Transpostion of the superior mesenteric artery
- Transposition of the left ovarian vein to the left external iliac vein

Endovascular Options

- Stenting of the left renal vein
- Coil occlusion of the left ovarian vein

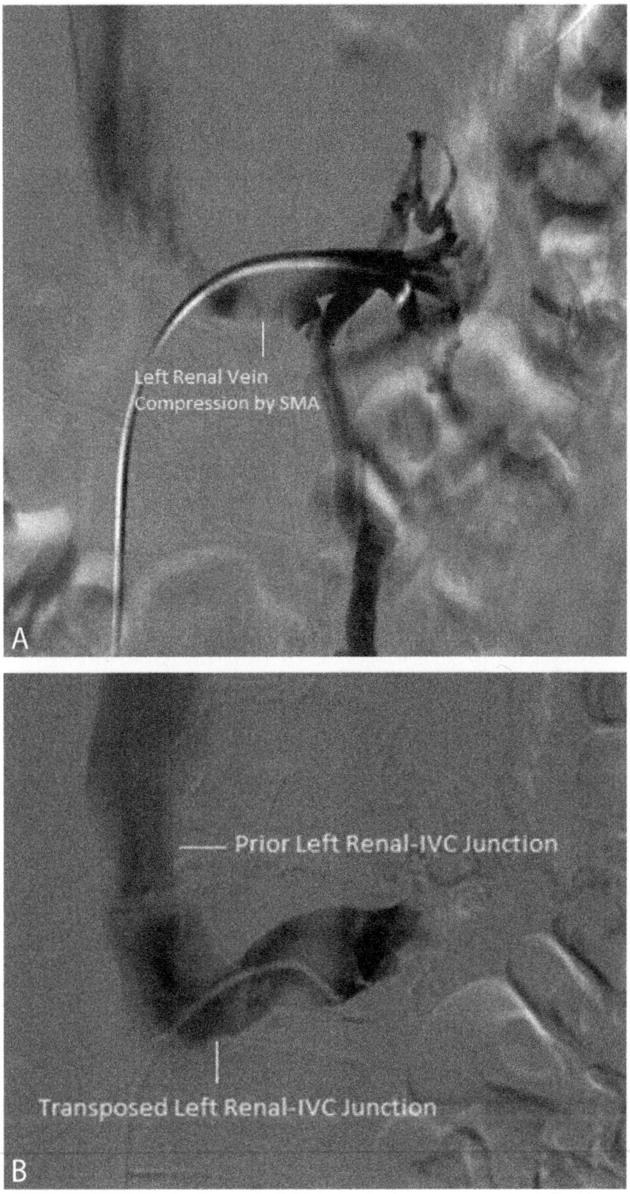

Figure 24-5. Before and after appearance of the left renal vein after transposition. (A) the left renal vein has a horizontal course from the hilum to the inferior vena cava with compression by the superior mesenteric artery evident in the midportion. (B) The angled course of the left renal vein after transposition to a site on the more distal inferior vena cava. Note that the compression has been eliminated.

renal vein by ligating and dividing its venous tributaries including the suprarenal vein superiorly and the lumbar and ovarian veins posteriorly. Once the left renal vein is isolated and free, heparin is administered intravenously, the renal vein is clamped in its hilar segment, the inferior vena cava is partially occluded with a side-biting clamp, and then the renal vein is removed with a small cuff from the

IVC. The inferior vena caval venotomy is primarily repaired. The left renal vein is then brought distally 2-3 cm and reattached to the IVC with an end-to-side anastomosis. We use a continuous suture posteriorly and interrupted sutures anteriorly to reduce the likelihood of stenosis. Care must be taken to avoid tension on the vein by forcefully stretching it to a too distal location on the inferior vena cava. A cuff of saphenous vein can be used to provide a small extension of the renal vein to reduce tension on the anastomosis.

Left renal vein transposition to the more distal IVC has the advantage of preserving direct left renal venous drainage into the IVC. The disadvantages are many, including the need for open abdominal surgery in a relatively young patient population and the risks of subsequent complications, such as stenosis of the anastomosis and late intestinal obstruction.

Alternative surgical approaches have been developed to reduce the risks associated with mobilization of the left renal vein and the inferior vena cava. Several of these have been performed using minimally invasive technique. The left ovarian vein has been transposed to other major abdominal veins to successfully reduce left renal vein pressures and reduce pelvic venous flow abnormalities.[14] The ovarian vein has been transposed to the inferior vena cava, the inferior mesenteric vein[15], and to the splenic vein[16]. When transposition or bypass to reduce left renal venous pressure are not possible, left renal venoplasty may be useful.[17] Each of these procedures is significantly complex and requires that the ovarian vein and other major veins be mobilized and their courses altered to accommodate the anastomosis. Nonetheless, if well performed, each of these procedures should promote improved drainage of the left renal vein.

It is our current preference, when treating women with Nutcracker Syndrome, especially those with pelvic congestion syndrome, to transpose the dilated left ovarian vein to the left external iliac vein and ligate pelvic varicosities using minimally invasive techniques.[18] This procedure differs from other surgical treatments largely in its simplicity. Women, especially those who are multiparous, often have dilated ovarian veins more than 5 mm in diameters. Since the left ovarian vein normally crosses over the left external iliac vein, very little dissection needs to be performed. By placing the patient in the right lateral decubitus position, both the left ovarian vein and external iliac veins can be exposed through a small incision. The anastomosis can be created with minimal mobilization of either the external iliac or ovarian veins (Figure 24-6). The construction of the ovarian-iliac vein anastomosis directs left renal venous flow into the left external iliac vein which is a high capacitance vein, reducing left renal vein pressures and the flow through other, smaller venous tributaries. Since left renal venous flow has already been directed down the ovarian vein, no additional alterations in flow patterns need to occur. The driving pressure to drain the left renal vein has already been established. By eliminating the reflux of blood into the pampiniform plexus of the ovary and into the myometrial uterine veins, pelvic pain resolves as does the menorrhagia that often accompanies pelvic congestion syndrome.

Endovascular stent placement has also been shown to be an effective method of improving left renal venous drainage although it does not relieve the direct compression of the anterior surface of the left renal vein.[19] The procedure, although simple in concept, can be technically challenging. Because the diameter of the left

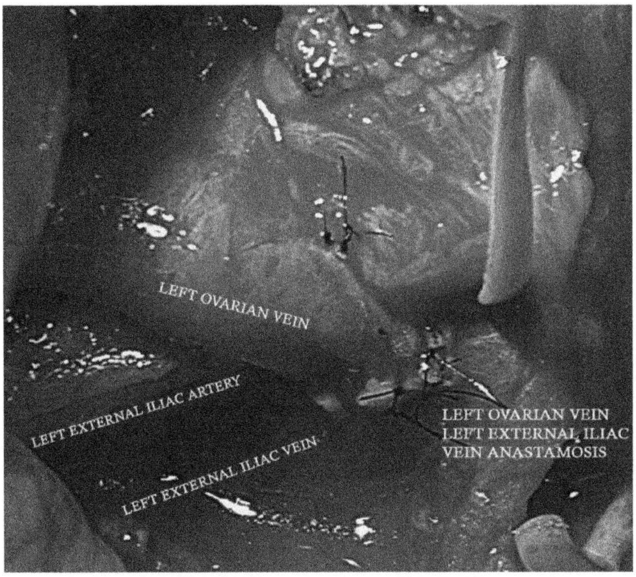

Figure 24-6. Transposition of the left ovarian vein to the left external iliac vein. The normal course of the left ovarian vein traverses the left external iliac vein so that little dissection is required for construction of the anastomosis.

renal vein, especially within the area of compression between the SMA and aorta, is difficult to measure, stent size is often difficult to determine. The compression of the renal vein during stent placement creates problems in achieving the appropriate position of the stent in the left renal vein so that it spans the area of compression but has the necessary proximal and distal extension to prevent dislodgment. A well placed stent is able to open the left renal vein within the mesoaortic space (Figure 24-7A,B). This should immediately improve venous outflow through the left renal vein to the inferior vena cava, manifesting with a spontaneous and significant reduction in flow through the collateral veins, such as the suprarenal and ovarian tributaries, on hand injection of contrast after stent placement (Figure 24-8A,B).

The continued cycles of compression and decompression of indeterminate length of the renal vein-stent complex may induce stent migration in 5% or more of the patients, at times creating a more critical problem than nutcracker syndrome[20–23] (Figure 24-9). Therefore, it is our preference to place a removable filter just above the level of the left renal vein stent to reduce the risks of uncontrolled stent migration (Figure 24-8A). The filter is removed 3 months after stent placement if the stent position has remained unchanged. While an endovascular approach has the advantage of avoiding open surgery and its long term attendant risks, it is difficult to imagine that the stent will remain patent and functional for the 7 to 8 decades of life many of these patients will have.

Because of the challenges of stent placement, some authors have recommended that the first approach be coil occlusion of the left gonadal vein to increase the driving pressure in the hilar portion of the left renal vein and promote drainage

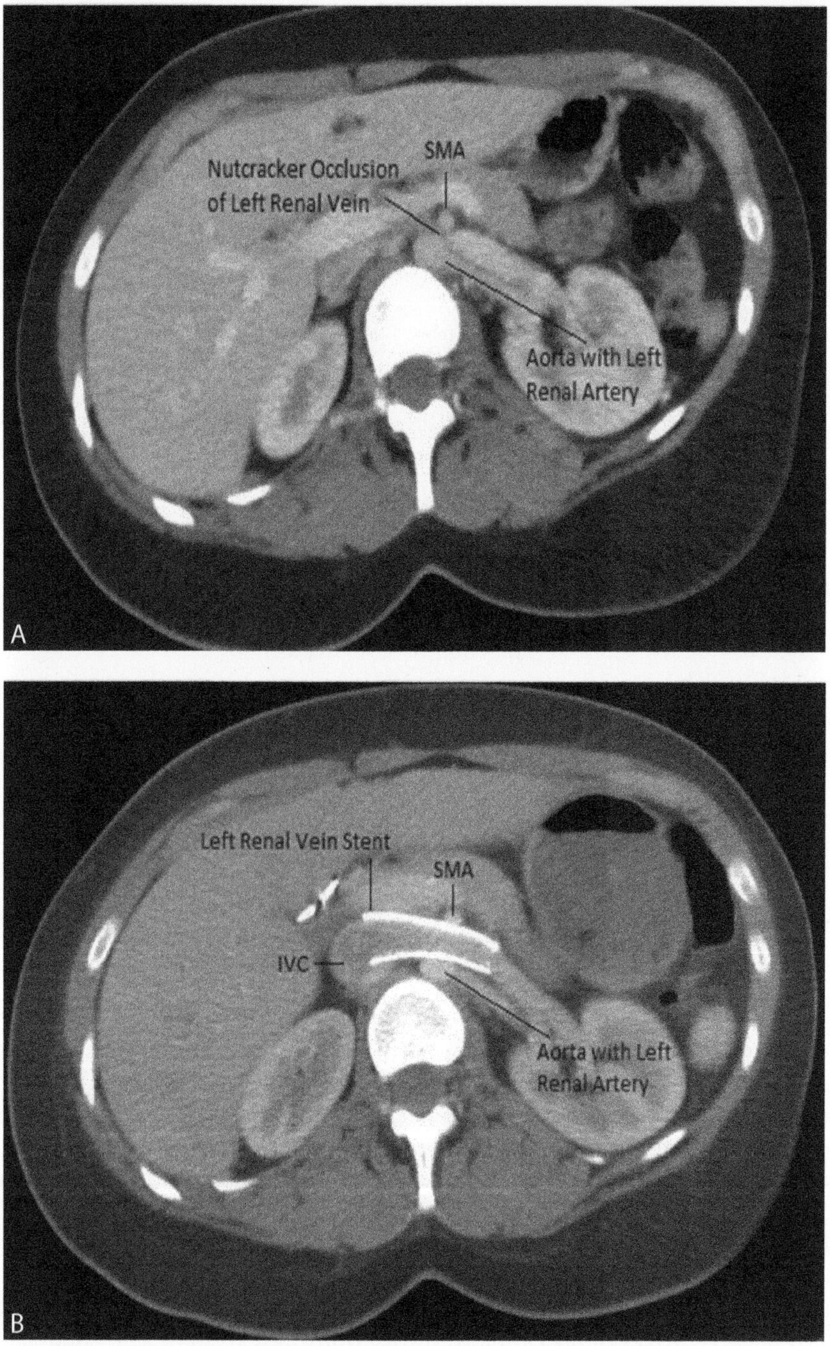

Figure 24-7. Endovascular treatment of Nutcracker Syndrome. (A) Note the near complete occlusion of the left renal vein as it traverses between the superior mesenteric artery and the aorta. (B) The left renal vein stent has widely opened the left renal vein in the area of prior occlusion.

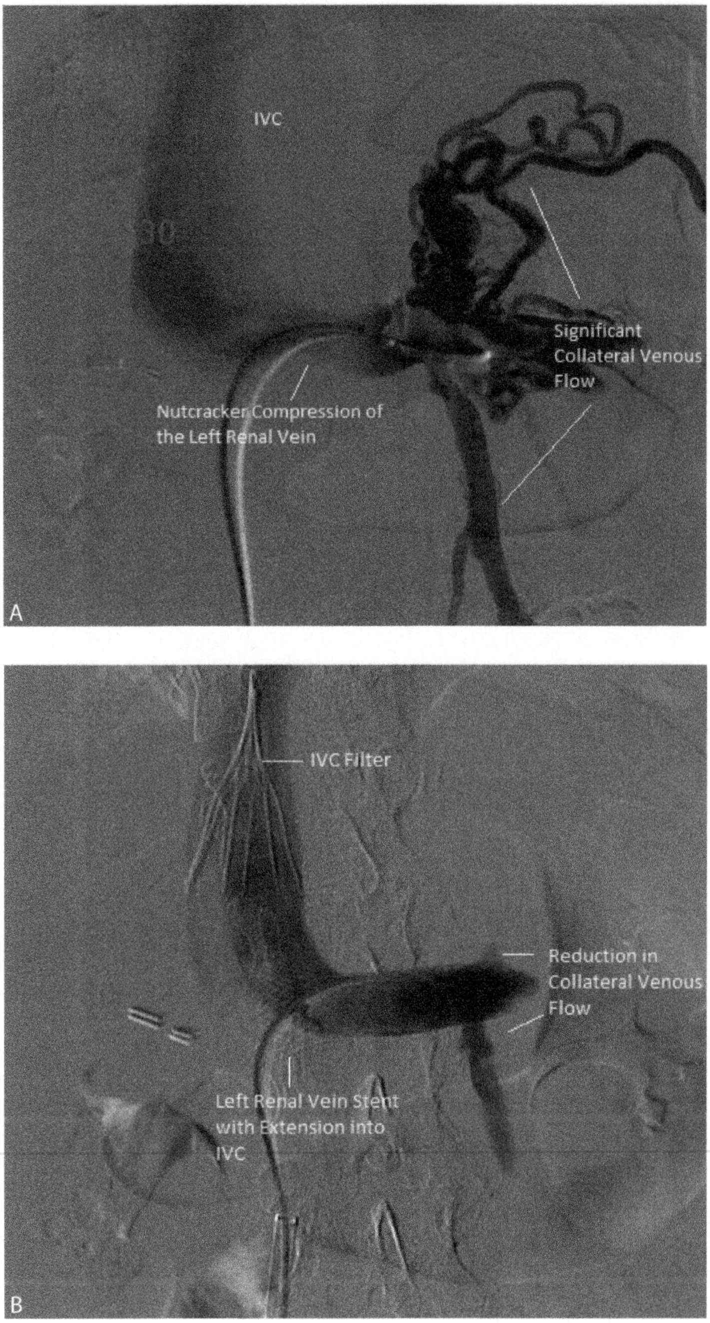

Figure 24-8. Normalization of venous flow patterns after stent placement. (A) Because of high left renal venous pressures blood is forced into smaller collateral vessels, such as the suprarenal vein and the ovarian vein. (B) After stent placement and the normalization of flow, there is a spontaneous and significant reduction is flow through smaller tributaries.

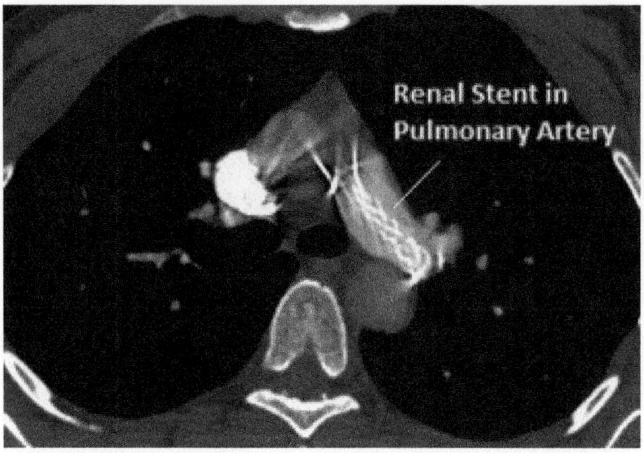

Figure 24-9. Stent migration. This patient had a stent placed successfully in her left renal vein for Nutcracker Syndrome. In a routine follow-up study, the stent was noted to have migrated to the pulmonary artery without causing injury to any of the intervening structures.

into the inferior vena cava. Such an approach may lead to further damage to the left kidney with little benefit to the patient (Figure 24-10 A,B). Clearly, the primary objective in Nutcracker Syndrome is a an improvement in left renal vein flow and a reduction in left renal vein pressure to avoid progressive hematuria and renal edema.

CONCLUSION

Nutcracker Phenomenon refers to compression of the left renal vein between the superior mesenteric artery and the aorta. Nutcracker Syndrome is the constellation of symptoms that may be caused by Nutcracker Phenomenon. These symptoms include left flank pain, intermittent hematuria, and the symptoms of pelvic congestion syndrome. Nutcracker phenomenon and Syndrome are based upon venous flow abnormalities. Our understanding of the principles of venous flow has improved our ability to establish the diagnosis through radiographic findings of renal vein varicosities, flow into small venous tributaries rather than the inferior vena cava, and significant reflux in a caudad direction. Once the diagnosis is made, procedures designed to reduce left renal venous pressure, enhance left kidney venous drainage, and eliminate reflux into small pelvic veins have been successful. Both endovascular and open surgical treatments have been used. In many patients, transposition of the left gonadal vein to the left external iliac vein is a simple treatment option that requires minimal surgical dissection, the avoidance of foreign material, and permits rapid recovery.

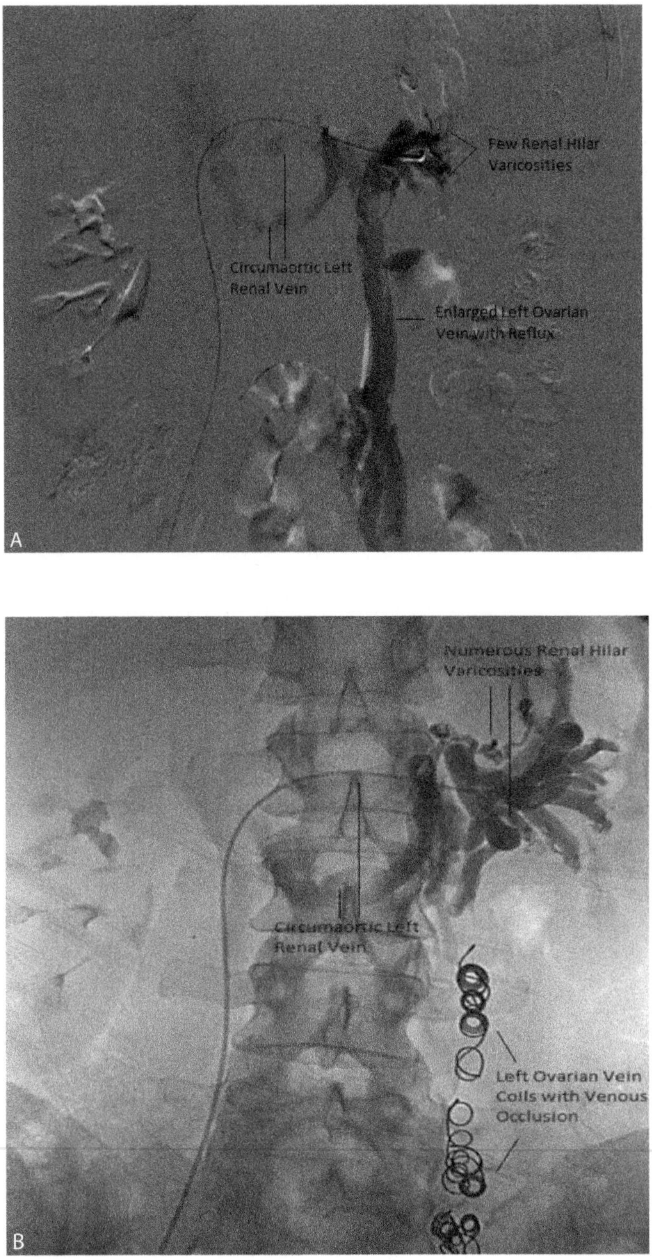

Figure 24-10. Coil occlusion of the left ovarian vein for treatment of Nutcracker Syndrome. (A) The patient underwent successful coil occlusion of her left ovarian vein for treatment of symptoms of pelvic congestion syndrome caused by Nutcracker Syndrome. (B) On follow-up venography 3 years later, the patient was noted to have formed numerous renal vein varicosities and collateral pathways of venous drainage because of the untreated renal venous hypertension.

REFERENCES

1. Grant JCB. *Method of Anatomy.* Baltimore, MD: Williams & Wilkins; 1937:158.
2. El-Sadr AR, Mina E. Anatomical and surgical aspects in the operative management of varicocele. *Urol Cutaneous Rev.* 1950;54(5):257–262.
3. Grimm LJ, Engstrom BI, Nelson RC, Kim CY. Incidental detection of nutcracker phenomenom on multidetector CT in an asymptomatic population: Prevalence and associated findings. *J Comput Assist Tomog.* 2013;37:414–418.
4. Beinart C, Sniderman KW, Tamura S, et al. Left renal vein to inferior vena cava pressure relationship in humans. *J Urol.* 1982;127:1070–1071.
5. Mugiya S, Nagata M, Ozono S. Experimental study on the pathogenesis of chronic unilateral hematuria in a porcine model: Focusing on the effect of an elevated blood pressure in the renal vein. *J Urol.* 2011;185(4) Supp:e559–e560.
6. White JV, Ryjewski C. Pelvic congestion syndrome. In Eskandari M, Pearce W, Yao J. (eds) *New Findings in Vascular Surgery.* Shelton, Connecticut: People's Medical Publishing House – USA; 2011:323.
7. Cheon JE, Kim WS, Kim IO, et al. Nutcracker syndrome in children with gross hematuria: Doppler sonographic evaluation of the left renal vein. *Pediatr Radiol.* 2006; 36:682–686.
8. Kurklinsky AK, Rooke TW. Nutcracker phenomenon and nutcracker syndrome. *Mayo Clin Proc.* 2010;85:552–559.
9. Kim KW, Cho JY, Kim SH, et al. Diagnostic value of computed tomographic findings of nutcracker syndrome: Correlation with renal venography and renocaval pressure gradients. *Eur J Radiol.* 2011;80:648–654.
10. Lamba R, Tanner DT, Sekhon S, et al. Multidetector CT of vascular compression syndromes in the abdomen and pelvis. *Radiographics.* 2014;34:93–115.
11. Park YB, Lim SH, Ahn JH, et al. Nutcracker syndrome: Intravascular stenting approach. *Nephrol Dial Transplant.* 2000;15:99–101.
12. Reed NR, Kalra M, Bower T, et al. Left renal vein transposition for nutcracker syndrome. *J Vasc Surg.* 2009;49:386–393.
13. Hartung O, Azghari A, Barthelemy P, et al. Laparoscopic transposition of the left renal vein into the inferior vena cava for nutcracker syndrome. *J Vasc Surg.* 2010;52:738–741.
14. Hartung O, Barthelemy P, Berdah SV, Alimi YS. Laparoscopy-assisted left ovarian vein transposition to treat one case of posterior nutcracker syndrome. *Ann Vasc.* 2009; 23: 413 e13–413 e16.
15. Xu D, Gao Y, Chen J, et al. Laparoscopic inferior mesenteric-gonadal vein bypass for the treatment of nutcracker syndrome. *J Vasc Surg.* 2013;57:1429–1431.
16. Chung BI, Gill IS. Laparoscopic splenorenal venous bypass for nutcracker syndrome. *J Vasc Surg.* 2009;49:1319–1323.
17. Said SM, Gloviczki P, Kalra M, et al. Renal nutcracker syndrome: Surgical options. *Semin Vasc Surg.* 2013;26:35–42.
18. White JV, Ryjewski C, Messersmith R, et al. Transposition of the left ovarian vein to the left external iliac vein for the treatment of nutcracker syndrome. *J Vasc Surg.* (in press)
19. Quevedo HC, Arain SA, Abi RN. Systematic review of endovascular therapy for nutcracker syndrome and case presentation. *Cardiovasc Revasc Med.* 2014 Apr 26. Pii:S1553-8389(14)00135-3. doi:10.1016/j.carrev.2014.04.008.
20. Hartung O, Grisoli D, Boufi M, et al. Endovascular stenting in the treatment of pelvic vein congestion caused by nutcracker syndrome: Lessons learned from the first five cases. *J Vasc Surg.* 2005;42:275–280.
21. Chen S, Zhang H, Shi H, et al. Endovascular stenting for the treatment of nutcracker syndrome: Report of 61 cases with long-term followup. *J Urol.* 2011; 186:570–575.
22. Wang X, Zhang Y, Li C, Zhang H. Results of endovascular treatment for patients with nutcracker syndrome. *J Vasc Surg.* 2012;56:142–148.
23. Chen S, Zhang H, Tian L, et al. A stranger in the heart: LRV stent migration. *Int Urol Nephrol.* 2009;41:427–430.

25

A Different Way of Thinking about Varicose Veins

Thom Rooke, MD and Cindy Felty, C-ANP

According to the Mayo Clinic, *"Varicose veins are gnarled, enlarged veins (including) ... spider veins*—a common, mild variation of varicose veins."*[1] "Common" is an understatement. The Edinburgh Vein Study demonstrates that roughly one-third of subjects between 18 and 64 years of age have large "trunk varicosities," and more than 80% have smaller reticular or intradermal varices.[2] These numbers suggest that varicose veins are not just "common"; they are (at least in a statistical sense) *normal*. Conversely, the absence of varicosities is actually *abnormal*. This is odd logic. We usually think of varicose veins as being "bad" or harmful, but in most situations "bad" things aren't arguably "normal." If varicosities are harmful (or even a "disease," as some have implied)[3] why hasn't natural selection removed them from the gene pool? Indeed, given the effects of natural selection, the high prevalence of varicose veins raises an obvious question. *Could varicosities be more benign than generally assumed—or perhaps even beneficial in certain circumstances?* If so, maybe varicose veins aren't a "disease" but rather a predictable (although undesirable) "side effect" caused by specific genetic traits that are normally associated with good health (i.e., traits that promote vascular growth and remodeling)?

CAUSES OF VARICOSE VEINS

Varicose veins are classically attributed to three factors: *venous hypertension*, *genetic factors*, and *acquired factors*.

Venous Hypertension

It is unclear whether venous hypertension is a cause or an effect of varicose veins.

* Where do you get information about "spider veins?" From a "Web site!"

Cause

Humans walk upright, and when we do the venous pressure in our legs and pelvis is relatively high. According to many theories on varicose vein formation, the high pressure contributes to *venous valve failure* with subsequent *dilatation and enlargement* of the veins; the role of venous hypertension explains why varicose veins develop in our legs but not our arms. But orthostatic pressure isn't the only factor that causes venous hypertension. For example, various venous pumps (such as the *calf muscle pump*) help decrease venous pressure during ambulation. If these pumps fail for any reason (venous obstruction, valvular damage from phlebitis, neuromuscular dysfunction, etc.) ambulatory venous pressure will be higher than normal.

Effect

Unspecified processes in the vein wall may cause veins to dilate and/or valves to become incompetent (*primary varicose veins*) leading to a vicious cycle of valvular reflux, pump failure, further impairment of venous emptying, venous hypertension, additional vein dilation, and progressive development of varicosities. Venous hypertension worsens over time.

Genetic Factors

Varicose veins can develop on a genetic basis.[4] For entities like the *Klippel-Trenaunay-Weber* (KTW) syndrome, the genetic basis is indisputable. The link between genes and vascular anomalies for other conditions may be less obvious, and in some cases the relationship has aspects that are puzzling (for example, why does someone with a genetic anomaly typically develop vascular manifestations only at certain sites—perhaps a single limb or organ—when the predisposing genetic defects presumably affect DNA everywhere?) Although varicose veins are not usually associated with identifiable genetic syndromes, most practitioners readily recognize the existence of a familial predisposition to varicose veins. Genetic factors associated with varicose veins have been identified[5] and include vascular endothelial growth factor, matrix metalloproteases (MMPs) and their inhibitors, FOXC2 genes, NOTCH3 genes, thrombomodulin promotor genes, transforming growth factors (TGFs), and many others.[6-10] Exactly how these factors affect collagen, elastin, and other basic elements of the vein wall are areas of active venous research.

Acquired Factors

Varicose veins may be due to etiologies like trauma, inflammation,[11] thrombosis with recanalization, and various non-genetic factors that induce or promote angiogenesis and vasculogenesis. These include factors such as estrogen; it is well-recognized that varicose veins may develop under the influence of various estrogens.[12] The effects of estrogen help to explain why pregnant and perimenopausal women, those with liver disease (who may not metabolize estrogen efficiently), and many others with abnormal estrogen metabolism are clearly prone to the formation of varicosities. Other poorly understood acquired factors (including certain cancers such as lymphoma) likewise appear to promote venous proliferation trough unexplained mechanisms.[13]

The relationship between venous hypertension, genes, acquired factors, and congenital syndromes with vascular features is poorly understood. For example, entities associated with the RASA 1 mutation (e.g., Parks-Weber syndrome) typically develop localized areas of venous proliferation downstream from fast-flow arteriovenous malformations (AVMs). Why? Perhaps the RASA 1 mutation exerts a direct effect on certain "normal" veins—an effect that causes them to enlarge and/or proliferate via the same mechanism(s) that promote the formation and growth of AVMs? Or is the influence of the RASA 1 mutation limited exclusively to the formation of AVMs? If so, the venous changes that occur distal to the AVM may simply reflect the subsequent response of veins to flow/volume overload. Other congenital conditions (including Paget-Schroetter syndrome, Hereditary Benign Telangiectasia, Sturge-Weber syndrome, KTW syndrome, and others) are also associated with high- or low-flow regional areas of varicose-like venous changes. How the genetic abnormalities associated with these conditions influence changes in venous structure remain incompletely understood.

The factors predisposing to the formation of varicose veins (venous hypertension, genetic tendencies, inflammation, thrombosis with recanalization, etc.) are generally considered to be "bad things" with regard to one's overall health. Of course, the varicosities they produce are likewise thought of as "bad things." Discussions about varicose veins typically use negative terms like "pathophysiology," "dysfunction," and even "incurable disease". For physicians, these terms can be useful when discussing varicose veins with patients, especially when the discussion turns to the exasperating tendency of varicosities to recur despite treatment. *"Don't blame me because your veins came back after I treated them—you're the one with an incurable disease...."*

But just how "bad" are varicose veins? The answer may depend, in part, on whether they are *primary* or *secondary* varicosities.

PRIMARY VERSUS SECONDARY VARICOSE VEINS

Primary-type varicose veins seemingly develop on a genetic basis, perhaps abetted by other factors like venous hypertension. In contrast, secondary varicose veins are typically blamed on specific precipitating factors—for example, varicosities that develop because of 1) recanalization of thrombotic veins, or 2) collateralization around a region of venous obstruction are both typically described as secondary "varicose veins" (Figure 25-1). However, the "secondary" varicose veins caused by phlebitis are clearly different entities from those arising from collateralization; for the purpose of further discussion, "secondary" varicose veins will refer to collateral-type veins. While primary varicose veins are always thought of as "bad" things (they cause problems such as cosmetic disfigurement, pain, swelling, and occasionally skin changes or ulceration), secondary varicose veins are usually treated as a healthy response to venous obstruction, and they are generally considered to be "good" things—even when they produce many of the same undesirable signs and symptoms associated with primary varicose veins. This is an important distinction; no one really wants varicose veins, but many people (for example, those with chronic venous obstruction) should welcome the appearance of secondary (collateral) varicose veins because they can relieve venous hypertension and prevent the development of a stasis ankle skin ulcer.

Are the factors that produce primary varicose veins (such as chronic venous hypertension, vein wall or valve damage, genes, and other factors leading to

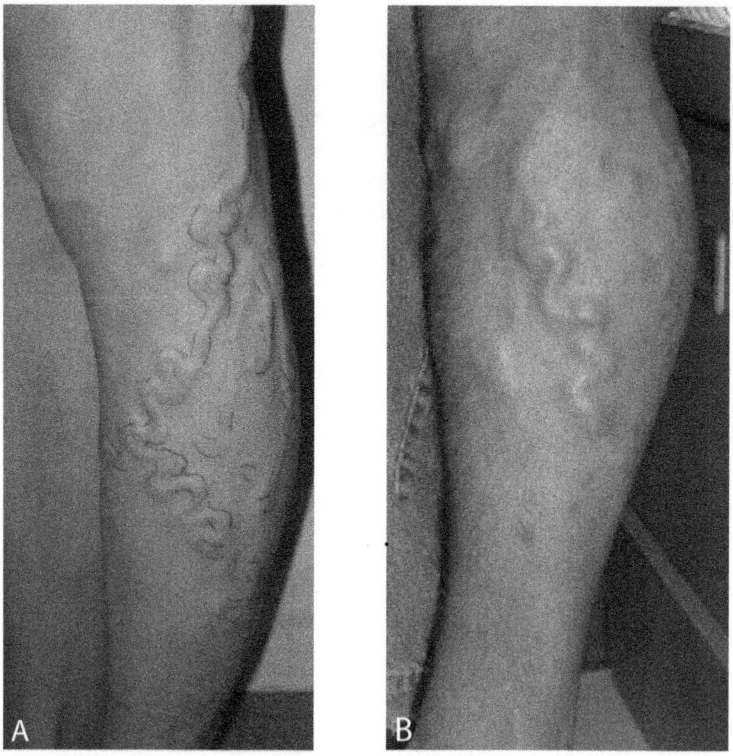

Figure 25-1. Primary and Secondary Varicose Veins. (A) Primary Varicose Veins. (B) Secondary Varicose Veins. Primary varicose veins (A) are clinically and pathologically similar to secondary baricos beins (B). In this case, the "varicosities" are caused by Klippel-Trenaunay syndrome; the enlarged skin veins are collateral veins that bypass the absent deep vein system. Conventional wisdom typically attributes the veins in Figure 25-1A to passive processes like "vein wall breakdown" and "degeneration" of the vein; in contrast, the veins in Figure 25-1B are usually considered to be an active process involving activities like "growth" and "remodeling." The end product, however, suggests that primary and secondary veins are more alike than unalike.

subsequent passive vein dilatation) different from the factors causing secondary varicose veins (i.e., those things that influence vein growth and/or remodeling of existing veins to produce collateral vessel development around a venous obstruction)? Maybe not. Insight into secondary varicose vein formation can be found in studies of collateral veins. A brief review of the literature (including studies that look at collateral vein formation, venous remodeling in arterial bypass vein grafts, and venous dialysis shunts)[14] confirms that the proposed mechanisms behind secondary varicose vein formation involve many of the same genetic and acquired factors associated with primary varicose vein formation including inflammation, MMPs, TGFs, estrogen, changes in elastin and collagen, and others.[15] Chronic venous hypertension likewise appears important in the formation of secondary varicosities, since collateral veins typically do not develop unless there is a pressure gradient across the obstructed vessels.

If people truly differ in their abilities to make secondary (collateral) veins just as they do in their tendency to make primary varicose veins, the implications are obvious and follow a logical progression: 1) Primary varicose veins develop because of identifiable biological factors, some of which are genetic in origin; 2) People differ in their possession/expression of these genetic factors and therefore differ in their ability to make primary varicose veins; 3) The same genetic factors that produce primary varicose veins also appear to contribute to the development of secondary or collateral varicose veins. It therefore follows that people who form primary varicose veins should also be good at making collateral (secondary) varicose veins when necessary. Although the observation that people who are *"the best makers of (primary) varicose veins should likewise be the best makers of (secondary) collateral veins"* is not well-described in the literature, in retrospect it seems almost obvious that this phenomenon should be true.

VARICOSE VEINS AND ARTERIAL COLLATERALS

If the idea that "people with primary varicose veins should also be good at making collateral veins" is plausible, can this reasoning can be extended to the formation of collateral arteries? Why not? Several lines of reasoning suggest an association between varicose veins and arterial collateral vessels. First, varicose veins occur less commonly in patients who undergo infrainguinal arterial bypass than in those who don't; this suggests that patients with primary varicose veins are better at making arterial collaterals and are therefore less likely to need bypass surgery than those with varicose veins.[16] Second, the literature suggests that inflammation, MMPs, TGFs, collagen changes, estrogen, and many of the other factors shown to be involved in varicose vein and collateral vein formation are also associated with the formation of collateral arteries.[17-21] Finally, other clinical scenarios point toward an association between varicose veins and the potential for arterial growth and remodeling; for example, patients with *coronary artery ectasia* (a pathological combination of unfettered arterial growth and remodeling) have an unusually high incidence of varicose veins.[22] The prospect of similar factors driving the production and growth of varicose veins, collateral veins, and collateral arteries may seem odd at first—but wouldn't it seem even odder if the development of different types of blood vessels didn't share a number of similar mechanisms?

VARICOSE VEINS AND LYMPHATIC COLLATERALS

Consider one last vascular conduit—the *lymphatic vessel*. Are the factors involved in the development and growth of lymphatics similar to those that promote varicose veins, venous collaterals, and arterial collaterals? Once again, the answer appears to be "yes." The literature reveals that many of the same factors (including vascular endothelial growth factor, FOXC2, growth hormone, and others) driving the growth of veins and arteries also play a role in the genesis and maturation of lymphatic vessels.[23] In addition, a clinical association exists between varicose veins and certain forms of lymphatic proliferation; for example, *lymphedema distichiasis* (a condition characterized by excessive lymphatic vessels proliferation) is associated with an increased tendency to form varicose veins. Both conditions may be influenced by the FOXC2 gene.[8]

DO THE GENETIC FACTORS THAT CAUSE VARICOSE VEINS HELP INDIVIDUALS IN OTHER WAYS?

The possibility that varicose veins share common genetic factors with collateral veins, arteries, and lymphatic vessels provides a rationale for even more speculation. If varicose veins derive from genetic factors that also promote the development of collateral veins, arteries, and lymphatics, then do patients with varicose veins have less (clinical) arterial and lymphatic obstructive disease? Put differently, if people with varicose veins can develop arterial collaterals when necessary, is their incidence of cardiovascular morbidity and mortality lower than it is for patients without varicose veins (i.e., can/will they develop collaterals that attenuate the effects of disease)? Do patients with varicose veins have less frequent/severe lymphedema (from lymphatic obstruction) than patients without varicose veins?

An initial look into the literature is not encouraging. Multiple reports suggest that those with varicose veins actually have a *higher* incidence of arterial atherosclerosis than those without varicose veins.[24,25] However, while people with primary varicose veins apparently have coronary artery disease more often than those without, they do not necessarily have more angina. This curious observation raises the possibility that those with varicose veins may be more inclined to create coronary collaterals (and thus experience less cardiac ischemia) than those without varicosities.[25] Further support for a relationship between varicose veins and arterial collateralization comes from the Normative Aging Study.[16] This investigation was spawned by the primary authors' clinical observation that "varicose veins are less frequent in patients undergoing... surgery for femoral artery disease"—it's an observation that makes sense if people with varicose veins are somehow better at developing arterial collaterals (and therefore less likely to require bypass surgery) than those without varicose veins. The study demonstrated 36% less symptomatic coronary disease in patients with varicose veins (compared with those without) along with a highly significant increase in "survival-free of coronary heart disease" in patients with varicose veins. Although explanations other than "improved collateralization" might explain why patients with varicose veins live longer and have less coronary symptoms than those without*, the possibility that varicose vein formation predicts a person's ability to form collateral arteries remains an intriguing one.

Is there a similar link between lymphedema and varicose veins? An association (or lack of association) between varicose veins and the development of lymphedema has not otherwise been described in the literature. However, my own personal experience suggests that patients with varicosities do not develop lymphedema of the arm after treatment for breast cancer as often as those without varicose veins. I've also observed that patients presenting with lymphedema (primary or secondary) seem to have far less varicosities than those without lymphedema (Figure 25-2).

---

* For example, patients without angina might be more active—and therefore spend more time in an upright position—than those with angina and other coronary symptoms; if so, perhaps the increased time spent upright (a sign of good health) contributes to varicose vein formation?

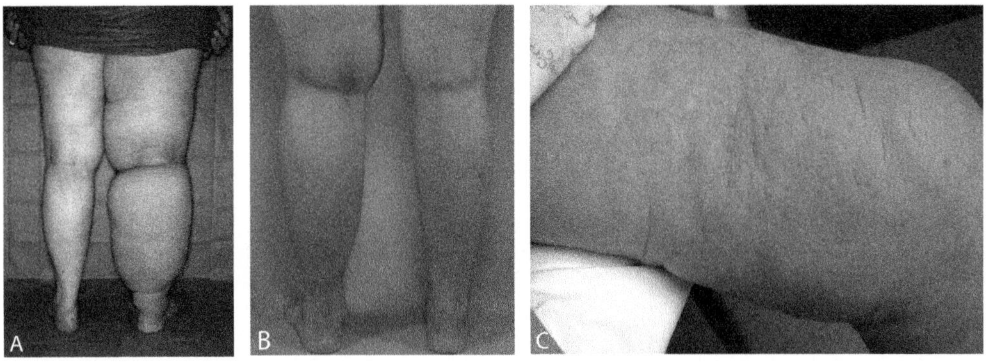

Figure 25-2. Lymphedema. (A) Primary LE of the right leg. (B) Secondary LE of the left leg. (C) Localized LE of the thigh with "peau d'orange" skin changes. The lack/absence of visible veins—especially varicose veins—is often striking in limbs with all types of lymphedema. Is it possible that those who are "bad" at making lymphatic vessels (and thus are prone to developing LE) are also "bad" at making normal (or varicose) veins?

CONCLUSIONS

Nobody wants (primary) varicose veins. They cause pain, are impossible to prevent, progress relentlessly, and inevitably recur after treatment; these characteristics have led some to designate them a "disease." Yet the conventional wisdom suggesting that varicose veins are pathological entities (caused by "degeneration" of normal veins) is challenged by their high prevalence in most populations (half or more of people have some type of varicose veins) and their well-established genetic nature (i.e., most heritable traits that are truly detrimental are removed from the gene pool by natural selection.) These apparent contradictions suggest that there may be alternative explanations for the high prevalence of varicose veins.

One potential explanation involves the idea that varicose veins result from the same mechanism(s) that lead to the production of other types of blood vessels. Based on the literature and personal observations, it appears that people who are "good" at forming varicose veins are often "good" at forming venous, arterial, and lymphatic collateral vessels. As a result, those with varicose veins may have lower morbidity/mortality from vascular diseases than do those without varicosities. Ultimately, varicose veins (which we neither need nor want) may be "the price we pay" in order to make collateral vessels (which we both need and want) when necessary.

REFERENCES

1. http://www.mayoclinic.org/diseases-conditions/varicose-veins/basics/definition/con-20043474. Accessed September 2, 2015.
2. Evans CJ, Fowkes FG, Ruckley CV, Lee AJ. Prevalence of varicose veins and chronic venous insufficiency in men and women in the general population: Edinburgh Vein Study *J Epidemiol Community Health.* 1999;53:49–153.
3. Beckman JA. Diseases of the veins. *Circulation.* 2002;106:2170–2.

4. Pappas PJ. Pathogenesis of varicose veins and cellular pathophysiology of chronic venous insufficiency. In P. Gloviczki, Ed. *Handbook of Venous Disorders* (3rd ed.), Boca Raton, FL: CRC press, 2008:56–9.
5. Jaoum JJ, Hunter GC. Pathogenesis of varicose veins and implications for clinical management. *Vascular.* 2007;15:242–9.
6. Hollingsworth SJ, Powell GL, Barker SGE, Cooper DG. Primary varicose veins: Altered transcription of VEGF and its receptors (KDR, flt-1, soluble flt-1) with sapheno-femoral junction incompetence. *Eur J Vasc Endovasc Surg*. 2004;27:259–68.
7. Ng MY, Andrew T, Spector TD, Jeffery S. Linkage to the FOXC2 region of chromosome 16 for varicose veins in otherwise healthy, unselected sibling pairs. *J Med Genet*. 2005;42:235–9.
8. Mellor RH, Brice G, Stanton AW, et al. Mutations in FOXC2 are strongly associated with primary valve failure in veins of the lower limb. *Circulation*. 2007;115:1912–20.
9. Saiki S, Sakai K, Saiki M, et al. Varicose veins associated with CADASIL result from a novel mutation in the Notch3 gene. *Neurology*. 2006;67:337–9.
10. Raffetto JD, Khalil RA. Mechanism of varicose vein formation: Valve dysfunction and wall dilation. *Phlebology*. 2008;23:85–98.
11. Nicolaides AN. Chronic venous disease and the leukocyte-endothelium interaction: From symptoms to ulceration. *Angiology*. 2005;56(Suppl 1):S11–S19.
12. Morales DE, McGowan KA, Grant DS, et al. Estrogen promotes angiogenic activity in human umbilical vein endothelial cells in vitro and in a murine model. *Circulation*. 1995;91:755–63.
13. Özgüro lu E, Büyülbabani N, Özgüro lu M, Baykal C. Generalized telangiectasia as the major manifestation of angiotropic (intravascular) lymphoma. *Br J Dermatol*. 1997;137:422–5.
14. Abeles D, Kwei S, Stavrakis G, et al. Gene expression changes evoked in a venous segment exposed to arterial flow. *J Vasc Surg*. 2006;44:863–70.
15. Anwar A, Georgiadis KA, Shalhoub J, et al. A review of familial, genetic, and congenital aspects of primary varicose veins disease. *Circ Cardiovasc Genet*. 2012;5:460–6.
16. Scott TE, Mendez MN, LaMorte WW, et al. Are varicose veins a marker for susceptibility to coronary disease? Results from the normative aging study. *Ann Vasc Surg*. 2004;18:459–64.
17. Haas TL, Doyle JL, Distasi MR, et al. Involvement of MMPs in the outward remodeling of collateral mesenteric arteries. *Am J Physiol Heart Circ Physiol*. 2007;293:H2429–H2437.
18. Van Royen N, Hoefer I, Buschmann I, et al. Exogenous application of transforming growth factor bête 1 stimulates arteriogenesis in the peripheral circulation. *FASEB J*. 2002;16:432–4.
19. Cai W, Schaper W. Mechanisms of arteriogenesis. *Acta Biochim Biophys Sin*. 2008;40: 681–92.
20. Kyriakides ZS, Petinakis P, Kaklamanis L, et al. Intramuscular administration of estrogen may promote angiogenesis and perfusion in a rabbit model of chronic limb ischemia. *Cardiovasc Res*. 2001;49:626–33.
21. Losordo DW, Isner JM. Brief reviews: estrogen and angiogenesis. *Arterioscler Thromb Vasc Biol*. 2001;21:6–12.
22. Androulakis AE, Katsaros AA, Kartalis AN, et al. Varicose veins are common in patients with coronary artery ectasia. Just a coincidence or a systemic deficit in the vascular wall? *Eur J Vasc Endovasc Surg*. 2004;27:519–24.
23. Kärpänen T. Lymphatic vessels in health and disease: Role of the VEGF-C/VEGFR-3 pathway and the transcription factor FOXC2. Helsinki University Biomedical Dissertations No. 79. 2006. Available at: http://ethesis.helsinki.fi/julkaisut/bio/bioja/vk/karpanen/lymphati.pdf (Accessed March 5, 2015.)
24. Brand FN, Dannenberg AL, Abbott RD, Kannel WB. The epidemiology of varicose veins: the Framingham study. *Am J Prev Med*. 1988;4:96–101.
25. Ducimetiere P, Richard JL, Pequignot G, Warnet JM. Varicose veins: A risk factor for atherosclerotic disease in middle-aged men? *Int J Epidemiol*. 1981;10:329–35.

26

Home-Based Exercise for Peripheral Artery Disease: Prescribing a Successful Regimen

Mary McGrae McDermott, MD

Lower extremity peripheral artery disease (PAD) affects eight million people in the United States and over 200 million men and women worldwide.[1,2] Patients with PAD have greater functional impairment and are at increased risk for cardiovascular events and mobility loss, compared to people without PAD.[3–5] Recently, improved treatments for cardiovascular disease have resulted in declining rates of cardiovascular death in the United States and in other high socioeconomic countries.[1] As cardiovascular death decreases, people with PAD in the United States and other high socioeconomic countries will survive longer with chronic debilitating diseases, such as PAD. Therefore, optimal management of PAD-related disability is essential to ensure that people with PAD survive longer with an optimal quality of life and without disability.

FUNCTIONAL IMPAIRMENT AND DECLINE IN PAD: MAGNITUDE OF THE PROBLEM

Patients with PAD have greater functional impairment, faster functional decline, and higher rates of mobility loss compared to people without PAD.[3–6] However, measuring decline in functional performance among people with PAD in clinical practice can be difficult unless a 6-min walk test is measured or patients are explicitly questioned about their ability to walk ¼ mile or climb a flight of stairs without assistance. This is because patients with PAD frequently limit their activity to avoid leg symptoms, as their PAD progresses. Thus, PAD patients may perceive improvement or stabilization of their leg symptoms over time.[7–9] However, prospective longitudinal studies document decline in walking performance over time in people with PAD.[6,10]

The Walking and Leg Circulation Study (WALCS) cohort was the first to objectively demonstrate rates of actual functional decline in people with PAD. The WALCS cohort consisted of 740 participants, including 460 with PAD, who were identified from Chicago-area vascular laboratories and followed prospectively with annual study visits.[3–6] At baseline and at each annual follow-up visit, the six-minute walk test was performed and participants were asked about their ability to walk ¼ mile and walk up and down a flight of stairs without assistance.

At baseline in the WALCS cohort, PAD participants with an ankle brachial index (ABI) < 0.50 walked 523 fewer feet in the 6-min walk test compared to those without PAD and were significantly less likely to be able to maintain a tandem stand for 10 sec, compared to individuals without PAD (odds ratio = 0.37, 95% Confidence Interval = 0.18–0.76). Across the entire cohort, lower ABI values were also associated with lower levels of physical activity and slower walking velocity.[3] At 2-year follow-up, PAD participants in the WALCS cohort were more likely to become unable to walk continuously for 6 min without stopping, compared to those without PAD.[6] Lower ABI values were associated with greater declines in 6-min walk distance.[6] At 5-year follow-up, PAD participants in the WALCS cohort had higher rates of mobility loss than those without PAD.[4] Lower ABI values were associated with higher rates of mobility loss.[10] In summary, a major therapeutic goal for clinicians is to maintain or improve functioning and prevent mobility loss in people with PAD. This challenge is increasingly common as the U.S. population survives longer with chronic disease.[2]

EXERCISE THERAPY TO PREVENT FUNCTIONAL DECLINE IN PAD

In 2015, only two medications, cilostazol and pentoxifylline, are FDA approved for treating walking impairment due to intermittent claudication.[11,12] Cilostazol confers modest improvement in walking ability.[11] Pentoxifylline may be no better than placebo. In contrast, supervised treadmill exercise therapy is well established as an effective therapy for improving treadmill walking performance in people who have PAD.[13] Multiple randomized clinical trials of supervised treadmill exercise have demonstrated clear benefits of treadmill walking exercise for improving treadmill walking performance in PAD patients.[13]

Home based walking exercise prescriptions are best understood in the context of evidence regarding supervised treadmill exercise. The benefits of exercise for PAD patients were first clearly established in a meta-analysis by Gardner et al, which was published in 1995.[14] Gardner et al performed a meta-analysis to address the question of whether exercise therapy improves treadmill walking performance in people with PAD.[14] The meta-analysis included studies of exercise rehabilitation conducted between 1966 and 1993 in people with PAD and intermittent claudication. All studies measured treadmill walking performance as a study outcome. Of the 21 studies included, only three (with a total of 23 participants) were randomized trials. Remaining studies were non-randomized studies or uncontrolled studies. The meta-analysis concluded that exercise rehabilitation in PAD patients with intermittent claudication improves pain-free treadmill walking distance by 179% and maximal treadmill walking distance by 122%. Gardner et al also used the meta-analysis to identify characteristics of exercise rehabilitation programs that are particularly beneficial for improving treadmill walking performance in PAD patients with intermittent claudication.[14] Exercise rehabilitation programs in which PAD patients walked for exercise (vs. an alternative form of exercise), exercised to maximal ischemic leg pain (rather than to onset of ischemic leg pain), and were enrolled for at least 26 weeks (vs. less than 26 weeks) were most effective.[14] Gardner et al also concluded that supervised exercise was more effective than unsupervised exercise and that programs with an exercise frequency of ≥ 3 times weekly were more effective than those in which participants exercised less than 3 times weekly.[14] In summary, these results by Gardner et al established supervised treadmill walking exercise as an important therapeutic modality for patients with PAD.

Since the original meta-analysis published by Gardner et al., many randomized clinical trials of supervised walking exercise in patients with PAD have been published. A 2012 meta-analysis by Fakhry et al. included 25 randomized controlled trials of supervised walking therapy, published between 1996 and February 2012. The meta-analysis by Fakhry et al. included 1054 PAD patients with intermittent claudication.[13]All of the randomized trials in the meta-analysis included outcomes of maximal and/or pain-free treadmill walking time or distance.[13] The included studies ranged in duration from four two 104 weeks. Overall, the meta-analysis demonstrated a 180 meter greater increase in maximal treadmill walking distance in the walking exercise groups as compared to the control group. The meta-analysis also demonstrated a 128-m greater increase in pain-free treadmill walking distance in the supervised walking therapy group relative to the control group.[13]

Fakhry et al performed analyses to determine whether greater intensity of walking therapy was associated with greater improvements in treadmill walking among PAD participants with intermittent claudication.[13] In contrast to the evidence from the meta-analysis by Gardner et al., Fakhry et al. reported that supervised walking therapy programs in which participants walked only to the onset of ischemic pain and walking programs that pushed participants to maximum ischemic pain each achieved significant gains in treadmill walking performance. This result suggests that the intensity of walking exercise may not be an important determinant of the efficacy of a supervised walking therapy program. In addition, Fakhry et al. studied the association of duration of walking exercise programs and walking outcomes. Increases in treadmill walking time were not different between exercise programs of 2- to 11-week duration and those that lasted up to 26 weeks. Fakhry et al. also reported that supervised walking therapy programs that included at least 1080 min of exercise over the course of the exercise program improved treadmill walking distance, while exercise programs with less than 1,080 min of exercise over the course of the exercise program did not improve treadmill walking distance. In summary, robust evidence demonstrates the benefits of supervised treadmill exercise therapy for improving treadmill walking performance in people with PAD.

THE IMPORTANCE OF HOME-BASED EXERCISE PROGRAMS IN PAD

Despite the well-established efficacy of supervised treadmill exercise for improving treadmill walking performance in people with PAD, most patients with PAD do not

TABLE 26-1. SUMMARY OF RANDOMIZED CLINICAL TRIALS OF HOME-BASED EXERCISE IN PERIPHERAL ARTERIAL DISEASE PUBLISHED SINCE 2011

Study and Year Published	Sample Size	Duration (weeks)	Study Groups	Home-based Exercise Intervention	Primary Outcome Results	Additional Outcome Results	Comments
Gardner et al. 2011	119	12	Supervised treadmill exercise. Home-based walking exercise. Control group	Home-based walking exercise intervention in which participants were provided with an activity monitor and asked to walk three days per week for 45 min/session. Participants received feedback on-site every 2 weeks.	Supervised exercise: Increase in treadmill walking time by 104 sec. Home-based exercise: Increase in treadmill walking time by 111 sec. Control: Increase in treadmill walking time by 22 sec.	The supervised and home-based exercise groups each had significantly improved pain-free treadmill walking time compared to the control group.	There was a 25% drop-out rate in the home-based walking exercise group.
Gardner et al. 2014	180	12	Supervised treadmill exercise. Home-based walking exercise. Control group	Home-based walking exercise intervention in which participants were provided with an activity monitor and asked to walk three days per week for 45 min/session. Participants received feedback on-site every 4 weeks.	Supervised exercise: Increase in treadmill walking time by 215 seconds. Home based exercise: Increase in treadmill walking time by 124 seconds. Control:Decrease in treadmill walking time by 10 seconds.	The supervised and home-based exercise groups each had significantly improved pain-free treadmill walking distance and significantly improved 6-min walk performance compared to the control group. Physical activity levels were not higher in the supervised or home-based exercise groups compared to control.	Participants randomized to supervised treadmill exercise had significantly greater improvement in treadmill walking compared to home-based exercise. Participants randomized to home-based exercise had greater improvement in 6-min walk compared to those randomized to supervised exercise.

(Continued)

TABLE 26-1. ***(Continued)***

Study and Year Published	Sample Size	Duration (weeks)	Study Groups	Home-based Exercise Intervention	Primary Outcome Results	Additional Outcome Results	Comments
McDermott et al. 2013	192	26 (primary outcomes) 52 (secondary outcomes)	Intervention vs. control	Group Mediated Cognitive Behavioral (GMCB) intervention in which participants met weekly at the medical center with a group of PAD patients a facilitator.	The 6-min walk increased by 42.4 m in the intervention group and declined by 11.4 m in the control group at 6-month follow-up.	Maximal treadmill walking time increased by 1.54 min in the intervention and by 0.53 min in the control group. Pain-free treadmill walking time increased by 1.43 min in the intervention group and by 0.43 min in the control group. Physical activity levels and patient-reported walking endurance and walking speed also significantly improved in the intervention, compared to the control.	The intervention benefits for improving the six-minute walk were sustained at 12-month follow-up, 6 months after the final intervention on-site visit.
Collins. et al 2011	145	26	Intervention vs. control	Participants in the intervention were instructed to walk three days/wk at home, working up to 50 min per session. Participants in the intervention were also asked to walk for exercise once weekly at the study exercise center with an instructor.	The intervention increased their maximal treadmill walking distance by 24.5 m, which was not significantly different from the increase in maximal treadmill walking distance of 39.2 m in the control group.	The intervention significantly improved their perceived walking speed and mental health, measured by the SF-36, compared to the control group. However, ten other secondary outcome measures showed no benefit in the intervention compared to the control group.	All participants had diabetes mellitus

participate in supervised exercise training programs.[15,16] There are at least two major barriers to participation in supervised exercise programs among people with PAD. First, most medical insurance companies, including Medicare, do not pay for supervised exercise for people with PAD and intermittent claudication. Thus, PAD patients interested in participating in supervised exercise programs frequently must pay out of pocket to participate. Second, travelling to an exercise center three times weekly may be burdensome for people with PAD and claudication. Therefore, developing effective home based exercise programs that are accessible to most patients with PAD has the potential to have a wide public health impact in people who have PAD. However, implementing a home-based exercise program in PAD is particularly challenging in part because PAD patients are limited by ischemic leg pain. Thus, PAD-related ischemic leg pain presents unique challenges in the adoption of home-based exercise programs by people who have PAD.

EVIDENCE REGARDING HOME-BASED EXERCISE IN PAD

The most recently published clinical practice guidelines for PAD state that evidence does not support advising patients with PAD to go home and walk.[17] However, these clinical practice guidelines were published in 2006. Since 2011, four randomized clinical trials have tested the ability of home-based exercise programs to improve walking ability in patients with PAD (Table 26-1).[18–21] Three of these four recently published randomized clinical trials demonstrate significantly improved walking endurance in PAD patients who have participated in a home-based exercise interventions. Thus, growing evidence suggests a role for home-based exercise to improve walking ability in people who have PAD. The following paragraphs summarize these studies and identify characteristics that may be important in developing a successful home-based walking program for people with PAD.

Gardner et al. randomized 119 men and women with PAD and intermittent claudication to one of three groups: supervised treadmill exercise, home-based walking exercise, or a control group for twelve weeks.[19] Participants randomized to supervised treadmill exercise attended exercise sessions three times per week and walked for up to 40 min at each supervised exercise session. Participants randomized to home-based walking exercise received step-counter activity monitors and were instructed to walk three times per week to maximal ischemic leg pain at a self selected pace, working up to 45 min of walking exercise per session. PAD participants were instructed to wear the step counter during exercise sessions and also to record their walking exercise activity on a log. Every two weeks during the 12-week intervention, participants in the home-exercise group returned to the medical center with their activity monitors and a walking exercise log. At these visits, an exercise physiologist reviewed the activity monitor data and the exercise log and provided feedback to the PAD participant about their home walking exercise program. Instructions were provided for walking exercise at home during the subsequent two weeks. Rates of completed exercise sessions during the study were 81.7% in the supervised exercise group and 80.6% in the home-exercise group. The home-based exercise group spent significantly more time engaged in walking exercise, compared to the supervised exercise group. The average time spent exercising per session was 24.6 min in the supervised exercise group and 41.6 min in the home-based exercise group. However, the total volume of exercise, measured as the product of the estimated intensity of exercise and the minutes spent exercising was not different between the two exercise groups.

At 12 week follow-up, the groups randomized to supervised treadmill exercise and home-based walking exercise each significantly improved their pain-free and maximal treadmill walking performance, compared to the control group. The home-based walking exercise group increased their pain-free treadmill walking time by 104 sec and their maximal treadmill walking time by 110 sec as compared to baseline. The supervised exercise group increased their pain-free walking time by 170 sec and their maximal treadmill walking time by 192 sec as compared to baseline. The control group increased their pain-free walking time by 17 sec and their maximal treadmill walking time by 22 sec as compared to baseline. There were no significant differences in the degree of improvement in pain-free or maximal treadmill walking time between the supervised treadmill exercise intervention group and the home-based exercise intervention group. The trial was limited, however, by a 28% drop-out rate in the home-based exercise group. The high dropout rate in the home-exercise group may represent evidence of the difficulties with adherence to home-based exercise in people with PAD.

A more recent randomized trial by Gardner et al randomized 188 participants with PAD and intermittent claudication to supervised treadmill exercise, home-based walking exercise, vs. an attention control group.[20] The study design was similar to the 2011 home-based exercise study by Gardner et al. but with fewer on-site visits. The supervised exercise group engaged in a typical supervised treadmill exercise program, as recommended by clinical practice guidelines for people with PAD.[14] Participants randomized to supervised exercise were asked to walk for exercise on the treadmill three days per week, working up to 40 min per session, and walking to maximal ischemic leg pain. Participants randomized to home exercise were asked to walk for exercise three days weekly, working up to 45 min per session. PAD participants were provided with an exercise step monitor to wear only during exercise sessions and track their walking exercise activity. PAD participants in the home-exercise group walked at a self-selected pace during exercise sessions. PAD participants in the home-based exercise program returned at one-week follow-up and subsequently at four, eight, and twelve- week follow-up. At each follow-up session, an exercise physiologist reviewed the exercise data measured by the step-counter and provided feedback. PAD patients were provided with instructions for exercise activity during the next four weeks. Participants randomized to the attention control group engaged in resistance training, predominately involving the upper extremities. Participants in the supervised exercise group completed 84.8% of their exercise sessions and participants in the home-based exercise group completed 82.5% of their exercise sessions. At 12 week follow-up, both the supervised exercise group and the home-exercise group significantly improved their pain-free and maximal treadmill walking performance, compared to the control group. The supervised exercise group increased their pain-free treadmill walking time by 165 seconds, the home-based walking exercise group increased their pain-free treadmill walking time by 134 seconds, and the control group declined by 16 seconds. The supervised exercise group increased their maximal treadmill walking time by 215 seconds, the home-based walking exercise group increased their maximal treadmill walking time by 124 seconds, and the control group had a 10 second decline in their maximal treadmill walking time. The supervised treadmill exercise group improved their six-minute walk performance by 15 meters, the home-based exercise group improved their six-minute walk performance by 45 meters and the control group improved their six-minute walk performance by four meters. Notably, participants randomized to home exercise had significantly greater improvement in the six-minute walk test compared to those randomized to supervised treadmill exercise, while those randomized to supervised treadmill exercise had greater improvement in treadmill walking performance compared to those randomized to home-based exercise. These two randomized trials by Gardner et al demonstrate that home-based exercise, in which participants receive a step-monitor and in-person feedback either bi-weekly or as infrequently as once per month, can significantly improve treadmill walking performance and the six-minute walk in people with PAD and intermittent claudication.[19,20] These studies provide new evidence that home-based exercise, with self-monitoring and use of a step counter, significantly improve walking performance in patients with PAD.

The Group Oriented Arterial Leg Study (GOALS) randomized trial tested the ability of a Group Mediated Cognitive Behavioral (GMCB) intervention to help 192 patients with PAD adhere to a home-based walking exercise program, thereby improving their walking endurance. The GMCB intervention employed methods that included social cognitive behavioral change theory and group support. For the first six months of the GOALS trial, PAD participants in the intervention group met weekly at the medical center with other PAD patients and a facilitator. The facilitator led discussions regarding goal setting, self-monitoring, and overcoming obstacles to exercise adherence. After the first six-months of the GOALS trial, baseline outcome measures were repeated. Between months seven and twelve of the GOALS trial, participants no longer returned to the medical center for weekly meetings, but were contacted by telephone at decreasing frequency, ranging from every one to two weeks during months 7-9 to once monthly during months 9-12. Outcome measures were repeated at twelve-month follow-up. In contrast to other home-based exercise trials in PAD, the GOALS trial included PAD participants both with and without symptoms of intermittent claudication.[21]

At six-month follow-up, the GMCB home-based exercise intervention significantly improved their six-minute walk performance, their pain-free treadmill walking time, and their maximum treadmill walking time relative to the control group. The intervention group had a 53.5 meter greater increase in six-minute walk performance, a 1.01 minute greater increase in maximal treadmill walking time, and a 1.02 minute greater increase in pain-free treadmill walking time compared to the control group. The GMCB home-based exercise intervention also significantly improved physical activity levels and patient-reported walking ability, compared to the control group. Furthermore, the benefits of the GMCB home-based exercise intervention on walking endurance persisted at 12-month follow-up, six months after the final on-site study intervention. Participants randomized to the GMCB intervention were also less likely to experience mobility loss, defined as becoming unable to either walk up and down a flight of stairs or walk ¼ mile, at 6-month and at 12-month follow-up, compared to the control group. For example at six-month follow-up, rates of mobility loss were 6.3% in the GMCB intervention group vs. 26.5% in the control group. At twelve-month follow-up, rates of mobility loss were 5.2% in the GMCB intervention vs. 18.5% in the control group. As compared to other home-based walking exercise trials in patients with PAD, the GOALS trial is the longest randomized trial to demonstrate benefits of home-based exercise in patients with PAD. In addition, the GOALS trial demonstrates that home-based exercise can be effective in PAD patients both with and without classical symptoms of claudication.

One randomized trial of home-based exercise demonstrated no benefit of home-based walking exercise in patients with PAD. Collins et al randomized 145 participants with PAD and diabetes to a six-month behavioral intervention vs. an attention control group.[18] The behavioral intervention consisted of one walking session per week at an exercise center with an instructor and other patients with PAD and three days of walking at home, working up to 50 min of exercise per session. Participants in the intervention group also received bi-weekly telephone calls, in which an instructor reviewed their walking progress and provided feedback. However, at six months follow-up, there were no differences in treadmill walking performance between the home-based behavioral intervention vs. the control group. It is unclear whether including only PAD participants with diabetes mellitus or whether aspects of the intervention resulted in lack of benefit of this home-based walking exercise intervention.

PRACTICAL ASPECTS OF PRESCRIBING HOME-BASED EXERCISE IN CLINICAL PRACTICE

Home-based walking exercise may be prescribed by practicing clinicians who treat PAD patients with intermittent claudication (Table 26-2). Prior to recommending or prescribing a home-based exercise program, PAD patients should undergo a baseline cardiac stress test to rule out coronary artery ischemia. The cardiac stress test serves to identify coronary ischemia that may develop during a new walking exercise program. Current clinical practice guidelines for patients with PAD indicate that a regular treadmill exercise stress test is sufficient for evaluating PAD patients for coronary ischemia prior to initiating a new exercise program.[17] PAD patients whose baseline treadmill exercise stress test shows no ischemia may proceed with exercise therapy. PAD patients whose baseline treadmill exercise stress test indicates ischemia require additional evaluation and appropriate treatment prior to proceeding with exercise therapy.

Based on published literature, PAD patients should be advised to walk for exercise at least three times weekly. The exercise program should be tailored for the individual patient. In general, PAD patients should be advised to begin with 15 to 20 min of walking exercise per day. Based on current evidence, PAD patients should be advised to walk to maximal leg pain, although it is possible that walking only to the onset of

TABLE 26-2. COMPONENTS OF SUCCESSFUL HOME-BASED EXERCISE PROGRAMS IN PATIENTS WITH PAD

Characteristics of successful programs
• Walking exercise at least three times weekly.
• Increase walking exercise sessions by 5 min each week, working up to 45 to 50 min per session.
• Walk to maximal leg pain.
• Monitor activity level, using a step-counter or log.
• Include feedback from a coach or physiologist at least once monthly.

ischemic pain may also be beneficial. PAD patients should be advised to walk at a speed that elicits leg ischemia symptoms within 10 min. They should be advised that stopping to rest is acceptable and typical for patients with PAD. Once leg pain subsides during a rest, the PAD patient should be advised to resume walking again. The duration of exercise should be increased by 5 min each week, until the PAD patient is walking at least 30 min per session and preferably 45 to 50 min per session, not including rest periods.

Home based exercise programs that have been effective for PAD patients have either used activity monitors and/or have incorporated principles of behavioral change theory including goal-setting and monitoring progress. Therefore, PAD patients should be advised to set walking goals each week and write them down. PAD patients should be specific about when and where and for how long they will walk for exercise. For example, they should record on which dates and at what time they will exercise. They should record their exercise activity each week and/or monitor it using an activity monitor. Their actual walking exercise activity should be compared to their walking exercise goals. Ideally, this information should be reviewed periodically by a coach or a clinician who can provide feedback to the patient. In the study by Gardner et al., participants' frequency and duration of walking exercise was reviewed as infrequently as every four weeks.[20] Further study is needed to determine whether even less frequent monitoring is also effective.

ALTERNATIVE FORMS OF HOME-BASED EXERCISE FOR PAD PATIENTS

In supervised settings, exercise modalities other than walking have been shown to improve walking ability in people who have PAD. For example, both upper and lower extremity ergometry exercise have been shown to increased walking endurance in patients with PAD.[24–26] In one study, a 40 minute exercise session, including 10 bouts of two minute arm ergometry, each bout separated by two min of rest, significantly improved walking endurance in PAD patients who had intermittent claudication.[24] However, these exercises were performed in a supervised setting, and there is no evidence that upper or lower extremity ergometry exercise carried out in a home-based setting improves walking endurance who people have PAD. Further study is needed to determine whether other forms of exercise that have been effective in a supervised setting may also be effective when carried out at home.

CONCLUSION

Supervised treadmill exercise significantly improves treadmill walking performance in people who have PAD. However, most PAD patients do not participate in supervised exercise programs because of lack of insurance coverage and because travelling to a center for exercise may be burdensome for people who have PAD. Growing evidence, published in the past five years, suggests that home based exercise can improve walking performance and prevent mobility loss in people who have PAD. Use of activity monitors and tracking progress appear to be important components of successful home-based exercise programs in people who have PAD.

REFERENCES

1. Go A, Mozaffarian D, Roger V, et al. AHA statistical update: Heart disease and stroke statistics, 2013 update. *Circulation.* 2013;127:e6–e245.
2. Fowkes FG, Rudan D, Rudan I, et al. Comparison of global estimates of prevalence and risk factors for peripheral artery disease in 2000 and 2010: a systematic review and analysis. *Lancet.* 2013;382:1329–40.
3. McDermott MM, Greenland P, Liu K, et al. The ankle brachial index is associated with leg function and physical activity: the Walking and Leg Circulation Study. *Ann Intern Med,* 2002;136:873–83.
4. McDermott MM, Guralnik JM, Tian L, et al. Baseline functional performance predicts the rate of mobility loss in persons with peripheral arterial disease. *J Am Coll Cardiol.* 2007;50:974–82.
5. McDermott MM, Greenland P, Liu K, et al. Leg symptoms in peripheral arterial disease: associated clinical characteristics and functional impairment. *JAMA.* 2001;286:1599–1606.
6. McDermott MM, Liu K, Greenland P, et al. Functional decline in peripheral arterial disease: associations with the ankle brachial index and leg symptoms. *JAMA.* 2004;292:453–61.
7. Imparato AM, Kim GE, Davidson T, et al. Intermittent claudication: its natural course. *Surgery.* 1975;78:795–9.
8. McAllister FF. The fate of patients with intermittent claudication managed nonoperatively. *Am J Surg.* 1976;132:593–5.
9. Boyd AM. The natural course of arteriosclerosis of the lower extremities. *Proc R Soc Med.* 1962;55:591–3.
10. McDermott MM, Guralnik JM, Tian L, et al. Associations of borderline and low normal ankle-brachial index values with functional decline at 5-year follow-up: the WALCS (Walking and Leg Circulation Study). *J Am Coll Cardiol.* 2009;53:1056–62.
11. Bedenis R, Stewart M, Cleanthis M, et al. Cilostazol for intermittent claudication. *Cochrane Database Syst Rev.* 2014;10:CD003748. doi: 10.1002/14651858.CD003748.pub4.
12. Salhiyyah K, Senanayake E, Abdel-hadi M, et al. Pentoxifylline for intermittent claudication. *Cochrane Database Syst Rev.* 2012;1:CD005262. doi: 10.1002/14651858.CD005262.pub2.
13. Fakhry F, van de Luijtgaarden KM, Bax L, et al. Supervised walking therapy in patients with intermittent claudication. *J Vasc Surg.* 2012;56:1132–42.
14. Gardner AW, Poehlman ET. Exercise rehabilitation programs for the treatment of claudication pain. A meta-analysis. *JAMA.* 1995;274:975–80.
15. Falcone RA, Hirsch AT, Regensteiner JG, et al. Peripheral arterial disease rehabilitation: A review. *J Cardiopulm Rehabil.* 2003;23:170–5.
16. Regensteiner JG. Exercise rehabilitation for the patient with intermittent claudication: a highly effective yet underutilized treatment. *Curr Drug Targets Cardiovasc Haematol Disord.* 2004;4:233–9.
17. Hirsch AT, Haskal ZJ, Hertzer NR, et al. ACC/AHA 2005 Practice Guidelines for the management of patients with peripheral arterial disease (lower extremity, renal, mesenteric, and abdominal aortic): a collaborative report from the American Association for Vascular Surgery/Society for Vascular Surgery, Society for Cardiovascular Angiography and Interventions, Society for Vascular Medicine and Biology, Society of Interventional Radiology, and the ACC/AHA Task Force on Practice Guidelines (Writing Committee to Develop Guidelines for the Management of Patients With Peripheral Arterial Disease): endorsed by the American Association of Cardiovascular and Pulmonary Rehabilitation; National Heart, Lung, and Blood Institute; Society for Vascular Nursing; TransAtlantic Inter-Society Consensus; and Vascular Disease Foundation. *Circulation.* 2006;113:e463–e654.
18. Collins TC, Lunos S, Carlson T, et al. Effects of a home-based walking intervention on mobility and quality of life in people with diabetes and peripheral arterial disease: a randomized controlled trial. *Diabetes Care.* 2011;34:2174–9.

19. Gardner AW, Parker DE, Montgomery PS, et al. Efficacy of quantified home-based exercise and supervised exercise in patients with intermittent claudication: a randomized controlled trial. *Circulation.* 2011;123:491–8.
20. Gardner AW, Parker DE, Montgomery PS, et al. Step-monitored home exercise improves ambulation, vascular function, and inflammation in symptomatic patients with peripheral artery disease: a randomized controlled trial. *J Am Heart Assoc.* 2014;3:e001107. doi: 10.1161/JAHA.114.001107.
21. McDermott MM, Liu K, Guralnik JM, et al. Home-based walking exercise intervention in peripheral artery disease: a randomized clinical trial. *JAMA.* 2013;310:57–65.
22. McDermott MM, Guralnik JM, Criqui MH, et al. Home-based walking exercise in peripheral artery disease: 12-month follow-up of the GOALS randomized trial. *J Am Heart Assoc.* 2014;3:e000711. doi: 10.1161/JAHA.113.000711.
23. McDermott MM, Guralnik JM, Criqui MH, et al. Unsupervised exercise and mobility loss in peripheral artery disease: a randomized controlled trial. *J Am Heart Assoc.* 2015;4. pii: e001659. doi: 10.1161/JAHA.114.001659.
24. Zwierska I, Walker RD, Choksy SA, et al. Upper- vs lower-limb aerobic exercise rehabilitation in patients with symptomatic peripheral arterial disease: a randomized controlled trial. *J Vasc Surg.* 2005;42:1122–30.
25. Zwierska I, Walker RD, Choksy SA, et al. Relative tolerance to upper- and lower-limb aerobic exercise in patients with peripheral arterial disease. *Eur J Vasc Endovasc Surg.* 2006;31:157–63.
26. Treat-Jacobson D, Bronas UG, Leon AS. Efficacy of arm-ergometry versus treadmill exercise training to improve walking distance in patients with claudication. *Vasc Med.* 2009;14:203–13.

27

Femoropopliteal In-stent Restenosis (FP-ISR): Classification, Prevention, and Treatment

Karen J. Ho, MD

Lower extremity endovascular procedures are commonly used alternatives to traditional bypass surgery for disabling claudication and critical limb ischemia. Between 1996 and 2006, endovascular interventions in the lower extremity tripled in the Medicare population, with peripheral angioplasty being the most frequently performed endovascular intervention. Femoropopliteal (FP) angioplasty procedures comprised approximately 40% of all lower extremity endovascular interventions in this cohort.[1] High technical success rates and low morbidity and mortality associated with superficial femoral artery angioplasty/stenting have made endovascular therapy the preferred treatment modality for patients with symptomatic and mild-to-moderate disease. However, despite advances in self-expanding stent structural integrity and conformability over the past three decades,[2] in-stent restenosis (ISR) remains a pervasive challenge to the long-term patency of superficial femoral artery (SFA) and popliteal artery stents. The goal of this review is to summarize current strategies for the classification, prevention, and treatment of in-stent restenosis in the femoropopliteal segment.

FP-ISR: DEFINITION AND ETIOPATHOLOGY

In-stent restenosis refers to restenosis within the area of a stented artery, in contrast to "in-segment" restenosis, which refers to restenosis in the stented area and 5 mm on either side of the stent. Quantification of ISR varies and can include net gain of lumen, percent diameter restenosis, and binary restenosis. The latter term refers to restenosis of the diameter by 50% or more, as defined by duplex ultrasonography or angiography.

In-stent restenosis is caused by neointimal proliferation, primarily due to medial vascular smooth muscle cell proliferation[3] in response to arterial "injury" represented by angioplasty and stent implantation. Overdistension of the angioplastied segment causes endothelial disruption, internal elastic lamina fracture, and medial dissection, which then incites an acute inflammatory cascade that leads to vascular smooth muscle and adventitial fibroblast proliferation and neointimal hyperplasia.[4] Lumen enlargement is caused by plaque compression/embolization, axial plaque redistribution towards the proximal and distal segments outside the stent, plaque extrusion, and vessel expansion.[5] Stent deployment after angioplasty minimizes early elastic recoil and compresses the dissection plane.[4] Stent implantation also influences arterial remodeling over time. An intravascular ultrasound study of stented arteries demonstrated that since stents prevent elastic recoil and negative remodeling in response to angioplasty, lumen loss over time is due to stent-related vascular injury and exaggeration in neointimal proliferation within and adjacent to the stent.[4,6] Histological examination of stented porcine coronary arteries demonstrated that intimal thickening over each strut correlated with the depth of strut penetration, and the extent of restenosis over arterial cross sections correlated with the average injury imposed by all struts.[7] Excessive stent oversizing also leads to ISR.[8] Of note, the SFA responds to stent implantation with an acute inflammatory response that is greater than that seen in other arteries,[9,10] which may be related to micromovements of the stent along the vessel wall that leads to persistent inflammation and endothelial activation. Finally, in addition to the biologic and inflammatory events that lead to ISR, anatomic and clinical risk factors that contribute to ISR include longer lesion lengths, small vessel diameters, and diabetes mellitus.[11]

CLASSIFICATION

A classification system for FP-ISR was proposed by Tosaka et al.[12] ISR lesions were classified by angiographic appearance (Figure 27-1):

- class I (focal ISR): includes lesions <50 mm in length that are positioned in the stent body, at the stent edge, or both
- class II (diffuse ISR): includes stent body lesions and stent edge lesions >50 mm in length
- class III: totally occluded ISR

As in coronary ISR, different angiographic classes of FP-ISR are independent predictors of outcomes after balloon angioplasty.[11,12] Kaplan-Meier analysis showed that the rate of recurrent ISR at 2 years after angioplasty was higher in patients with class

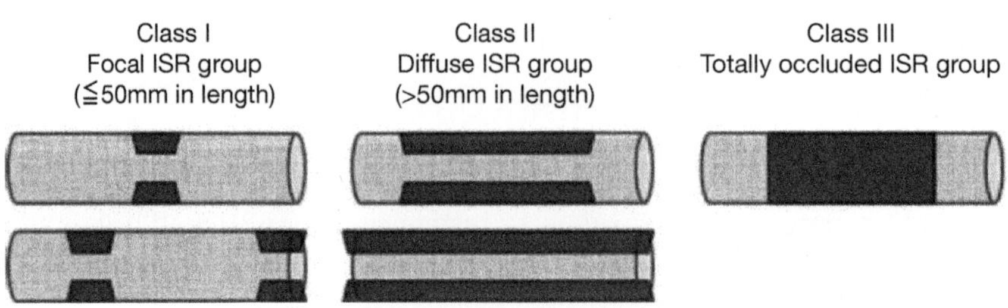

Figure 27-1. Classification of FP-ISR based on angiography. (Modified from Tosaka et al.)[12]

III lesions than patients with lesions in class I or class II (84.8%, class III vs. 49.9%, class I vs. 53.3%, class I; $p < .001$). The rate of recurrent occlusion at 2 years was also higher in class III compared to the other classes (64.6%, class III vs. 15.9%, class I vs. 18.9%, class II; $p < .001$). While this classification system could provide a framework for treatment strategies for FP-ISR, all FP-ISR lesions were treated with balloon angioplasty alone. Since no other adjunctive modalities (e.g. laser, atherectomy, stents, stent-grafts, or drug-eluting devices) were used, it is unclear if this classification scheme is relevant to the "real-world" setting.

INCIDENCE

Early studies demonstrated that patency of percutaneous transluminal balloon angioplasty (PTA) alone was inferior to stenting for longer lesions in the SFA.[13–17] However, the SFA presents unique challenges to achieving durable long-term stent patency due to mechanical forces that include axial compression and extension, radial compression, bending, and torsion.[18] The presence of diffuse and/or heavy calcific disease, long lesion length, small caliber vessel, and concomitant popliteal and tibial disease all compromise the long-term patency of endovascular interventions in the SFA. Several randomized trials comparing self-expanding nitinol stents to PTA alone in the SFA (Table 27-1A) and registries of self-expanding nitinol stents (Table 27-1B) provide estimates of the incidence of FP-ISR. Overall, ISR rates remain high despite advances in stent technology, ranging from 15% to 40% in lesions of moderate length (up to 150 mm) at 1 year.

ENDOVASCULAR TREATMENT OPTIONS

Endovascular treatment options include balloon angioplasty, cutting balloon angioplasty, repeat stenting, drug-eluting stent (DES) placement, drug-coated balloons (DCB), stent grafting, excisional or laser atherectomy, or a combination of these. Each of these treatment modalities is briefly discussed below.

Balloon Angioplasty or Cutting Balloon Angioplasty

Despite high rates of technical success after balloon angioplasty for FP-ISR, recurrence rates of restenosis and reocclusion are high.[12] Cutting balloons offer the theoretical advantage of less vessel wall trauma due to controlled incisions by balloon-mounted microtomes that lead to smooth lumen gain, less vascular inflammation, and reduced neointima formation. However, an early small study demonstrated no benefit to cutting balloons over conventional balloons in the 6-month restenosis rate (65% conventional vs. 73% cutting balloon, $P = .73$), ABI, or maximum walking capacity.[19]

Drug-coated Balloons and Drug-eluting Stents

The concept of preventing neointimal hyperplasia development with local delivery of antiproliferative drugs has proven to be safe and effective in coronary arteries in certain

TABLE 27-1A. PRIMARY PATENCY OF BARE METAL STENTS IN RANDOMIZED TRIALS USING SELF-EXPANDING NITINOL STENTS IN THE SFA

Study name	Treatment groups	Cohort size	Lesion length (bare metal stent group) (mm)	Primary endpoint	Study period	Primary patency (bare metal stent group)	Ref.
ABSOLUTE	Absolute vs. PTA	104	132±71	Binary restenosis	6 mo	76%	15
					12 mo	63%	15
ASTRON	Astron vs. PTA	73	98±54	Binary restenosis	6 mo	78%	17
					12 mo	66%	17
RESILIENT	LifeStent vs. PTA	206	71±44	TLR	12 mo	81%	16
SUPER	SMART vs. PTA	150	123±54	Binary restenosis	12 mo	53%	40

TABLE 27-1B. REGISTRIES OF SELF-EXPANDING NITINOL STENTS IN THE SFA

Study name	Treatment groups	Cohort size	Lesion length	Primary endpoint	Study period	Primary patency	Ref.
DURABILITY I and II	EverFlex	151, 287	96±27, 89±45	In-stent restenosis	12 mo	72%, 77.2%	41 42
COMPLETE SE	Complete SE	196	60.7	In-stent restenosis	12 mo	72.6%	43
STROLL	SMART	250	77.3±35.3	In-stent restenosis	12 mo	81.7%	44
SUPERA	SUPERA	107	111±50	In-stent restenosis	12, 24 mo	85% (12 mo), 76% (24 mo)	45
PEACE I	Pulsar-18	200	182±52	In-stent restenosis	12 mo	85.4%	46
SUMMIT	EPIC	100	69.5±40.5 mm	In-stent restenosis	12 mo	85.1%	47

patient and lesion subsets. Sirolimus (Rapamycin) and paclitaxel (Taxol) have both been used for SFA applications. Clinical trials comparing DES to self-expanding nitinol stents for the treatment of *de novo* SFA occlusive disease are shown in Table 27-2.

SIROCCO I and II, the earliest trials of DES in the SFA, showed an early advantage to the sirolimus DES in binary restenosis, but there was no difference between the bare metal stent (BMS) and DES groups by 18 months. In addition, there was a high stent fracture rate and the loading dose and elution profile of sirolimus in the DES used were lower and faster, respectively, than was utilized for the more successful sirolimus-eluting Cypher stent. The Zilver® PTX® stent (Cook Medical Inc., Bloomington, IN) is the only FDA-approved DES for use in the SFA. It has a self-expanding nitinol platform with a polymer-free paclitaxel coating at 3 μg/mm^2 dose density. Paclitaxel is a highly lipophilic drug that alters microtubule formation and inhibits vascular smooth muscle cell migration and proliferation. It has a narrow therapeutic range and, at higher concentrations, can disrupt the internal elastic lamina.[20,21] The stent was evaluated in the pivotal Zilver PTX trial, which randomized patients with relatively short SFA lesions (mean lesion length 54±41 mm, 29.6% total occlusions) to either the Zilver PTX stent or PTA. The trial allowed use of only one stent per patient.[22] The primary endpoint at 12 months was primary patency, defined by a peak systolic velocity ratio of less than 2.0 by duplex ultrasonography or a stenosis of >50% on angiography. Primary patency at 12 months was significantly better in the Zilver PTX group than the PTA group (83.1%, DES vs. 32.8%, PTA; $P < 0.01$). These benefits were maintained at 2 years with superior event-free survival and primary patency (74.8%, DES vs. 26.5%, PTA; $P < 0.01$) in the Zilver PTX group.[23] Analysis of the subgroup with suboptimal initial PTA results who underwent a second randomization before provisional stenting, found the 12-month primary patency rate to be better in the PTA and Zilver PTX group than in the PTA and BMS group (89.9% versus 73%; $P = 0.01$). The provisional DES group exhibited a trend toward superior primary patency at 2 years over the provisional BMS group (83.4% versus 64.1%; $P = 0.05$). Some criticisms of the trial were that the lesions treated were relatively short and not typical of those seen in clinical practice, that the comparison group was PTA rather than BMS, and that the use of a single stent may have aided in minimizing stent fracture rates.

TABLE 27-2. SUMMARY OF TRIALS COMPARING DES TO SELF-EXPANDING NITINOL STENTS FOR *DE NOVO* SFA LESIONS

Study name	Treatment groups	Cohort size	Lesion length	Primary endpoint	Study period	Primary patency	Ref.
SIROCCO	Sirolimus-eluting SMART vs. bare metal stent	57	86.5±37 DES 76.3±46 BMS	In-stent restenosis	6 mo	100% (DES) vs. 93% (BMS), $P = .49$	48
		93	85±44 DES 81±52 BMS	In-stent restenosis	2 yr	77% (DES) vs. 79% (BMS), $P > .05$	49
Zilver PTX	Zilver PTX (Paclitaxel eluting PTX) vs. bare metal stent or PTA	238	54±41	Patency	12 mo	83.1% (DES) vs. 32.8% (PTA); 89.9% (provisional DES) vs. 73% (provisional BMS)	22

DES have also been used for treatment of FP-ISR. The Zilver PTX Registry included 108 patients who were treated for FP-ISR. Mean lesion length in this subgroup was 133 mm with 31% stent occlusions. Primary patency after DES placement was 78.8% at 12 months and clinically driven freedom from target lesion revascularization was 81% at 12 months and 80.5% at 24 months. Interestingly, a multivariate analysis of patient and anatomic factors associated with recurrent ISR showed that stent occlusion was not a predictor of recurrent restenosis or reocclusion.[24,25]

Drug-coated balloons for the treatment of SFA ISR are also promising. Stabile et al.[26] used a paclitaxel-eluting balloon (IN.PACT® Admiral® (Medtronic, Inc., Minneapolis, MN) in 39 patients with SFA ISR and observed a 12-month patency rate of 92.1%. Two-year primary patency rate was 70.3%,[27] but complex ISR lesions (classes II and III) were associated with a higher rate of recurrent restenosis compared with class I lesions (33.3%, II and 36.3%, III vs. 12.5%, I; $P = 0.05$). The DEBATE-ISR trial of 44 patients with diabetes and FP-ISR treated with the IN.PACT observed a 12-month primary patency rate of 80.5%, which was improved from historical controls of patients with diabetes and FP-ISR (71.8%, $P < .0001$).[28] Completed and ongoing trials for DCB for treatment of FP-ISR include FAIR, Lutonix, and Cotavance.

Stent Grafting

Stent grafts such as a polytetrafluoroethylene-covered nitinol stent (Viabahn®, W. L. Gore, Inc., Flagstaff, AZ) offer the advantage of excluding the neointima from the vessel lumen.[29] A small series of 22 patients with FP-ISR (mean lesion length 214 mm) treated with a Viabahn stent graft demonstrated 85.1% primary patency rate at 12 months.[30] The RELINE trial, which is a multicenter trial of 100 patients with SFA ISR (mean lesion length 190 mm) randomized to Viabahn stent grafting or PTA, demonstrated a primary patency rate of 28% in the PTA group vs. 72% in the Viabahn group ($P < .001$). There were no stent fractures at one year in the Viabahn group.[31]

Excimer Laser Atherectomy

Laser atherectomy, which ablates and debulks neointimal tissue and suppresses platelet aggregation,[32,33] has been examined for the treatment of FP-ISR in two recent studies. The PATENT trial employed the Turbo Elite® laser catheter and Turbo Booster® (Spectranetics, Inc., Colorado Springs, CO) for FP-ISR (mean lesion length 123±95.9 mm) in 90 patients. Adjunctive balloon angioplasty was performed in 87.8% lesions. Primary patency at 6 and 12 months was 64.1% and 37.8%, respectively.[34] The EXCITE ISR trial randomized 250 patients to Turbo-Tandem® laser atherectomy with PTA vs. PTA alone for the FP-ISR. Mean lesion length was 196±120 mm with total occlusions in 30.5% and 36.8% of patients in the laser+PTA and PTA groups, respectively. Six-month freedom from target lesion revascularization was 73.5% (laser) vs. 51.8% (PTA; $P < 0.005$), and 30-day major adverse event rates were 5.8% (laser) vs. 20.5% (PTA; $P < 0.001$), respectively.[35]

Laser-assisted angioplasty and stent-grafting was studied in the SALVAGE trial, which included 27 patients with FP-ISR (mean lesion 207±103) length. In theory, debulking of the neointimal hyperplasia prior to stent-graft implantation improves the cross-sectional area of the artery to reduce stent-graft infolding and the risk of acute or subacute thrombosis. VIABAHN stent-grafts were used in all patients. Technical success was 100%. Primary patency was 48% at 12 months and target lesion revascularization was 17.4% at 12 months.[36] Reduced patency was attributed to edge restenosis, potentially due to stent oversizing. Newer models of VIABAHN have a proximal contoured edge to reduce proximal edge restenosis. Future studies will determine if laser atherectomy combined with stent grafting are a durable treatment strategy for FP-ISR.

Excisional Atherectomy and DCB

The combination of catheter-based atherectomy with DCB angioplasty offers the advantages of combined lesion debulking and the anti-restenotic effect of DCB. In a retrospective analysis of 29 patients with FP-ISR treated with excisional atherectomy with DCB vs. excisional atherectomy with PTA, 12-month restenosis rates were 15.3% in the DCB group vs. 56.2% in the PTA group. Multivariable analysis for restenosis demonstrated that DCB treatment was independently associated with decreased restenosis compared to PTA (hazard ratio 0.28, 95% confidence interval 0.120–.66; P = .004).[37] The ongoing PHOTOPAC randomized trial will further evaluate safety and efficacy of laser atherectomy prior to DCB angioplasty vs. DCB angioplasty alone.

SURGICAL TREATMENT OPTIONS

There is notably little data on surgical bypass outcomes for FP-ISR. As restenosis lesions often extend beyond the stent, bypass options often involve a below-knee anastomosis. Furthermore, repeated endovascular reinterventions may lead to diminished distal runoff and more severe ischemia. There is also increasing evidence that "endovascular first" may be associated with poorer options for secondary lower extremity bypass. In a retrospective analysis of patients undergoing infrainguinal bypass, patients with prior ipsilateral endovascular interventions had higher rates of one-year amputation (31% vs. 20%; P = .046) and one-year graft occlusion (28% vs. 18%; P = .009) than those without.[38] Furthermore, the BASIL trial demonstrated that patients who underwent bypass surgery after failed or suboptimal balloon angioplasty had a lower amputation-free survival rate than those who underwent primary bypass surgery.[39]

SUMMARY

In summary, the prevention and treatment of FP-ISR are among the greatest unmet challenges in vascular surgery. Endovascular treatment for advanced femoropopliteal occlusive disease continues to have high treatment failure rates and current available strategies for prevention and treatment of FP-ISR, though improving with time, continue to be limited. Trials involving currently available technologies have been heterogeneous in terms of angiographic patterns of ISR and other anatomic factors, comparison groups, and primary endpoints, which makes evaluation of these technologies and development of treatment algorithms difficult. At this time, DCB and DES are particularly promising, but larger scale randomized trials with long-term follow-up are warranted to further define their role in the treatment of FP-ISR.

REFERENCES

1. Goodney PP, Beck AW, Nagle J, et al. National trends in lower extremity bypass surgery, endovascular interventions, and major amputations. *J Vasc Surg.* 2009;50:54–60.
2. Scheinert D, Scheinert S, Sax J, et al. Prevalence and clinical impact of stent fractures after femoropopliteal stenting. *J Am Coll Cardiol.* 2005;45:312–5.
3. Kearney M, Pieczek A, Haley L, et al. Histopathology of in-stent restenosis in patients with peripheral artery disease. *Circulation.* 1997;95:1998–2002.
4. Edelman ER, Rogers C. Hoop dreams. Stents without restenosis. *Circulation.* 1996;94:1199–202.
5. Bennett MR. In-stent stenosis: pathology and implications for the development of drug eluting stents. *Heart.* 2003;89:218–24.
6. Hoffmann R, Mintz GS, Dussaillant GR, et al. Patterns and mechanisms of in-stent restenosis. A serial intravascular ultrasound study. *Circulation.* 1996;94:1247–54.
7. Schwartz RS, Huber KC, Murphy JG, et al. Restenosis and the proportional neointimal response to coronary artery injury: results in a porcine model. *J Am Coll Cardiol.* 1992;19:267–74.
8. Zhao HQ, Nikanorov A, Virmani R, et al. Late stent expansion and neointimal proliferation of oversized Nitinol stents in peripheral arteries. *Cardiovasc Intervent Radiol.* 2009;32:720–6.
9. Schillinger M, Exner M, Mlekusch W, et al. Balloon angioplasty and stent implantation induce a vascular inflammatory reaction. *J Endovasc Ther.* 2002;9:59–66.
10. Schillinger M, Exner M, Mlekusch W, et al. Inflammatory response to stent implantation: differences in femoropopliteal, iliac, and carotid arteries. *Radiology.* 2002;224:529–35.
11. Mehran R, Dangas G, Abizaid AS, et al. Angiographic patterns of in-stent restenosis: classification and implications for long-term outcome. *Circulation.* 1999;100:1872–8.
12. Tosaka A, Soga Y, Iida O, et al. Classification and clinical impact of restenosis after femoropopliteal stenting. *J Am Coll Cardiol.* 2012;59:16–23.
13. Capek P, McLean GK, Berkowitz HD. Femoropopliteal angioplasty. Factors influencing long-term success. *Circulation.* 1991;83:I70–80.
14. Laird JR, Katzen BT, Scheinert D, et al. Nitinol stent implantation vs. balloon angioplasty for lesions in the superficial femoral and proximal popliteal arteries of patients with claudication: three-year follow-up from the RESILIENT randomized trial. *J Endovasc Ther.* 2012;19:1–9.
15. Schillinger M, Sabeti S, Loewe C, et al. Balloon angioplasty versus implantation of nitinol stents in the superficial femoral artery. *N Engl J Med.* 2006;354:1879–88.
16. Laird JR, Katzen BT, Scheinert D, et al. Nitinol stent implantation versus balloon angioplasty for lesions in the superficial femoral artery and proximal popliteal artery: twelve-month results from the RESILIENT randomized trial. *Circ Cardiovasc Interv.* 2010;3:267–76.
17. Dick P, Wallner H, Sabeti S, et al. Balloon angioplasty versus stenting with nitinol stents in intermediate length superficial femoral artery lesions. *Catheter Cardiovasc Interv.* 2009;74:1090–5.
18. Cheng CP, Wilson NM, Hallett RL, et al. In vivo MR angiographic quantification of axial and twisting deformations of the superficial femoral artery resulting from maximum hip and knee flexion. *J Vasc Interv Radiol.* 2006;17:979–87.
19. Dick P, Sabeti S, Mlekusch W, et al. Conventional balloon angioplasty versus peripheral cutting balloon angioplasty for treatment of femoropopliteal artery in-stent restenosis: initial experience. *Radiology.* 2008;248:297–302.
20. Pires NM, Eefting D, de Vries MR, et al. Sirolimus and paclitaxel provoke different vascular pathological responses after local delivery in a murine model for restenosis on underlying atherosclerotic arteries. *Heart.* 2007;93:922–7.
21. Axel DI, Kunert W, Goggelmann C, et al. Paclitaxel inhibits arterial smooth muscle cell proliferation and migration in vitro and in vivo using local drug delivery. *Circulation.* 1997;96:636–45.

22. Dake MD, Ansel GM, Jaff MR, et al. Paclitaxel-eluting stents show superiority to balloon angioplasty and bare metal stents in femoropopliteal disease: twelve-month Zilver PTX randomized study results. *Circ Cardiovasc Interv.* 2011;4:495–504.
23. Dake MD, Ansel GM, Jaff MR, et al. Sustained safety and effectiveness of paclitaxel-eluting stents for femoropopliteal lesions: 2-year follow-up from the Zilver PTX randomized and single-arm clinical studies. *J Am Coll Cardiol.* 2013;61:2417–27.
24. Dake MD, Scheinert D, Tepe G, et al. Nitinol stents with polymer-free paclitaxel coating for lesions in the superficial femoral and popliteal arteries above the knee: twelve-month safety and effectiveness results from the Zilver PTX single-arm clinical study. *J Endovasc Ther.* 2011;18:613–23.
25. Zeller T, Dake MD, Tepe G, et al. Treatment of femoropopliteal in-stent restenosis with paclitaxel-eluting stents. *J Am Coll Cardiol Interv.* 2013;6:274–81.
26. Stabile E, Virga V, Salemme L, et al. Drug-eluting balloon for treatment of superficial femoral artery in-stent restenosis. *J Am Coll Cardiol.* 2012;60:1739–42.
27. Virga V, Stabile E, Biamino G, et al. Drug-eluting balloons for the treatment of the superficial femoral artery in-stent restenosis: 2-year follow-up. *J Am Coll Cardiol Interv.* 2014;7:411–5.
28. Liistro F, Angioli P, Porto I, et al. Paclitaxel-eluting balloon vs. standard angioplasty to reduce recurrent restenosis in diabetic patients with in-stent restenosis of the superficial femoral and proximal popliteal arteries: the DEBATE-ISR study. *J Endovasc Ther.* 2014;21:1–8.
29. Doomernik DE, Golchehr B, Lensvelt MM, et al. The role of superficial femoral artery endoluminal bypass in long de novo lesions and in-stent restenosis. *J Cardiovasc Surg. (Torino)* 2012;53:447–57.
30. Al Shammeri O, Bitar F, Ghitelman J, et al. Viabahn for femoropopliteal in-stent restenosis. *Ann Saudi Med.* 2012;32:572–82.
31. Adams GL, Bersin RM, George JC, Subramanianm V, Soukas PA. Data-driven Treatment Approach to In-Stent Restenosis. *Endovascular Today.* 2015:6.
32. Topaz O, Bernardo NL, Shah R, et al. Effectiveness of excimer laser coronary angioplasty in acute myocardial infarction or in unstable angina pectoris. *Am J Cardiol.* 2001;87:849–55.
33. Topaz O, Minisi AJ, Bernardo NL, et al. Alterations of platelet aggregation kinetics with ultraviolet laser emission: the "stunned platelet" phenomenon. *Thromb Haemost.* 2001;86:1087–93.
34. Schmidt A, Zeller T, Sievert H, et al. Photoablation using the turbo-booster and excimer laser for in-stent restenosis treatment: twelve-month results from the PATENT study. *J Endovasc Ther.* 2014;21:52–60.
35. Dippel EJ, Makam P, Kovach R, et al. Randomized controlled study of excimer laser atherectomy for treatment of femoropopliteal in-stent restenosis: initial results from the EXCITE ISR trial (EXCImer Laser Randomized Controlled Study for Treatment of FemoropopliTEal In-Stent Restenosis). *JACC Cardiovasc Interv.* 2015;8:92–101.
36. Laird JR, Jr., Yeo KK, Rocha-Singh K, et al. Excimer laser with adjunctive balloon angioplasty and heparin-coated self-expanding stent grafts for the treatment of femoropopliteal artery in-stent restenosis: twelve-month results from the SALVAGE study. *Catheter Cardiovasc Interv.* 2012;80:852–9.
37. Sixt S, Carpio Cancino OG, Treszl A, et al. Drug-coated balloon angioplasty after directional atherectomy improves outcome in restenotic femoropopliteal arteries. *J Vasc Surg.* 2013;58:682–6.
38. Nolan BW, De Martino RR, Stone DH, et al. Prior failed ipsilateral percutaneous endovascular intervention in patients with critical limb ischemia predicts poor outcome after lower extremity bypass. *J Vasc Surg.* 2011;54:730-735; discussion 735–6.
39. Bradbury AW, Adam DJ, Bell J, et al. Bypass versus Angioplasty in Severe Ischaemia of the Leg (BASIL) trial: Analysis of amputation free and overall survival by treatment received. *J Vasc Surg.* 2010;51:18S–31S.

40. Chalmers N, Walker PT, Belli AM, et al. Randomized trial of the SMART stent versus balloon angioplasty in long superficial femoral artery lesions: the SUPER study. *Cardiovasc Intervent Radiol.* 2013;36:353–61.
41. Bosiers M, Torsello G, Gissler HM, et al. Nitinol stent implantation in long superficial femoral artery lesions: 12-month results of the DURABILITY I study. *J Endovasc Ther.* 2009;16:261–9.
42. Matsumura JS, Yamanouchi D, Goldstein JA, et al. The United States StuDy for EvalUating EndovasculaR TreAtments of Lesions in the Superficial Femoral Artery and Proximal Popliteal By usIng the Protege EverfLex NitInol STent SYstem II (DURABILITY II). *J Vasc Surg.* 2013;58:73–83 e71.
43. Laird JR, Jain A, Zeller T, et al. Nitinol stent implantation in the superficial femoral artery and proximal popliteal artery: twelve-month results from the complete SE multicenter trial. *J Endovasc Ther.* 2014;21:202–12.
44. Gray WA, Feiring A, Cioppi M, et al. S.M.A.R.T. self-expanding nitinol stent for the treatment of atherosclerotic lesions in the superficial femoral artery (STROLL): 1-year outcomes. *J Vasc Interv Radiol.* 2015;26:21–8.
45. Scheinert D, Grummt L, Piorkowski M, et al. A novel self-expanding interwoven nitinol stent for complex femoropopliteal lesions: 24-month results of the SUPERA SFA registry. *J Endovasc Ther.* 2011;18:745–52.
46. Lichtenberg M, Kolks O, Hailer B, et al. PEACE I all-comers registry: patency evaluation after implantation of the 4-French Pulsar-18 self-expanding nitinol stent in femoropopliteal lesions. *J Endovasc Ther.* 2014;21:373–80.
47. Werner M, Piorkowski M, Thieme M, et al. SUMMIT registry: one-year outcomes after implantation of the EPIC self-expanding nitinol stent in the femoropopliteal segment. *J Endovasc Ther.* 2013;20:759–66.
48. Duda SH, Bosiers M, Lammer J, et al. Sirolimus-eluting versus bare nitinol stent for obstructive superficial femoral artery disease: the SIROCCO II trial. *J Vasc Interv Radiol.* 2005;16:331–8.
49. Duda SH, Bosiers M, Lammer J, et al. Drug-eluting and bare nitinol stents for the treatment of atherosclerotic lesions in the superficial femoral artery: long-term results from the SIROCCO trial. *J Endovasc Ther.* 2006;13:701–10.

28

Endoscopic Vein Harvesting in Lower Extremity Bypass: Technique, Outcomes, and Concerns

Raymond E. Eid, MD and Rabih A. Chaer, MD, MSc

Saphenous vein grafts have been established as the gold standard conduit for lower extremity bypass grafting.[1] Conventionally, the great saphenous vein (GSV) is typically harvested via a long continuous or "skip" incisions that may extent form the groin to the ankle, before its use as an arterial conduit. This approach, however, is associated with significant morbidities including surgical site infections, ischemic skin flaps, fat necrosis, lymph leak, increased postoperative pain, and longer hospital stay for as many as 24% to 43% of patients.[2,3] Although these complications are reported extensively in the cardiac literature, wound complications in patients with peripheral vascular disease are even further compounded by arterial and venous insufficiency, diabetes, and redo operations, common comorbidities in this patient population.

Minimally invasive vein harvesting techniques were introduced in 1994 and have been developed in an attempt to reduce the wound morbidity associated with open vein harvest (OVH).[4] Further technical and technological refinements have allowed minimally invasive conduit harvesting to become a routine practice in cardiac surgery, especially in the United States. The Society of Thoracic Surgeons' National Cardiac Database reported that 70% of CABG procedures performed in 2008 used EVH.[5]

Initial studies have shown promising results with reduced rates of postoperative wound complications, decreased hospital length of stay, and reduced overall cost following endoscopic vein harvest (EVH) compared with traditional vein harvest.[6–10] However, concerns of coronary vein graft patency when harvested endoscopically have been raised in some reports, questioning the widespread applicability of EVH.

The patency of lower extremity bypass grafts harvested endoscopically were initially reported to parallel that of standard open technique, with a 5-year primary patency rates ranging from 51% to 73% and secondary patency from 68% to 81%.[11–15]

Nevertheless, several recent reports raised concerns about the potential safety of the endoscopic technique for vessel procurement, especially in terms of vein graft patency in the mid and long-term and clinical outcomes.[16,17]

The purpose of this chapter is to review the currently available vein harvesting techniques and devices, as well as the outcomes of OVH and EVH in patients with peripheral vascular disease.

TYPES OF ENDOSCOPIC VEIN HARVESTING

There are predominantly two distinct types of disposable and reusable EVH systems on the market, that is, sealed and open systems. Sealed systems (Vasoview System, Maquet Cardiovascular, Wayne, NJ) use carbon dioxide (CO_2) at a set pressure to assist in the endoscopic tunnel dissection. A blunt dissector and a multipurpose instrument are used for tissue sealing and division of side branches. On the other hand, open systems (such as Karl Storz, Tuttlingen, Germany, and Sorin Group, Milan, Italy) do not use CO_2 or any positive pressure to create the endoscopic tunnel. A retractor and the endoscopic camera provide the mechanical traction for the vein exposure. Several devices are used for tissue sealing and side branches division such as Harmonic Scalpel (Ethicon, Somerville, NJ), Ligasure (Covidien, Mansfield, MA), Enseal (Ethicon, Somerville, NJ) or Starion (Microline Surgical, Beverly, MA). CO_2 is only used for smoke evacuation and visual flush.

There have been a number of reports demonstrating differences in vein quality and outcomes between the two EVH approaches, as will be outlined in the following sections. Consequently, the distinction between these approaches is of paramount importance. Unfortunately, the majority of published literature fails to indicate or clearly disclose the approach utilized making interpretation more challenging.

SURGICAL TECHNIQUES

During endoscopic vein harvesting, patients are placed in a supine position and the operator identifies the location of GSV through palpation, osseous landmarks or a portable ultrasound machine. A stab incision is made at the medial tibial condyle, just above the knee. Sharp dissection is then carried to identify the GSV, which is then elevated with a vessel loop. A separate incision is usually made in the groin to disconnect the saphenous vein at the saphenofemoral junction. This is usually sufficient to harvest the entire thigh GSV. If the entire length of the GSV is needed, the system can be redirected caudally, and a separate incision is made at the medial calf or ankle to disconnect and ligate the vein distally.

The vein conduit is bluntly dissected under direct videoscopic visualization, proper traction, and hemostasis minimizing vein trauma as much as possible. Side branches are identified and dissected thoroughly to allow adequate length for branch division using previously mentioned sealing devices. By providing an adequate margin and keeping heat energy settings on the lowest possible settings, the risk of thermal injury is theoretically minimized.

Once the vein is extracted, it is prepared in the usual fashion as conduits harvested using open techniques. The proximal end is cannulated and gently dilated and flushed to avoid endothelial trauma. The branches are ligated and lacerations are repaired with fine monofilament sutures. The vein is gently flushed to remove any clots that may have accumulated and then preserved in solution until ready to be used.

OUTCOMES

A large amount of evidence has emerged in recent years in the form of randomized controlled trials, observational studies, as well as systematic reviews and meta-analyses comparing EVH to OVH in both CABGs and lower extremity bypass surgery. We will be focusing primarily on the vascular literature in this chapter.

Wound Complications

Infectious wound complications associated with long incisions used to harvest the GSV are common and well documented. The incidence of infectious wound complications following traditional OVH ranges from 3%–40%, resulting in a significant economic and clinical burden. A recent meta-analysis of eighteen studies (12 cohorts studies, comparing EVH to OVH in lower extremity bypasses reported no significant improvement in wound complication rates with EVH, with a pooled relative risk 0.808 (95% CI 0.61–1.08; $p = .15$). The different cohort studies showed different results with most of them demonstrating lower vein harvest incision complications in the EVH group compared to OVH.[18]

Another meta-analysis has looked at rates of wound complications in cardiac surgery patients. It showed a significant reduction in wound infection using endoscopic techniques (OR 0.22, 95% CI; 0.14–0.37, $P < 0.00001$), for a number needed to treat of 14.[19] Sastry et al.[20] in a more recent meta-analysis of 31 studies [15 prospectively randomized (PR), 7 prospective non-randomized (PNR) and 9 retrospective non-randomized (RNR)] also indicated less surgical site wound infection in the EVH groups (SRRisk 0.31, 95% CI; 0.23–0.42, $P < 0.0001$).

The UPMC Experience

At the author's institution EVH has been associated with a significant reduction in donor site wound infection compared to OVH. A recently published retrospective study of EVH from the author's institution confirms that adoption of EVH significantly lowered wound complication rates (0% vs. 20.0%, $P < .001$).[16] The reduction in donor site infections likely occurs because of preserved tissue perfusion and a lower likelihood of creating vital tissue flaps than with open saphenectomy. This may be of particular importance in patients with high risk of wound complications such as with diabetes, obesity, and peripheral vascular disease.

Postoperative Pain, Mobility, and Patient Satisfaction

Several studies have demonstrated improved quality of life indices, including postoperative pain, time to mobilization, and patient satisfaction following EVH. The incidence of pain (23.1% versus 6.7%), neuralgia (24.3% versus 7.1%), and patient satisfaction (49% versus 75%) was significantly improved with EVH compared with OVH.[21] Using a visual analogue scale, patients undergoing EVH rated their experience of pain two points lower on a 0–10 scale throughout the entire postoperative period and labeled themselves pain-free days earlier than their OVH.[22] A number of studies have also reported earlier mobility for patients undergoing EVH as well as improved mobility at hospital discharge and six weeks after surgery.[23] Patient satisfaction with the cosmetic result is initially higher with EVH than after traditional harvest, although the cosmetic outcome is equivalent six weeks after surgery.[22]

Hospital Length of Stay (LOS) and Costs

Earlier mobilization of patients and a reduction of wound complications may result in a reduction of recovery time and therefore hospital LOS. The results in small series have not been consistent, although two meta-analyses have reported a reduction in hospital LOS by EVH with weighted mean difference ranging from –0.85 to –1.04 days; 95% CI: –1.92 to –0.16.[21,24]

Other studies have evaluated the cost effectiveness of endoscopic saphenous vein harvesting for patients undergoing infra-inguinal or cardiac bypass, compared with open harvesting.[25–27] In all cases, there are methodological limitations that compromise the validity of the results. Most of the available studies performed cost analyses, without accounting for the effectiveness of the treatment. Such studies, often termed "partial economic evaluation studies," are less useful in guiding decision making, because they only measure the costs of technologies and not their effectiveness. Thus, in light of the current literature, available evidence does not allow conclusions to be made on the cost-effectiveness of EVH. More evidence is needed on the efficacy and long-term effectiveness of this technique, with studies measuring final outcomes, such as vein graft failure, myocardial infarction, mortality or need for repeat revascularization and other interventions.

GRAFT QUALITY AND EFFECT OF EVH APPROACHES

The issue of potential vein injury during endoscopic harvesting has been largely investigated during the past decade: however, to date, there are no standard parameters to report the degree of damage occurring during the vein procurement. In general, it is possible to consider a macroscopic injury (i.e., visually detected) or a microscopic injury (i.e., assessed by means of histology or functional evaluations such as vasoreactivity or expressions of interleukins, vascular cell adhesion molecules, intracellular adhesion molecule) occurring during harvesting. Of note, it should be stressed that the impact of storage solution during harvested conduit could also play an important role in its preservation, albeit having being poorly investigated to date. Finally, the operator's experience may also consistently influence the quality of the harvested conduit.

Several retrospective and systematic reviews have looked at graft quality following open and endoscopic approaches. At the macroscopic level, both approaches had comparable vein quality score ("good," "fair," or "poor") and vein length. However, vein harvested endoscopically required a higher number or repairs.[20,28,29] Moreover, sealed EVH systems (such as Vasoview) are associated with increased incidence of graft thrombosis compared to open systems, likely related to flow stasis, external compression form gas inflation, and possibly thermal injury.[28] This has led some surgeons to administer systemic heparin prior to endoscopic vein harvesting.

When conduits are evaluated microscopically, Hussaini et al. demonstrated attenuated vasomotor function using the minimally invasive technique with preservation of graft endothelium.[30] This was also supported by few other reports,[21,31] primarily with the sealed systems, indicating potential intimal injuries and tears at the origin of side branches.

VEIN GRAFT STENOSIS AND REINTERVENTION

In a recent systematic review, Jauhari et al. evaluated 18 cohort studies and case series assessing graft patency in lower extremity arterial bypass following open or endoscopic technique. This included 2343 patients with considerable clinical heterogeneity. In their analysis, the authors found a significant difference in primary patency rates for EVH compared to OVH with a pooled HR of 1.294 (95% CI: 1.03–1.63; $p = .028$).[18] In a subgroup patency analysis by Julliard et al., patients with diabetes and limb-threatening ischemia had significantly worse patency rates following EVH when compared to OVH.[32]

THE UPMC EXPERIENCE

We recently reviewed our experience comparing graft patency between different harvesting techniques specifically in patients with critical limb ischemia. Patency rates were significantly better in the open group compared the minimally invasive group. The primary patency rate was 43.2% in the EVH group and 69.4% in the OVH group ($P = .007$) at a mean follow-up of 30 months. Primary assisted and secondary patency rates were also superior in the open group. In addition to differences in patency rates, both groups demonstrated significant disparities in the etiology of graft failure. The most common reason for loss of primary patency in the OVH group was graft occlusion (OVH = 57.2%, EVH = 22.7%, $P = .04$), whereas the most reason for lost of primary patency in the EVH group was mid-graft stenosis (EVH = 54.5%, OVH = 0%, $P < .001$) (Figure 28-1). This raised the concern of vein graft injury related to the harvest technique, resulting in stenoses in unusual locations, possibly related to the thermal injury at branch points.

The average number of vascular reinterventions per bypass graft was significantly lower in the OVH group compared to the EVH group (OVH = 0.37, EVH = 1.28, $P < .001$). Limb salvage was not different between the two groups.

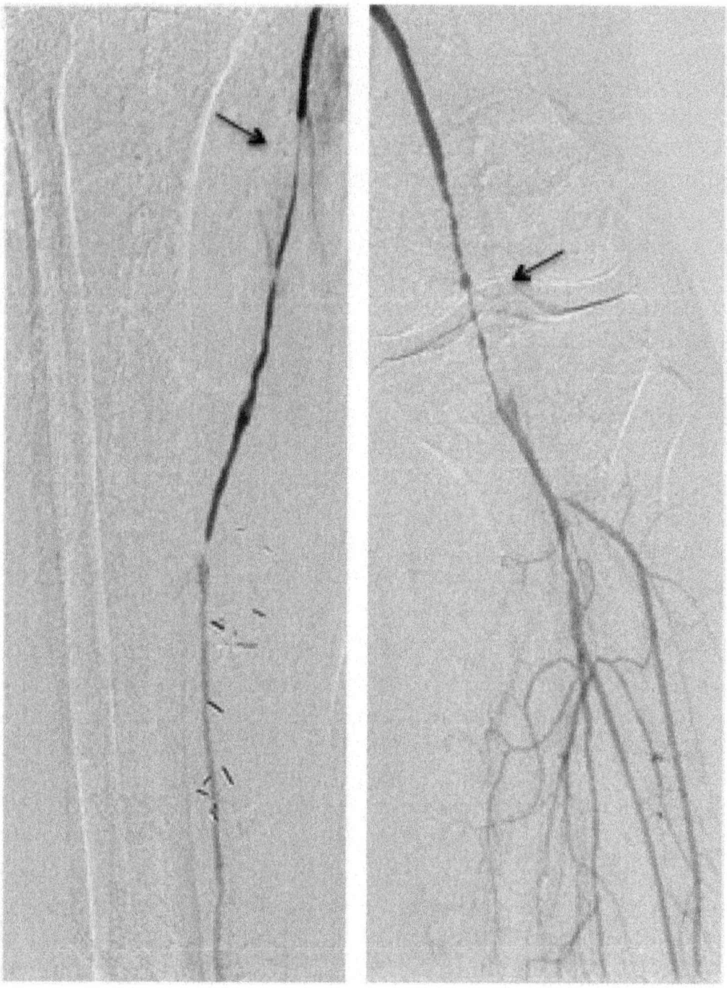

Figure 28-1. Representative angiogram of two different bypass grafts harvested endoscopically with stenosis in the body of the vein. Arrows are pointing to the area of stenosis.

LEARNING CURVE

With the adoption of new techniques, there is a significant institutional as well as personal learning curve. Macroscopic vein injuries (holes or torn side branches) are reported to occur 3–5 times more often after EVH compared to OVH, raising concerns regarding the overall quality of the vein conduit.[33]

In a well-designed study, Desai et al. compared conduits harvested by an open technique to those harvested by EVH performed by experienced versus novice technicians. Veins were evaluated at time of surgery using optical coherence tomography (OCT) and postoperatively by computed tomographic angiography (CTA).[34] Vein injury was more common and significant in novice operators (<100 EVH cases) compared to more experienced technicians (>900 EVH cases). Additionally, they demonstrated that the number of isolated graft injuries correlated with early graft failure.

Vein grafts with at least 4 intimal or medial dissections showed significantly worse patency (67% versus 96% patency; P = .05).

The impact of learning curve on vein quality and function was further evaluated by Kinai and colleagues.[35] Veins harvested by experienced (>900 cases, n = 55 patients) or "novice" (<100 cases, n = 30 patients) technicians were examined for vascular injury using optical coherence tomography and gene expression using a tissue injury array. The authors concluded that grafts harvested by inexperienced technicians had increased number of graft injuries and higher level of tissue injury genes expression. This further correlated with a greater degree of late lumen loss when these grafts were followed with CTA at 6 months. Both of these studies confirm that vein graft quality is dependent on the harvester experience, stressing the importance of adequate and reliable training of technicians at the beginning of their learning curve. This is more significant in the lower extremity bypasses where longer conduits are used, requiring longer segments of intact harvested veins.

CONCLUSIONS

Endoscopic vein harvesting is associated with reduced primary patency rates after lower extremity bypass surgery and does not clearly demonstrate a reduction in post-operative wound complication rates. However, the available data are heterogeneous and of poor quality. Further ambiguity is introduced by the evolution and improvement in EVH technologies over time, the impact of variation in case selection, and the effect of the learning curve on EVH outcomes with increasing technical experience. There is a need for a high quality prospective study of EVH in LEAB with modern equipment, experienced operators, defined reporting criteria, and strict inclusion criteria. The authors recommend that EVH should be used with caution in routine vascular clinical practice, with careful selection based on patient characteristics and clinical comorbidities.

REFERENCES

1. Pereira CE, Albers M, Romiti M, et al. Meta-analysis of femoropopliteal bypass grafts for lower extremity arterial insufficiency. *J Vasc Surg.* 2006;44:510–7.
2. Kent KC, Bartek S, Kuntz KM, et al. Prospective study of wound complications in continuous infrainguinal incisions after lower limb arterial reconstruction: Incidence, risk factors, and cost. *Surgery.* 1996;119:378–83.
3. Wengrovitz M, Atnip RB, Gifford RRM, et al. Wound complications of autogenous subcutaneous infrainguinal arterial bypass surgery: Predisposing factors and management. *J Vasc Surg.* 1990;11:156–63.
4. Lumsden AB, Eaves FF III, Ofenloch JC, Jordan WD. Subcutaneous, video-assisted saphenous vein harvest: Report of the first 30 cases. *Cardiovasc Surg.* 1996;4:771–6.
5. Raja SG, Rochon M, Sproson C, Bahrami TT. 4-year outcome analysis of endoscopic vein harvesting for coronary artery bypass grafting. *ISRN Vascular Medicine,* vol. 2013, Article ID 517806, 8 pages, 2013. doi:10.1155/2013/517806.
6. Baddour LM, Bisno AL. Recurrent cellulitis after coronary bypass surgery. *JAMA.* 1984;251:1049–52.

7. Wengrovitz M, Atnip RG, Gifford RR, et al. Wound complications of autogenous subcutaneous infrainguinal arterial bypass surgery: Predisposing factors and management. *J Vasc Surg*. 1990;11:156–63.
8. Illig KA, Rhodes JM, Sternbach Y, et al. Reduction in wound morbidity rates following endoscopic saphenous vein harvest. *Ann Vasc Surg*. 2001;15:104–9.
9. Illig KA, Rhodes JM, Sternbach Y, Green RM. Financial impact of endoscopic vein harvest for infrainguinal bypass. *J Vasc Surg*. 2003;37:323–30.
10. Black EA, Campbell K, Channon KM, et al. Minimally invasive vein harvesting significantly reduces pain and wound morbidity. *Eur J Cardiothorac Surg*. 2002;22:381–6.
11. Jordan WD, Alcocer F, Voellinger DC, Wirthlin DJ. The durability of endoscopic saphenous vein grafts: A 5-year observational study. *J Vasc Surg*. 2001;34:434–9.
12. Erdoes LS, Milner TP. Encouraging results with endoscopic vein harvest for infrainguinal bypass. *J Vasc Surg*. 2005;42:442–8.
13. Gazoni LM, Carty R, Skinner J, et al. Endoscopic versus open saphenous vein harvest for femoral to below the knee arterial bypass using saphenous vein graft. *J Vasc Surg*. 2006;44:282–7.
14. Hines GL, Wain RA, Montecalvo J, Feuerman M. Femoral-popliteal bypass with endoscopically harvested saphenous vein in patients with TASC D disease of the superficial femoral artery. *Ann Vasc Surg*. 2010;24:615–20.
15. Dacey LJ, Braxton JH Jr, Kramer RS, et al. Long-term outcomes of endoscopic vein harvesting after coronary artery bypass grafting. *Circulation*. 2011;123:147–53.
16. Eid RE, Wang L, Kuzman M, et al. Endoscopic versus open saphenous vein graft for lower extremity bypass in critical limb ischemia. *J Vasc Surg*. 2014;59(1):136–44.
17. Santo VJ, Dargon PT, Azarbal AF, et al. Open versus endoscopic great saphenous vein harvest for lower extremity revascularization of critical limb ischemia. *J Vasc Surg*. 2014;59(2):427–34.
18. Jauhari YA, Hughes CO, Black SA, et al. Endoscopic vein harvesting in lower extremity arterial bypass: A systematic review. *Eur J Vasc Endovasc Surg*. 2014;47(6):621–39.
19. Markar SR, Kutty R, Edmonds L, et al. A meta-analysis of minimally invasive versus traditional open vein harvest technique for coronary artery bypass graft surgery. *Interact Cardiovasc Thorac Surg*. 2010;10(2):266–70.
20. Sastry P, Rivinius R, Harvey R, et al. The influence of endoscopic vein harvesting on outcomes after coronary bypass grafting: A meta-analysis of 267 525 patients. *Eur J Cardiothorac Surg*. 2013;44(6):980–9.
21. Cheng D, Allen K, Cohn W, et al. Endoscopic vascular harvest in coronary artery bypass grafting surgery: A meta-analysis of randomized trials and controlled trials. *Innovations (Phila)*. 2005;1(2):61–74.
22. Bonde P, Graham A, MacGowan S. Endoscopic vein harvest: Early results of a prospective trial with open vein harvest. *Heart Surg Forum*. 2002;5 Suppl 4:S378–91.
23. Kiaii B, Moon BC, Massel D, et al. A prospective randomized trial of endoscopic versus conventional harvesting of the saphenous vein in coronary artery bypass surgery. *J Thorac Cardiovasc Surg*. 2002;123(2):204–12.
24. Athanasiou T, Aziz O, Al-Ruzzeh S, et al. Are wound healing disturbances and length of hospital stay reduced with minimally invasive vein harvest? A meta-analysis. *Eur J Cardiothorac Surg*. 2004;26(5):1015–26.
25. Rao C, Aziz O, Deeba S, et al. Is minimally invasive harvesting of the great saphenous vein for coronary artery bypass surgery a cost-effective technique? *J Thorac Cardiovasc Surg*. 2008;135(4):809–15.
26. Brandt CP, Greene GC, Pollard TR, et al. Review of efforts to decrease costly leg wound complications in the Medicare population following coronary revascularization. *Heart Surg Forum*. 2003;6(4):258–63.
27. Illig KA, Rhodes JM, Sternbach Y, Green RM. Financial impact of endoscopic vein harvest for infrainguinal bypass. *J Vasc Surg*. 2003;37(2):323e30.

28. Burris N, Schwartz K, Brown J, et al. Incidence of residual clot strands in saphenous vein grafts after endoscopic harvest. *Innovations (Phila).* 2006;1:323–7.
29. Schultz SC, Stapleton D, D'Ambra P, et al. Prospective randomized study comparing the Teleflex Medical SaphLITE Retractor to the Ethicon CardioVations Clearglide Endoscopic System. *J Cardiothorac Surg.* 2006;1:24.
30. Hussaini BE, Lu HG, Wolfe JA, Thatte HS. Evaluation of endoscopic vein extraction on structural and viability of saphenous vein endothelium. *J Cardiothorac Surg.* 2011;10(6):82.
31. Campanella A, Berqamasco L, Macri L, et al. Endoscopic saphenous harvesting with an open CO_2 system (ESOS) trial for coronary artery bypass grafting surgery: study protocol for a randomized trial. *Trials.* 2011;12(12):243.
32. Julliard W, Katzen J, Nabozny M, et al. Long-term results of endoscopic versus open saphenous vein harvest for lower extremity bypass. *Ann Vasc Surg.* 2011;25(1):101–7.
33. Ouzounian M, MacPherson C, Ali IS. Endoscopic versus open vein harvesting for coronary artery bypass grafting. In: Raja SG, Amrani M. eds. *Off-pump coronary artery bypass grafting: Outcomes, concerns & controversies.* Nova: New York, 2012: 331–42.
34. Desai P, Kiani S, Thiruvanthan N, et al. Impact of the learning curve for endoscopic vein harvest on conduit quality and early graft patency. *Ann Thorac Surg.* 2011;91(5):1385–91.
35. Kiani S, Desai PH, Thirumvalavan N, et al. Endoscopic venous harvesting by inexperienced operators compromises venous graft remodeling. *Ann Thorac Surg.* 2012;93(1):11–7.

29

Hemodynamic Adaptation of Vein Grafts and Treatment of Vein Graft Failure

Christopher D. Owens, MD, MSc

THE VENOUS BYPASS

Vein bypass surgery is a technically challenging procedure performed predominantly on a geriatric population with cardiovascular comorbidities for ischemia of the leg. The goal of course is to increase tissue oxygenation, relieve ischemia, and maintain a functional extremity. Diabetes mellitus and tobacco abuse, both resulting in decreased tissue oxygenation, are the two most common risk factors for lower extremity ischemia and each impairs wound healing through many mechanisms. Indeed, wound healing is one of the single biggest drawbacks to bypass surgery and is commonly reported at 30%, which is likely to be underreported depending on the definition of wound complication used.[1] Offsetting this, however, is the increased patency that lower extremity bypass surgery offers, which is largely independent of the length of the bypass or the level of the distal anastomosis. The successful vein bypass is a living and functional organ configured within the arterial circulation and capable of responding to local and distant chemical and mechanical signals. It is extremely versatile and can function with very low blood flow conditions such as a bypass to the isolated popliteal segment where outflow is provided only through collaterals. By contrast, it can be used in high flow conditions such as a renal bypass or a common iliac artery to superficial femoral artery through the obturator foramen. It can be used to salvage foot necrosis and is resistant to infection; its patency is not influenced by either diabetes mellitus or chronic kidney disease. The vein bypass can dilate to accommodate an increased blood flow in response to an increased oxygen demand such as during vigorous walking, climbing a hill, or healing a wound. Yet despite this versatility, very little is known regarding the stages of healing following implantation, the vein's adaptive process in the arterial circulation, or the recovery time of a functional endothelial lining.

Experimental vein graft models in any individual animal species are generally poor representations of the physiology in the human.[2] However by examining experimental models in several different species, common universalities can be determined. For instance, low shear stress conditions have been found to be associated with an increase in intimal hyperplasia in the rabbit, swine, canine, and mouse models firmly establishing the shear–hyperplasia relationship. However, the exuberant, flow-limiting, vein bypass stenosis that is seen in 30%–40% of human bypass grafts cannot be reproduced in any animal; and, as previously stated, vein bypasses often function perfectly well despite very low flow and shear conditions. Systematic, longitudinal study of human vein bypass adaptation must complement experimental models to gain a better understanding of the (patho) physiology that produces vein graft stenosis. In this chapter, I will outline about a decade's worth of research we have conducted studying bypass grafts at multiple time points following surgery with ultrasound and magnetic resonance imaging protocols and the required precedent research. From these studies, three temporally distinct phases of venous adaptation, along with defining characteristic features of each phase, can be described.[2] Areas that are discordant with animal data will be highlighted, and potential mitigating therapies described. With no FDA-approved therapies to treat vein bypass failure, however, speculation substitutes for evidence. Research resources and interest into the study of venous bypass failure have waned recently. As the limitations of endovascular treatment of ischemia become more visible, research resources are likely return to this important area. These resources would be well spent, as recent epidemiological studies estimate that 202 million individuals are afflicted with peripheral artery disease (PAD) worldwide. Prior to discussing venous bypass in particular, a brief overview of the forces produced by flowing blood in general should provide the requisite background. This material is intended as a supplement to the lecture and not a complete treatment of the topic.

Remodeling Is Required to Offset the Stresses Produced by Pressurized, Flowing Blood

The adult cardiovascular system is dynamic and adaptive, capable of acute and chronic structural changes, i.e. lumen dimeter, wall thickness, total vessel area, etc., made in response to changes in blood flow and pressure. This natural plasticity of the vascular system is clinically obvious in different normal and abnormal physiologies such as a dilated radial–cephalic arteriovenous fistula, visible venous collaterals crisscrossing the shoulder to bypass a chronically thrombosed subclavian vein, or a dilated arc of Riolan in a patient with mesenteric artery occlusion. Infra-renal aortic occlusion can present as severe buttock and thigh pain with impotence in the setting of thrombosis of a severely narrowed atherosclerotic vessel or as complete paralysis of the lower extremities when an embolism lodges in the aortic bifurcation in the patient with atrial fibrillation. The event by which the disease is brought to a clinical horizon is the sudden cessation of blood flow to the lower extremities but the time course over which the underlying pathologic process develops is dramatically different: The first develops slowly over years to decades as atherosclerotic plaque produces a progressively narrowed blood vessel lumen to the point of thrombosis while the second is acute occlusion of a relatively normal aorta. These examples highlight the importance of vascular plasticity in response to a change in hemodynamics. Arteriogenesis, or collaterogenesis, can be life- and limb-saving in the patient with ischemic heart disease or critical limb ischemia where dilation of pre-existing, small channels that can span long distances to connect remote vascular territories. The geometric enlargement of a blood vessel results from a choreographed rearrangement of cellular and fibrous components of the blood vessel to offset stresses exerted on the blood vessel. Cytokines, growth factors, and chemotaxins produced by invading inflammatory cells but acting locally on vascular intrinsic cells help to accomplish this. These stress response changes are known as vascular remodeling. By contrast, angiogenesis is the production of new vascular channels from preexisting blood vessels in response to a proliferative stimuli such as vascular endothelial growth factor (VEGF) and low oxygen tension.[3]

Of course, here in Chicago, one can never discuss remodeling without mentioning the pioneering work of two giants in the field, Seymour Glagov (1925–2008) and Philip B. Dobrin (1934–2011) from the University of Chicago's Pritzker School of Medicine and Loyola University's Stritch School of Medicine, respectively. Glagov, a prolific writer and inquisitive researcher, was most famous for his "partial blockage" studies conducted throughout the 1980s of an artery's response to atherosclerotic plaque growth.[4] Before this time, it was thought that the vessel was essentially a fixed cylinder in which luminal narrowing proceeds at a rate commensurate with plaque growth in a one-to-one exchange. In contrast to this model, Glagov demonstrated that arteries underwent enlargement in response to plaque growth to maintain a normal luminal area. However, when the plaque growth became excessive, > 40% luminal area, further enlargement was not possible, and luminal area became compromised. This observation became known as Glagovian remodeling or compensatory enlargement and brought about a flurry of research to identify the hemodynamic forces that allowed the blood vessel to "sense" what the atherosclerotic plaque was doing.[5] While Glagovian remodeling preserves luminal area, the plaque may appear insignificant on coronary angiography. Despite its angiographic appearance, however, the blood vessel is far from normal, and the patient may remain at risk for devastating clinical events such as myocardial infarction (MI). Such remodeling in the coronary artery may create what is known as a vulnerable plaque, which is characterized by the thin fibrous cap fatty atheroma (TFCA). The luminal enlargement acts to stretch the fibrous cap over an ever-enlarging lipid core. Inflammation generated at the edge of the fibrous cap liberates the matrix proteinases necessary for luminal expansion, but in so doing may inadvertently cause plaque rupture or simply plaque erosion and intraluminal thrombosis. While the concept of a remodeled artery harboring a vulnerable TFCA is heuristic, it has recently been challenged.[6,7] Nevertheless, this highlights the notion that not all vascular remodeling serves the purpose of the vascular surgeon.

Of course we now know the predominant force that regulates acute luminal caliber is shear stress, one of many forces the vessel is subject to by pulsatile pressurized blood flow.[4,8] By the liberation of endothelium-derived relaxing factors (EDRF) such as nitric oxide (NO), prostacyclin (PGI2), and hyperpolarizing factor, luminal dilation occurs in response to an acute increase in shear stress. This phenomenon is exploited clinically and is described as flow-mediated, endothelium-dependent, vasodilation (FMD). In human brachial arteries, this is mediated predominantly by NO, and decreased FMD is regarded as a sign of endothelial dysfunction, the earliest evidence of atherosclerosis. FMD is an acute response to an increase in flow but once the flow stimulus is removed, the artery returns to baseline dimensions without any evidence of structural change. But the exact mechanism by which vascular remodeling occurs as the result of a chronically imposed elevation of shear stress is less known. FMD is functional while remodeling is structural.

Philip Dobrin, trained in engineering, was not the first to describe blood flow forces, but he offered the most complete analysis of the differential effects of pressure and flow on different layers in the vessel wall. Prior to his experiments, the intima/media was regarded as a single entity because there was no ability to distinguish between the two under experimental conditions. The ideal arterialized vein graft should have a functional endothelial layer, a minimal neointima area, and a normal or slightly thickened tunica media capable of dilating and constricting in response to vasoactive stimuli. Dobrin highlighted these important limitations and designed experiments capable of separating individual components of the multidimensional effects of blood pressure and correlate each parameter to histological changes to vessels. Fortunate for us, he was a vascular surgeon, so he principally studied vein grafts.[9,10] When a blood vessel is subjected to intraluminal pressure, it deforms simultaneously in three orthogonal directions, with little or no torsion. Clinically, torsion can result in vein graft failure by technical errors during tunneling of the graft or by creating the distal anastomosis with rotational error. Pressurizing the vein graft should never result in torsion. The circumferential deformation produces luminal enlargement, the longitudinal deformation produces a stretch and the radial deformation produces wall compression. When deformed, tissues exert opposing or retractive forces that resist further deformation and the vessel dimensions become stable and considered to be in equilibrium. Despite being in a state of equilibrium, there are residual stresses along the graft, which becomes apparent when a vessel ring is cut longitudinally and it springs open as the energy of the bending stress is released. Another example is the retraction of a vessel once it has been divided and removed from the patient. The harvested saphenous vein conduit often appears much too short to stretch from proximal to distal anastomosis to the uninitiated. Dividing the retractive forces by the cross-sectional area over which they are exerted, one obtains the stresses exerted by the wall in each direction. The stress in the circumferential direction is the largest, the stress in the longitudinal direction is about one-half as great, and the stress in the radial direction is one-twelfth as great. Hence, by pressurizing a vein graft, one obtains simultaneous deformations, forces, and stresses in three directions, and with blood flow comes the development of shear stress across the endothelium. Through elegant experimental vein graft models utilizing a series of supporting cuffs and/or flow constrictors, individual components of the nine parameters of intraluminal pressure were able to be separated, and the effects of these forces were studied by quantitative histology on pressure-perfused sections. In this way, he was able to determine that low blood flow is most closely associated with intimal thickening, whereas circumferential stress is associated with medial thickening.

It is common to describe the venous system as a highly compliant reservoir for blood. For example, nitroglycerin relieves angina by reducing venous return to the heart and reducing cardiac output through the distension of systemic capacitance veins.[11,12] This is due to the elastin componentof the wall. Elastin is a fibrous protein that behaves mechanically and thermodynamically like a folded chain. As the vein is pressure-loaded, the elastin can elongate by 50 to 70% of its resting length as the links in the chains are unfolded and then return to its normal folded state once the load is removed. Interestingly, like rubber, elastin shrinks when heated as it assumes a higher entropy state. However, arteries and veins behave vastly differently under increased loaded conditions. The artery, while less compliant at low pressures, retains its compliance throughout a pressure range up to 200 mmHg. By contrast, the vein becomes extremely rigid at pressures above 50 mmHg. At these pressures, the elastin fibers are stretched and become stiff, and collagen fibers are recruited to bear the load. To quantify the relative stiffness of these fibrous proteins, the elastic modulus for each is compared. The elastic modulus is an engineering term for stiffness and is about 4.5×10^6 dynes/cm^2 for elastin while that of collagen is 1.0×10^{10} dynes/m^2. So collagen is about 10,000 times the stiffness of elastin.

Remodeling of the Vein Graft and Its Implications for Vein Graft Failure

While the autogenous vein bypass remains the most effective and durable revascularization strategy for patients with lower extremity ischemia, 30 to 40% of vein bypasses will yield one or more flow-limiting stenosis within the first year of implantation. Unlike coronary bypass grafts, duplex surveillance of lower extremity vein grafts can detect hemodynamically significant stenosis due to the vein graft's superficial location within the leg. The distribution of ultrasound-detected stenosis is diffuse in 12% of vein grafts, but most stenotic lesions are focal, often occurring in the peri-anastomotic regions or at valve sites. It is not clear why these areas are predisposed to stenosis, but it is likely that flow disturbances may be a factor. However, another factor may be a deficit of outward remodeling in response to implantation into the arterial environment. The idea of human vein graft remodeling is hardly novel, as Szilagyi et al. noted over 50 years ago from studying autopsy specimens. He saw that mature vein grafts increased their pre-implantation dimensions by as much as 50% to 75%, implying that remodeling was critical to successful vein graft function.[13]

With the benefit of this background, we hypothesized that successful early remodeling of the vein graft was important to its long-term success.[14] To test this hypothesis, we initiated a prospective cohort study to systematically determine remodeling characteristics of lower extremity bypass grafts during the first year of implantation. High-resolution ultrasound images were used to characterize luminal diameter and wall thickness changes from a defined region of the vein graft. Because it was impractical to map the entire bypass graft, we used a 5-cm segment (no branches or valves) of the graft as a surrogate for the behavior of the entire graft. High-resolution M-mode ultrasound was used to conduct vein graft lumen measurements at predetermined times, beginning in the operating room after the anastomoses were complete and then at 1, 3, 6, 9, and 12 months thereafter. We used ECG-gated doppler-spectral waveform analysis to determine the pulse-wave velocity (PWV) along the length of the bypass graft. PWV is the speed at which the flow pulse propagates through the conduit and is one measure of stiffness that is relatively independent of the outflow. In these same patients, we collected demographic information and cardiovascular risk factors. Preoperative blood samples were obtained to measure routinely tested and experimental blood chemistries to assess their clinical value and to provide insights into mechanisms of vein graft failure. To ensure that these markers were not spuriously elevated, any patient with active infection, a recent procedure, or concurrent systemic illness was excluded from biomarker evaluation.

While the study design was relatively simple, the collective information on each patient studied included vein bypass graft morphometry and stiffness (compliance) and systemic biomarkers of the innate immune system, including acute-phase reactants, markers of endothelial dysfunction, inflammatory cytokines, and adipokines. Controlling for cardiovascular risk factors and routinely measured laboratory chemistry values such as lipid fractions, endpoints for patient-level, vein graft-related, limb-related outcomes were assessed. These patients were therefore well phenotyped, and this study represented one of the first to employ multiple data sources in a bioinformatics approach to model vein graft failure.[15]

Our early findings of this study were largely descriptive in nature.[14, 16] We determined that most of the luminal and wall remodeling occurred in the first 30 days following implantation, after which the vein morphometry remained relative stable. On average, there was an increase of 25% in lumen diameter of the vein graft between the operating room and 30 days later, but the luminal remodeling response varied substantially. Although the lumens of most of the grafts increased, about one-quarter decreased in size. Over this same time period, the venous wall thickness increased an average of 35%. For example, if the vein had an initial lumen diameter of 3.7 mm and wall thickness of .8 mm, the lumen-to-wall ratio would be 4.6 at the time of implantation. By 30 days, the lumen would have grown to 4.6 mm and the wall to 1.1 mm, maintaining a lumen-to-wall ratio of 4.7, a value remarkably similar to baseline.

As expected from our previous discussion, the initial shear stress at the time of implantation was the parameter most closely associated with luminal remodeling, but still only explained 10% of luminal remodeling. Luminal diameter change was found to be directly associated with the initial shear stress at the time of implantation and with the change in outer graft diameter while it was negatively associated with initial vein diameter.[14,17] Our PWV studies determined that bypass grafts on average developed a 65% increase in stiffness that was temporally delayed in comparison to the wall thickness changes. In fact, during the time wall thickness was increasing, stiffness actually decreased before rebounding and peaking at 6 months. We believe that the decrease followed by an increase reflects matrix metalloproteinase activity and reorganization of fibrous proteins. Considering the vein wall consists of three principal components, cells and proteoglycans, elastin, and collagen, only collagen production could account for this. That early luminal and wall thickness changes were followed by a period of stiffening in a dynamic process lasting six months demonstrates that remodeling in humans is significantly longer than in animals where the 30-day time point is most often referenced as the end of healing.

The variability in lumen caliber remodeling was not sufficiently explained by shear stress or by the grafts inflow, outflow, or runoff. So we sought other factors that may affect the normal expected remodeling response. One possibility was inflammation. At the time, emerging data suggested that baseline inflammation, assessed by C-reactive (CRP) protein measured with a high sensitivity assay, was associated with increased cardiovascular risk.[18] We found that CRP was related to major adverse cardiac events and mortality even in patients with advanced PAD undergoing bypass surgery.[19] We also noted that CRP was inversely associated with the magnitude of luminal remodeling. Specifically, veins placed in patients who had elevated preoperative CRP levels (≥5 mg/L) dilated substantially less than those with CRP <5 mg/L and were an average of 0.5-mm smaller by the end of the first month. This was true despite having similar initial size at the time of implantation to those patients with CRP <5 mg/L.[20] Surprisingly, clinical factors were also found to be associated with vein graft remodeling including race and statin use, both of which were independent of starting diameter and CRP levels. Vein grafts placed in African Americans did not remodel to the same extent as their white counterparts, and they remained smaller throughout the study period. This striking finding may, in part, explain the racial disparity in revascularization outcomes. By contrast, diabetes mellitus, hypertension, hyperlipidemia, or renal failure, were not associated with remodeling, nor have they been found to be important in vein graft failure.[2,20]

That early remodeling was associated with known parameters of vein graft failure—inflammation, race, and statin use—but not with risk factors that are not associated with bypass failure, suggests that early vein remodeling to the arterial circulation was important to maintaining a patent graft. However, the direct link still eluded us until the study was complete. Only then, by linking bypass outcome data (patency) with serial imaging data, was it determined that remodeling was associated with vein graft patency independent of initial vein size or other risk factors.[20] Veins that do not enlarge or negatively remodel, referred to by us as poor remodelers, have a 13-fold increased risk of failure compared with more "robust remodelers." To put this in perspective, the use of small veins for bypass, <3.0 mm, carries only a 2.5-fold increased risk of failure at 1 year, suggesting that the remodeling of the vein in the first 30 days is at least as important as vein implantation size.[21]

These data suggest that vein graft failure cannot be thought of as simply a segmental hyperproliferative disease that develops within a static tube. But rather, intimal hyperplasia develops within a dynamic conduit, molded by hemodynamics under the influence of systemic and regional factors. Thus, inflammation, race, gender, and genetics can act globally on the entire vein graft to influence its adaptation in the arterial circulation. However, should local vascular response to the dominant hemodynamic forces the vein is subject to upon implantation, shear stress and circumferential stress be impeded from offsetting these stresses and reaching or reestablishing baseline conditions due to local environmental conditions, flow disturbances, or intrinsic vein disease, the proliferative intimal reaction would be expected to continue and stenosis to supervene. Therefore one explanation for segmental stenosis may be a hyperproliferative response superimposed on a restrictive pattern of inadequate outward remodeling.

The final phase of vein graft remodeling is recovery of endothelial function. By employing a cuff-occlusion hyperemic flow model at several time points after bypass surgery, we determined that endothelial recovery did not occur until 6 months after implantation, when vein grafts, free of stenosis, become capable of NO-mediated dilation. Thus full adaptation to pulsatile arterial flow occurs over 6 months: luminal dilation and wall thickening occur within 30 days, after which the vein undergoes matrix reorganization characterized by increased collagen and stiffening. The final phase is biochemical remodeling of a functional endothelial layer. These phases correspond to clinical failure; most occur within the first 6 months and then less frequently. If a vein is stenosis-free and the patient is walking significantly better or the wound is healing well, that patient will likely enjoy long-term patency of her bypass graft without further intervention.

In conclusion, vein graft failure is a multidimensional problem involving systemic and local factors. But perhaps the most important factor has not yet been touched on: the surgeon. Vein quality, surgical judgment, and technical finesse, in that order, dictate success or failure of the procedure. Vein bypass surgery is where the rubber meets the road, as my mentor used to say, requiring intra-operative decision-making and shifting of the surgical plan when necessary, stamina, and patience. The operation rests solely in the domain of the vascular surgeon, and we have led the way in its technical and experimental model development as well as supporting molecular and clinical research. Its future is secure so long as we seek ways to improve our craft and perform this operation with the diligence and precision of our teachers.

REFERENCES

1. Ozaki CK, Hamdan AD, Barshes NR et al. Prospective, randomized, multi-institutional clinical trial of a silver alginate dressing to reduce lower extremity vascular surgery wound complications. *J Vasc Surg*. 2015;61:419–27 e411.
2. Owens CD, Gasper WJ, Rahman AS, Conte MS. Vein graft failure. *J Vasc Surg*. 2015;61:203–16.
3. Liebson PR. Stem-cell angiogenesis and regeneration of the heart: Review of a saga of 2 decades. *Clin Cardiol*. 2015;38:309–16.
4. Glagov S, Weisenberg E, Zarins CK et al. Compensatory enlargement of human atherosclerotic coronary arteries. *N Engl J Med*. 1987;316:1371–5.
5. Korshunov VA, Schwartz SM, Berk BC. Vascular remodeling: hemodynamic and biochemical mechanisms underlying glagov's phenomenon. *Arterioscler Thromb Vasc Biol*. 2007;27:1722–8.
6. Toutouzas K, Benetos G, Karanasos A et al. Vulnerable plaque imaging: Updates on new pathobiological mechanisms. *Eur Heart J* (2015) ehv508 DOI: http://dx.doi.org/10.1093/eurheartj/ehv508 First published online: 29 September 2015.
7. Libby P, Pasterkamp G. Requiem for the "vulnerable plaque." *Eur Heart J*. ehv349 DOI: http://dx.doi.org/10.1093/eurheartj/ehv349 First published online: 23 July 2015.
8. Zarins CK, Zatina MA, Giddens DP, Ku DN, Glagov S. Shear stress regulation of artery lumen diameter in experimental atherogenesis. *J Vasc Surg*. 1987;5:413–20.
9. Dobrin PB, Littooy FN, Endean ED. Mechanical factors predisposing to intimal hyperplasia and medial thickening in autogenous vein grafts. *Surgery*. 1989;105:393–400.
10. Dobrin PB, Littooy FN, Golan J, Blakeman B, Fareed J. Mechanical and histologic changes in canine vein grafts. *J Surg Res*. 1988;44:259–65.
11. Grund E, Muller-Ruchholtz ER, Lapp ER, Losch HM, Lochner W. Comparative study of nitroglycerin and molsidomine. Effects on the integrated systemic venous bed and the arterial pressure in dogs. *Arzneimittelforschung*. 1978;28:1624–8.
12. Mitchell A, Buhrmann S, Seifert A et al. Venous response to nitroglycerin is enhanced in young, healthy carriers of the 825t allele of the g protein beta3 subunit gene (gnb3). *Clin Pharmacol Ther*. 2003;74:499–504.
13. Szilagyi DE, Smith RF, Elliott JP. Venous autografts in femoropopliteal arterioplasty. Observations in the treatment of occlusive disease. *Arch Surg*. 1964;89:113–25.
14. Owens CD, Wake N, Jacot JG et al. Early biomechanical changes in lower extremity vein grafts—distinct temporal phases of remodeling and wall stiffness. *J Vasc Surg*. 2006;44:740–6.
15. Owens CD, Ho KJ, Conte MS. Risk factors for failure of lower-extremity revascularization procedures: Are they different for bypass and percutaneous procedures? *Semin Vasc Surg*. 2008;21:143–53.
16. Owens CD, Rybicki FJ, Wake N et al. Early remodeling of lower extremity vein grafts: Inflammation influences biomechanical adaptation. *J Vasc Surg*. 2008;47:1235–42.
17. Jacot JG, Abdullah I, Belkin M et al. Early adaptation of human lower extremity vein grafts: Wall stiffness changes accompany geometric remodeling. *J Vasc Surg*. 2004;39:547–55.
18. Ridker PM. High-sensitivity c-reactive protein: Potential adjunct for global risk assessment in the primary prevention of cardiovascular disease. *Circulation*. 2001;103:1813–8.
19. Owens CD, Ridker PM, Belkin M et al. Elevated c-reactive protein levels are associated with postoperative events in patients undergoing lower extremity vein bypass surgery. *J Vasc Surg*. 2007;45:2–9; discussion 9.
20. Gasper WJ, Owens CD, Kim JM et al. Thirty-day vein remodeling is predictive of midterm graft patency after lower extremity bypass. *J Vasc Surg*. 2013;57:9–18.
21. Schanzer A, Hevelone N, Owens CD et al. Technical factors affecting autogenous vein graft failure: Observations from a large multicenter trial. *J Vasc Surg*. 2007;46:1180–90.

30

Indications for Treatment of Isolated Degenerative Femoral Aneurysms

Juan Carlos Jimenez, MD and Peter F. Lawrence, MD

True aneurysms of the femoral artery (FAA) and its branches are rare. The incidence of FAA is estimated to be approximately five patients per 100,000.[1] Due to its infrequent presentation, the majority of publications consists of retrospective heterogeneous patient cohorts, which include: degenerative, anastomotic, pseudoaneurysms and mycotic aneurysms.[2–4] Because the natural history of FAA has not been truly determined due to the rarity of the disorder, clear, evidence-based management guidelines have not been universally established. Over the past decade, advances in diagnostic imaging modalities and the use of multi-institutional databases have shed light on both the natural history and optimal treatment for this low-frequency disease.

INCIDENCE AND DEMOGRAPHICS

Femoral artery aneurysms are much less common than other more frequently encountered aneurysms (i.e., aortic, popliteal), however their true incidence is likely underreported.[5] Many FAA's are diagnosed during work up or repair of concomitant arterial aneurysms. Synchronous and metachronous arterial aneurysms are frequently encountered in these patients (Figure 30-1).[6] The presence of an abdominal aortic aneurysm (AAA) in patients with FAA has been reported in up to 40% of cases.[7] In a review of 313 patients with AAA, Diwan and colleagues found 11 patients with unilateral FAA and one patient with 1 bilateral FAA.[8] In addition, there appears to be a significant male preponderance for development of FAA. A male predilection for development of FAA has been reported to be approximately 15:1.[9–11]

Synchronous aneurysms

Location	n	
Bilateral FAAs	45	25%
Aorta	113	62%
Iliac	109	60%
Popliteal	86	47%

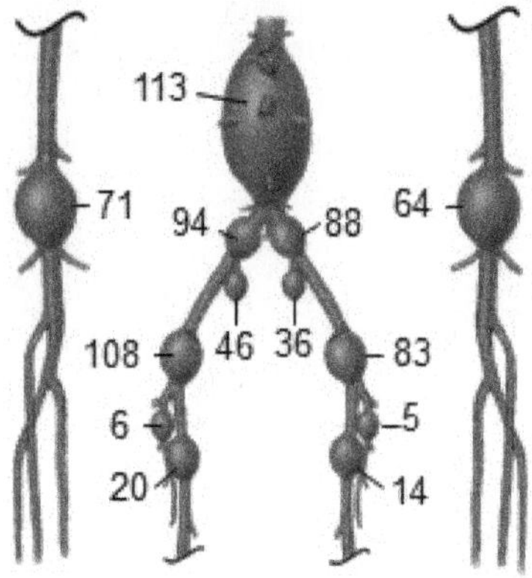

Figure 30-1. The presence of synchronous and metachronous aneurysms in other anatomic locations is common in patients with femoral aneurysms in our series.

PATHOPHYSIOLOGY AND CLINICAL PRESENTATION

True femoral aneurysms involve all three layers of the arterial wall, regardless of the underlying pathology. *False* (or "pseudo-aneurysms") are differentiated from true aneurysms by the presence of blood flow outside of the normal layers of the arterial wall. The risk factors for development of degenerative FAA appear to be similar to the traditional comorbidities that predispose to atherosclerosis and other arterial aneurysms.[6] However, distinctions between true FAA and other arterial aneurysms suggest that all the risk factors for development of these aneurysms are not yet clearly identified.

Several studies have suggested that the natural history of true FAA is more benign than that of arterial aneurysms in other anatomic locations.[6,8] In a recent multi-institutional study of the Vascular Low-Frequency Disease Consortium (VLFDC), 66% of patients who underwent FAA repair were asymptomatic at presentation.[6] Following initial evaluation, 114 patients with 156 FAA were observed without definitive treatment. Of these patients managed conservatively initially, 64% underwent operative repair. Indications for repair included: development of intraluminal thrombus, increase in size to > 2.5 cm, rapid enlargement, and acute complications. Twelve patients developed acute complications during the period of conservative treatment. These complications included: FAA rupture (n = 7, mean FAA diameter, 5.7 + 1.3 cm), FAA thrombosis (n = 3), and FAA embolization (n = 2). This study suggests that patients with asymptomatic degenerative FAA rarely develop a complication unless they are > 3.5 cm and have intraluminal thrombus.

Our study demonstrated that the presence of intraluminal thrombus might increase the risk of thrombotic and/or embolic complications in patients with FAA. Multivariate analysis in our cohort demonstrated that FAA's larger than 4 cm with intraluminal thrombus are at significant risk for complications and that the presence of aneurysm related thrombus may indicate the need for earlier repair.

A prior study by Graham and colleagues also demonstrated a low incidence of major complications associated with untreated FAA.[9] In their series of 172 FAA, forty patients were asymptomatic at presentation. Eight presented with evidence of peripheral arterial embolization. However, 5 of these patients had concomitant popliteal artery aneurysms (PAA) and treatment of the PAA eliminated further embolic phenomena. Three FAA thromboses occurred, five demonstrated rapid growth and two patients experienced rupture requiring operative treatment.

A recent 20-year review by Piffaretti and colleagues suggested a less benign clinical presentation with 30% of patients presenting with symptoms. In 31 patients, rupture, localized pain, and acute thrombosis were observed in 10%, 10%, and 6%, respectively. Although the patients who presented with these symptoms had a significantly higher operative risk and required prolonged postoperative stay, no differences were noted in early complications and/or mortality rates.

DIAGNOSIS

Vascular surgeons evaluating patients with aortic and popliteal aneurysms should have a low index of suspicion for the presence of a synchronous FAA. Physical examination may demonstrate a pulsatile femoral mass, however distal profunda femoris and superficial femoral artery aneurysms may not be detected by palpation until they are larger in size, due to their location deeper in the leg. B-mode and Duplex ultrasound can reveal the presence of a FAA, provide accurate sizing and determine the extent of intraluminal thrombus (Figures 30-2A, 2B and 2C). Ankle-brachial indices may denote the presence of prior embolic disease and/or compromised runoff vessels.

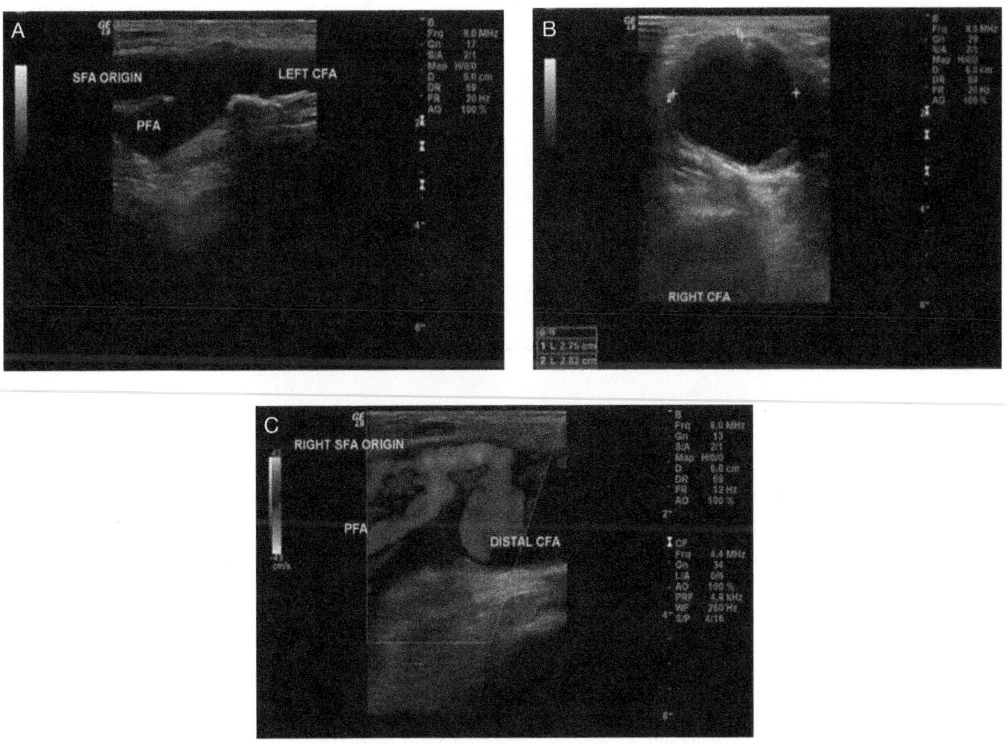

Figures 30-2A, 2B and 2C. B-mode and duplex ultrasound demonstrate the presence of a common femoral artery aneurysm.

Improvements in computed tomography (CT) and magnetic resonance angiography (MRA) over the past decade have also helped to characterize these aneurysms prior to invasive treatment (Figure 30-3). The use of these imaging modalities in the abdomen, pelvis and extremities aid in the identification of synchronous and metachronous aneurysms and are essential prior to surgical intervention. Accurate preoperative evaluation of aneurysm size, associated thrombus, relation to adjacent soft tissue structures, and evaluation of arterial runoff can also be achieved. In our series of 182 patients with 236 FAA, CT imaging was used in 127 (70%), duplex ultrasound imaging in 70 (38%), conventional angiography in 57 (31%), and MRA in 18 (10%).[6] Routine conventional angiography is no longer recommended as the initial diagnostic modality for these aneurysms.

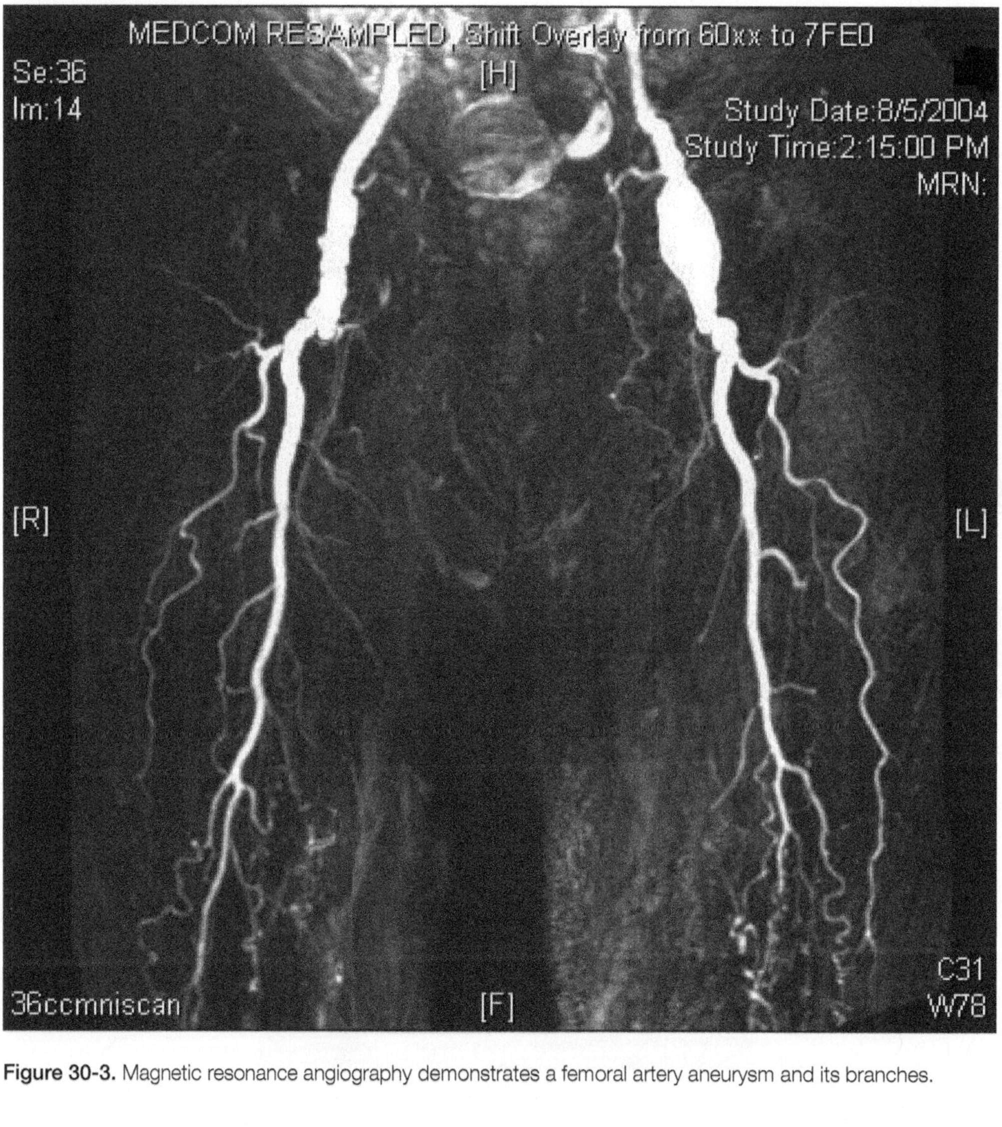

Figure 30-3. Magnetic resonance angiography demonstrates a femoral artery aneurysm and its branches.

INDICATIONS FOR TREATMENT

The recent VLFDC multi-institutional review of patients with degenerative FAA is the largest contemporary series reported and demonstrates that the currently accepted treatment algorithm may be too aggressive for their natural history.[6] Prior studies, which have included heterogeneous cohorts of patients and small case series, have recommended repair of asymptomatic FAA's with diameters of > 2.5 cm and all symptomatic aneurysms. We noted that complications from FAA's ≥ than 3.5 cm and without intraluminal thrombus were rare. The location of the aneurysm and whether they originated in the CFA, PFA or SFA was also not significant with regard to natural history and presentation. Based on our data, FAA's have a more benign natural history than popliteal artery aneurysms, which contradicts those who advocate that they should be treated with the same indications. In our series, only 4% of FAA's ruptured and thrombosis and/or embolization occurred in 7%. Our conclusion is that FAA's < 3.5 cm with minimal associated intraluminal thrombus may be managed safely and conservatively with serial imaging.

The data supports aggressive surgical treatment for patients where intraluminal thrombus is present. The presence of increased intraluminal thrombus was correlated with symptomatic patients and asymptomatic patients who then developed an acute embolic or thrombotic complication. Thus patients with thrombus need to be evaluated distinctly and the size threshold for repair may be lower in order to prevent embolic or thrombotic complications.

TREATMENT OUTCOMES

The results of surgical treatment for FAA across several series are favorable with low rates of postoperative complications and amputation (Tables 30-1A and 1B).[6,9] In the VLFDC cohort, surgical repair was performed in 141 patients with 180 aneurysms. Open surgical approach was used in all but three patients (98%), who underwent endovascular repair of SFA aneurysms (2%). Interposition graft was used to repair 142 aneurysms (80%) and bypass was performed in 35 (20%) (Figures 30-4A, 4B and 4C). The most common distal target for bypass was the CFA (34%) followed by the SFA (26%), PFA (23%) and the tibial arteries (6%). The mean diameter for FAA's that were surgically repaired was 3.3 + 1.5 cm. One patient died intraoperatively of multi-system organ failure.

The 30-day mortality in the series was 1.1%.[6] Major postoperative complications included: wound infection/seroma/hematoma (12%), respiratory failure (3%), acute lower extremity ischemia (1.5%), acute renal failure (1.5%), compartment syndrome (1%) and deep venous thrombosis (1%). Patients with symptomatic FAA demonstrated no correlation with the development of perioperative complications. The mean length of follow up was 49 months and the life-table cumulative survival rate was 94.5% at 6 months and 61.1% at 5 years. There was no difference in survival between symptomatic and asymptomatic patients.

TABLE 30-1A. EARLY RESULTS OF ELECTIVE FEMORAL ARTERY ANEURYSM REPAIR IN VLFDC MULTI-INSTITUTIONAL SERIES

	n = 4	%
Wound complications	4	5%
Acute lower extremity ischemia	0	0%
Respiratory failure	0	0%
Acute renal insufficiency	0	0%
Compartment syndrome	0	0%
Deep venous thrombosis	0	0%

TABLE 30-1B. EARLY RESULTS OF EMERGENT FEMORAL ARTERY ANEURYSM REPAIR IN VLFDC MULTI-INSTITUTIONAL SERIES

	n = 23	%
Wound complications	13	14%
Acute lower extremity ischemia	2	2%
Respiratory failure	4	4%
Acute renal insufficiency	2	3%
Compartment syndrome	1	1%
Deep venous thrombosis	1	1%

A smaller contemporary series by Piffaretti demonstrated similar favorable outcomes following surgical repair of FAA's.[12] Interventions included: resection with interposition graft (65%), ligation and bypass graft (29%), endograft repair of SFA aneurysms (7%), and ligation alone for a PFA aneurysm (1%). Open repair of PFA aneurysms was associated with longer operative times and postoperative hospitalizations. Conversely, repair of SFA aneurysms were associated with shorter operative times and decreased blood loss compared with CFA and PFA aneurysms. No primary or postoperative complications were performed in this cohort. Major respiratory complications developed in 2 patients and one patient required re-exploration for wound hematoma. Mean follow up was 56 months. Actuarial survival at one and five years was 93% and 77.6%, respectively.

Outcomes following endovascular treatment of SFA and PFA aneurysms are limited to case reports and small case series. Methods described include endovascular exclusion of SFA aneurysms with covered stent-grafts and transcatheter coil embolization of distal PFA aneurysms.[13,14] Technical success was achieved in the small number of SFA aneurysms treated with an endograft in Piffaretti's series and in our recent cohort.[6,12] The long-term durability and outcomes associated with this type of repair are unknown.

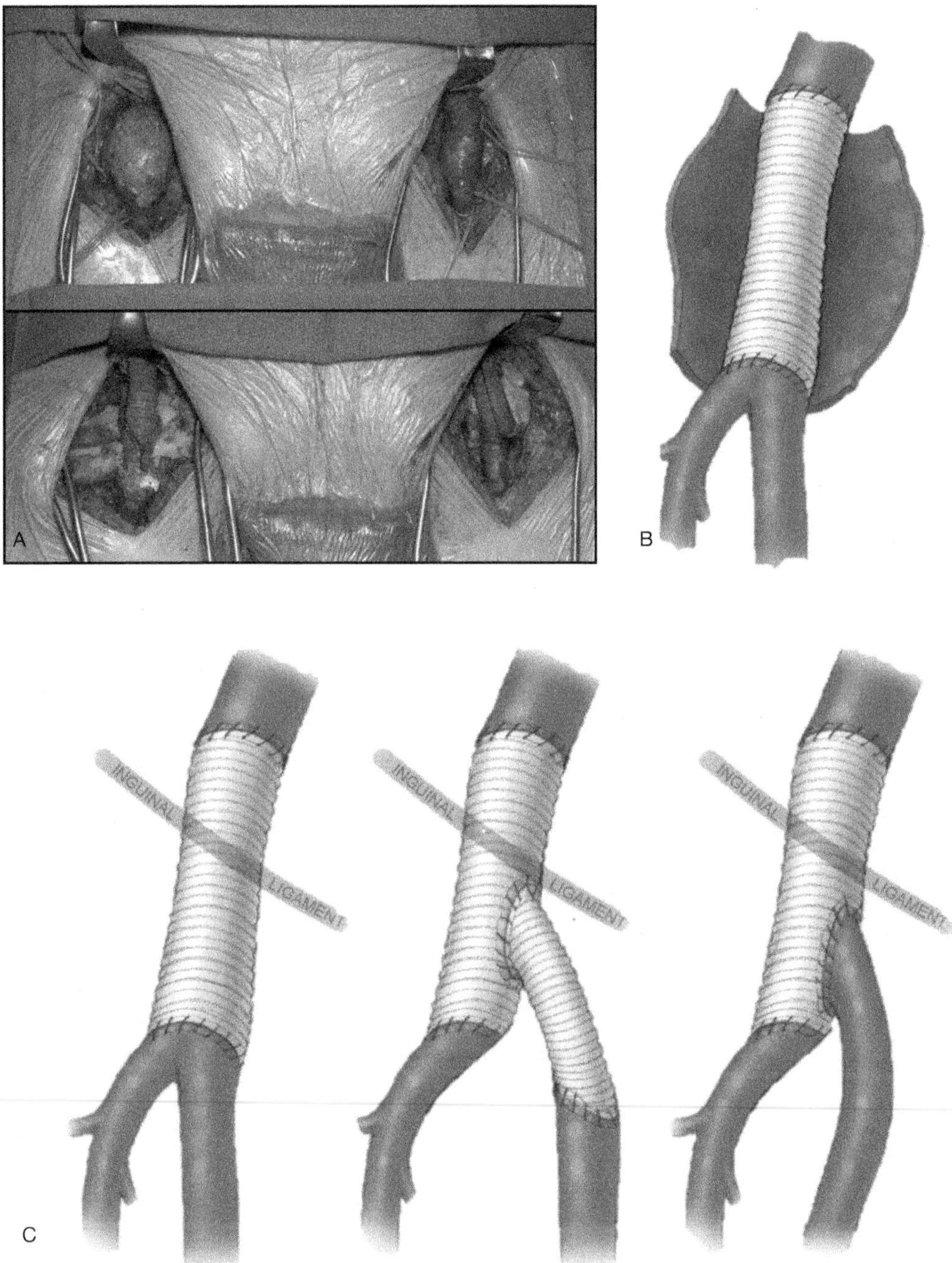

Figures 30-4A, 4B and 4C. Interposition graft repair of common femoral artery aneurysm—intra-operative photo and diagram. Figure 4C demonstrates surgical options for managing the superficial femoral and profunda femoris arteries.

CONCLUSION

Established criteria based on historical, small and heterogeneous cohorts, advocating repair at 2.5 cm, likely overestimate the likelihood of FAA related complications. Asymptomatic true FAA's can be managed conservatively with serial imaging to a diameter of 3.5 cm in the absence of significant intramural thrombus. The presence of associated thrombus should lower the size threshold for repair. Patients with symptomatic FAA's should undergo surgical treatment with resection and interposition grafting or ligation and surgical bypass. Development of consensus guidelines for management of low-frequency vascular diseases like FAA continues to present a challenge to clinicians, and unanswered questions will likely not be answered by additional single-institution series. The use of multi-institutional databases may reveal much needed insight into management of similar low frequency vascular diseases.

REFERENCES

1. Lawrence PF, Lorenzo-Rivero S, Lyon JL. The incidence of iliac, femoral, and popliteal artery aneurysms in hospitalized patients. *J Vasc Surg.* 1995;22:409–16.
2. Cho YP, Choi SJ, Kwon TW, et al. Deep femoral artery aneurysm presenting as lower limb swelling: a case report. *YMJ (Yonsei Medical Journal).* 2006;47(1):148–51.
3. Sharma S, Nalachandran S. Isolated common femoral artery aneurysm: a case report. *Cases J*;2:7522.
4. Igari K, Kudo T, Toyofuku T, et al. Surgical treatment for profunda femoris artery aneurysms: Five case reports. *Case Rep Vasc Med.* 2015;2015:375278.
5. Levi N, Schroeder TV. Arteriosclerotic femoral artery aneurysms. A short review. *J Cardiovasc Surg.* 1997;38:335–8.
6. Lawrence PF, Harlander-Locke MP, Oderich GS, et al. The current management of isolated degenerative femoral artery aneurysms is too aggressive for their natural history. *J Vasc Surg.* 2014;59:343–9.
7. Rigdon EE, Monajjem N. Aneurysms of the superficial femoral artery: A report of two cases and review of the literature. *J Vasc Surg.* 1992;16:790–793.
8. Diwan A, Sarkar R, Stanley JC, et al. Incidence of femoral and popliteal artery aneurysms in patients with abdominal aortic aneurysms. *J Vasc Surg.* 2000;31:863–869.
9. Graham LM, Zelenock GB, Whitehouse WM, Jr., et al. Clinical significance of arteriosclerotic femoral artery aneurysms. *Arch Surg.* 1980;115:502–7.
10. Adiseshiah M, Bailey DA. Aneurysms of the femoral artery. *Br J Surg.* 1977;64:174–6.
11. Tolstedt GE, Radke HM, Bell JW. Late sequelae of arteriosclerotic femoral aneurysms. *Angiology.* 1961;12:602–2.
12. Piffaretti, G, Mariscalco, G, Tozzi, M, et al. Twenty-year experience of femoral artery aneurysms. *J Vasc Surg.* 2011;53:1230–1236.
13. Keskin S, Koc O, Keskin Z, et al. Radiolgical findings and endovascular treatment in giant deep femoral artery aneurysms. *BMJ.* Case Rep 2014. In Press.
14. Ramus JR, Gibson M, Magee T, et al. Spontaneous rupture of the superficial femoral artery treated with endovascular stent-grafting. *Cardiovasc Intervent Radiol.* 2007;30:1016–9.

31

Visceral Artery Dissection

Armando Cardenas, MD, Courtney Morgan, MD, William H. Pearce, MD, and Heron Rodriguez, MD

Isolated Visceral artery dissections (VAD) are infrequent. More commonly, they present as incidental findings during computed tomography (CT) or magnetic resonance (MR). When symptoms are present, they vary from chronic unspecific pain, weight loss, acute abdomen, abdominal angina, renal dysfunction, rupture and death. Due to the rarity of this condition, there are no consensus guidelines regarding management of patients presenting with VAD. The intent of this chapter is to review the existing literature and provide a general understanding on how to approach and treat VADs.

CELIAC ARTERY DISSECTIONS

About 100 cases of isolated celiac artery (CA) dissections have been reported in the literature during the past 12 years.[1] The etiology of this condition remains unknown. Some authors have suggested that vasculitides like Marfan syndrome, Ehlers-Danlos, giant-cell arteritis, Takayasu arteritis, fibromuscular dysplasia (FMD), segmental arterial mediolysis (SAM) and polyarteritis nodosa may be associated with CA dissections. Some case reports have documented CA dissection following motor vehicle accidents and falls. We treated a patient with a CA dissection occurring after a spell of severe cough.

In most series, the majority of patients are asymptomatic. The remaining present with upper abdominal, back or flank pain. In rare cases when the dissection involves branch vessels, hepatic failure and splenic rupture have been reported.[2] In a report by Amabile (which included multiple vessel dissections) all of the patients were male, all were smokers, and all had symptoms for more than 10 days. In this report, 75% of patients did not require operative treatment and were treated medically.[3] A recent single-institution series found 19 patients with celiac artery dissection during a period of 8 years.[4] The majority of patients were male (75%) and asymptomatic (63%). The mean age of diagnosis was 54 years. All patients were initially treated conservatively with observation alone. Only 4 required interventions: 3 patients received a stent for persistent abdominal pain and one patient was treated surgically for aneurismal degeneration of the dissected celiac artery.

Based on the available evidence, it appears reasonable to treat most patients conservatively. Anticoagulation can be used to preserve flow when severe luminal compromise is evident. Intervention should be reserved for patients who present initially with complications (ischemia, rupture) and for those with persisting pain or with aneurismal dilation. The size threshold for intervention once aneurysms develop is controversial, but most authors suggest that CA smaller than 2–3 cm rarely rupture.

SUPERIOR MESENTERIC ARTERY DISSECTION

Dissections of the superior mesenteric artery (SMA) are the most common type of spontaneous visceral artery dissection. Similar to other locations, detection has become more common with increasing use of CT however the majority present as symptomatic lesions with abdominal or back pain.[1] In an extensive review of the literature on SMA dissection by Oppat et al. in 2009,[5] most cases presented in the fifth decade of life with the majority of patients being male. Male preponderance has also been observed in other series.[1,6] Although most patients had known risk factors such as hypertension or smoking history, some did not and presented after either trauma of strenuous exercise.[7] Other potential causes include cystic medial necrosis, SAM,[3,8] vasculitis, and congenital connective tissue disorders.

CT is the preferred imaging modality.[9] The distance between the SMA ostium and the origin of the dissection tends to fall between 2–3 cm in the majority of cases.[10] Several classification schemes based on the characteristics of the true and false lumen have been proposed (Figure 31-1).[11] In the largest series of patients reported, most

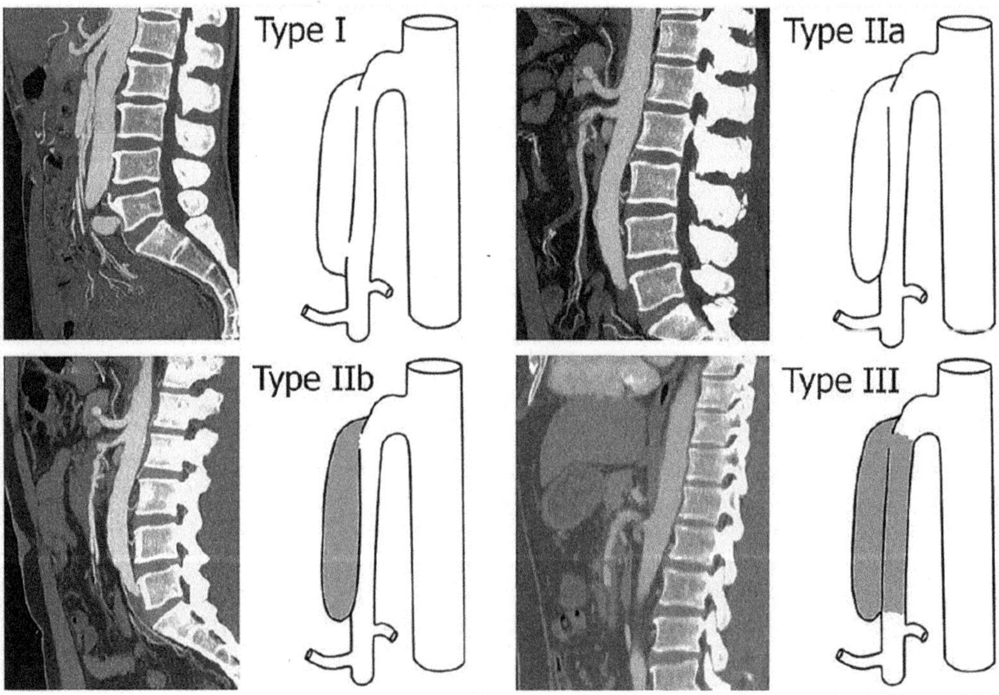

Figure 31-1. Angiographic classification of SMA dissections.

symptomatic patients were observed to have a patent true lumen with no re-entry from the false lumen (Type II) on CT angiography.[11]

Although there are no guidelines regarding management of SMA dissection, several treatment algorithms have been suggested. The majority of patients can be managed conservatively; however the definition of conservative or medical management differs between studies. Most studies recommend managing patients with no clinical signs of bowel ischemia or SMA branch rupture with bowel rest, anti-impulse control and either anticoagulation or antiplatelet therapy (Figure 31-2).[3,6,7,12,13] Several other studies have also reported successful management without anticoagulation.[1,9,14] An argument to withhold anticoagulation is that this form of therapy prevents thrombosis of the false lumen and thus perpetuates the dissection. On the other hand, anticoagulation may preserve flow in cases of severely compromised true lumen.

Indications for revascularization in the reported series include: signs or symptoms of intestinal ischemia, progression of dissection or aneurysm size, narrowing or thrombosis of the true lumen, and saccular aneurysm formation that is likely to rupture or embolize.[5] Revascularization options include both endovascular stenting, and surgical revascularization. The first reported case for endovascular stenting for SMA

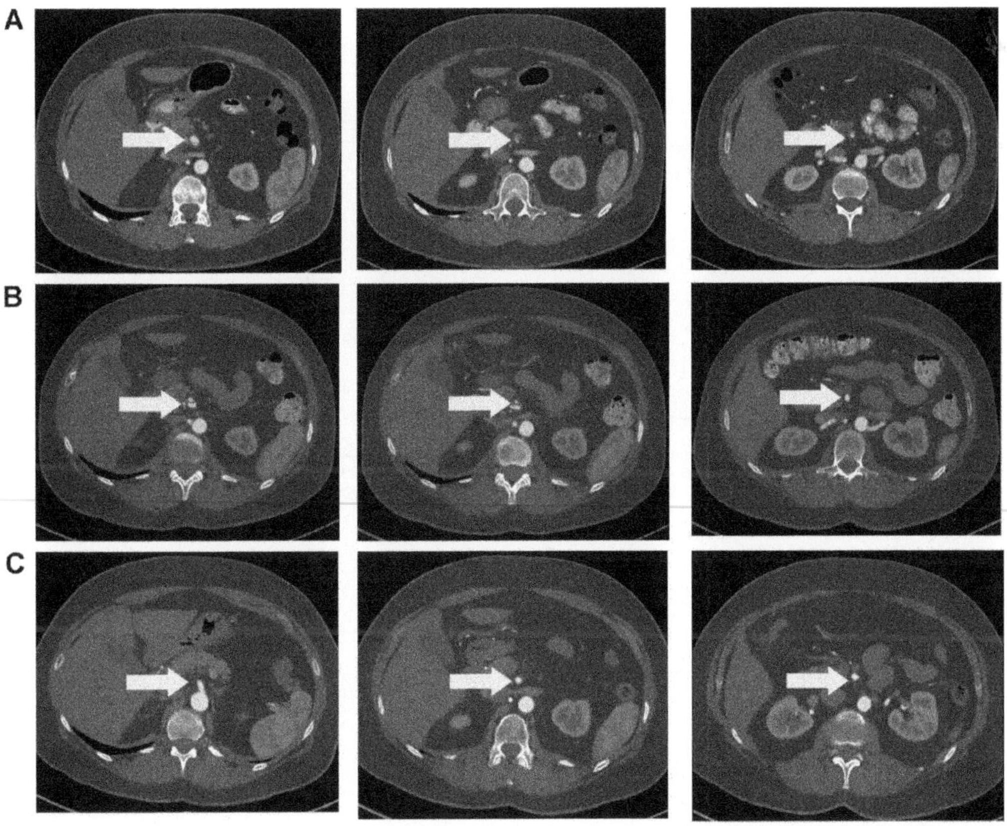

Figure 31-2. Spontaneous isolated SMA dissection treated with bowel rest and anticoagulation. CT scan during acute presentation (A) after 10 months of anticoagulation (B) and 2 years after (C) showing complete remodeling of the very narrowed true lumen. Arrows denote SMA.

dissection was by Leung in 2000.[15] Anatomy which is favorable for stenting involves localized intimal flaps, or short segments of dissection. Stents need to have good flexibility, minimal shortening, and minimal migration due to the continuous motion of the mesenteric arteries.[1] Surgical revascularization is indicated for bowel infarction or arterial rupture. Numerous options for surgical revascularization have been described including bypass or intimectomy with patch angioplasty closure.[5] When choosing a conduit, saphenous vein, radial artery, superficial femoral artery, cryopreserved conduit, or prosthetic grafts may be used, however in the setting of gross bowel spillage, prosthetic grafts should be avoided.

RENAL ARTERY DISSECTIONS

Spontaneous renal artery (RA) dissection is a rare occurrence with less than 200 cases reported in the literature (Figure 31-3). The overall incidence of spontaneous RA dissection was found to be between 0.036% and 0.049% in a large angiographic study.[16] While it has been suggested that spontaneous RA dissections occur as an underlying manifestation of (FMD), recent literature suggests that it is an independent entity not associated with FMD.

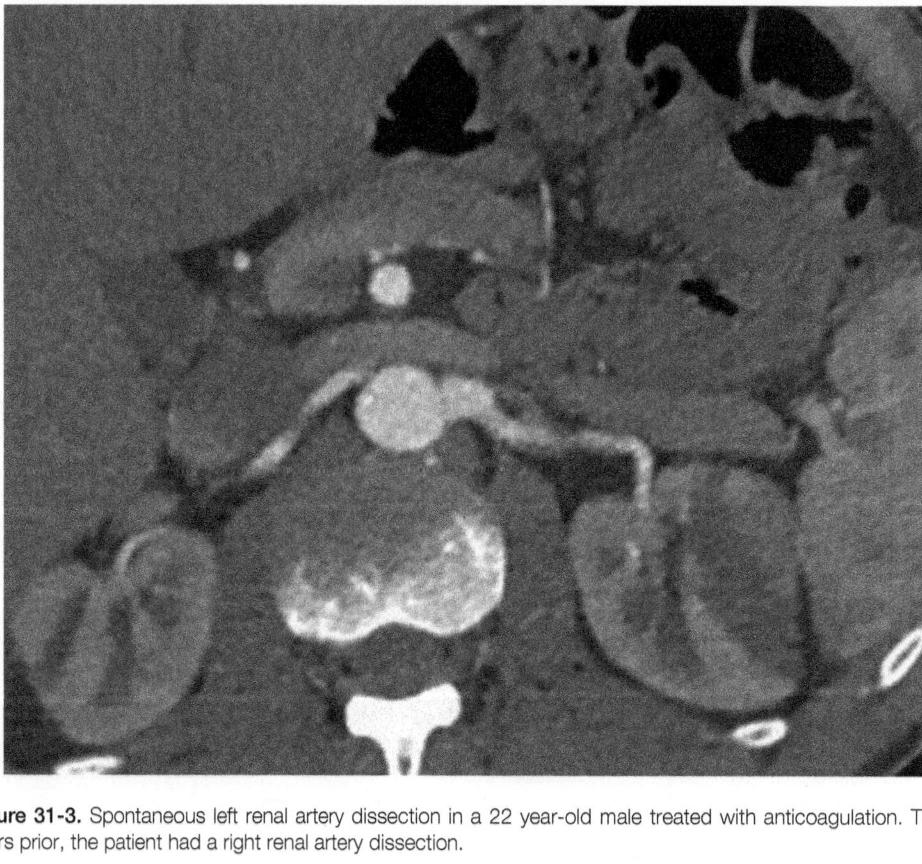

Figure 31-3. Spontaneous left renal artery dissection in a 22 year-old male treated with anticoagulation. Three years prior, the patient had a right renal artery dissection.

Spontaneous RA dissections occur in the fourth and fifth decades of life and have a male preponderance (4:1). This is unlike FMD, which affects women in the second and third decades of life. Bilateral dissections occur in 10% to 15% of cases. Furthermore, there is no evidence that one artery is more susceptible to dissections. Conditions that have been associated with spontaneous RA dissection include FMD, malignant hypertension, atherosclerosis and inherited connective tissue disease such as Marfan's or Ehlers-Danlos, cystic medial necrosis, SAM and extreme physical activity.[16–18] There is one case report of bilateral RA dissection following marathon running.[16]

Initial presentation is non-specific and can suggest a renal colic. The most common symptom is severe pain, occurring unilaterally in the upper abdomen or flank with radiation to the epigastrium. Hypertension, renal dysfunction and hematuria can also be present. With these non-specific findings, high clinical suspicion and early imaging are the only ways to detect RA dissection. CTA or MRA are effective in determining the diagnosis. Initial treatment and long term management are poorly defined. There are no guidelines and the limited available information make this condition a therapeutic challenge. A thorough clinical and angiographic assessment must be done to determine management. If the RA dissection is stable with no deterioration of renal function conservative treatment may be the best option. This is especially true in complex dissections with branch involvement for which endovascular options are limited. As it occurs with carotid and other visceral dissections, anticoagulation may be of value when true lumen compromise exists. Anticoagulation alone is advocated by some authors as the best initial strategy.[19]

If the dissection is unstable or renal function is compromised, a more aggressive treatment should be considered. Endovascular treatment with placement of intraluminal stents has been used with success. In one series, 16 patients were treated successfully with no restenosis or occlusion with the use of intraluminal stents.[20] This treatment modality appears attractive in RA dissections that occur in the main renal artery with no branch vessel involvement and with significant luminal compromise.

Surgical approaches have a more limited role in the management of acute RA dissection and are reserved for late stages with aneurismal degeneration in cases where endovascular options are poor. Surgical repair has been associated with 8% and 27% risk of nepherectomy, 6% to 12% of renal artery stenosis, and a 15% risk of anastomotic restenosis.[21,22]

COMMENT

Given the widespread use of CT and MR imaging, VAD are being detected more frequently. The etiology of VAD remains unknown. There appears to be some relationship with trauma and extraneous physical activity. It also appears feasible that some of these dissections are associated with SAM. Slavin and Gonzalez-Vitale in 1976[23] were the firsts to describe SAM; this condition has a predilection for visceral arteries. It is a non-atheroclerotic, non-inflammatory disease with unknown etiology. The characteristic lesion is mediolysis in the outer media, which may extend inward to involve almost all the inner media. The mediolysis is produced by expanding vacuoles within the cytoplasm of the smooth muscle cells.[24,25] The vacuoles enlarge to a point that the cell ruptures and the media is lost. Slavin and colleagues have described a process of healing following this injury. Granulation tissue fills the areas of media, which may lead to hemorrhage from ruptures, dissecting hematomas, and aneurismal enlargement. In addition there may be separation of the outer media from the adventitia that fills the vessel with granulation tissue forming a fibrous organization that is not dissimilar from FMD. Slavin and colleagues believe that SAM is a precursor for fibromuscular dysplastic disease. The arterial lesions are segmental and may involve part of the entire arterial wall circumference. The early phases of the process are asymptomatic and only become evident when a complication occurs. Several reports have detailed multiple artery involvement. Ro described a 70-year-old gentleman who had rupture of a gastroepiploic aneurysm, but was also found to have recent arterial dissections in the left gastric artery and both intracranial vertebral arteries.[26] While it appears that in many instances the disease is self-limiting, one report by Hashimoto describes a 59-year-old male with a rupture of a splenic artery aneurysm who developed a superior mesenteric artery dissection 1½ years later, a gastroepiploic aneurysm 3 weeks later, a right internal carotid artery aneurysm one month later, and splenic artery aneurysms 3 weeks later.[27]

Mechanisms that produce SAM are unknown. Arterial vasopasm plays a predominant role in the etiology. The visceral circulation is known for its vasoreactivity. The application of norepinepfhrine to the surface of the vessel may produce experimental SAM, which demonstrated identical histologic findings. In a histologic study, Slavis reported the presence of endothelin one (ET-1) surrounding these vessels and in adjacent veins.[22] He suggests that the segmental nature of the lesions is related to the location of visceral nerves. He suggests ET-1 potentiates the vasoconstriction effect of the neurotransmitters. His theory would account for why the lesion is scattered and may explain why dissections occur after marathon running. Marathon running produces marked intestinal Ischemia from intense vasoconstriction.

Slavin believes that this lesion is a precursor to FMD. However, it is difficult to reconcile the fact that FMD is much more common in young women than in elderly to middle-aged men. He suggests that with aging the arterial structure changes, which allows easier separation between the media and adventitia than in the younger individuals. Thus the disruption of the arterial wall is less likely to occur in the young than it does in the old. However, he does not have an explanation why female patients are more common in the young.

In the last several years, we have diagnosed a number of VAD at Northwestern. Unless there is clear evidence of severe end organ ischemia, our current preference is for initial conservative management. If the true lumen shows significant reduction, intravenous anticoagulation and serial imaging is pursued. In only one patient this strategy failed. In this middle aged male, SMA thrombosis occurred 4 days after initial presentation despite therapeutic anticoagulation. He was then treated with an aortomesenteric bypass to a branch of the SMA (Figure 31-4), and remains asymptomatic 2 years later. Patients with uncontrolled hypertension, renal failure, bowel ischemia, and hemorrhage mandate immediate intervention. Endovascular approaches are favored unless anatomy precludes them.

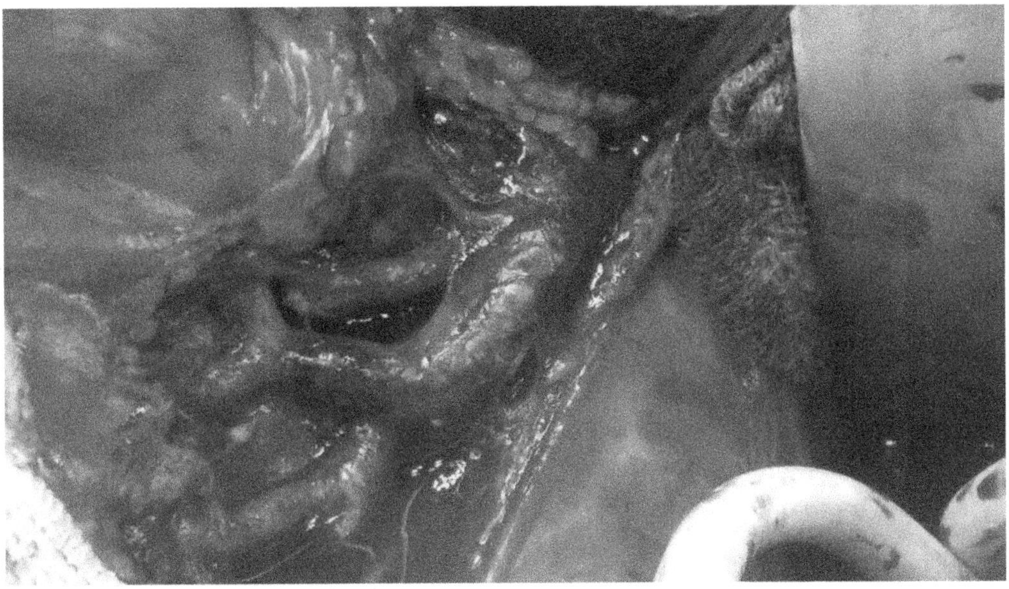

Figure 31-4. Acute SMA thrombosis after failed conservative management of a spontaneous SMA dissection. An aorto-mesenteric bypass was performed to a patent branch of the SMA.

REFERENCES

1. Ko SH, Hye R, Frankel DA. Management of spontaneous isolated visceral artery dissection. *Ann Vasc Surg*. 2015;29(3):470–474.
2. Nordanstig J, Gerdes H, Kocys E. Spontaneous isolated dissection of the celiac trunk with rupture of the proximal splenic artery: a case report. *Eur J Vasc Endovasc Surg*. 2009;37(2):194–197.
3. Amabile P, Ouaissi M, Cohen S, Piquet P. Conservative treatment of spontaneous and isolated dissection of mesenteric arteries. *Ann Vasc Surg*. 2009;23(6):738–744.
4. DiMusto PD, Oberdoerster MM, Criado E. Isolated celiac artery dissection. *J Vasc Surg*. 2015;61(4):972–976.
5. Subhas G, Gupta A, Nawalany M, Oppat WF. Spontaneous isolated superior mesenteric artery dissection: a case report and literature review with management algorithm. *Ann Vasc Surg*. 2009;23(6):788–798.
6. Takach TJ, Madjarov JM, Holleman JH, et al. Spontaneous splanchnic dissection: application and timing of therapeutic options. *J Vasc Surg*. 2009;50(3):557–563.
7. Zhang WW, Killeen JD, Chiriano J, et al. Management of symptomatic spontaneous isolated visceral artery dissection: is emergent intervention mandatory? *Ann Vasc Surg*. 2009;23(1):90–94.
8. Tameo MN, Dougherty MJ, Calligaro KD. Spontaneous dissection with rupture of the superior mesenteric artery from segmental arterial mediolysis. *J Vasc Surg*. 2011;53(4):1107–1112.
9. Gobble RM, Brill ER, Rockman CB, et al. Endovascular treatment of spontaneous dissections of the superior mesenteric artery. *J Vasc Surg*. 2009;50(6):1326–1332.
10. Solis MM, Ranval TJ, McFarland DR, Eidt JF. Surgical treatment of superior mesenteric artery dissecting aneurysm and simultaneous celiac artery compression. *Ann Vasc Surg*. 1993;7(5):457–462.

11. Yun WS, Kim YW, Park KB, et al. Clinical and angiographic follow-up of spontaneous isolated superior mesenteric artery dissection. *Eur J Vasc Endovasc Surg.* 2009;37(5):572–577.
12. Morris JT, Guerriero J, Sage JG, Mansour MA. Three isolated superior mesenteric artery dissections: update of previous case reports, diagnostics, and treatment options. *J Vasc Surg.* 2008;47(3):649–653.
13. Kang TL, Teich DL, McGillicuddy DC. Isolated, spontaneous superior mesenteric and celiac artery dissection: case report and review of literature. *J Emerg Med.* 2011;40(2):e21–e25.
14. Min S-I, Yoon K-C, Min S-K, et al. Current strategy for the treatment of symptomatic spontaneous isolated dissection of superior mesenteric artery. *J Vasc Surg.* 2011;54(2):461–466.
15. Leung DA, Schneider E, Kubik-Huch R, et al. Acute mesenteric ischemia caused by spontaneous isolated dissection of the superior mesenteric artery: treatment by percutaneous stent placement. *Eur Radiol.* 2000;10(12):1916–1919.
16. Iqbal FM, Goparaju M, Yemme S, Lewis BE. Renal artery dissection following marathon running. *Angiology.* 2009;60(1):122–126.
17. Kanofsky JA, Lepor H. Spontaneous renal artery dissection. *Rev Urol.* 2007;9(3):156–160.
18. Soga Y, Nose M, Arita N, et al. Aneurysms of the renal arteries associated with segmental arterial mediolysis in a case of polyarteritis nodosa. *Pathol Int.* 2009;59(3):197–200.
19. Ramamoorthy SL, Vasquez JC, Taft PM, et al. Nonoperative management of acute spontaneous renal artery dissection. *Ann Vasc Surg.* 2002;16(2):157–162.
20. Pellerin O, Garcon P, Beyssen B, et al. Spontaneous renal artery dissection: long-term outcomes after endovascular stent placement. *JVIR.* 2009;20(8):1024–1030.
21. Reilly LM, Cunningham CG, Maggisano R, et al. The role of arterial reconstruction in spontaneous renal artery dissection. *J Vasc Surg.* 1991;14(4):468–477; discussion 477–469.
22. Slavis SA, Hodge EE, Novick AC, Maatman T. Surgical treatment for isolated dissection of the renal artery. *J Urol.* 1990;144(2 Pt 1):233–237.
23. Slavin RE, Gonzalez-Vitale JC. Segmental mediolytic arteritis: a clinical pathologic study. *Lab Iinvest.* 1976;35(1):23–29.
24. Slavin RE, Inada K. Segmental arterial mediolysis with accompanying venous angiopathy: a clinical pathologic review, report of 3 new cases, and comments on the role of endothelin-1 in its pathogenesis. *IJSP.* 2007;15(2):121–134.
25. Slavin RE. Segmental arterial mediolysis: course, sequelae, prognosis, and pathologic-radiologic correlation. *Cardiovasc Pathol.* 2009;18(6):352–360.
26. Ro A, Kageyama N, Takatsu A, Fukunaga T. Segmental arterial mediolysis of varying phases affecting both the intra-abdominal and intracranial vertebral arteries: an autopsy case report. *Cardiovasc Pathol.* 2010;19(4):248–251.
27. Hashimoto T, Deguchi J, Endo H, Miyata T. Successful treatment tailored to each splanchnic arterial lesion due to segmental arterial mediolysis (SAM): report of a case. *J Vasc Surg.* 2008;48(5):1338–1341.

32

One- Versus Two-Vessel Mesenteric Artery Bypass for Chronic Mesenteric Ischemia

Gustavo S. Oderich, MD and Thomas C. Bower, MD

Endovascular therapy has changed the management of patients with acute and chronic mesenteric ischemia. Stenting of the superior mesenteric artery (SMA) now is offered as first line therapy for most patients with chronic mesenteric ischemia (CMI) and favorable lesions.[1,2] The introduction of covered stents seems to have reduced the risk of recurrent stenosis.[3] The primary role for single or two vessel mesenteric artery bypasses includes symptomatic patients with flush occlusions of the celiac or SMA at the aortic origin; those with thick, calcified lesions; long segment stenosis; individuals who fail angioplasty and stenting, and young patients with non-atherosclerotic lesions.[4,5]

SURGICAL TREATMENT

The primary goals of treatment are to alleviate symptoms, prevent bowel infarction, allow weight gain and improve nutritional status.[5] Mesenteric bypass to treat CMI can be done to reconstruct the SMA alone, or both the celiac and SMA.[4–7] In contrast to the dictum that CMI requires two of three mesenteric arteries to be occluded or have high-grade stenoses because of the normally rich collateral network between visceral artery beds, between 2% and 10% of patients have single vessel disease, usually the SMA.[4,6,8] Such patients have poor collaterals between the visceral artery territories.[8] It is for these reasons that some surgeons focus solely on SMA revascularization.[7] Antegrade bypass implies graft origin from the supraceliac aorta while retrograde bypass originates from the infrarenal aorta, common or external iliac arteries. Retrograde bypass can be done with the graft position straight or as a C-shape.[4,5,7,9–11] Both antegrade and retrograde reconstructions, and two vessel versus single vessel bypass, provide excellent symptom relief and are durable.[5–7,9–21] The conduit for bypass most often is prosthetic, but saphenous vein, femoral vein or rarely cryopreserved artery can be utilized.

Antegrade versus retrograde bypass, the need for single versus two vessel reconstructions, and graft orientation are based on patient risk for operation and the ability to tolerate an aortic cross-clamp, calcification or stenosis in the aorta or iliac arteries, and whether the patient has acute or chronic symptoms.[4,5,9,17] In our practice, most patients undergo antegrade bypass from the supraceliac aorta.[4–6,9,11,12,15,17] High risk patients or those with calcification of the supraceliac aorta are better treated with a retrograde bypass from a common iliac artery, more often the right one. If the common iliac arteries are heavily calcified, the external iliac artery can be used for inflow. We have treated a rare patient who is not a candidate for stenting, too high risk for aortic clamping, but has iliac artery disease. These patients have been treated with common iliac artery stents, followed by a single retrograde bypass from the external iliac.

Technique and Exposure

Exposure is everything in open vascular surgery. Isolation of the supraceliac aorta for antegrade bypass is done through an upper midline or bilateral subcostal incision, depending on the body build and costal flare of the patient.[4,9] Either incision is applicable for a transperitoneal approach or a left medial visceral rotation to isolate the aorta or visceral arteries. If medial visceral rotation is planned, a small bump placed under the left side of the patient, and securing of the knees and/or legs so that the operating table can be rotated, facilitates exposure. The xiphoid process is the linchpin to expose the upper abdominal aorta and its branches when a midline incision is chosen. A 2 cm incision along the side of the xiphoid side releases 6 muscular and aponeurotic attachments and allows for upward and lateral retraction of the body wall.[4] The patient is positioned slightly head up. Transperitoneal isolation of the supraceliac aorta begins by taking down the left triangular ligament of the liver and opening the lesser sac (Figure 32-1). The crura of the diaphragm are divided longitudinally, though portions of the muscle may require resection to adequately isolate the aorta. Care must be taken to protect the esophagus, and having an NG tube in place is helpful. In most patients, 5 to 6 cm of lower descending thoracic or supraceliac aorta can be dissected free.[4] Thin patients have little soft tissue alongside the aorta, so it is easy to make a pleural rent. The pleura can be closed using a red rubber suction catheter to remove air from the pleural space.

The celiac artery is isolated before the SMA if antegrade bypass of each is planned. Laparotomy pads or a folded towel is laid over the pancreas so it and the bowel can be gently retracted caudally for isolation of the celiac and its branches. If the celiac artery is the target for bypass, the artery can be identified at its origin and circumferentially dissected free toward the common hepatic and splenic branches. This requires resection of periarterial ganglionic and fibrous tissue, and ligation and division of the occasional small side branch. Often, the left gastric artery is ligated and divided, which helps in creating a retropancreatic tunnel for the SMA graft limb. Alternatively, if there is scarring around the celiac, the common hepatic artery can be isolated and dissected

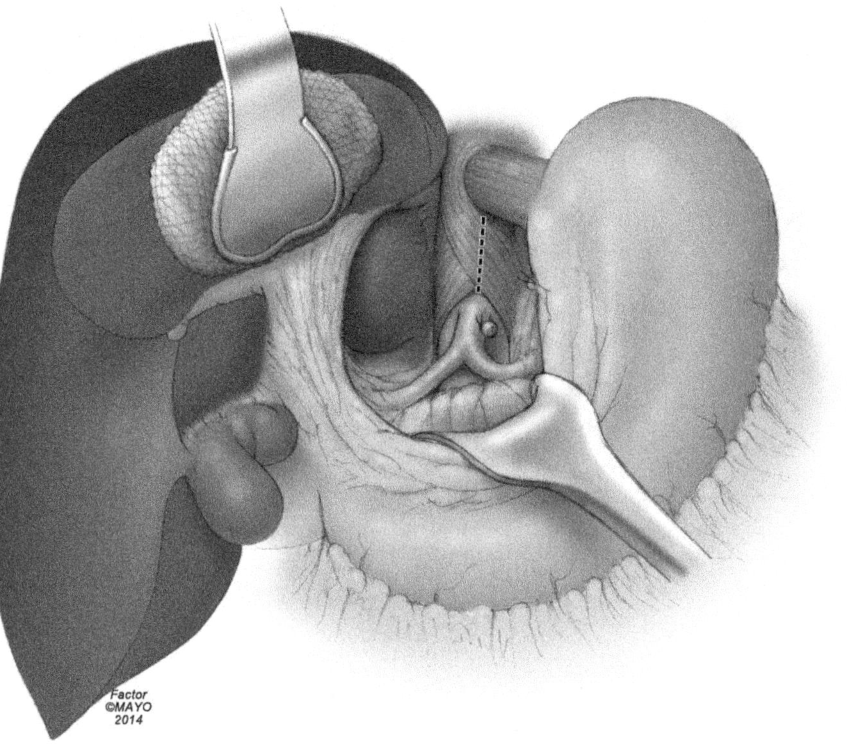

Figure 32-1. Transperitoneal exposure of the supraceliac aorta and celiac artery or branches begin by dividing the left triangular ligament of the liver and gently retracting it; and opening the lesser sac and dividing the crura of the diaphragm overlying the aorta. The celiac artery can be identified at its origin and dissected free distally, or the common hepatic artery can be isolated and traced proximally to find the celiac.

free toward the celiac bifurcation. One or more small veins which run alongside the artery may need to be ligated. Isolation of the splenic artery origin then allows the surgeon to dissect free the celiac trunk. If the celiac is occluded, the common hepatic artery becomes the target for revascularization. In this case, the celiac trunk does not to be freed.[4]

The SMA can be isolated above the pancreas if disease is confined to the first centimeter or two of the artery; or at the base of the transverse mesocolon, which is the more common exposure. For the latter, the transverse colon is retracted cephalad and the small intestine is retracted to the right side. The ligament of Treitz is taken down so that the SMA can be palpated in the mesentery. Lymphatic and fibro-fatty tissues are ligated and divided along the left side near the base of the duodenal sweep as part of the dissection to isolate the SMA trunk. Jejunal branches which arise along the side, or sometimes the posterior wall of the SMA, can be isolated with vessel loops (Figure 32-2). These branches tear easily and cause troublesome bleeding if injured. Care should be taken to not injure a replaced right hepatic artery if one is present. Extensive calcification and long segment stenosis in the SMA warrants dissection further into the mesentery. The most challenging patients are those with diffuse calcification from prior abdominal radiation, which affects almost every SMA branch. A retropancreatic tunnel anterior to the left renal vein and along the left anterolateral

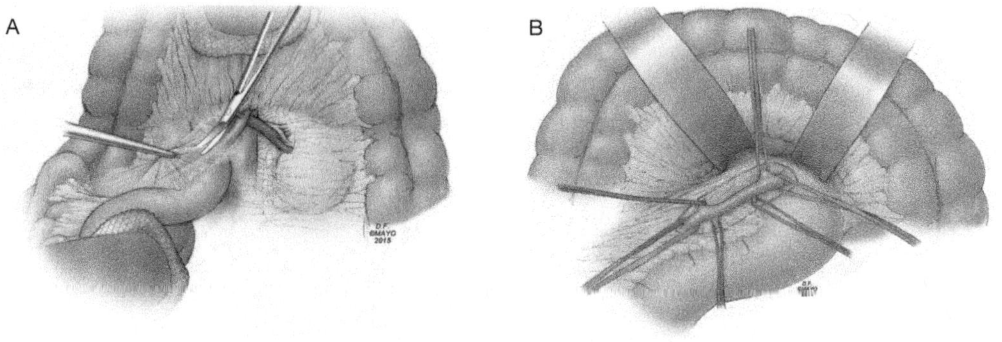

Figure 32-2. Isolation of the SMA can be done above the pancreas for patients with very focal disease, or the artery and its branches can be isolated near the base of the transverse mesocolon, as illustrated here (A). The latter exposure is more common. Side branches must be carefully dissected free (B).

aorta is created by blunt and sharp dissection for an antegrade SMA bypass. The tunnel must be free of fibrous bands and large enough to avoid compression of the graft.[4]

The infrarenal aorta and iliac arteries are isolated in the same way as a transperitoneal approach used to perform open aorto-iliac reconstructions. We rarely use the infrarenal aorta as an inflow source because it is too easy to misjudge the length of the graft and have it kink or buckle. There are steps to create a short stovepipe bypass from the infrarenal aorta to the SMA, a useful technique described later.

Transaortic visceral endarterectomy is infrequently used in current practice, but an effective technique for individuals with atherosclerotic lesions isolated to the origins of the arteries.[4,18] Endarterectomy may be appealing in the select patient with acute ischemia and feculent spillage in which prosthetic should be avoided.[18] This technique also is useful for the rare symptomatic patient who has high-grade orificial visceral and renal atherosclerotic lesions. The aorta and visceral arteries are isolated via left medial visceral rotation with the kidney kept down. Care is needed to avoid injury to the spleen and pancreas. Dissection extends from the supraceliac to the juxtarenal aortic segment. For most patients, the adrenal branch of the left renal vein is ligated and divided and the renal vein is mobilized and gently retracted caudally. Several centimeters of the celiac and SMA are dissected free to their origins, to allow for an eversion endarterectomy. The left renal artery origin is identified to facilitate clamp position on the upper infrarenal aorta. Phrenic and other side branches may require ligation and division.[4]

Patients who undergo antegrade reconstruction based on the supraceliac aorta are given between 50 and 100 units per kg of intravenous heparin and 12.5 gm of mannitol before placement of the aortic cross clamp. The aortic anastomosis either is done with a partial occlusion clamp (all- purpose clamp), or full aortic clamping. If the aorta is 18 mm or larger in diameter and not calcified, partial occlusion works well. Patients who are deep or have a thick aortic wall are better served with a double clamp technique (Figure 32-3A). A straight aortic clamp is applied to the proximal supraceliac aorta. A hypogastric clamp can be placed on the distal supraceliac aorta or from behind the celiac artery so that it occludes the aorta and the intercostal arteries. It is important to have a good view of the interior aortic walls when suturing the graft. Since the aortic anastomosis can be done within 15 minutes in most patients, it is preferable to fully cross clamp the aorta if it is small diameter or diseased than to struggle using a partial occlusion clamp and risk an imperfect anastomosis which has to be redone. Moreover, close communication with the anesthesiology team lessens the adverse effects of cardiac afterload during complete aortic cross clamping, and reduces declamping hypotension with restoration of blood flow to the kidneys and lower extremities. A slight oblique aortotomy is made on the anterolateral left anterolateral wall of the aorta. A stay stitch is placed as needed. Patients with an aortic diameter of at least 16 mm have a small ellipse of the anterior wall excised which obviates the need for a stay stitch. Two vessel reconstructions are done with a 12 × 7 mm or 14 × 7 mm knitted polyester grafts most often. The bifurcated graft can be cut so that the limbs either sit side by side or on top of one another. Choice of graft orientation is based on patient anatomy. If a single antegrade bypass is done, the bifurcated graft is cut leaving a small part of the graft body as a flange. This allows the graft to sit off the aorta so there is no flattening of the heel which can cause stenosis or graft failure. This is why we rarely use saphenous vein as a conduit from the supraceliac aorta unless a pantaloon configuration is used. We avoid graft limbs less than 7-mm diameter because the pseudointima that forms within smaller diameter limbs has led to failures in our experience. The aortic anastomosis is tested, once completed, by infusing saline into the graft limbs with clamps still in place. If hemostatic, blood flow is slowly restored through the native aorta after back-bleeding and fore-bleeding through the limbs has been done. The limbs are clamped at their origins. If ischemia time exceeds 20 minutes during complete aortic cross-clamp, additional mannitol and Lasix are given to stimulate urine output.[4]

The distal anastomosis to the celiac artery is done end-to-end or end-to-side. For the latter, ligation of the artery immediately proximal to the heel creates a functional end-to-end anastomosis (Figure 32-3B). If the celiac is occluded, diffusely stenotic, or calcified, the target artery is the common hepatic with the anastomosis done end-to-side. An end-to-end anastomosis to the celiac is challenging for two reasons. First, there is a tendency to cut the graft too long so that it buckles and kinks when retraction is released. Second, the artery can be fragile, and if the graft is too taught, the artery will tear. An end-to-side celiac anastomosis makes it easier to gauge graft length in the authors' opinions. Back-bleeding is allowed prior to completion of the anastomosis. Fore-bleeding is done through the SMA graft limb, after which the limb is irrigated and suctioned to be sure it is clean. A clamp is placed at the origin of that limb, the clamp on the celiac limb is released, and blood flow established into the celiac branches.[4]

A ringed forceps is placed on the distal plasma tubing which had been passed through the retropancreatic tunnel (Figure 32-3C). With an assistant gently lifting up on the transverse colon, the tubing is gently pulled cranially and the clamp guided through the tunnel. The SMA graft limb is grasped, brought through the tunnel, straightened and secured with a clamp at the base of the transverse mesocolon in an infracolic position (Figure 32-3D). This maneuver fixes graft length and keeps blood or debris from collecting inside the graft during the distal anastomosis. The retractors on the liver and intestine are released, and exposure reset for the SMA anastomosis. The SMA is opened vertically on its left lateral or anterolateral side. The graft is cut to length after retraction on the small bowel is relaxed. The anastomosis is done end-to-side (Figure 32-3D). Backbleeding is allowed, the anastomosis is completed and blood flow established through the graft into the SMA. Some patients require a focal endarterectomy of the SMA as part of the reconstruction. If needed, we close the arteriotomy with a patch, which makes for an easier graft anastomosis.[4]

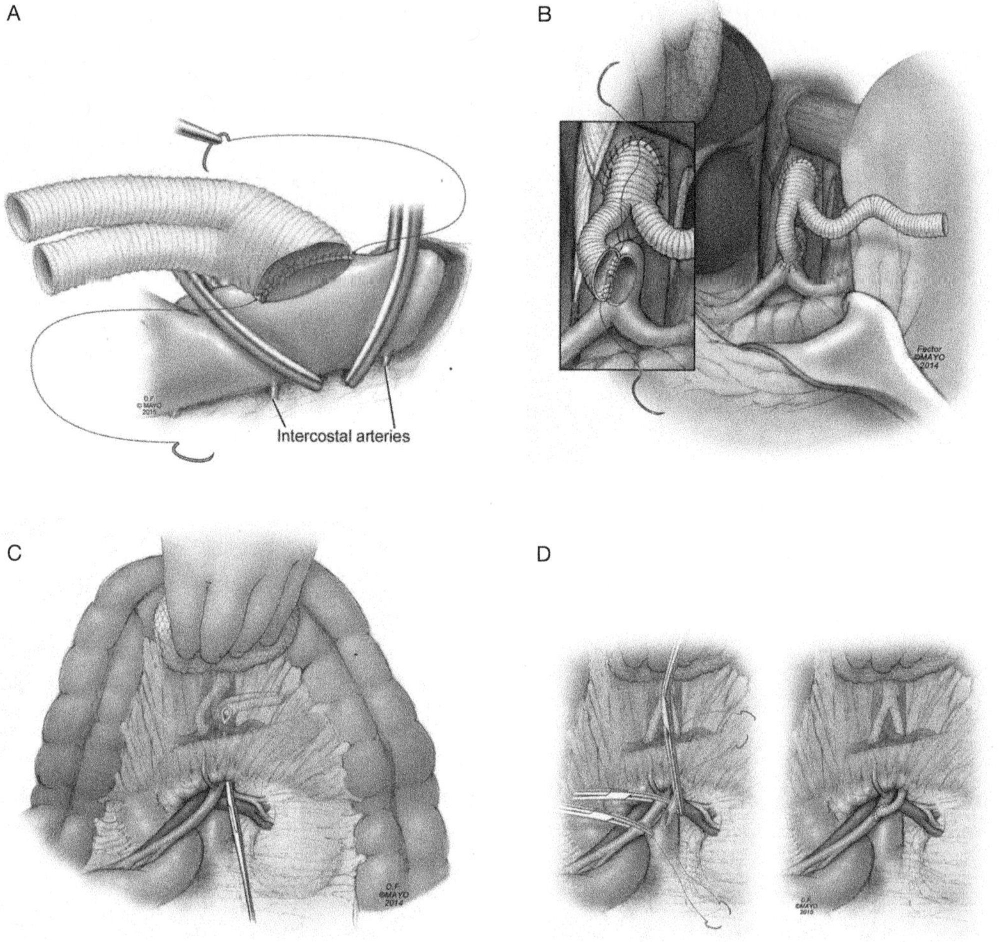

Figure 32-3. The steps of an antegrade bypass to the celiac artery and SMA are shown. The aortic anastomosis is done with a partial occlusion clamp or a two clamp technique as in (A). The limbs of the bifurcated graft can be oriented one on top of the other, or side by side. The celiac anastomosis is easier done end-to-side than end-to-end because it is simpler to cut the graft limb the appropriate length (B). Alternatively, this limb can be sewn to the common hepatic artery (not shown). The SMA limb is passed through a retropancreatic tunnel and fixed at the base of the mesocolon with a straight clamp (C, D). The SMA anastomosis is performed end-to-side for most patients (D).

Retrograde bypass can be done with prosthetic or vein with revascularization of the SMA alone, or the SMA and common hepatic.[4,7,9] If two vessels are reconstructed, which is done rarely, we do a side-to-side anastomosis to the SMA, and carry the graft behind or on top of the pancreas with a gentle curve and perform an end-to-side anastomosis to the common hepatic. Choice of conduit is based on size of the target artery and saphenous vein; and the course of the graft to the common hepatic is dictated by patient anatomy so that the graft does not kink. Our group prefers the common iliac artery for inflow, more often the right one because a bypass graft to the SMA lies better (Figure 32-4).[4,9] If the common iliacs are circumferentially calcified, an external iliac artery is used for inflow. A 7- or 8-mm polyester graft is chosen and is either sewn directly to the SMA or configured in a C-shape as popularized by the Oregon Health

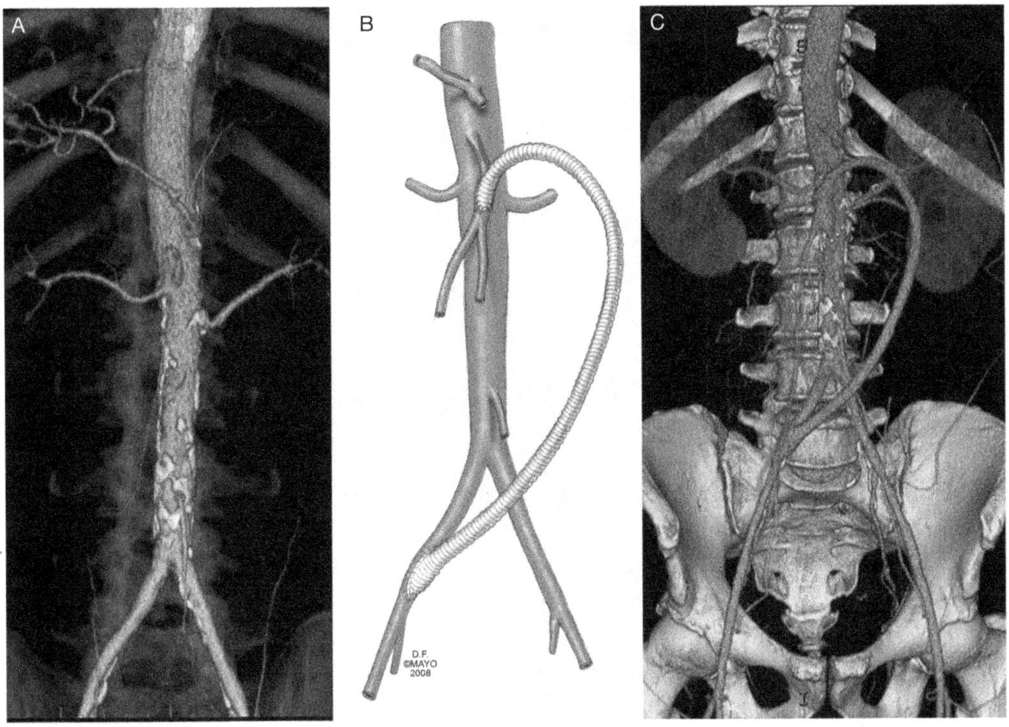

Figure 32-4. Example of a retrograde prosthetic bypass to the SMA, taken from the right common iliac artery in a high risk patient with infrarenal aortic calcification on CT angiography (A, B). The configuration often is done with the graft in a C-shape to allow antegrade blood flow vis-a vis the SMA. The postoperative CTA shows a widely patent graft.

Sciences University group.[7] For a direct ilio-SMA bypass, the iliac artery anastomosis is done first. If a C-shape is chosen, either the iliac or SMA anastomosis can be done first based on surgeon preference. The authors often sew the graft to the SMA first, let the bowel relax, fill the graft with saline, and lay the graft in a C-shape to be confident that there is no redundancy in the graft when it is cut to length and sewn to the iliac.[4,9] Use of the infrarenal aorta for inflow is hampered by buckling of the graft from redundancy that occurs after the small bowel is returned to its normal position. One solution is to perform a short 1.5 cm to 2 cm stove-pipe bypass graft between the aorta and SMA (Figure 32-5).[4,9] The SMA anastomotic site is chosen and the graft sewn to the posterior or left posterolateral side of the artery. Retraction on the mesentery and bowel is relaxed and the aorta is marked where the graft wants to sit. The infrarenal aorta is fully or partially cross-clamped and opened vertically or with a 6-mm coronary punch. The graft is cut short and beveled according to whether there will be a slight retrograde or antegrade position of it. The anastomosis begins by placing a running polypropylene suture in the center of the right side of the aortotomy and graft. A parachute technique is used for this side, and the suture tied on each end to another corner suture after the bowel is relaxed. The left side of the anastomosis is completed by sewing the new suture on each end toward the center. At times, the anastomosis is done with a combination of running and interrupted suture.

Transaortic visceral artery endarterectomy requires full aortic clamping after administration of intravenous heparin and mannitol; and occlusion of the celiac,

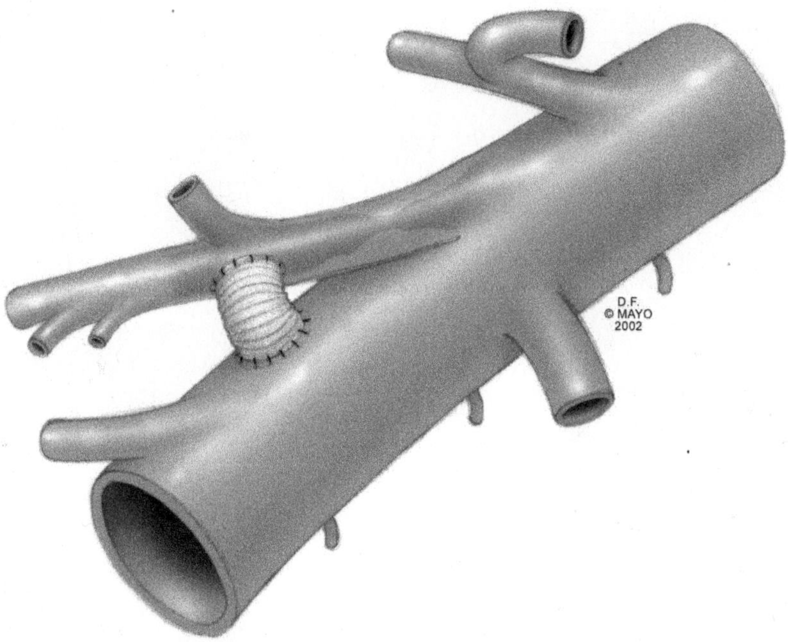

Figure 32-5. Schematic representation of a short stove-pipe graft to the SMA from the infrarenal aorta. This configuration obviates kinking of the graft, the bane of other infrarenal aortic-based grafts. It is a rarely used but good technique to know.

SMA and sometimes the left renal artery with atraumatic clamps or large vessel loops (Figure 32-6).[4,9] Lumbar arteries are controlled with small vessel loops or bull dog clamps. A curvilinear trapdoor aortotomy is made around the visceral arteries from above the celiac to below the SMA. An endarterectomy plane is developed with a freer, and the aortic plaque is circumferentially freed around the orifices of the SMA and celiac. An eversion technique is used to remove the plaque from each artery. Sometimes it is better to create separate buttons of plaque around each visceral artery to facilitate ease of eversion rather than try to remove the endarterectomy specimen as one piece. The distal endpoint in the aorta can be secured as necessary, and the aortotomy closed with running 4-0 polypropylene suture. Backbleeding and fore-bleeding are allowed prior to removal of the aortic clamps. If concomitant renal endarterectomy also is planned, the aortotomy is carried distally on the anterior wall beyond the renal artery origins and an eversion technique is used to remove the occlusive plaque from them. If aortic replacement is necessary, a padded clamp is placed in an infrarenal position once the aortotomy closure goes distal to the renal artery origins. Diuresis is induced with Lasix and mannitol after the cross clamp period. Endarterectomy can be done for lesions that extend 2 cm or more into the artery. However, the surgeon must be prepared to do a completion endarterectomy of any residual plaque if it all cannot be removed from inside the aorta. This is accomplished by making a transverse or longitudinal arteriotomy in the visceral artery and closing the artery primarily or with a patch.

Completion intraoperative duplex ultrasound imaging is routinely done in our practice after any mesenteric or renal reconstruction to assess technical outcome and blood flow velocities. It is important to let the bowel return to normal position to alleviate stretch on the celiac and SMA which otherwise can cause falsely high elevation

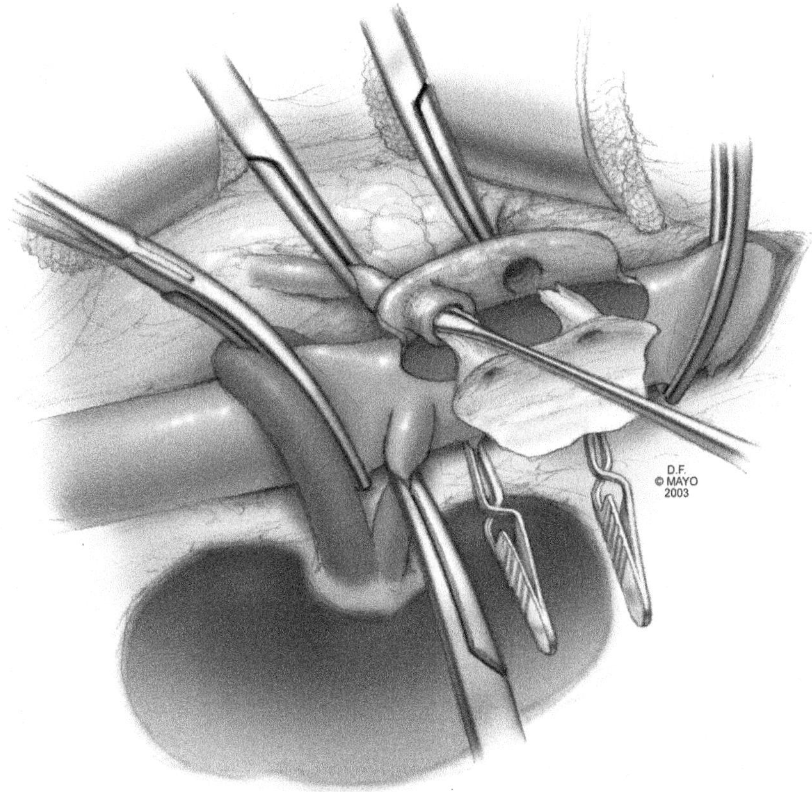

Figure 32-6. Transaortic visceral endarterectomy is done though a retroperitoneal exposure of the aorta using a left medial visceral rotation. The left kidney often is kept down as shown. The supraceliac and juxtarenal aorta have to be isolated over enough length to allow for a trapdoor aortotomy and good visualization.

in flow velocities. Identification and immediate correction of technical defects in the operating room lowers early bypass graft failure or arterial thrombosis.[22]

OUTCOMES

Outcome measures for open surgical and endovascular treatment of CMI include mortality and morbidity, symptom relief, and freedom from restenosis, symptom recurrence and re-intervention. Reporting standards, stratification of patient risk and methods to compare anatomic severity of disease must be created in order to compare effectiveness of open and endovascular treatments.[1,5,17] Interpretation of data and comparison of outcomes between published reports remains difficult because studies mix patients with acute and chronic presentations, include median arcuate ligament syndrome in the analysis, and cover long periods of time.[1] Furthermore, definition of technical success varies, and analyses lack objective determinants of both patency and data regarding symptom recurrence, restenosis and re-intervention.

Patient outcome after open mesenteric artery reconstruction depends on many factors.[1,17] Anatomy, patient comorbid conditions, surgeon experience, and perioperative management impact choice of reconstruction and the risk of patient death or major adverse events. The extent of atherosclerosis in the visceral arteries, target artery size, aortic aneurysm or symptomatic aorto-iliac occlusive disease, and calcification of the supraceliac aorta or iliac arteries must be considered in operative planning. Moreover, old patients, those with cardiopulmonary, liver or renal dysfunction, and individuals with malnutrition or inanition are factors which affect outcome. The more those conditions are present, the higher the operative risk. The Mayo Clinic group reported risk-stratified outcomes in 229 patients with CMI treated by open or endovascular procedures using the Society for Vascular Surgery comorbidity scoring system.[1] Each patient was deemed high or low risk. While the overall mortality was similar between the open (2.7%) and endovascular (2.4%) groups, peri-operative mortality was only 1% for low-risk but 6.7% for high-risk patients treated by open bypass. Operative mortality correlated with the number of high risk criteria present. For instance, patients with no high risk factors had a 30 day operative mortality of 0.7%. This contrasts to mortality rates of 3.1% with one high risk criterion, and at least 25% with four criteria present. Concomitant aortic reconstruction imparted an 8.9% mortality, which corroborated our previous observations.[6,12] Therefore, we believe aortic replacement should be done only if it is absolutely needed for inflow, and the mesenteric revascularization be the sole focus of operation and tailored to what the anatomy and patient risk allow. In contrast to prior years, patients with diffuse aortoiliac disease precluding inflow can now be offered hybrid retrograde mesenteric revascularization.[5,9] Importantly, not every patient needs complete revascularization or a supra-celiac aortic based bypass.

Surgeon experience matters, as does good intraoperative anesthetic management and perioperative critical care. While low mortality rates are achieved at high-volume centers where the operations are done by high-volume surgeons, mortality as high as 13%–20% is reported in lower volume community hospitals.[5,16,19] Isolated open surgical bypass can be done with low mortality in good risk patients operated by experienced surgeons, and even for redo open reconstruction.[1,6,10,12–15,18,23] Operative planning, execution and attention to technical and postoperative care detail are keys to successful outcome. Outcomes based on single-center reports and a systematic review is shown in Table 32-1.

Surgeons should anticipate fluid shifts during the first 48 postoperative hours because of the loss of mesenteric arteriolar autoregulation. Some patients with subacute on chronic mesenteric ischemia develop a systemic inflammatory response which may not only require fluid support, but the use of intravenous pressors to maintain adequate perfusion pressures. Pressors which cause splanchnic vasoconstriction should be used with caution. Close monitoring of the intravascular volume, cardiac function, and acid-base status are imperative, and may best be done in an intensive care unit.[9,17] The risk of perioperative complications can be high, and ranges between 20% to 40%.[1,6,9–10,12–18] The Mayo Clinic group had an overall complication rate of 36%.[1] The most common problems are pulmonary (15%), gastrointestinal (14%), cardiac (10%) and renal (4%). Prolonged ileus occurs in 8% of patients. Peri-operative graft occlusion and intestinal ischemia occur rarely (<2%) if the intraoperative ultrasound imaging showed a widely patent reconstruction.[22] However, this complication can be catastrophic and lead to patient death. Early signs of these problems include an increase in fluid volume requirements and a drop in urine output, thrombocytopenia and/or leukocytosis, a narrowing of the A-aO2 gradient and/or pulse pressure, and metabolic acidosis which may be subtle at first.[17] Such signs should prompt CT angiography in our opinion. Ultrasound imaging of the bypass graft also is an option,

TABLE 32-1. SELECT SERIES OF PATIENT OUTCOME AFTER MESENTERIC ARTERY REVASCULARIZATION

Author (Year)	*n*	Vessels	Mortality	Morbidity	Recurrence	Re-intervention	Primary Patency	Follow-up
					%			Months
Leke (2002)	17	25	6	41	0	0	100 at 34 months	34
Cho (2002)	25	41	4	–	32	20	57 at 5 years	64
Kruger (2007)	39	67	2.5	12	5	3	92 at 5 years	39
Mell (2008)	80	120	3.8	26	11	11	90	46
Oderich (2009)	146	265	2.7	36	6	5	88 at 5 years	36
Low risk	101	–	0.9	37	6	6	94 at 5 years	–
High risk	45	–	6.7	38	11	11	90 at 5 years	–
Concomitant aortic reconstruction	23	–	8.4	–	–	–	–	–
Ryer (2012)	116	203	2.5	50	14	16	86 at 5 years	43
Total	339	721	3.6	33	11.3	9.2	–	44

but visualization may be hampered by bowel gas. In addition to a technical problem, which is the most common cause of early graft occlusion, a hypercoagulable state may contribute to early graft failure.[3] Monitoring platelet counts to detect heparin-induced thrombocytopenia, or checking a serum hypercoagulable profile are considerations if the clinical index of suspicion for these problems is high.[1,9] Wound-related complications range between 4% and 8%.[9] Ascites may occur postoperatively in patients with subacute on chronic ischemia because the bowel weeps so much fluid and these patients are often hypoproteinemic. Rarely does the ascites cause an abdominal compartment syndrome in this patient subgroup.[1,9]

Intravenous nutrition with vitamins and trace elements is given to patients who are malnourished until bowel function allows for oral intake.[1,3] We avoid preoperative central parenteral nutrition for days or weeks prior to operation because there is a risk of clinical deterioration and catheter-related complications.[3] Some patients experience diarrhea for several weeks after hospital dismissal, and on occasion, this problem is recalcitrant to treatment. In these cases, patient weight and volume status should be closely monitored as an outpatient. Hospital stay and recovery time are longer after open operations by comparison to patients treated by endovascular therapy.[1,3] Length of stay averages 14 days with open surgery and 3 days after endovascular treatment.[21] Postoperative care should include smoking cessation, cholesterol-lowering agents, particularly a statin, and an anti-platelet medication which often is aspirin. Duplex ultrasound surveillance imaging is done at 6 month intervals the first year or two, then annually.[9]

SYMPTOM RELIEF AND RECURRENCE, AND RE-INTERVENTION

Open revascularization provides better symptom relief and durability than endovascular therapy. Symptom improvement averaged 93% with open bypass and 88% with endovascular revascularization in one systematic review.[20] In addition, most single center series show higher patency, lower rate of restenosis, better freedom from recurrent symptoms and fewer re-interventions for open reconstruction compared to mesenteric angioplasty and stenting. In a Mayo Clinic report, patients treated by endovascular therapy were five times more likely to develop stenosis in the treated artery, seven times more likely to have recurrent symptoms, and needed re-intervention four times more often than patients who had open surgical revascularization.[1] Primary patency following open bypass averaged 89% at 5 years in a recent review of the pooled literature (57% to 92%), and freedom from re-intervention was 93%.[19] Antegrade and retrograde bypass have similar patency rates in some series.[1,7] Although endovascular therapy is first-line treatment at most centers because of its low mortality and morbidity, and short hospital stay, the systematic review by van Petersen et al.,[21] showed open bypass to have better primary (86% versus 51%) and secondary patency rates (87% versus 83%), lower restenosis (15% versus 37%), less symptom recurrence (13% versus 30%) and fewer re-interventions (9% versus 20%). A contemporary report from Ryer et al.,[15] found open bypass to be increasingly performed in high risk patients with worse anatomy compared to those treated with endovascular therapies. Open surgery had a respectable 76% five-year primary patency rate despite the need for more difficult reconstructions. One theoretic advantage of two vessel revascularization is that occlusion of one graft limb does not always cause recurrent symptoms or require re-intervention.[1,6]

Reoperation for Failed Open Mesenteric Reconstructions

Redo open reconstruction for symptomatic patients with a failed bypass pose challenges. Reoperation is technically more difficult because of bowel adhesions and periarterial scar tissue. The atherosclerotic disease in the target artery may be more extensive, requiring dissection further along the SMA. Important intestinal arterial collaterals are at risk of injury during exposure of the artery. Moreover, patients with chronic graft occlusions or graft occlusion causing acute mesenteric ischemia are not candidates for endovascular intervention.[17] Retrograde stenting or an iliac artery-based bypass is an option to be considered in these patients.[3,7,9] Giswold and colleagues reported an operative mortality rate of 6% among 22 patients who needed redo mesenteric revascularization.[23] Primary patency at 4 years was 62%. In the patient where inflow cannot be obtained from the abdominal aorta or iliac arteries, mesenteric bypass has been done using the thoracic aorta for its origin.[17,24]

PATIENT SURVIVAL

Long-term patient survival after mesenteric revascularization is influenced by advanced age and poor preoperative cardiac, pulmonary or renal function.[1] Survival impact based on whether a patient has open bypass or a mesenteric stent is affected by selection bias, because open bypass is typically done for good risk patients and stenting for higher risk ones.[17] The Mayo Clinic group[25] analyzed long-term survival among a cohort of 343 patients with CMI, using propensity matched scores. Nearly identical 5-year survival rates were found for patients treated by open (57%) or endovascular techniques (60%). Five-year patient survival was affected by patient comorbidity and risk score, and averaged 71 ± 4% for low-risk, 49 ± 6% for intermediate-risk, and 38 ± 7% for high-risk patients. Open bypass and endovascular treatment had similar 5-year freedom from mesenteric-related death, being 91 ± 2% after open surgery and 93 ± 4% after endovascular revascularization. Age over 80 years (OR 3.3, CI 1.03–1.06, P = <0.001), stage IV or V chronic kidney disease (OR 5.5, CI 1.4–16.6, $P < 0.01$), diabetes (OR 1.7, CI 1.2–2.6, $P < 0.01$) and home oxygen therapy (OR 3.7, CI 1.2–9.1, $P < 0.001$) were independent markers of all-cause mortality. Mesenteric-related death was independently impacted by Stage IV or V chronic kidney disease (OR 3.4, CI 3.3–345, $P = 0.003$) and diabetes (OR 4.2, CI 1.7–10.5, $P = 0.005$). The most common causes of late death were cardiac events, followed by cancer, respiratory problems and mesenteric-related complications. The combined early and late mesenteric-related death rate was 8% for patients treated by open bypass and 6% for those with endovascular intervention.[17,25]

SUMMARY

Our management of patients with CMI has evolved over the years. Open mesenteric revascularization continues to play an important role in the endovascular era. Surgical bypass or endarterectomy is applicable to patients with unfavorable anatomy for endovascular treatment. Low-risk patients with flush or long segment occlusions or stenosis, heavily calcified lesions or atheromatous debris seem better suited for open repair. Moreover, young patients or women with small vessels may also be better candidates for open repair. Our preference is to bypass the celiac artery and SMA from the supraceliac aorta, though a single bypass to the SMA works well whether done antegrade or retrograde. Data show that mesenteric bypass performed by experienced surgeons carries a comparable mortality rate to endovascular treatment, even for reoperation. Surgical treatment should focus on mesenteric artery revascularization as the primary goal, and not be combined with aortic replacement because of the higher mortality with the latter.

REFERENCES

1. Oderich GS, Bower TC, Sullivan TM, et al. Open versus endovascular revascularization for chronic mesenteric ischemia: risk-stratified outcomes. *J Vasc Surg*. 2009;49:1472–9.
2. AbuRahma AF, Campbell JE, Stone PA, et al. Perioperative and late clinical outcomes of percutaneous transluminal stentings of the celiac and superior mesenteric arteries over the past decade. *J Vasc Surg*. 2013;57:1052–61.
3. Oderich GS, Erdoes LS, LeSar C, et al. Comparison of covered stents versus bare metal stents for treatment of chronic atherosclerotic mesenteric arterial disease. *J Vasc Surg*. 2013;58:1316–24.

4. Bower TC. Techniques of open mesenteric reconstructions. In: Oderich GS, *Mesenteric vascular disease: Current therapy*. Springer, New York, 2015:145–56.
5. Oderich GS. Mesenteric vascular disease: Chronic ischemia. In: Shermerhorn, Marc. Es. 8th Edition of Rutherford's Textbook of Vascular Surgery. Elsevier, 2013:2373–97.
6. McAfee MK, Cherry KJ, Naessens JM, et al. Influence of complete revascularization on chronic mesenteric ischemia. *Am J Surg*. 1992;164:220–4.
7. Foley JI, Moneta GL, Abou-Zamsam AM, et al. Revascularization of the superior mesenteric artery alone for treatment of intestinal ischemia. *J Vasc Surg*. 2000;32:37–47.
8. De Martino RR. Normal and variant mesenteric anatomy. In: Oderich GS, *Mesenteric vascular disease: Current therapy*. Springer, New York, 2015:9–23.
9. Bower TC, Oderich GS. Acute and chronic mesenteric ischemia. In: Hallett JW Jr., Mills JL Sr., Earnshaw JJ, Reekers JA, Rooke TW. *Comprehensive Vascular and Endovascular Surgery*. 2nd Ed. Mosby Elsevier, 2009 p.339–50.
10. Leke MA, Hood DB, Rowe VL, et al. Technical consideration in the management of chronic mesenteric ischemia. *Am Surg*. 2002;68(12):1088–92.
11. Oderich GS, Gloviczki P, Bower TC. Open surgical treatment for chronic mesenteric ischemia in the endovascular era: when it is necessary and what is the preferred technique? *Semin Vasc Surg*. 2010;23(1):36–6.
12. Park WM, Cherry KJ Jr, Chua HK, et al. Current results of open revascularization for chronic mesenteric ischemia: a standard for comparison. *J Vasc Surg*. 2002;35(5):853–9.
13. Cho JS, Carr JA, Jacobsen G, et al. Long-term outcome after mesenteric artery reconstruction: a 37-year experience. *J Vasc Surg*. 2002;35(3):453–60.
14. Kruger AJ, Walker PJ, Foster WJ, et al. Open surgery for chronic atherosclerosis mesenteric ischemia. *J Vasc Surg*. 2007;46:941–45.
15. Ryer EJ, Oderich GS, Bower TC, et al. Differences in anatomy and outcomes in patients treated with open mesenteric revascularization before and after the endovascular era. *J Vasc Surg*. 2011;53:1611–8.
16. Schermerhorn ML, Giles KA, Hamdan AD, et al. Mesenteric revascularization: management and outcomes in the United States, 1988–2006. *J Vasc Surg*. 2009;50:341–8.
17. Bower TC. Results of open mesenteric reconstructions. In: Oderich GS, *Mesenteric vascular disease: Current therapy*. Springer, New York, 2015:157–64.
18. Mell MW, Acher CW, Hoch JR, et al. Outcomes after endarterectomy for chronic mesenteric ischemia. *J Vasc Surg*. 2008;48:1132–8.
19. Oderich GS, Malgor R, Ricotta JJ Jr. Open and endovascular revascularization for chronic mesenteric ischemia: a tabular review of the literature. *Ann Vasc Surg*. 2009; 23(5):700–12.
20. Gupta PK, Horan SM, Turaga KK, et al. Chronic mesenteric ischemia: endovascular versus open revascularization. *J Endovasc Ther*. 2010;17:540–549.
21. van Petersen AS, Kolkman JJ, Beuk RJ, et al. Open or percutaneous revascularization for chronic splanchnic syndrome. *J Vasc Surg*. 2010;51:1309–16.
22. Oderich GS, Panneton JM, Macedo TA, et al. Intraoperative duplex ultrasound of visceral revascularizations: optimizing technical success and outcomes. *J Vasc Surg*. 2003;38:684–91.
23. Giswold ME, Landry GJ, Taylor LM, et al. Outcomes after redo procedures for failed mesenteric revascularization. *Vasc Endovas Surg*. 2004;38:315–9.
24. Farber MA, Carlin RE; Marston WA, et al. Distal thoracic aorta as inflow for the treatment of chronic mesenteric ischemia. *J Vasc Surg*. 2001;33:281–7; Discussion: 287–8.
25. Tallarita T, Oderich GS, Gloviczki P, et al. Patient survival after open and endovascular mesenteric revascularization for chronic mesenteric ischemia. *J Vasc Surg*. 2013;57:747–55.

33

Inferior Pancreaticoduodenal Artery Aneurysms

Julia Glaser, MD and Ronald Fairman, MD

Inferior pancreaticoduodenal artery aneurysms (IPDAA) are a rare subset of visceral artery aneurysms. They comprise an estimated 2% of visceral artery aneurysms[1] and 0.1%–0.2% of all aneurysms discovered at autopsy.[2] As they are rare, their optimal management is the subject of numerous case reports, and increasingly, case series.

ETIOLOGY AND ASSOCIATION WITH CELIAC STENOSIS

True IPDAA can be associated with a number of systemic conditions. Fibromuscular dysplasia, arteritis, and atherosclerosis have all been associated with their development.[3–5] An association with celiac axis stenosis or occlusion was first described by Sutton and Lawson 1973[6] and has since been the subject of numerous case reports and small series.[7–10] One study estimated that 61% of patients with an IPDAA have a celiac axis stenosis or occlusion.[11] Furthermore, rapid development and rupture of an IPDAA has been described in the setting of a type B dissection involving the celiac origin.[12] Theoretically, a celiac stenosis or occlusion produces an increase in flow through the collaterals between the SMA and celiac axis, including the inferior pancreaticoduodenal arteries; this increase in flow may lead to changes within the arterial wall that predispose to aneurysm formation. Interestingly, despite their association with celiac axis stenosis or occlusion, IPDAA may not recur if they are treated without treating the celiac axis disease.[13]

Consensus about management of IPDAA is confounded by the fact that many series include both true and pseudoaneurysms as one entity. Pseudoaneurysms are associated with a history of trauma, infection, instrumentation or surgery, and pancreatitis.[14] Pancreatitis is known to be associated with the formation of pseudodaneurysms; an estimated 30%–40% of all aneurysms found in the pancreactioduodenal arteries (PDA) are associated with pancreatitis.[15] Furthermore, 10% of patients with chronic pancreatitis have PDA aneurysms. It is not clear that the management of the two should be similar, and here we primarily discuss the management of true IPDAA.

PRESENTATION

The presentation of IPDAA is variable. Due to the small sizes of case series within the literature, the published rates of various presentations also varies (Table 33-1). Between 50% and 64% of IPDAA present following rupture.[3,16] True IPDAA tend to rupture into the retroperitoneum, whereas pseudoaneurysms tend to rupture into the GI tract.[17] Rupture into the biliary pancreatic ducts has also been described.[13] Their presentation prior to rupture is protean, and symptoms can include nausea, vomiting, abdominal fullness, and as an abdominal mass.[17,18] Reports exist of their presentation as a hematoma mimicking pancreatic cancer.[19] The most common presenting symptom is abdominal pain, seen as the sole symptom in 29% of patients;[17] this pain may mimic mesenteric ischemia as well as biliary or pancreatic disease.[13] Following rupture, patients can present with stable vital signs due to tamponade of the bleeding within the retroperitoneum; an estimated 73% are stable at the time of presentation.[1] Figure 33-1 illustrates a patient who presented to our institution with chronic right upper quadrant pain who was found to have a 5-cm IPDAA.

RISK OF RUPTURE

Given their scarcity as well as variable etiology, the overall risk of rupture has not been quantified for IPDAA. Reports of rupture at various sizes, both large and small, exist.[4,5] Overall, the risk of rupture does not correlate with size (Figure 33-2).[11,17] Mortality for those who present with rupture is estimated to be 21-65%, with most studies reporting rates between 49 and 65%.[1,11]

MANAGEMENT—OBSERVATION

Conservative management of IPDAA can include observation alone, or simply addressing the celiac axis stenosis. Reports exist of spontaneous IPDAA regression with correction of the celiac stenosis, either with median arcuate ligament release[20] or

TABLE 33-1. IPDAA: RATES OF SYMPTOMS AT PRESENTATION

Symptom at Presentation[a]	Percent
Abdominal pain	29
Abdominal pain and shock	18
Abdominal pain and GI bleeding	15
Bilary colic	10
Abdominal pain and jaundice	7
Hematemesis	7
Hematochezia	7
Incidental finding	3
Anemia	3

[a]Symptoms at presentation of IPDAA. Adapted from Coll et al. *Annals of Vascular Surgery*. 1998;12:286-91.

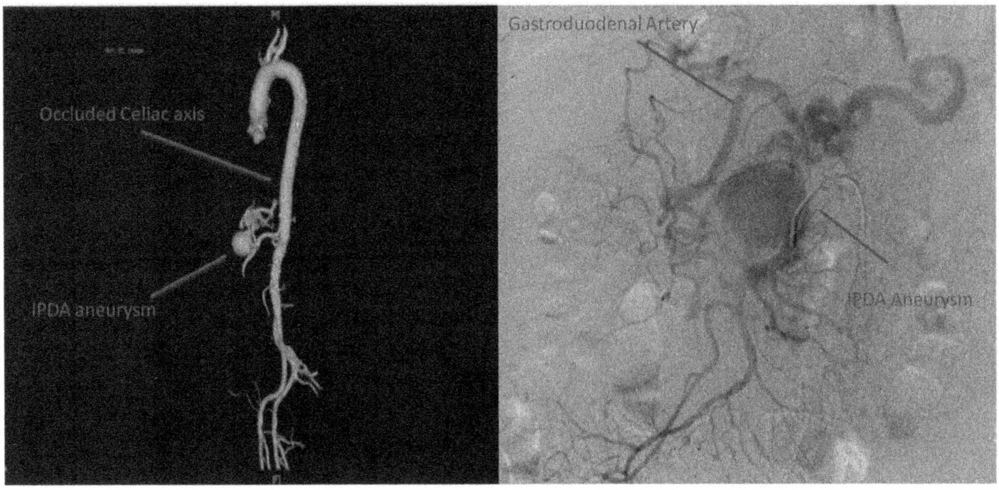

Figure 33-1. A 72-year-old male with a history of obesity, hypertension, diabetes, and alcoholism presented to our institution with abdominal pain. He was found to have a 5-cm aneurysm arising from a branch of the SMA on CT scan (top). Selective angiography confirmed that this was an IPDAA and that he had an associated occlusion of the celiac axis. Because of the large size of the aneurysm and its proximity to the SMA, he was treated with a hepato-renal bypass rather than embolization.

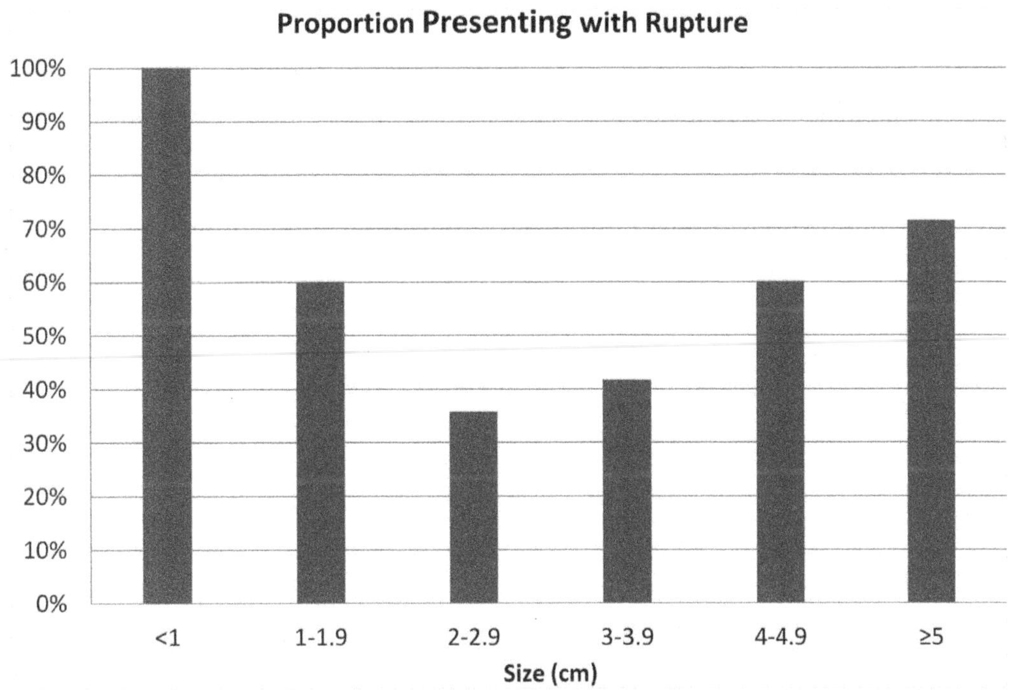

Figure 33-2. Risk of rupture as related to aneurysm size in peri-pancreatic arterial aneurysms (GDA and PDA). Adapted from Moore et al., *Journal of Vascular Surgery*. 2004;40:247–53.

bypass of a celiac artery stenosis.[21] Given the mortality associated with rupture as well as the lack of factors that predict rupture, conservative management involving either treating the celiac stenosis alone or simple observation is risky.

MANAGEMENT—ENDOVASCULAR REPAIR

Selected IPDAA may be amenable to endovascular repair. Certainly, angiography should be performed whenever possible to identify the vascular anatomy and identify the sources of collateral flow. In any repair, decreasing the risk of ischemia to organs fed by the celiac axis is vital. We advocate limiting endovascular repair to aneurysms that are small with a narrow neck that arise from adequate caliber vessels with minimal tortuosity. Those that arise from the predominant source of collateral flow to the celiac axis are less suitable for endovascular repair, due to the risk of ischemia from inadvertent embolization.

Endovascular techniques used to address IPDAA vary. Coils have been used successfully,[12,22,23] as well as stents.[22,23] N-butyl cyanoacrylate, which is often used in cerebral aneurysms, has also been described as used for IPDAA as well as other visceral aneurysms.[24] Endovascular techniques have been successful in both elective cases, as well as rupture.[14] Follow-up is variable in the literature. Although the rate of complications reported is generally low, there are reports of devastating consequences such as the occlusion of the right hepatic artery following embolization of an IPDAA.[11]

MANAGEMENT—OPEN REPAIR

Open surgical repair remains the gold standard of treatment. Various approaches have been described, including resection and exclusion with bypass (aorto-hepatic,[5] aorto-gastroduodenal,[25] and reno-hepatic[8]), placement of an interposition graft, and aneurysmorrhapy. Pancreaticoduodenectomy has been performed rarely in unstable patients.[4]

SELECTION OF MANAGEMENT STRATEGY

As endovascular techniques have become more advanced, it follows that more IPDAA may be suitable for endovascular repair; however, more complex endovascular techniques may also be accompanied by more complications. A widely-cited series by Coll reports a 20% mortality rate for open repair and 0% for endovascular techniques in all reported cases between 1980 and 1995.[17] While the series is excellent, it contains only 82 patients and may not reflect how rates of mortality and success have changed as endovascular techniques have advanced.

We recommend a treatment strategy as illustrated in Figure 33-3. In all patients, an attempt to stabilize them enough to undergo angiography for further characterization of the anatomy should be pursued. Based on the angiographic results, IPDAA will be suitable for either embolization or surgery. In patients who present with unstable, ruptured IPDAA and cannot be resuscitated, emergent open repair should be performed.

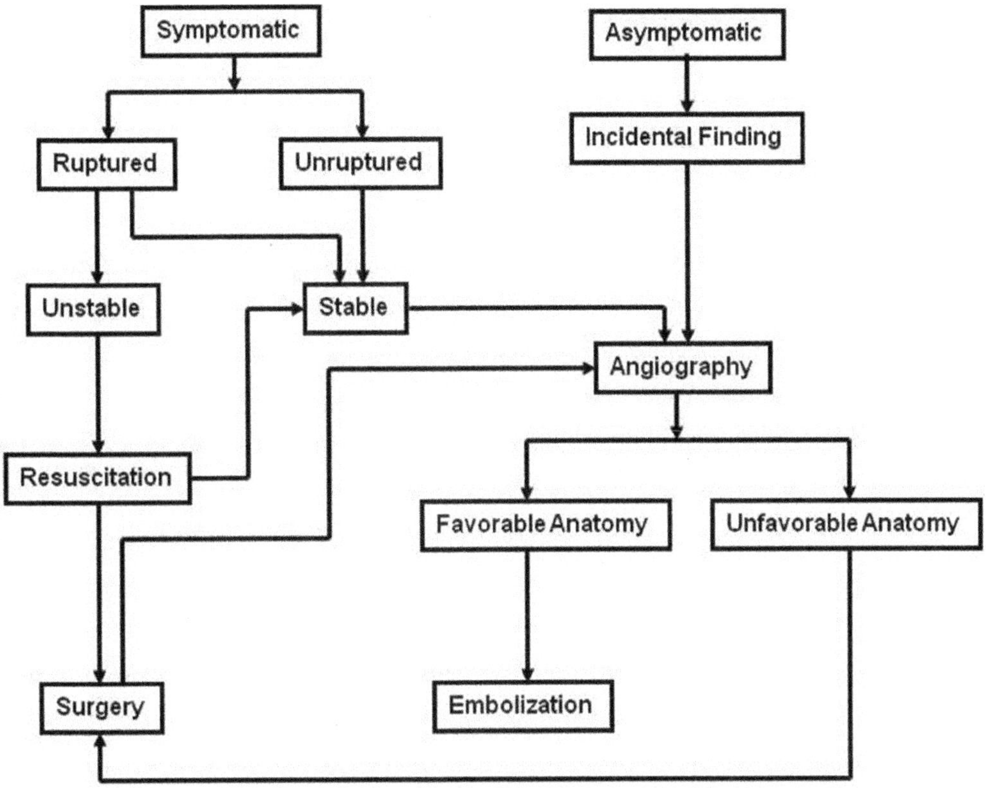

Figure 33-3. We recommend a treatment strategy that incorporates both angiography and open surgery depending on the stability of the patient as well as the anatomy of the aneurysm.

REFERENCES

1. Neschis DG, Safford SD, Golden MA. Management of pancreaticoduodenal artery aneurysms presenting as catastrophic intraabdominal bleeding. *Surgery.* 1998;123:8–12.
2. Ikeda O, Tamura Y, Nakasone Y, et al. Nonoperative management of unruptured visceral artery aneurysms: Treatment by transcatheter coil embolization. *J Vasc Surg.* 2008; 47(6):1212–9. doi:10.1016/j.jvs.2008.01.032.
3. Paty PS, Cordero JA Jr, Darling RC 3rd, et al. Aneurysms of the pancreaticoduodenal artery. *J Vasc Surg.* 1996; 23(4):710–3. doi:10.1016/S0741-5214(96)80054-1.
4. De Perrot M, Buhler L, Deleaval J, et al. Management of true aneurysms of the splenic artery. *Am J Surg.* 1998: 175(6):466–8. doi:10.1016/S0002-9610(98)00082-8.
5. Bageacu S, Cuilleron M, Kaczmarek D, Porcheron J. True aneurysms of the pancreaticoduodenal artery: Successful non-operative management. *Surgery.* 2006: 139(5):608–16. doi:10.1016/j.surg.2005.10.015.
6. Sutton D, Lawton G. Coeliac stenosis or occlusion with aneurysm of the collateral supply. *Clin Radiol.* 1973;24:49–53.
7. Suzuki K, Tachi Y, Ito S, et al. Endovascular management of ruptured pancreaticoduodenal artery aneurysms associated with celiac axis stenosis. *Cardiovasc Intervent Radiol.* 2008; 31(6):1082–7. doi:10.1007/s00270-008-9343-3.
8. Bowens NM, Woo EY, Fairman RM. Reno-hepatic artery bypass for an inferior pancreaticoduodenal artery aneurysm with associated celiac occlusion. *J Vasc Surg.* 2011;53(6):1696–8. doi:10.1016/j.jvs.2011.02.022

9. Ikeda O, Tamura Y, Nakasone Y, et al. Coil embolization of pancreaticoduodenal artery aneurysms associated with celiac artery stenosis: report of three cases. *Cardiovasc Intervent Radiol.* 2007;30(3):504–7. doi:10.1007/s00270-006-0083-y
10. Sugiyama K, Takehara Y. Analysis of five cases of splanchnic artery aneurysm associated with coeliac artery stenosis due to compression by the median arcuate ligament. *Clin Radiol.* 2007;62(7):688-93. Epub 2007 Apr 30. doi:10.1016/j.crad.2007.02.002
11. Moore E, Matthews MR, Minion DJ, et al. Surgical management of peripancreatic arterial aneurysms. *J Vasc Surg.* 2004 ;40(2):247–53. doi:10.1016/j.jvs.2004.03.045
12. Miyayama S, Terada T, Tamaki M. Ruptured pancreaticoduodenal artery aneurysm associated with median arcuate ligament compression and aortic dissection successfully treated with embolotherapy. *Ann Vasc Dis.* 2015;8(1):40–2. doi:10.3400/avd.cr.14-00117
13. Flood K, Nicholson A. Inferior pancreaticoduodenal artery aneurysms associated with occlusive lesions of the celiac axis: Diagnosis, treatment options, outcomes, and review of the literature. *Cardiovasc Intervent Radiol.* 2013;36:578–587.
14. Ohira S, Kimura T, Takeuchi K, et al. Pancreaticoduodenal artery aneurysm involving papilla of vater successfully treated with endovascular approach despite intraoperative rupture. *Ann Vasc Surg.* 2013;27:802.e9–802.e12.
15. Ducasse E, Roy F, Chevalier J, et al. Aneurysm of the pancreaticoduodenal arteries with a celiac trunk lesion: Current management. *J Vasc Surg.* 2004;39(4):906–11. doi:10.1016/j.jvs.2003.09.049
16. Takao H, Nojo T, Ohtomo K. True pancreaticoduodenal artery aneurysms: A decision analysis. *Eur J Radiol.* 2010;75(1):110–3. doi:10.1016/j.ejrad.2009.03.041
17. Coll DP, Ierardi R, Kerstein MD, et al. Aneurysms of the pancreaticoduodenal arteries: A change in management. *Ann Vasc Surg.* 1998;12:286–91.
18. Ikeda O, Nakasone Y, Yokoyama K, et al. Simultaneous coil embolization and angioplasty using a self-expanding nitinol stent to treat pancreaticoduodenal artery aneurysms associated with celiac artery stenosis. *Acta Radiol.* 2013;54:949–53.
19. Scheflan M, Kadir S, Athanasoulis C, Hedberg SE. Pancreaticoduodenal artery aneurysm simulating carcinoma of the head of the pancreas. *Arch Surg.* 1977;112:1201–3.
20. Proud G, Chamberlain J. Aneurysm formation on the small pancreatic arteries in association with coeliac axis compression. *Ann R Coll Surg Engl.* 1978;60:294–7.
21. Mora JD. Coeliac-axis artery stenosis with aneurysmal calcification of the collateral supply. *Australas Radiol.* 1976;20:252–4.
22. Cochennec F, Riga CV, Allaire E, et al. Contemporary Management of Splanchnic and Renal Artery Aneurysms: Results of Endovascular Compared with Open Surgery from Two European Vascular Centers. *Eur J Vasc Endovasc Surg.* 2011;42:340–6.
23. Sgroi MD, Kabutey NK., Krishnam M, et al. Pancreaticoduodenal artery aneurysms secondary to median arcuate ligament syndrome may not need celiac artery revascularization or ligament release. 2015;29(1):122.e1-7. doi:10.1016/j.avsg.2014.05.020
24. Won Y, Lee SL, Kim Y, KY. Clinical efficacy of transcatheter embolization of visceral artery aneurysms using n-butyl cyanoacrylate (NBCA). *Gastrointest. Imaging* 2015;S2211–5684.
25. Ritter JC, Johnston M, Caruana MF, Laws PE. Aorto-gastroduodenal bypass grafting for an inferior pancreaticoduodenal aneurysm and celiac trunk thrombosis. *Interact Cardiovasc Thorac Surg.* 2010;10(1):125–7. doi:10.1510/icvts.2009.219949

34

How to Approach Aortic Aneurysms with a Horseshoe Kidney

Karthik Mikkineni, MD and Satish Muluk, MD

First described by Berenger de Carpi in 1552 and a century later in detail by Botallus in 1665, horseshoe kidney (HSK), also known as crossed renal ectopia, is the most common fusion anomaly of the kidneys (Figure 34-1). It is seen in roughly 1 in 400 births (0.15%–0.25% among all new births),[1] with males twice as commonly affected as females.

Julian first described the association of abdominal aortic aneurysm (AAA) and HSK in 1956. Phelan et al. described the first successful repair of AAA with HSK in 1957.[2] Association of HSK with AAA is found in about 1 in every 710 autopsied cases and about 0.12%–0.25% of all aortic operations.[1] The incidence of aneurysm in people with HSK is similar to that seen among general population.

The presence of such a renal anomaly with AAA poses a challenge to vascular surgeons. However with proper understanding of the anatomy and vascularization of the abnormal organ, the characteristics of the isthmus portion, and modern imaging, the unique task or repairing AAA in HSK patients can be achieved with good outcomes.

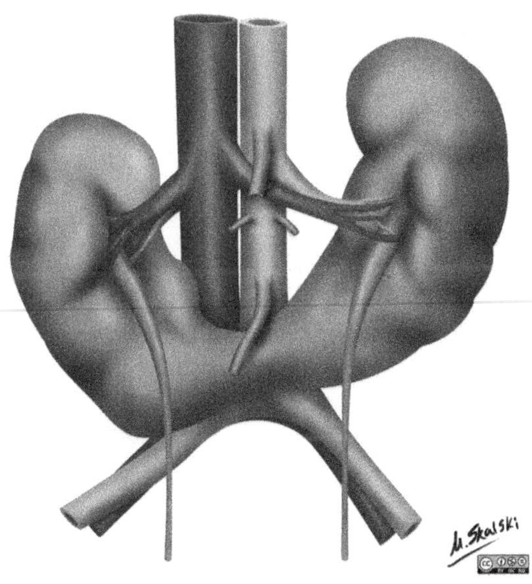

Figure 34-1. Artist's rendering of a horseshoe kidney. The isthmus is located below the takeoff of the inferior mesenteric artery in 40% of cases. For the sake of clarity, multiple renal arteries, which are typically-present, are not shown.

EMBRYOLOGY AND VASCULATURE

HSK is the term used when the two kidneys fuse in the midline, connected by an isthmus resulting in so called horseshoe shape.

Development of the urogenital system begins early in the fourth week of gestation from the intermediate mesoderm, which forms a urogenital ridge on either side of the aorta (Figure 34-2). The urogenital ridge develops into pronephros, mesonephros and metanephros. The pronephros and mesonephros eventually regress, and the kidneys and collecting system develop from the metanephros. The metanephros forms from an outgrowth of caudal mesonephric duct, the ureteric bud, and a condensation of renogenic intermediate mesoderm, the metanephric blastemia.

The metanephros is initially situated in the pelvis opposite sacral somites. Rapid growth caudally leads to the migration of the kidneys from pelvis to retroperitoneal fossa on either side of the second lumbar vertebra by eighth week of gestation. As the kidneys ascend, they rotate through 90 degrees such that the renal hilum is directed medially as kidney reaches the final position.

During the process of ascent, if the two kidneys come into contact, crossed renal ectopia, or HSK, will result. The fusion of embryonic kidneys occurs early in gestation, when they are in close proximity and is the result of abnormal migration of nephrogenic cells.[3] The kidneys are joined by an isthmus, which links lower poles in 95% of cases and upper poles in 5% of cases.[4] The isthmus may be fibrotic, dysplastic, or normal renal parenchyma. The position of isthmus is variable. In about 40% of cases, it lies below the origin of IMA. The presence of IMA may restrict further ascent during early embryogenesis. In another 40% isthmus is located above the IMA with kidneys in normal location. Finally, in 20% of HSK cases, the kidneys lie in the pelvis. Horseshoe kidneys are almost always malrotated with anterior renal pelvises and ureter crossing anterior to the isthmus. This configuration is attributed to early fusion prior to normal rotation.

While ascending, the kidneys derive blood supply sequentially from vessels that are closest to them, initially the median sacral, then common iliac, IMA, and finally aorta. Ectopic kidneys usually contain numerous small vessels, reflecting continuous changes in blood supply to the developing kidney during ascent.

The blood supply to the HSK is extremely variable. About 30% have a normal anatomical pattern with two renal arteries, one on each side arising from the aorta.

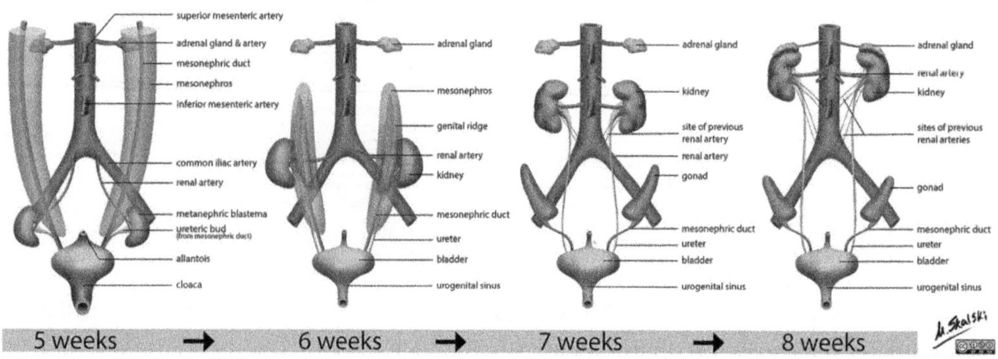

Figure 34-2. Normal embryology of kidneys and the renal arteries. Note that multiple renal arteries develop and regress over the course of gestation. HSK occurs because of fusion of the renal parenchyma early in development (prior to 7 weeks).

The remaining 70% are supplied by a combination of vessels entering from the aorta, renal, mesenteric, iliac or sacral vessels.[4] Venous return may also be abnormal. The major venous return in patients with HSK is by main right and left renal veins draining directly into the inferior vena cava. Accessory veins draining either into vena cava or iliac veins may also be present. Because these structures do not arise from the aorta and are not directly involved in aortic operations, the venous abnormalities have not been extensively described. Regardless, preservation of venous drainage is considered important and should be studied in each case.

The arterial supply of the crossed ectopic kidney is the most important factor in determining the best treatment approach. In the current era of endovascular repair, knowing this anatomy in detail is crucial in making therapeutic decisions. It is imperative to have a good preoperative knowledge of the anomalous vascularization of the HSK and its relationship with aneurysm.

Various classifications are described in literature by authors for elucidating the anatomy of the abnormal vasculature of the HSK. These classifications aid in understanding the anatomy and making appropriate decisions for operative intervention. Four major classifications described in the literature are: (1) Papin's classification, (2) Crawford's classification, (3) Eisendrath's classification, and (4) Boatman's classification.

Papin's Classification[5]: According to Papin's classification, which is based on the number of renal arteries, there are three types of HSK vascularization. In Papin I, seen in 20% of cases, there are no abnormal renal arteries; in Papin II, which accounts for 66%, there are three to five renal arteries; and in Papin III, which accounts for 14%, there are more than five renal arteries.

Crawford's Classification[1]: This classification is based on the origin of the renal arteries. In Crawford I, there are two renal arteries of normal origin. In Crawford II, there are two normal renal arteries and one to three anomalous renal arteries arising from infrarenal aorta or iliac arteries; in Crawford III: all renal arteries have an anomalous origin.

Eisendrath's Classification[6]: This classification, dating to 1925, is the oldest. It presents five types of HSK vascularization. Type I includes subjects who have one renal artery for each side of the HSK (20%). Type II has one renal artery for each side and one artery for HSK (30%); Type III has two renal arteries for each side and one artery for renal isthmus (15%); Type IV presents two renal arteries for each side with one or more arising from iliac arteries for renal isthmus (15%). Type V includes multiple renal arteries originating from aorta and iliac or mesenteric arteries (20%).

Boatman's classification[7] consists of six types of vascularization (types A to F). In type A, there is one renal artery supplying each side of the HSK; in type B, two renal arteries supply each side of the kidney; in type C, one renal artery supplies each side of the kidney and a separate isthmus branch; in type D, two renal arteries supply each side of the kidney and one isthmus branch; in type E, the renal arteries supply each side of the kidney and renal arteries arising from the iliac arteries supply the isthmus; and in type F, two renal arteries supply each side of the kidney, with an isthmus branch and renal arteries arising from the iliac arteries.

Papin's classification seems to be more appropriate from the endovascular point of view because of its simplicity. Papin's type I vascularization is a good indication for endovascular treatment, whereas Papin's type II and III vascularization should be evaluated individually. Crawford's classification has more significant surgical impact in open repair in regards to clamping and revascularization options.

PREOPERATIVE PLANNING

The key to success in dealing with the challenging association of HSK with AAA is preoperative planning. Imaging plays a pivotal role in therapeutic decisions and management options.

Historical reports describe aneurysms that were detected and operated on the basis of physical examination and/or plain radiographs.[8] In those situations HSK was almost always revealed as a surprising and challenging intraoperative finding. In the present day with modern imaging modalities, HSK might not pose as much of a diagnostic challenge as a therapeutic challenge. The unexpected finding of HSK, however, remains an issue for unstable patients with ruptured aneurysm and limited available imaging.

CT scan with contrast is the most important imaging modality in operative planning. CT angiogram (CTA) on a 64-slice scanner with thin-cut images is most diagnostic. This modality identifies both HSK and AAA very effectively. Although some minor renal accessory arteries may be missed, the accuracy of the CTA is reported to be 90%,[2] whereas catheter angiography has a reported accuracy of only 67%.[2] A diagnostic angiogram is almost never indicated or advised as a part of routine preoperative planning.

A 3D workstation (e.g., Aquarius WS, Terarecon Inc., San Matteo, CA) with multiplanar reconstruction, maximum intensity projection, 3D Volume rendering and curved planar images will provide information needed for operative planning, especially when endovascular therapy is contemplated.

Magnetic resonance angiography (MRA), though sensitive enough and free of radiation, does not offer substantive advantage over a CTA. MRA is associated with added cost, claustrophobia, and inferior delineation of calcification. Gadolinium, the contrast agent for MRA, has lost its place of preference over iodinated dyes for patients with renal insufficiency because of the risk of nephrogenic systemic fibrosis.

Ultrasonography can detect HSK, which presents as an isthmus of renal tissue in front of the aorta, but a narrow isthmus or the presence of excess bowel gas can cause it to be missed. Apart from routine AAA screening and fetal surveillance, ultrasonography will not be accurate in assessing the vasculature of the HSK and the operative anatomy of the AAA. However, there are reports showing contrast-enhanced ultrasound is as effective as CTA for routine post-EVAR detection of endoleaks.

Excretory intravenous pyelography is rarely, if at all, necessary preoperatively. It might have clinical significance in patients with recurrent UTI/obstructive symptoms, because it is 88% sensitive in revealing anomalies of urinary tract.[2]

Morphological evaluation with associated functional information can be gained from nuclear scintigarphic study that is able to give information about parenchymal renal function through capture and excretion of radionucleotide. Some authors recommend use of this modality to assess the functional status of the isthmus and the main renal parenchyma in advance of surgery.[9]

Renal function tests are the single most important laboratory work required in dealing with renal anomalies. As a matter of fact routine renal function tests are obtained for any operative intervention involving the aorta. Abnormal preoperative renal function test is a crucial indicator of negative prognosis. It is associated with fivefold increase in mortality after any type of aortic surgery independent of renal malformations. Abnormal renal function tests and its impact on therapeutic decisions are enormous.

Apart from the imaging modalities, patients should also undergo appropriate cardiac and pulmonary evaluation and optimization just as with any elective aortic intervention.

DECISION-MAKING AND TREATMENT OPTIONS

Adequate preoperative diagnosis of the HSK and its vascular anatomy is important in choosing the best surgical approach in each individual patient. In the emergency setting of a ruptured aneurysm with patient in shock there is no time for extensive diagnostic study. This has little significance, however, in the choice of surgical approach, because a transabdominal approach is advised for rapid control and maximal overview.

In more stable patients, the HSK is normally discovered during preoperative workup, and detailed knowledge of the vascular anatomy is essential to determine the choice of approach. When aortic morphology is suitable and renal artery pattern allows, the first choice of operation is endovascular repair.

As noted earlier, CTA delineates the anatomy and feasibility of an endovascular repair. If the scan reveals an aneurysm with reasonable neck length and angulation and adequate seal zones, the next important factor to consider is the presence of aberrant vessels. A significant body of literature indicates that any accessory vessel less than 3 mm in size can be safely covered with minimal renal consequences if the baseline renal function is good.[2,10,11] The accessory arteries are in theory end arteries and risk of endoleak is minimal. There are only rare reports in the literature about type II endoleak from accessory renal arteries.[12] If there are multiple significant (>3 mm in diameter) accessory arteries arising from the aneurysm itself or from the iliac, open repair is the preferred approach.

When open repair is necessary, a left-sided retroperitoneal approach is advised in the elective setting. In situations where the patient is acutely unstable or when technical issues require open conversion from endovascular repair, however, a transperitoneal approach is recommended. Transabdominal approach is also advised in cases with concomitant right iliac aneurysm or accessory renal arteries arising from the right iliac, due to the technical difficulty in reaching the right iliac from a retroperitoneal approach.

TRANSPERITONEAL APPROACH

The patient is prepped from the nipples to the knees. An incision is made from the xiphoid to the symphysis pubis along the midline. After the fascial layers are cauterized, the peritoneum is identified and entered. After careful inspection of the intra-abdominal contents, the greater omentum and transverse colon are elevated superiorly, and the small bowel is mobilized to the right side with the help of appropriate blades using the Omni self-retaining retractor (Omni-Tract surgical, St. Paul, MN). This exposes the retroperitoneum. The posterior peritoneum is incised, starting just below the bifurcation of the aorta inferiorly and extending superiorly to the level of the ligament of Treitz. The aorta and the HSK isthmus, lying anterior to the aorta, are exposed. If necessary, the inferior mesenteric vein can be divided to allow better exposure. The left renal vein is usually identified at the neck of the aneurysm, but careful examination of the CT scan for venous anomalies must be done preoperatively to look for left-sided IVC, retro-aortic renal vein or other venous anomalies that may be found in association with HSK. If the aneurysm extends to the level of the renal arteries and will require suprarenal clamping, the left renal vein should be mobilized to the level of its confluence with the inferior vena cava (IVC). During the procedure, the key dilemma is whether to sacrifice the isthmus in order to improve the approach to the aorta. The isthmus connecting the lower poles may be a fibrous band or may contain functional parenchyma. The renal pelvis may be asymmetric and extend across the midline region of the isthmus. These latter anatomic configurations make the division of renal isthmus potentially hazardous, as inadvertent entry into the collecting system may result in a urinary fistula and the dire consequence of graft infection.[2] In a meta-analysis of 176 patients with HSK and AAA, division of the renal isthmus was associated with increased post-operative renal insufficiency.[8] In addition, division of the isthmus might also lead to increased morbidity, including hemorrhage, renal fistula, and potential sepsis. Division of the renal isthmus is also associated with higher chance of dividing the arteries supplying the isthmus, which leads to further risk of necrosis and fistulas. Furthermore, the blood supply may be asymmetric relative to the isthmus, with isthmus feeder arteries crossing the midline. Even with the main renal parenchymal segments can be supplied predominantly and unpredictably from one side or the other. As a consequence, the effect of ligation one or more aberrant/accessory renal arteries may result in unpredictable renal ischemia. For these reasons, the isthmus should be preserved whenever technically feasible. The isthmus is carefully mobilized anteriorly from the aneurysm from bottom upwards. The can also be facilitated by shifting the HSK via right or left retro colic access. When short vessels prevent the dissection or when the HSK is tightly adherent to the anterior wall of the aneurysm, assessment of the vessels should be done after the proximal and distal clamp with assessment of vessels from within the aneurysm sac. Blind dissection can result in ischemia of the isthmus and increase the chances of post-operative renal failure and increased morbidity. These anatomic difficulties suggest that the anterior approach should be attempted only when other options are not feasible. Many of the renal artery and isthmus problems can be avoided with a retroperitoneal approach using a lumbar or thoracolumbar incision.

Proximal control is obtained by aortic cross clamp, usually at a suprarenal location. Distal control is obtained at the distal aorta or bilateral common iliac arteries. Circumferential dissection of the common iliac is to be avoided to prevent venous injury. During the dissection of the aorta and the common iliac arteries, great care is to be taken to identify the ureters and preserve them. Once proximal and distal control is obtained and after systemic heparinization, the aortic sac is entered, and the thrombus is evacuated. Careful examination of the accessory renal arteries is done from within the sac. Any vessel supplying the kidneys with diameter greater than 3 mm should be preserved.[13] In addition to orifice location, the lack of back-bleeding may help to distinguish the accessory renal arteries, which are end arteries, from the lumbar arteries. Small accessory vessels and lumbar arteries are suture ligated within the aneurysm sac. An end-to-end anastomosis between prosthetic graft and aorta or the iliac arteries is performed with polypropylene suture. The graft is tunneled behind the anteriorly mobilized isthmus prior to the distal anastomosis.

Two surgical options are available to deal with anomalous renal arteries during aneurysm repair[13]: preservation, usually demanding their reattachment into the vascular graft, or simple ligation. The consensus is that anomalous renal arteries larger than

3 mm in diameter should be preserved. This is done by implanting the renal arteries into the graft or using a Carrell's patch technique. Aortorenal bypass can also be performed if needed. Small accessory renal arteries can be ligated and small renal infarcts are anticipated with minimal clinical consequences. The aneurysmal sac is closed over the graft with running absorbable suture as much as possible. The graft may have to be left exposed in areas with anastomosis to the renal arteries. The isthmus will lie with the graft tunneled posterior to it. The posterior peritoneum is closed with an absorbable suture. The abdominal wall is then closed in the standard manner with running nonabsorbable sutures.

In case of rupture with a rapid need for supraceliac control, the supraceliac aorta can be exposed at the diaphragm by retracting the left lobe of the liver to the right and the gastrohepatic omentum opened to allow entry into the lesser sac. The nasogastric tube is used to identify and avoid injury to the esophagus and proximal part of the stomach, which are both retracted to the left. The aorta is identified between the crura of the diaphragm, which may be split with an electrocautery device for rapid accurate placement of a clamp. Supraceliac clamping should be as brief as possible.

RETROPERITONEAL APPROACH

Retroperitoneal approach to aneurysm repair with concomitant HSK is advisable[2,8,13] in an elective scenario if the patient requires an open repair. Thoracoabdominal or juxta-pararenal aneurysms with associated HSK should receive a thoracolumbar incision to facilitate reaching the thoracic and visceral aorta. However, standard infrarenal AAAs can be managed through flank incisions through the bed of the 11th or 12th rib.

The retroperitoneal approach has several advantages. It avoids interference with the renal isthmus, the ureters, most renal arteries, and the renal veins. This is particularly advisable when major renal vessels arise from the AAA, because it enables the simultaneous reimplantation of one or more renal arteries, using a single cuff of the anterior aortic wall. However, the approach to right iliac artery is more difficult if the iliac artery is aneurysmal or when important renal vessels originate from the right iliac artery. For the retroperitoneal approach, after intubation, the patient is placed in the supine position on a deflated beanbag apparatus. The left arm is elevated and rotated way from the operating table, keeping the hips flat, so that the torso is twisted. The arm is placed on a support and the bean bag is inflated. The exact location of the incision is based on the area of aorta that needs to be exposed. The appropriate interspace level of the thoracic portion of the incision is based on the proximal extent of the aneurysm. For Crawford Type II and I thoracoabdominal aneurysms, optimal exposure of the aorta is achieved through the fifth interspace. The descending thoracic aneurysm is best exposed through the sixth through eighth interspaces for exposure of the aorta at the level of the diaphragm (Crawford type IV). For repair of an infrarenal aneurysm, an incision is made extending from the 11th or 12th rib to the midline. The incision is extended further towards the pubis symphysis if exposure of the iliacs is required. The 11th or 12th rib may be partially removed for better exposure and to avoid inadvertent fracture due to excessive traction.

The incision is opened using an electrocautery device, carefully separating the layers of the abdominal wall, following which the retroperitoneum is entered in the lateral wound. This is achieved by stripping the peritoneum and transversalis fascia from the posterior surface of the abdominal wall musculature. A plane is developed by initially mobilizing the transversalis fascia posteriorly and to the right. Once the midaxillary line is crossed, the peritoneal contents are pulled anteriorly and to the right. The HSK, its collecting system and vasculature are also mobilized anteriorly along with the peritoneal contents. The aorta is exposed from the left renal vein to the left iliac bifurcation. The left gonadal vein may be divided near its junction with renal vein to aid in exposure of the infra renal neck. With this exposure, the need for dissection of the kidneys and its associated arterial supply and collecting system is generally avoided. For infrarenal AAAs, proximal control of the aorta is obtained at the level of the renal vein. The exposure of the right common iliac can be difficult and its control can be obtained with an intraluminal balloon. Accessory renal arteries are accessed from within the aorta. They can be cold-perfused using a Pruitt balloon catheter, but in general, rapid renal reimplantation is a better strategy than attempting to perfuse the renal arteries. After systemic heparinization, the aorta is clamped and opened along the posterolateral wall. Proximal anastomosis with tube graft is done with polypropylene suture; after the proximal anastomosis, the significant accessory renal arteries (>3 mm) can be reimplanted to the aortic graft as a patch within the aneurysm sac, or less commonly, using an aorto-renal bypass.[13] The distal anastomosis is then performed either to the distal aorta or bilateral iliac arteries. If the right common iliac artery is aneurysmal the exposure may be challenging. It may be facilitated with a counterincision in right lower quadrant. The fascia and abdominal wall are closed in the usual fashion after ensuring hemostasis.

ENDOVASCULAR REPAIR

Aneurysms with suitable neck morphology and normal renal vasculature should be approached with an endograft in the standard fashion. No data support a different AAA size threshold for AAA associated with HSK. As noted earlier, aneurysms with HSK have accessory/aberrant renal vasculature in 70% of cases, and the average number of renal arteries has been reported to be in the range of 3.1 to 3.98. Careful planning is required with accessory arteries arising from the aneurysm or within the neck region. As mentioned above, accessory renal arteries less than 3 mm in diameter can be safely covered without long-term clinical consequences. If the accessory renal arteries are larger than 3 mm and originate within the aneurysm, the proximal landing zone, or from the iliac artery, complex endovascular strategies may be necessary if the patient is not a good candidate for open repair. These complex endovascular approaches require careful preoperative planning and, possibly, customized devices. Thus, expertise in catheter and wire skills and an adequate endovascular inventory become essential.

In endovascular management of complex strategies, the target vessel can be tackled in different ways. When a target vessel lies within the proximal or distal landing zone, an endograft with a scallop or fenestration (opening in the endograft sometimes reinforced by a nitinol ring) is an option.[15] When using a scallop, stent-grafting of the target vessel is optional. Fenestrations should always be stented with appropriately sized balloon expandable covered stents, however, and a proximal "riveting balloon" technique is highly desirable to minimize endoleak and graft migration.

If the target vessel origin is located within the aneurysmal sac or if the gap between deployed graft and vessel orifice is more than 10mm, a customized endo-branch should be considered. Such customized devices can be manufactured for some non-US sites and in research settings. These grafts can also be created from modification of approved devices. These modifications, which are off-label, require back-table unsheathing and resheathing of existing devices. The patient should be advised about the off-label nature of the modification during the consent process. Radio-opaque markers and precannulation of the branches can be extremely helpful in these situations. Accurate diameter evaluation of accessory vessels and screening for early bifurcation are critical to selecting the correct stent-graft to bridge the gap between the endograft branch and target vessel.

Another possible endovascular technique is to use snorkel or chimney grafts to maintain flow to significant accessory arteries arising from the aneurysm or from within the seal zones. There are not enough data at this time to determine which of the various endovascular options is superior. The choice is often made in accordance with the operator's experience and other factors, such as the feasibility of access from the arm or axilla.

It should be emphasized that these are highly complex endovascular procedures with steep learning curves; the operators must be well versed with guidewire and catheter skills. These cases are not without complications, as technical difficulties can lead to prolonged operative times, high doses of radiation, and increased morbidity. Most of the accessory arteries for HSK usually come at acute angles and originate behind the organ low in the aorta, factors that may preclude groin-based cannulation, instead requiring brachial access. The major risk of renal revascularization in conjunction with endovascular aneurysm repair is an increased risk of renal dysfunction.

CONCLUSION

AAA with HSK is a true surgical challenge. Careful preoperative planning and case by case approach is advised. Endovascular option is to be considered as a procedure of choice avoiding the anatomic difficulties of aortic exposure. Renal vasculature, however, plays a key role in dictating the modality of approach. When open surgery is needed, the retroperitoneal approach is advised in elective setting, but transabdominal approach may be necessary in acute settings or with right iliac aneurysm. Preservation of perfusion to the abnormal organ is the primary challenge with either open or endovascular therapy, and avoidance of renal isthmus injury is a significant additional concern with open surgery.

REFERENCES

1. Crawford ES, Coselli JS, Safi HJ, et al. The impact of renal fusion and ecotpia on aortic surgery. *J Vasc Surg*. 1988; 18(4):375–83.
2. O'Hara PJ, Hakaim AG, Hertzer NR, et al. Surgical management of aortic aneurysm and coexistent HSK: review of a 31-year experience. *J Vasc Surg*. 1993; 18(4):586.
3. Domenech-Mateu JM, Gonzalez-Compta X. HSK: a new theory on its embryogenesis based on the study of a 16mm human embryo. *Anat Rec*. 1988; 222: 408–17.

4. Cambell MF. Renal ectopy. *J Urol.* 1930; 24:187–98.
5. Papin E., Chirugurgie du Rein E. Anomalies du rein. *Paris: G. Dion;* 1928. P. 205–20.
6. Eisendrath DN, Phifer FM, Culvier HB. HSK. *Ann Surg.* 1925; 82:735–64.
7. Boatman DL, Cornell SH, Kolln CP. The arterial supply of horseshoe kidneys. *Am J Roentgenol Radium THer Nucl Med.* 1971; 113(3):447–51.
8. Stroosma OB, kootstra G, Schrunik GW. Management of aortic aneurysm in the presence of a horsehoe kidney. *Br J Surg.* 2001; 88(4): 500–9.
9. PieroV, Giovanni N, Ilias D, et al. Endovascular repair of an abdominal aortic aneurysm in a patient with HSK: report of a case. *Surg Today.* 2006;36:623–8.
10. Aquino RV, Rhee RY, Muluk SC, et al. Exclusion of accessory renal arteries during endovascular repair of abdominal aortic aneurysms. *J Vasc Surg.* 2001; 34(5): 878–84.
11. Jackson RW, Fay DM, Wyatt MG, Roser JD. The renal impact of aortic stent-grafting in patients with a HSK. *Cardio Vasc Intervent Radiol.* 2004; 27(6): 632–6.
12. Ruppert V, Umscheid T, Rieger J, et al. Endovascular aneurysm repair: Treatment of choice for abdominal aortic aneurysm coincident with horseshoe kidney. Three case reports and review of literature. *J Vasc Surg.* 2004; 40(2):367–70.
13. Davidovic L, Markovic M, Ilic N, et al. Repair of abdominal aortic aneurysms in the presence of HSK. *Int Angiol.* 2011;30:534–40.
14. Spear R, Maurel B, Sobocinski J, et al. Technical note and results in the management of anatomical variant of renal vascularization during endovascular aneurysm repair. *Eur J Vasc Endovasc Surg.* 2012.01.003.
15. Greenburg RK, Haulon s, O'Neill S, et al. Primary endovascular repair of juxtarenal aneurysms with fenestrated endovascular grafting. *Eur J Vasc Endovasc Surg.* 2004;27(5);484–91.

35

Ex Vivo Renal Artery Reconstruction

Sung Wan Ham, MD and Fred A. Weaver MD, MMM

Management of complex renal artery pathology involving the distal renal artery, segmental branch vessels, or renal hilum presents a surgical challenge. Aneurysm, occlusive disease, dissection, or mass due to variety of etiologies including atherosclerosis, medial fibrodysplasia, arteritis, arteriovenous fistulas and tumor can involve the renal arterial tree. A number of techniques for renal salvage in the treatment of complex renal artery pathology have been reported.[1–7] Many kidneys with segmental renal branch disease, once treated by nephrectomy, are now preserved by a variety of reconstructive techniques and adjuncts.

A number of modifications have been made to the original description of ex situ renal artery reconstruction as described by Ota in 1967.[8] Modifications include ex vivo repair, in situ repair with or without cold preservation, and orthotopic or heterotopic autotransplantation of the repaired kidney. Hybrid approaches combining laparoscopic nephrectomy with ex vivo bench repair and pelvic auto-transplantation have also been described.[9] In addition, catheter-based interventions using coils and stents have increasingly been used as a primary treatment for complex renal artery lesions.

Many studies have demonstrated the safety, durability and clinical benefits on blood pressure and renal function when using open reconstructive and renal parenchymal protective strategies in the management of complex renal artery pathology.[1–5,7,10] These reports come from select centers with a focused interest in the management of renal artery disease. We recently reported our own institutional experience over a 25-year period with the ex vivo technique. The results both short and long term demonstrated excellent durability and favorable effects on blood pressure and renal function with minimal perioperative morbidity.

COMPLEX RENAL ARTERY PATHOLOGY

Complex renal artery pathology involves the distal renal artery with extension to the primary, secondary, or tertiary segmental branches. Examples of segmental branch involvement include aneurysms originating from a major branch point, saccular aneurysm of a branch vessel, or branch occlusive disease. Specific underlying etiologies encountered include non-atherosclerotic renal artery disease such as fibromuscular dysplasia (FMD), Takayasu arteritis (TA), and dissection as well as atherosclerotic degenerative lesions and neoplasms.

Preoperative Considerations

Indications for renal reconstructive surgery vary depending on the underlying etiology and include aneurysm, abdominal/flank pain, and resistant hypertension. Baseline parameters to measure include resting blood pressure in both arms, the number and duration of antihypertensive medications, laboratory assessment of renal function including serum creatinine (SCr), blood urea nitrogen (BUN) and electrolytes. Calculation of glomerular filtration rate is estimated from SCr, and known body mass index using the Cockcroft-Gault equation.

Imaging Studies

Renal artery duplex ultrasonography is performed early in the evaluation. Renal duplex ultrasonography provides important information on the existing renal artery disease, renal blood flow and velocity, associated renal size and intra-parenchymal renal blood flow indices. Renal artery stenosis (>60%) is documented by elevated (> 220 cm/sec) peak systolic velocity measurements across existing lesions. Baseline functional characteristics (i.e., velocity, spectral waveforms, resistive index) and morphologic parameters including renal size in length measured pole-to-pole and cortical thickness over a medullary pyramid, perpendicular to the capsule in the sagittal plane, serves as a reference for surveillance imaging after renal revascularization.

Conventional abdominal aortography with selective renal artery catheterization is routinely used for all patients. Angiography is critical in defining renal artery anatomy including the presence of multiple renal arteries as well as evaluating the extent of the renal artery disease.

Liberal use of CT imaging provides information on extent of disease not appreciated on angiography in addition to anatomic relationships between the lesion and surrounding structures (i.e. ureter, renal vein). CT imaging is complementary to the information provided by catheter-based angiography and is critical to a successful operative strategy. Reconstructive planning is predicated on identifying inflow and outflow bypass target vessels unaffected by disease, which is particularly imperative for arteritic/inflammatory pathologies.

SURGICAL TECHNIQUE

General aspects of the ex vivo renal artery repair are well described.[1,2,5,10,11,12] We preferentially perform ex vivo renal vascular reconstruction with orthotopic placement of the reconstructed kidney. A subcostal incision extending from the midline to the tip of the 12th rib is used for unilateral renal artery exposure. In large or obese patients, the medial extent of the incision can be extended across the midline as a chevron. A midline transperitoneal approach is employed for patients who require a more extensive exposure. The preferred conduit is autogenous greater saphenous vein with a prosthetic graft being used only in patients without suitable saphenous vein. Operations are staged for patients with bilateral renal artery disease (Figure 35-1).

Exposure of the renal artery begins by mobilizing the main renal artery/vein. On the left this requires the identification and ligation of the lumbar, gonadal and adrenal branches of the left renal vein. All arterial segmental branch vessels are identified and encircled with a silastic loop. The ureter is left intact and mobilized to permit elevation of the kidney to the level of the abdominal wall. Once the kidney is mobilized from the renal fossa and systemic heparin given, the renal vein is divided and the proximal renal artery divided and ligated at the stump (Figures 35-2 and 35-3). We employ ex vivo repair with renal vein division to address all pathology involving the terminal renal artery with segmental branch involvement. Alternative techniques such as in situ repair or total renal mobilization without renal vein transection with cold perfusion has been reported by others but has not been used at our institution.

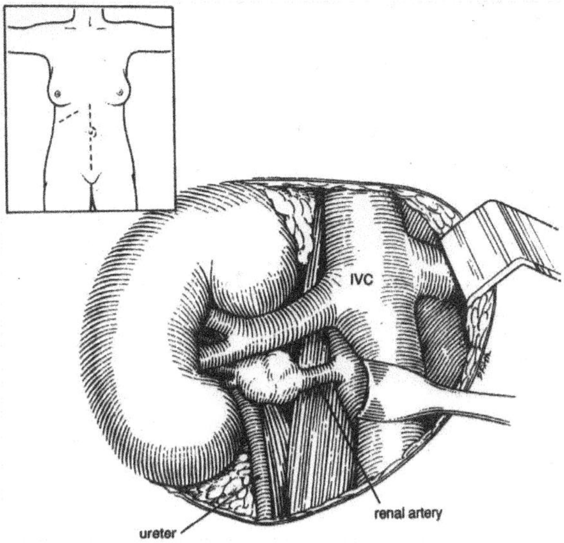

Figure 35-1. Exposure of the right kidney and renal vascular pedicle.[1] (Taken from Hood and Weaver[11]; used with permission from *The American Surgeon*.)

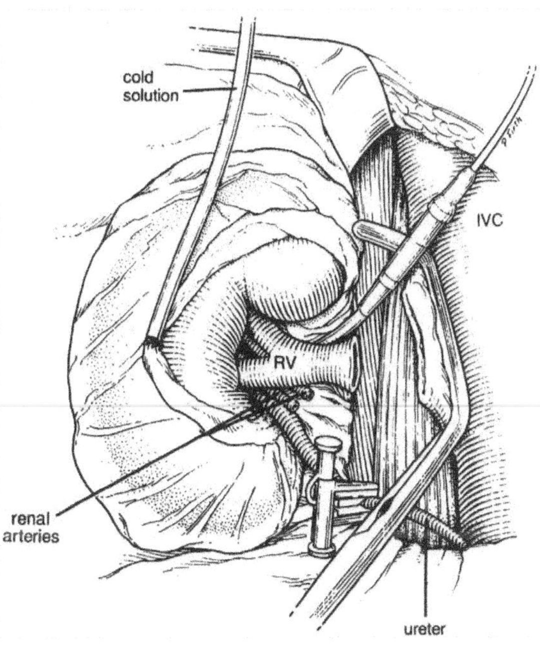

Figure 35-2. The ex vivo right kidney under hypothermic cold preservation. Right renal artery and vein transected. Note the Fogarty soft jaw clamp placed on the ureter to prevent rewarming of the kidney during cold perfusion.[1] (Taken from Ham and Weaver[10]; used with permission from the *Journal of Vascular Surgery*.)

Hypothermic renal preservation

Profound renal parenchymal hypothermia is established through external and internal parenchymal cooling. For internal parenchymal hypothermia, approximately 500 cc of University of Wisconsin (UW) solution chilled to 4°C is flushed through the renal artery until the effluent of the renal vein is clear. Collin's solution modified with the addition of heparin 2000 units and

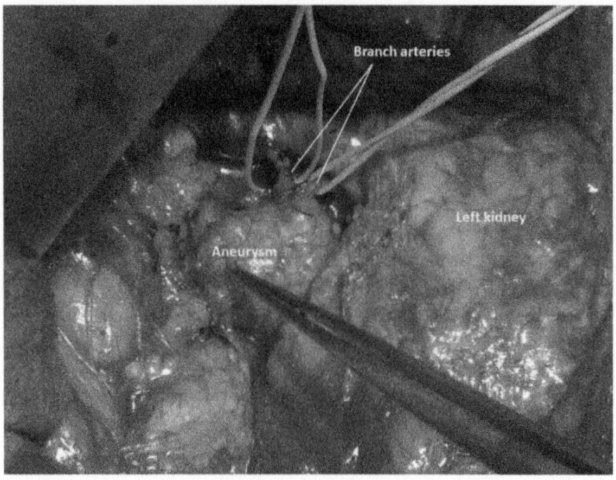

Figure 35-3. Intraoperative photo of a left renal artery aneurysm with segmental branch vessel involvement. All segmental branch vessels are individually controlled with silastic loops.[2] (Taken from Ham and Weaver[10]; used with permission from the *Journal of Vascular Surgery*.)

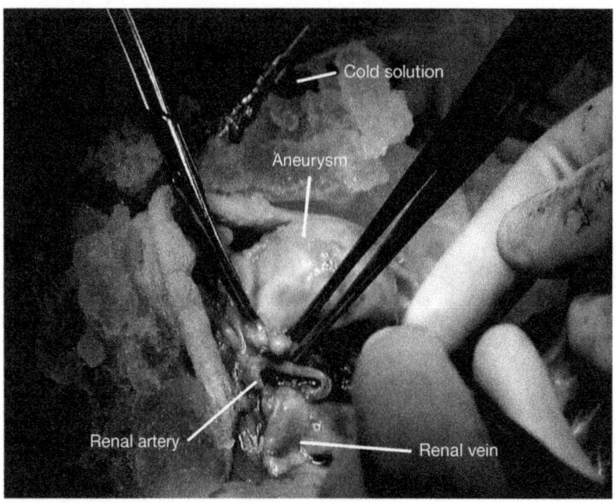

Figure 35-4. Intraoperative photo of an ex vivo renal artery aneurysm repair. Aneurysm repair and branch reconstruction are performed first.[2]

50 mL of 10% dextrose was used in the earlier part of our experience. For external renal cooling, the kidney is brought out of the renal fossa to level of the abdominal incision. A sterile bag of ice slush is placed around the kidney along with chilled laparotomy pads to provide external cooling. To maintain surface hypothermia, cold saline is continuously irrigated onto the surface of the kidney. A soft jaw noncrushing clamp is placed on the ureter to prevent rewarming of the kidney from retrograde periureteral collateral perfusion. At this point, complex renal artery lesions at the hilum are explored and reconstructed in a bloodless field.

Reconstructive Technique

The reconstructive technique varies depending on the type and extent of renal artery involvement. For aneurysmal disease with branch vessel involvement, aneurysm resection is followed by branch repair using a variety of techniques. For aneurysms with a fistulous communication to the renal vein, both aneurysm and fistula resection is followed by branch repair and primary repair of the renal vein. In most cases, branch repair involves the joining of multiple segmental vessels at their origin thereby creating a common patch that is used for the vein graft distal anastomosis. Branch vessels that cannot be combined into the common patch are reimplanted individually on the bypass graft (Figure 35-4).

Once branch reconstruction and the distal anastomosis are finished, the kidney is placed back into the orthotopic renal bed. The proximal vein graft to infrarenal aorta anastomosis is performed first followed by the renal vein anastomosis to the vena cava. Soft jaw noncrushing clamps placed on the completed arterial and venous reconstructions are released simultaneously at the time of renal reperfusion. An intraoperative renal duplex is routinely performed with revision of any technical defects. Once the reconstruction is deemed satisfactory, Gerota's fascia is reapproximated to prevent renal torsion (Figure 35-5).

RESULTS

Since 1987, 23 patients have undergone ex vivo repair for complex renal artery pathology at the University of Southern California. This experience over a 25-year period includes 24 kidneys with a mean follow-up of 44 months. Longitudinal observation of this clinical experience has provided important information on the benefits of the ex vivo technique on blood pressure, renal function and renal structure preservation.

The majority of patients were women (74%) and relatively young (mean age 45). Seventy-eight percent of patients had pre-existing hypertension and none were dialysis dependent (Table 35-1). The underlying etiology included FMD (12), atherosclerotic aneurysm (6), TA (3), dissection (2), and renal carcinoma (1). Aneurysm of the renal artery was the most common indication for ex vivo repair (Table 35-2).

All 24 kidneys underwent successful ex vivo aorta-renal revascularization with orthotopic replacement. Reversed saphenous vein was used in 22 of the 24 repairs. Procedure details are summarized in Table 35-3.

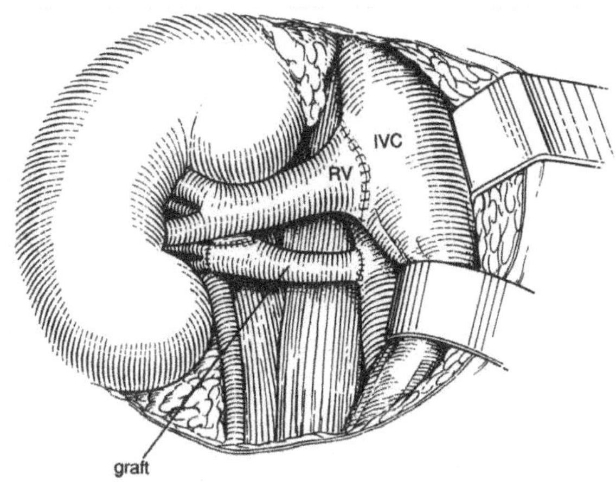

Figure 35-5. Illustration of a right renal artery aneurysm repair at completion with the kidney replaced in its orthotopic position.[1]

TABLE 35-1. DEMOGRAPHIC AND PATIENT CHARACTERISTICS

Characteristics	Number (%)
Total number of patients	23
Women	17 (74%)
Age in years (mean ± SD)	45 ± 15
Diabetes mellitus	2 (8.7%)
Tobacco (history or current)	4 (17%)
CAD/MI	0
CHF	1 (4.3%)
Hypertension	18 (78%)
COPD	0
Renal Insufficiency†	5 (22%)
Dialysis dependent	0
Follow-up (mo)	
Mean ± SD	44.4 ± 53.8
Median	29.7
Range	0.2 – 193

SD, standard deviation; CAD, coronary artery disease; MI, myocardial infarction; CHF, congestive heart failure; COPD, chronic obstructive pulmonary disease.
†Serum creatinine ≥1.5 mg/dL; mo, months.

TABLE 35-2. RENAL ARTERY PATHOLOGY

	Number of kidneys N = 24 (%)
Fibromuscular dysplasia	12 (50%)
aneurysm	12
Atherosclerotic aneurysm	6 (25%)
Takayasu arteritis	3 (12.5%)
branch occlusive	2
aneurysm	1
Other	3 (12.5%)
dissection	2
renal cell cancer*	1

*Solitary kidney.

TABLE 35-3. PROCEDURE DETAILS

Procedure	Number of kidneys N = 24 (%)
Ex vivo repair with orthotopic placement into renal fossa	24 (100%)
Branch repair with saphenous vein graft	21 (88%)
Branch repair with cephalic vein graft	1 (4%)
Branch repair with re-implant	1 (4%)
Partial nephrectomy, saphenous vein graft*	1 (4%)

*Solitary kidney.

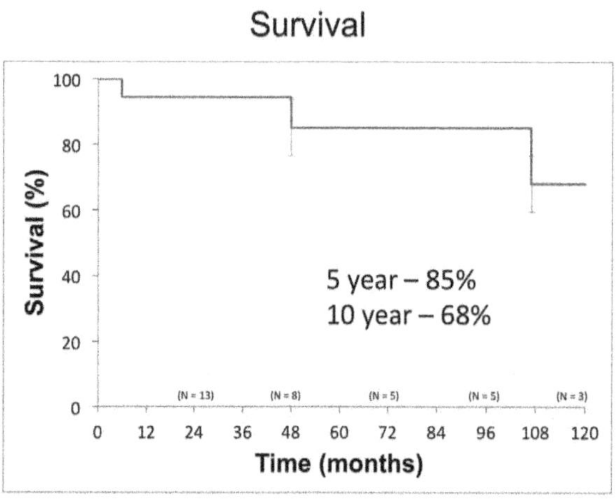

Figure 35-6. Patency curve using life table methods for all interventions. Primary, primary assisted, and secondary patency are shown. Standard error is >10% indicated by standard error bars. Standard error is < 10% for all other data points.[2]

No nephrectomies were performed for either primary or remedial procedures and no renal artery graft occlusions occurred in the perioperative period. There were no operative deaths. Two patients required reoperation for bleeding and one patient had postoperative nonoliguric acute tubular necrosis, which resolved by discharge. There were three late deaths; none related to the renal procedure. Five- and 10-year survival by Kaplan-Meier analysis was 85% and 68%, respectively (Figure 35-7).

Over a mean follow up of 44 months, one bypass graft in which reversed cephalic vein was used, developed a stenosis at 8 months and underwent transluminal angioplasty. A month later the patient developed severe hypertension due to an occluded graft. An iliac to renal bypass with prosthetic was successfully performed with preservation of the kidney. The profound intimal hyperplastic reaction we observed in in the cephalic vein conduit over a relatively short period of time was most likely due to the high flow rates in the aortorenal position. Consequently, our current preference when greater saphenous vein is not available is a prosthetic conduit. Overall, primary, primary assisted, and secondary graft patency rates were 94% at 5 and 10 years (66). A number of institutional case series have demonstrated similar durability and survival rates following ex vivo renal artery reconstruction.[1–5]

With regards to hypertension, 94% of all patients with pre-existing hypertension were either cured or had statistically significant improvement in blood pressure and antihypertensive medication requirements on follow-up (Tables 35-4 and 35-5). Furthermore, renal function was preserved with no statistically significant change in baseline mean SCr and eGFR when compared to post-revascularization values (Table 35-6).

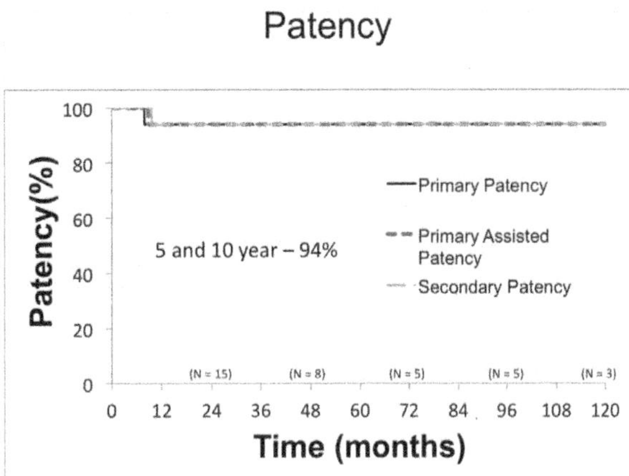

Figure 35-7. Survival curve using life table methods for all patients. Standard error is < 10% for all data points[2]

TABLE 35-4. CHANGE IN BLOOD PRESSURE AND MEDICATION REQUIREMENT

	Pre-intervention	Post-intervention	*P* value
Blood Pressure (mmHg)	166 ± 22/100 ± 21	133 ± 16/81 ± 12	= 0.002
Number of Medications	2.3 ± 1.2	1.2 ± 1	= 0.001

TABLE 35-5. BLOOD PRESSURE CLINICAL RESPONSE

N = 18	Cure	Improvement	No Improvement
Patients with HTN*	5 (28%)	12 (67%)	1 (5%)

*HTN, hypertension.

TABLE 35-6. PRESERVATION OF RENAL FUNCTION AND RENAL MASS

	Pre-intervention	Post-intervention	*P* value
SCr* (mg/dL)	1.1 ± 0.6	0.9 ± 0.6	= 0.25
eGFR* (mL/min/1.73m²)	94.6 ± 45	103 ± 40	= 0.35
Renal length‡ (cm)	10.9 ± 1.3	11.3 ± 1.7	= 0.15
Cortical‡ thickness (cm)	1.4 ± 0.4	1.4 ± 0.4	= 0.62

SCr, serum creatinine; eGFR, estimated glomerular filtration rate.

*Data available for 20 patients.

‡Data available for 15 patients: mean follow-up 68 months (range 7.7–192.7 months).

Finally, renal mass using morphologic parameters obtained by ultrasonography was quantified during follow-up. Serial ultrasonography demonstrated that renal mass as measured by mean kidney length (11.3 cm) and cortical thickness (1.4 cm) was preserved compared to pre-intervention values ($P = .15$, $P = .62$, respectively) (Table 35-6).

DISCUSSION

The experience reported above demonstrates the value of open renal artery reconstruction and the ex vivo technique and is consistent with other reports which demonstrate the value of open renal artery reconstruction. A single institutional series of 500 patients with atherosclerotic renal artery disease who underwent open renal artery revascularization had cure or improvement in blood pressure in 85% of those who survived. In the same series, 57% of patients with ischemic nephropathy and atherosclerotic renovascular hypertension had improved renal function following revascularization.[13] Furthermore, a recent study by the Vascular Low-Frequency Disease Consortium reported outcomes for 213 patients with renal artery aneurysms who underwent open reconstructive surgery. In this report of pooled data from multiple institutions, open renal artery aneurysm repair was associated with significant minor morbidity, but rarely major morbidity and mortality. Although only 10% of patients had difficult-to-control hypertension, >50% of this group had cure or improvement following open renal artery aneurysm repair.[14] Finally, we reported in 2010 an experience with open renal revascularization performed in 46 patients with non-atherosclerotic renal artery disease. In this series, renal revascularization demonstrated a cure or improvement in blood pressure in 90% of patients.[15]

Numerous experiments have demonstrated the relationship between aging and renal function and mass.[16–18] The normal aging process is associated with a steady decline in renal function.[16,17] Classic insulin clearance studies by Davies and Shock demonstrated that GFR declines by about 8 mL/min/1.73 m^2 per decade starting in the fourth decade.[18] Moreover, renal senescence is associated with a progressive reduction in kidney weight with cortex being affected more than the medulla.[19] The decrease in renal mass with aging is also consistent with thinning of the cortical ribbon and the reduction in the number of glomeruli.[20–22] Up to 10% of glomeruli may be sclerotic in the healthy person younger than the age of 40.[23]

Given the normal steady deterioration in renal function and mass with aging, coupled with the adverse consequences of renal function due to chronic systemic diseases such as hypertension and atherosclerosis, renal preservation is paramount in patients with renal artery pathology; particularly in young patients with an otherwise normal life expectancy. The vast majority of patients included in published studies that specifically evaluated outcomes of complex renal artery lesions treated with surgical revascularization were young woman, in relatively good health with a normal life expectancy.[1–5,7,24] The demographic of this patient population not only underscores the importance of renal preservation over their lifetime, but mandates the surgical modality to be safe, efficacious, and durable. Our experience with the ex vivo technique for complex renal artery pathology meets these requirements by demonstrating preservation of renal function as well as renal mass.

Alternative approaches to complex renal artery pathology have been described. A small series was reported successfully utilizing laparoscopic nephrectomy modeled after live-donor transplant techniques with backbench ex vivo reconstruction and heterotopic implantation in the pelvis. Claimed advantages of this technique include less incisional morbidity and optimal surgical visualization at the back table allowing meticulous dissection and complex reconstruction of branch vessels. However, the putative advantages of this technique require an additional anastomosis between the ureter and bladder and the potential complications of leak or stricture formation. Furthermore, the potential development and progression of atherosclerotic occlusive disease of the iliac vessels in the relatively young population of patients requiring complex renal artery repair may compromise long term durability.

Recently, a primary use of endovascular repair for complex renal artery disease has been proposed.[25,26] Data with acceptable technical and clinical outcomes using endovascular approaches for lesions of the main renal artery due to atherosclerotic stenosis or fibromuscular dysplasia has been reported.[27–30] These results have led to several case reports and small series demonstrating technically successful treatment of more anatomically complex lesions. Though technically feasible, endovascular repair for complex renal artery lesions can be associated with post embolization syndrome, segmental renal ischemia, a decline in renal function and on occasion nephrectomy.[31–34] Zhang reported a series of 15 patients, 9 renal artery aneurysms and 6 renal artery arteriovenous fistulas, who were treated using coil embolization, stent grafting, or a combination of the two with a technical success of 100% and no mortality or major morbidity. However, 60% of patients experienced post-embolization syndrome and radiologic evidence of segmental renal infarct was found in 33% of patients over a mean imaging follow-up of 16 months. At a mean clinical follow up of 24 months; no evidence of renal insufficiency was detected based on serum creatinine levels.[31] A more sophisticated analysis of renal function and imaging data on preservation of renal mass were lacking. A more recent study of 40 patients compared endovascular intervention with open repair of renal artery aneurysms. Over a mean follow up of 36 months, both groups had equivalent perioperative morbidity and mortality, and similar freedom from reintervention. An adjusted mixed linear analysis of the rate of GFR change over time, however, demonstrated a significant decline in renal function (a decrease of 15 $mL/min/1.73\ m^2$ in GFR at 36 months) following endovascular intervention when compared to open repair (no decline).[26] These reports suggest additional data on late renal function and renal structure preservation is necessary before an endovascular approach is employed as the first-line strategy for complex renal artery disease.

CONCLUSION

This review describes the surgical repair of 24 kidneys with complex renal artery pathology in 23 consecutive patients over a 25-year period. Using ex vivo cold preservation techniques, complex renal artery lesions were repaired and reconstructed safely with minimal perioperative morbidity and no mortality. Anatomic durability was achieved with a 5 and 10-year primary patency rates of greater than 90% and over 90% of all patients with pre-existing hypertension were either cured or improved while antihypertensive medication requirements decreased. Finally, renal function and mass were preserved. This longitudinal experience documents the value of the ex vivo reconstructive technique for patients with complex renal artery pathology and argues for its preferential use in in the management of this challenging patient population.

REFERENCES

1. Dean RH, Meacham PW, Weaver FA. Ex vivo renal artery reconstructions: indications and techniques. *J Vasc Surg*. 1986;4(6):546–52.
2. Crutchley TA, Pearce JD, Craven TE, et al. Branch renal artery repair with cold perfusion protection. *J Vasc Surg*. 2007;46(3):405–12; discussion 12.
3. Barral X, Gournier JP, Frering V, et al. Dysplastic lesions of renal artery branches: late results of ex vivo repair. *Ann Vasc Surg*. 1992;6(3):225–31.
4. Murray SP, Kent C, Salvatierra O, Stoney RJ. Complex branch renovascular disease: management options and late results. *J Vasc Surg*. 1994;20(3):338–45; discussion 46.
5. Anderson CA, Hansen KJ, Benjamin ME, et al. Renal artery fibromuscular dysplasia: results of current surgical therapy. *J Vasc Surg*. 1995;22(3):207–15; discussion 15–6.
6. van Bockel JH, van den Akker PJ, Chang PC, et al. Extracorporeal renal artery reconstruction for renovascular hypertension. *J Vasc Surg*. 1991;13(1):101–10; discussion 10–1.
7. English WP, Pearce JD, Craven TE, et al. Surgical management of renal artery aneurysms. *J Vasc Surg*. 2004;40(1):53–60.
8. Ota K, Mori S, Awane Y, Ueno A. Ex situ repair of renal artery for renovascular hypertension. *Arch Surg*. 1967;94(3):370–3.
9. Gallagher KA, Phelan MW, Stern T, Bartlett ST. Repair of complex renal artery aneurysms by laparoscopic nephrectomy with ex vivo repair and autotransplantation. *J Vasc Surg*. 2008;48(6):1408–13.
10. Ham SW, Weaver FA. Ex vivo renal artery reconstruction for complex renal artery disease. *J Vasc Surg*. 2014;60(1):143–50.
11. Hood DB, Weaver FA. Orthotopic ex vivo renal artery reconstruction. *Am Surg*. 1994;60(10): 804–8.
12. Brekke IB, Flatmark A, Albrechtsen D, eds. *Extracorporeal Renal Surgery and Autotransplantation. Illustrated ed.* University of Michigan: Springer Verlag; 1997.
13. Cherr GS, Hansen KJ, Craven TE, et al. Surgical management of atherosclerotic renovascular disease. *J Vasc Surg*. 2002;35(2):236–45.
14. Klausner JQ, Lawrence PF, Harlander-Locke MP, et al. The contemporary management of renal artery aneurysms. *J Vasc Surg*. 2015;61(4):978–84.
15. Ham SW, Kumar SR, Wang BR, et al. Late outcomes of endovascular and open revascularization for nonatherosclerotic renal artery disease. *Arch Surg*. 2010;145(9):832–9.
16. Rodriguez-Puyol D. The aging kidney. *Kidney Int*. 1998;54(6):2247–65.
17. Zhou XJ, Rakheja D, Yu X, et al. The aging kidney. *Kidney Int*. 2008;74(6):710–20.
18. Davies DF, Shock NW. Age changes in glomerular filtration rate, effective renal plasma flow, and tubular excretory capacity in adult males. *JCI*. 1950;29(5):496–507.
19. Zhou XJ, Saxena R, Liu Z, et al. Renal senescence in 2008: progress and challenges. *Int Urol Nephrol*. 2008;40(3):823–39.
20. Hughson MD, Douglas-Denton R, Bertram JF, Hoy WE. Hypertension, glomerular number, and birth weight in African Americans and white subjects in the southeastern United States. *Kidney Int*. 2006;69(4):671–8.
21. Newbold KM, Sandison A, Howie AJ. Comparison of size of juxtamedullary and outer cortical glomeruli in normal adult kidney. *Virchows Arch A Pathol Anat Histopathol*. 1992;420(2):127–9.

22. Nyengaard JR, Bendtsen TF. Glomerular number and size in relation to age, kidney weight, and body surface in normal man. *Anat Rec.* 1992;232(2):194–201.
23. Kaplan C, Pasternack B, Shah H, Gallo G. Age-related incidence of sclerotic glomeruli in human kidneys. *Am J Pathol.* 1975;80(2):227–34.
24. Robinson WP, 3rd, Bafford R, Belkin M, Menard MT. Favorable outcomes with in situ techniques for surgical repair of complex renal artery aneurysms. *J Vasc Surg.* 2011;53(3):684–91.
25. Hislop SJ, Patel SA, Abt PL, et al. Therapy of renal artery aneurysms in New York State: outcomes of patients undergoing open and endovascular repair. *Ann Vasc Surg.* 2009;23(2):194–200.
26. Tsilimparis N, Reeves JG, Dayama A, et al. Endovascular vs open repair of renal artery aneurysms: outcomes of repair and long-term renal function. *JACS.* 2013;217(2):263–9.
27. Bush RL, Najibi S, MacDonald MJ, et al. Endovascular revascularization of renal artery stenosis: technical and clinical results. *J Vasc Surg.* 2001;33(5):1041–9.
28. Davies MG, Saad WE, Peden EK, et al. The long-term outcomes of percutaneous therapy for renal artery fibromuscular dysplasia. *J Vasc Surg.* 2008;48(4):865–71.
29. Kim HJ, Do YS, Shin SW, et al. Percutaneous transluminal angioplasty of renal artery fibromuscular dysplasia: mid-term results. *Korean J Radiol.* 2008;9(1):38–44.
30. Slovut DP, Olin JW. Fibromuscular dysplasia. *N Engl J Med.* 2004;350(18):1862–71.
31. Zhang Z, Yang M, Song L, et al. Endovascular treatment of renal artery aneurysms and renal arteriovenous fistulas. *J Vasc Surg.* 2013;57(3):765–70.
32. Gutta R, Lopes J, Flinn WR, Neschis DG. Endovascular embolization of a giant renal artery aneurysm with preservation of renal parenchyma. *Angiology.* 2008;59(2):240–3.
33. Altit R, Brown DB, Gardiner GA. Renal artery aneurysm and arteriovenous fistula associated with fibromuscular dysplasia: successful treatment with detachable coils. *JVIR.* 2009;20(8):1083–6.
34. Carmo M, Bower TC, Mozes G, et al. Surgical management of renal fibromuscular dysplasia: challenges in the endovascular era. *Ann Vasc Surg.* 2005;19(2):208–17.

36

Incidence and Treatment of Central Venous Catheter-Associated Upper Extremity DVT

Timothy K. Liem, MD, MBA and Jeffrey D. Crawford, MD

Peripherally inserted central catheters (PICC) and central venous catheters (CVC) provide reliable access for the administration of parenteral nutrition, long-term antibiotics, chemotherapy, and numerous other medications. They also provide convenient access for patients who require dialysis or frequent laboratory testing. These multiple utilities have led to the placement of over 5 million CVCs every year.[1] Over the past decade, many hospitals have developed specialized nursing teams, whose primary function has been the placement and maintenance of intravenous catheters and PICC lines. The ease with which these PICC line may be ordered, and the added convenience for patients, have contributed to the rapid expansion of PICC line usage as well.

The use of CVCs and PICC lines may be complicated by arterial injury and hemorrhage, pneumothorax and lymphatic injury, deep or superficial vein thrombosis, central-line-associated blood stream infection (CLABSI), and central vein stenosis (potentially compromising options for future dialysis access). Some of these complications may be reduced with the use of a variety of best practices for insertion and maintenance. For example, ultrasound-guided CVC insertion reduces the rate of arterial injury and pneumothorax, and the use of "central line bundles" for insertion and maintenance may decrease the rate of CLABSI.[2,3] More recently, several professional societies also have made attempts to reduce the rate of catheter-associated upper extremity deep vein thrombosis (CA-UEDVT). This chapter will focus on the incidence, prevention, and treatment of CA-UEDVT.

INCIDENCE AND CLINICAL SIGNIFICANCE OF CATHETER-ASSOCIATED UPPER EXTREMITY DVT

The reported incidence of CA-UEDVT varies significantly (2% to 67%), and depends upon many factors, including the study methodology. Prospective evaluations are more likely to perform routine upper extremity venous duplex scans, which will identify symptomatic and asymptomatic CA-UEDVT. However, only a small percentage of patients develop clinical manifestations (0% to 12%).[4,5] In contrast, retrospective studies demonstrate a lower rate of CA-UEDVT, since in this setting, duplex scans are more likely to be performed after patients develop symptoms of pain and edema. We performed a recent review, identifying that retrospective studies had a PICC-associated UEDVT incidence ranging from 1.6% to 3.9%, while prospective studies had a higher rate, ranging from 3.0% to 19.4%.[6] In addition, the incidence of CA-UEDVT will depend on the presence or absence of certain co-morbidities. Malignancy and chemotherapy, increased age, and prior DVT are associated with an increased risk for CA-UEDVT.[5,6] The more common inherited hypercoagulable conditions (Factor V Leiden and prothrombin gene mutation) also may have an association, but studies remain inconsistent, suggesting that any association with CA-UEDVT is likely to be mild.[7–9]

Several technical factors, and the clinical setting in which the central line was inserted also affect the incidence of CA-UEDVT. Technical factors such as increased catheter size, increased lumen number, tip location (brachiocephalic versus caval-atrial), insertion site (left > right, femoral > subclavian), catheter material (polyethylene), and catheter duration all have been associated with an increased risk of CA-UEDVT.[5,10,11] PICC lines that are place in the ICU are associated with a significantly higher rate of CA-UEDVT, when compared with lines that are placed in the non-ICU setting (13.91% vs 3.44%).[12] In addition, when evaluating only studies that directly compared the incidence of PICC versus centrally-inserted CVCs, the CA-UEDVT was significantly higher with PICCs (Odds Ratio 2.55, 95% CI: 1.54 – 4.23).[12] Numerous other risk factors for CA-UEDVT are shown in Table 36-1.

In recent studies, we defined catheter-associated UEDVT as a deep vein thrombus in the same vein as, or immediately adjacent to, a recently placed CVC or PICC (≤ 30 days). Using this definition, we found that 35% of all UEDVTs during a 12-month period were associated with a recent PICC line, and 20% were associated with a CVC.[6] Figure 36-1. Conversely, since over 2,000 PICC lines were placed during that same 12-month period, the rate of symptomatic PICC-associated UEDVT averaged 2.6%. This rate falls well within the 1.6% to 3.9% incidence that was seen in numerous other retrospective clinical studies.

The natural history of treated and untreated lower extremity DVT is better known than that of upper extremity DVT. The limited available data suggests that after treatment with 3 months of anticoagulation, upper extremity DVT has a lower likelihood of causing pulmonary embolization and recurrent thromboembolism. However, the rate of developing UEDVT-associated post-thrombotic syndrome remained significant, ranging from 7% to 46%. There is some suggestion that catheter-associated UEDVT may be associated with a slightly decreased risk for post-thrombotic syndrome.[13–16]

TABLE 36-1. RISK FACTORS FOR CATHETER-ASSOCIATED UPPER EXTREMITY DEEP VEIN THROMBOSIS

High Risk	Low-Moderate Risk
Critically ill in ICU	Tip not at cavoatrial junction
Active malignancy	Small vein caliber accessed by PICC
Prior VTE	Surgery with catheter in place
Hypercoagulable disorders	Prior catheterization
PICCs	No pharmacoprophylaxis (PICCs)
Prior chest radiation therapy	CVCs (Hickman > port; femoral v. > subclavian > IJ)
PICC in paretic arm	Diabetes
Triple or double lumen catheter	Renal failure
Vancomycin/amphotericin B/chemotherapy	COPD
	Obesity (BMI >30)
	Recent trauma
	Catheter associated infection
	Catheter tip not at caval-atrial junction
	Inflammatory bowel disease
	Longer catheter dwell time

ICU, intensive care unit; PICC, peripherally inserted central catheter; VTE, venous thromboembolism; v, vein; IJ, internal jugular; CVCs, central venous catheters; COPD, chronic obstructive pulmonary disease.

Infusates with extremes of pH (<5 or >9) or caustic medications are higher risk for upper extremity deep vein thrombosis.

Source: Adapted from Crawford JD, Liem TK, and Moneta GL. Management of catheter-associated upper extremity deep venous thrombosis. JVS Ven Lym Dis 2015; August [ePub ahead of print].

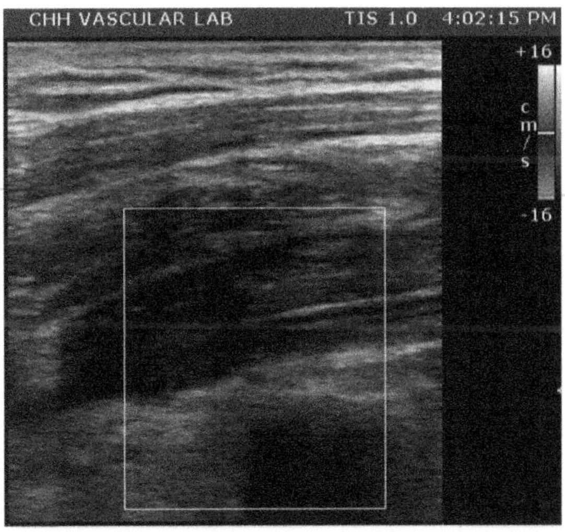

Figure 36-1. Duplex image of a subclavian vein with a PICC line and visible surrounding deep vein thrombosis.

PROPHYLAXIS AGAINST CATHETER-ASSOCIATED UEDVT

Prevention against CA-UEDVT begins with the judicious use of CVCs and PICC lines, and prompt removal when these catheters are no longer needed or functional. The Choosing Wisely® campaign, an initiative by the American Board of Internal Medicine in collaboration with various professional societies, has attempted to disseminate evidence-based recommendations for a variety of diagnoses and treatments.[17] The recommendations for the use of PICC lines are shown below:

1. Don't place, or leave in place, peripherally inserted central catheters for patient or provider convenience. (Society of General Internal Medicine).
2. Don't place peripherally inserted central catheters (PICC) in stage III-V CKD patients without consulting nephrology. (American Society of Nephrology).

Similarly, a position statement from the American Society of Diagnostic and Interventional Nephrology recommends to avoid PICC lines and subclavian-inserted CVCs in patients with chronic kidney disease stages III-V.[18] In these patients, the internal jugular (IJ) and external jugular veins are suggested for central access, and dorsal hand veins are suggested for phlebotomy and peripheral IVs. They also recommend that dialysis access should be coordinated with nephrology to minimize the need and duration of dialysis catheters.

If a PICC line is indicated, careful consideration should be given to the type of catheter to be used. The evidence is consistent that smaller catheter diameter and smaller lumen number are associated with lower rates of CA-UEDVT.[6,19–22] In addition, some preliminary data from our series of over 2000 PICC lines suggests that a cephalic PICC insertion site is associated with a higher rate of superficial vein thrombosis, but a lower rate of DVT.[6] However, the basilic and brachial veins still remain the most common sites for PICC insertion, probably related to several factors, including a greater ease of puncturing a larger target vein on ultrasound imaging, and a more direct route for passage of the catheter tip to the caval–atrial junction.

Some prospective trials demonstrate a mild benefit of thromboprophylaxis [fixed low-dose warfarin, prophylactic unfractionated heparin (UH) or low-molecular-weight heparin (LMWH)] compared to no prophylaxis, for prevention of *all* CVC-related UEDVT (symptomatic and asymptomatic). These same authors did not identify any benefit for prevention of *symptomatic* CVC-related UEDVT.[23] However, a Cochrane review of 12 randomized controlled trials (RCTs) failed to show a reduction in CVC-related UEDVT with prophylactic UH or low-dose warfarin, and thromboprophylaxis, therefore, is not recommended for CVCs.[24] The Jupiter trial in non-cancer patients and other studies in cancer patients have demonstrated decreased LEDVT with the use of statins by as much as 50%.[25,26] Statins reduce LEDVT by suppressing inflammatory mediators, but there is currently insufficient evidence to recommend statins for CA-UEDVT prevention.

TREATMENT OF CATHETER-ASSOCIATED UEDVT

The treatment of catheter-associated UEDVT is not well studied, and recommendations are largely based on extrapolation from data regarding lower extremity DVT (LEDVT). To date, there are no randomized clinical trials that have evaluated anticoagulation for initial and long-term therapy of CA-UEDVT. Because patients with UEDVT also may be at high risk for LEDVT, screening for LEDVT in patients with UEDVT may identify a clinically proven indication for short-term and intermediate-term anticoagulation. Based on the best available data, the 2012 American College of Chest Physicians (ACCP) Evidence-Based Clinical Practice Guidelines provide recommendations for the management of *acute* CA-UEDVT (Table 36-2).[27]

Of particular note, the Guidelines recommend *against* removal of the offending catheter unless it is no longer needed or nonfunctional (Grade 2C). This recommendation is in agreement with our experience, regarding the common reflex to remove the catheter and replacement it at a new access site. Although catheter removal is associated with improved thrombus resolution, the placement of a catheter at a different site is associated with an 86% incidence of developing CA-UEDVT at that new site.[28] This is a strong argument in favor of leaving the catheter in place, if it is functional and if there is ongoing need. A second caveat from the ACCP Guidelines also recommends continued anticoagulation, as long as the catheter remains in place, as opposed to a fixed-duration of therapy.[27]

New oral anticoagulants are FDA approved for VTE prophylaxis and treatment, but have not been studied for CA-UEDVT. Bleeding risk in CA-UEDVT specifically is not well-studied. However, small retrospective and prospective cohort studies suggest that major bleeding risk is slightly lower in the treatment of UEDVT compared to LEDVT with a rate of 2.0%–4.1% with either dalteparin or warfarin, compared to 4.9% for LEDVT.[29–31] Catheter-directed thrombolysis (CDT) for acute UEDVT has been evaluated only in retrospective and small prospective studies, and is not generally recommended except for patients with severe, acute (<14 days) symptoms and low bleeding risk (Grade 1C).[27] We rarely offer CDT to patients with catheter-associated UEDVT, since most patients usually have some relative or absolute contraindication to thrombolysis (e.g. recent surgery, active or recent malignancy, active infection). In addition, the rate of post-thrombotic syndrome seems to be lower with CA-UEDVT, when compared with non-catheter-associated thrombosis. There is no role for SVC filters in the management of CA-UEDVT as the risk of death from PE is believed to be extremely low and SVC filters carry significant risk of complications.[32]

TABLE 36-2. SUMMARY OF AMERICAN COLLEGE OF CHEST PHYSICIANS RECOMMENDATIONS REGARDING THE MANAGEMENT OF *ACUTE CATHETER-ASSOCIATED UPPER EXTREMITY DEEP VEIN THROMBOSIS*. LMWH, LOW-MOLECULAR-WEIGHT HEPARIN; IV, INTRAVENOUS; SC, SUBCUTANEOUS

1. **Acute UEDVT that involves the axillary or more proximal veins:** we recommend acute treatment with parenteral anticoagulation (LMWH, fondaparinux, IV unfractionated heparin, or SC unfractionated heparin) over no such treatment (Grade 1B).
2. **Most patients with UEDVT that is associated with a central venous catheter:** we suggest that the catheter NOT be removed if it is functional and there is an ongoing need for the catheter (Grade 2C).
3. **UEDVT that is associated with a central venous catheter that is removed:** we recommend 3 months of anticoagulation over a longer duration of therapy in patient with no cancer (Grade 1B), and we suggest this in patient with cancer (Grade 2C).
4. **UEDVT that is associated with a central venous catheter that is NOT removed:** we recommend that anticoagulation is continued as long as the central venous catheter remains in patients with cancer (Grade 1C), and we suggest this in patients with no cancer (Grade 2C).

Source: Adapted from Kearon C, et al. Antithrombotic Therapy for VTE Disease: Antithrombotic Therapy and Prevention of Thrombosis, 9th ed: American College of Chest Physicians Evidence-Based Clinical Practice Guidelines. Chest 2012; 141: e419S–e494S.

CONCLUSIONS

Upper extremity DVT is a common complication in patients who receive CVCs and PICC lines, with PICC lines having a slightly greater association with thrombosis. These catheters must be used judiciously, and not just for patient or provider convenience. Physicians and surgeons should be well versed with the various sizes and types of catheters which are being placed in their patients, and they should be familiar with clinical and technical factors that are associated with the development of UEDVT. Treatment consists of anticoagulation for at least 3 months, longer if the CVC or PICC line is left in place. If central venous access still is needed, and the catheter is functional, the access should NOT be removed, since a policy of remove and replace at another site is associated with a very high rate of thrombosis at the new access site.

REFERENCES

1. Radd I. Intravascular-catheter-related infections. *The Lancet*. 1998;351(9106):893–8.
2. Hind D, Calvert N, McWilliams R, et al. Ultrasonic locating devices for central venous cannulation: Meta-analysis. *BMJ*. 2003;327:361.
3. Guidelines for the prevention of intravascular catheter-related infections, 2011. http://www.cdc.gov/hicpac/pdf/guidelines/bsi-guidelines-2011.pdf. Updated 2011. Accessed June 2015.
4. Periard D, Monney P, Waeber G, et al. Randomized controlled trial of peripherally inserted central catheters vs. peripheral catheters for middle duration in-hospital intravenous therapy. *J Thromb Haemost*. 2008;6:1281–8.
5. Van Rooden CJ, Tesselaar MET, Osanto S, Rosendaal FR, Huisman MV. Deep vein thrombosis associated with central venous catheters – a review. *J Thromb Haemost*. 2005;3:2409–19.
6. Liem TK, Yanit KE, Moseley SE, et al. Peripherally inserted central catheter usage pattersn and associated symptomatic upper extremity venous thrombosis. *J Vasc Surg*. 2012;55(3):761–7.
7. Van Rooden CJ, Rosendaal RF, Barge RM, et al. Central venous catheter related thrombosis in haematology patietns and prediction of risk by screening with Doppler-ultrasound. *Br J Haematol*. 2003;123:507–12.
8. Fijnheer R, Paijmans B, Verdonck LF, et al. Factor V Leiden in central venous catehter-associated thrombosis. *Br J Haematol*. 2002;118:267–70.
9. Riordan M, Weiden P. Factor V Leiden mutation does not account for central venous catheter-related thrombosis. *Am J Hematol*. 1998;58:150–2.
10. De Cicco M, Matovic M, Balestreri L, et al. Central venous thrombosis: an early and frequent complication in cancer patients bearing long-term silastic catheter. A prospective study. *Thromb Res*. 1997;86:101–13.
11. Gould JR, Carloss HW, Skinner WL. Groshong cathteter-associated subclavian venous thrombosis. *Am J Med*. 1993;95:419–23.
12. Chopra V, Anand S, Hickner A, et al. Risk of venous thromboembolism associated with peripherally inserted central catheters" a systematic review and meta-analysis. *Lancet*. 2013;382:311–25.
13. Prandoni P, Polistena P, Bernardi E, et al. Upper-extremity deep vein thrombosis. Risk factors, diagnosis, and complications. *Arch Intern Med*. 1997;157(1):57–62.
14. Prandoni P, Bernardi E, Marchiori A, et al. The long term clinical course of acute deep vein thrombosis of the arm: prospective cohort study. *BMJ*. 2004;329(7464):484–5.
15. Kahn SR, Elman EA, Bornais C, et al. Post-thrombotic syndrome, functional disability and quality of life after upper extremity deep venous thrombosis in adults. *Thromb Haemost*. 2005;93(3):499–502.

16. Elman EE, Kahn SR. The post-thrombotic syndrome after upper extremity deep venous thrombosis in adults: A systematic review. *Thromb Res.* 2006;117:609–14.
17. American Board of Internal Medicine. Choosing Wisely®. http://www.choosingwisely.org. Updated June 2015. Accessed June 15, 2015.
18. Hoggard J, Saad T, Schon D, et al. Guidelines for venous access in patients with chronic kidney disease. A Position Statement from the American Society of Diagnostic and Interventional Nephrology, Clinical Practice Committee and the Association for Vascular Access. *Sem Dialysis.* 2008;21(2):186–91.
19. Grove JR, Pevec WC. Venous thrombosis related to peripherally inserted central catheters. *J Vasc Interv Radiol.* 2000;11(7):837–40.
20. Evans RS, Sharp JH, Linford LH, et al. Risk of symptomatic DVT associated with peripherally inserted central catheters. *Chest.* 2010;138(4):803–10.
21. Evans RS, Sharp JH, Linford LH, et al. Reduction of peripherally inserted central catheter-associated DVT. *Chest.* 2013;143(3):627–33.
22. O'Brien J, Paquet F, Lindsay R, Valenti D. Insertion of PICCs with minimum number of lumens reduces complications and costs. *JACR.* 2013;10(11):864–8.
23. Kirkpatrick A, Rathbun S, Whitsett T, Raskob G. Prevention of central venous catheter-associated thrombosis: a meta-analysis. *Am J Med.* 2007;120(10):901.e1–13.
24. Akl EA, Karmath G, Yosuico V, et al. Anticoagulation for thrombosis prophylaxis in cancer patients with central venous catheters. *The Cochrane database of systematic reviews.* 2007(3):CD006468.
25. Glynn RJ, Danielson E, Fonseca FA, et al. A randomized trial of rosuvastatin in the prevention of venous thromboembolism. *N Eng J Med.* 2009;360(18):1851–61.
26. Lotsch F, Konigsbrugge O, Posch F, et al. Statins are associated with low risk of venous thromboembolism in patients with cancer: a prospective and observational cohort study. *Thromb Res.* 2014;134(5):1008–13.
27. Kearon C, Akl EA, Comerota AJ, et al. Antithrombotic therapy for VTE disease: Antithrombotic therapy and prevention of thrombosis, 9th ed: American college of chest physicians evidence-based clinical practice guidelines. *Chest.* 2012;141(2 Suppl): e419S–94S.
28. Jones MA, Lee DY, Segall JA, et al. Characterizing resolution of catheter-associated upper extremity deep venous thrombosis. *J Vasc Surg.* 2010;51(1);108–13.
29. Rathbun SW, Stoner JA, Whitsett TL. Treatment of upper-extremity deep vein thrombosis. *J Thromb Haemost.* 2011;9(10):1924–30.
30. Savage KJ, Wells PS, Schulz V, et al. Outpatient use of low molecular weight heparin (Dalteparin) for the treatment of deep vein thrombosis of the upper extremity. *Thromb Haemost.* 1999;82(3):1008–10.
31. Munoz FJ, Mismetti P, Poggio R, et al. Clinical outcome of patients with upper-extremity deep vein thrombosis: results from the RIETE Registry. *Chest.* 2008;133(1):143–8.
32. Owens CA, Bui JT, Knuttinen MG, Gaba RC, Carrillo TC. Pulmonary embolism from upper extremity deep vein thrombosis and the role of superior vena cava filters: a review of the literature. *JVIR.* 2010;21(6):779–87.

37

Surgical Management of Lymphedema

Amanda K. Silva, MD and David W. Chang, MD

Lymphedema is a chronic, debilitating disease affecting up to 250 million people worldwide. It is caused by an accumulation of lymphatic fluid leading to progressive fibrosis, fat hypertrophy, and destruction of lymphatic vessels. Affected skin becomes prone to ulcerations and infections. It may be classified as primary due to abnormal development of the lymphatics or secondary due to damage to the lymphatic system. Globally, the most common cause is filariasis, but in the United States and developing countries, cancer and its treatments are the most common cause. There is currently no cure for this disease and we are still searching for the "gold" standard treatment for lymphedema. One of the current, most common treatments for lymphedema is complex decongestive lymphatic therapy including compression garments. These therapies are not ideal given they are labor intensive, time consuming, expensive, and often not covered by insurance. They also require strict lifetime compliance, which leads to high rates of non-compliance and patient dissatisfaction. Surgery is indicated when conservative measures fail. Goals of surgical intervention include weight reduction of the affected region, reduced frequency of infections, prevention of disease progression, and improvement in limb function and cosmesis.

EVALUATION TECHNIQUES

There are many modalities in place to evaluate lymphedema. The International Society of Lymphology has created a clinical staging system to help document disease progression. In stage I the limb is swollen, feels heavy, and has pitting edema partially reversible with elevation. In stage II the limb is swollen, the skin is brawny, and tissue fibrosis has started, leading non-pitting edema not reversible with elevation. In stage III there is enormous swelling of the involved extremity with fibrosis and hardening of the dermal tissues. Skin papillomas, acanthosis, fat deposits, and warty overgrowths may be present. The most common tool for evaluation of lymphedema is lymphoscintigraphy, in which a radioactive dye is injected into the affected limb to visualize the lymphatics and quantify the lymphatic flow by calculating a lymphatic transport index. The index ranges from 0 (optimal flow) to 45 (no flow). A transport index below 10 is considered normal. Indocyanine green (ICG) lymphangiography is a newer technology to help us visualize superficial lymphatics and determine the severity of the disease. ICG is a fluorescent dye that is activated when it binds to protein and imaged using near-infrared technology. A staging system has been proposed based on ICG lymphangiography findings.[1] In stage 1 disease, there are many patent lymphatic vessels, with minimal, patchy dermal backflow. Stage 2 disease shows a moderate number of patent lymphatic vessels, with segmental dermal backflow. Stage 3 disease shows few patent lymphatic vessels, with extensive dermal backflow involving the entire arm. Stage 4 disease shows no patent lymphatic vessels, with severe dermal backflow involving the entire arm and extending to the dorsum of the hand. Knowing the lymphedema disease stage helps guide appropriate surgical intervention. Postoperatively, one of the most common and simple methods to determine improvement is to perform serial circumferential measurements or limb volumes. Other means to measure outcomes include bioimpedence and quality of life questionnaires.

SURGICAL MANAGEMENT

There are two major categories of lymphatic surgery: reductive or excisional and physiologic.

Reductive/Excisional Techniques

Excision

In 1912, Charles wrote a book chapter entitled "Elephantiasis Scroti" in which he described a treatment for scrotal lymphedema that he had learned while spending time in Calcutta with his mentor McLeod. This procedure involved excision of the lymphedematous scrotal tissue and coverage with thigh advancement flaps. Charles suggested this technique could be applied to treat lymphedema in other areas of the body including the lower extremities, but would require preoperative arrangements for skin graft coverage. This idea of treating lower extremity lymphedema with radical excision down to deep fascia and covering with a skin graft wasn't actually reported until 1940, when Macey from the Mayo Clinic published his experience. What we currently consider the "Charles Procedure" was reported in 1947 by Poth from Galveston, who reported utilizing the skin from the excised specimen to cover the exposed limb.[2] Although this procedure does effectively treat lymphedema, it is an extensive surgery that comes with a high level of co-morbidity including significant blood loss and fluid shifts, chronic infections, poor skin graft take; and poor cosmesis with contour irregularities and severe scarring (Figure 37-1). It is still used today, but it is for reserved for severe cases not amenable to other techniques. An alternative, more safe method is to perform staged excisions.

Liposuction

Another reductive technique to treat lymphedema was proposed in 1989, when O'Brien reported the treatment of lower extremity lymphedema with liposuction in a series of patients. He noted an approximately 20% volume reduction at about 10 months follow-up.[3] In 1998, Brorson and Svensson used this technique to treat clinical stage II upper extremity lymphedema and noted a 104% versus 47% reduction when liposuction was combined with compression therapy versus compression therapy alone. This result was maintained at 4 years follow-up. The patients who received liposuction also had a significant decease in the number of cellulitis episodes.[4] Liposuction carries the theoretical risk of damaging the remaining lymphatics, but cadaveric and imaging studies have shown performing liposuction in a longitudinal direction to the affected limb reduces this risk.[5] In general, liposuction for lymphedema is safe and patients can expect a quick recovery. There is less evidence for efficacy in lower extremity cases and the major disadvantage of this technique is patients must continuously wear compression garments otherwise there is rapid reaccumulation of fluid.[4] Indications for liposuction to treat lymphedema include later stage lymphedema with fibrosis that has failed conservative management. Patients must also be aware of and compliant with the need for continued compression garments postoperatively.

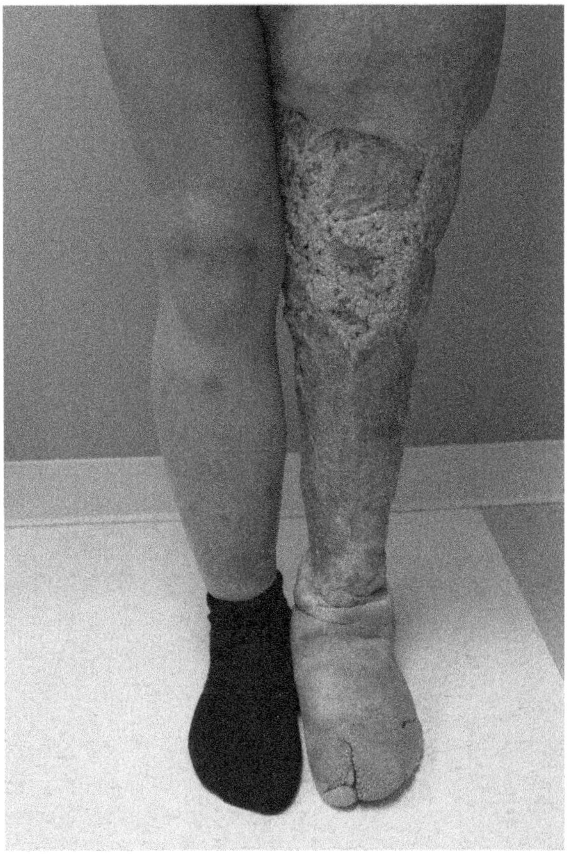

Figure 37-1. While the Charles procedure does effectively treat lymphedema, it is an extensive surgery that comes with a high level of co-morbidity, including significant blood loss and fluid shifts, poor skin graft take, and poor cosmesis with contour irregularities and severe scarring.

Physiologic Techniques

Another approach to surgically treat lymphedema is to create a new path for lymphatic drainage or repair the lymphatic dysfunction. This concept was first described by Kondoleon in 1912 and expounded upon by Sistrunk in 1927. The technique they described was an attempt to form a spontaneous connection between the superficial and deep lymphatic vessels by excising tissue on the affected limb including extensive removal of the deep fascia.[6] Thompson further developed this idea by burying de-epithelialized skin flaps from the excision along the neurovascular bundle to promote lymphangiogenesis.[7] Although these reports displayed new concepts and successfully treated lymphedema in many patients, there was no objective evidence that these procedures were in fact successful in creating a bridge between the superficial and deep lymphatic systems.

Flap interposition

In 1935, Gilles and Fraser described a two-staged procedure that involved moving healthy tissue from the arm to the groin of the affected lower extremity.[8] In 1974, Goldsmith further applied this concept by using pedicled omentum flaps tunneled through the subcutaneous tissue in the torso to treat upper or lower extremity lymphedema. He reported good subjective results in about 50% of his cases, but no objective evidence, and this procedure was fraught with many complications.[9] Many other flap interpositions have been described using various donor sites, but none have gained popularity due to unpredictable outcomes.

Lymphatic bypass

In 1962, Jacobson first described the idea of creating a lymphovenous shunt, which he performed in a canine model.[10] A few years later, Sedlacek performed end to side lymphovenous bypasses using the saphenous vein in patients with lymphedema due to filariasis.[11] His results, as well as others, highlighted the issue of too high back flow in large recipient veins. Later, Yamada reported a series of canine model cases and one human patient where microsurgery techniques were used to perform lymphovenous anastomosis to the saphenous vein and saphenous vein branches were ligated to reduce back flow. This highlighted the importance of using microsurgical technique for anastomosis and anastomosing to low flow venules instead of high flow systems.[12]

Another approach to attempt to bypass the diseased lymphatics was suggested by Ho in which the saphenous vein and accompanying lymphatics were harvested and transferred to the affected limb. Proximal and distal lymphatic anastomoses were made to bypass the damaged extremity lymphatics.[13] Baumeister and Suida, used a similar technique, and they showed an 80% volume reduction at 3 years follow-up. Additionally, lymphoscintigraphy showed new patterns of lymph flow and a 30% faster clearance.[14] Of note, this technique was thought to only be successful if it was performed prior to permanent damage to the lymphatic system from chronic high lymphatic pressure and recurrent infections. Eventually, due to the risk of donor site lymphedema, this method fell out of favor.[15]

Overtime, lymphovenous bypass has proved to be the preferred method of lymphatic bypass. As with other methods of treatment for lymphedema, it has been difficult to standardize objective outcomes data. Most studies have quoted a decreased cellulitis rate, volumetrics have shown at best a 75% decrease in 73% of patients to at worst no change in 50% of patients, with an average volume reduction of 55%.[1] A recent meta-analysis identified 22 studies that have reported outcomes using lymphovenous bypass. Two of these studies reported level III evidence and the remaining were level IV. Pooled results have shown 89% of patients report a subjective improvement, 88% experience a quantitative improvement, and 56% of patients were able to discontinue compression therapy. In addition to the reported benefits, the surgery has low complication rates including the need for an additional procedure (10%), lymphorrhea (4%), and cellulitis (4%).[16] Although helpful in summarizing outcomes, these results should be interpreted with scrutiny given the great amount of heterogeneity between the studies. In a recent report of the senior author's experience with 100 patients undergoing lymphovenous bypass (89 upper extremity, 11 lower extremity) symptom improvement was reported in 96% of patients and quantitative improvement was noted by 74%. The overall mean volume differential reduction at 12 months follow-up was 42%. This reduction was significantly larger in patients with earlier stage (stage 1 or 2) versus later stage (stage 3 or 4) lymphedema as determine with indocyanine green (61% versus 17%).[1] Lymphovenous bypass alone is best indicated in patients with mild to moderate upper extremity lymphedema where there are still some functioning lymphatic vessels and there is minimal tissue fibrosis.

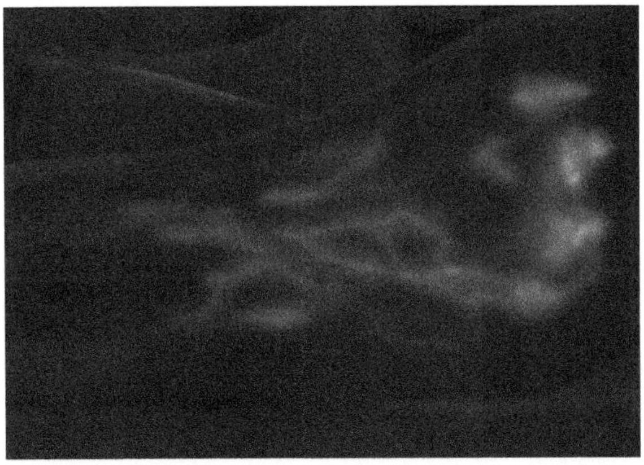

Figure 37-2. ICGN is injected into the dermis of the web space and superficial lymphatics are evaluated with near-infrared fluorescence. ICGN lymphangiography is useful in identifying functioning lymphatic channels for potential bypass.

The following is the author's preferred method for lymphovenous bypass. After the patient is anesthetized, indocyanine green (ICG) is injected into the dermis of the web space and superficial lymphatics are evaluated with near-infrared fluorescence. In early stage disease, it is easy to identify discrete functioning lymphatic channels. In late stage disease significant dermal back flow is present. Veins are identified as dark segments crossing over lymphatics and marked as good potential bypass sites (Figure 37-2). Dissection is performed under the microscope in the superficial subcutaneous plane to locate a good venule and lymph channel. Lymphatics are confirmed with isosulfan blue and ICG. Once a bypass site is determined, the lymphatic is anastomosed to the venule using 11-0 nylon under high magnification. If possible, it is preferable to perform the anastomosis in an end-to-side manner. It is thought that this is a more favorable flow pattern for the lymph to empty into the venule than end-to-end. After the anastomosis is complete the patency is confirmed with isosulfan blue and ICG (Figure 37-3). The incision is closed under the microscope as well to ensure no damage to the delicate superficial anastomosis. Postoperatively, the patient's limb is wrapped by the lymphedema physical therapist. Wrapping is performed in lieu of compression garments for about 1 month postoperatively to avoid shear injury to the delicate anastamoses.[1]

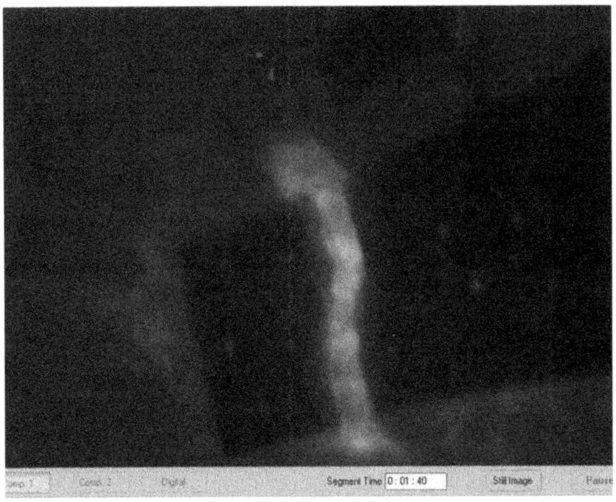

Figure 37-3. After the anastomosis is complete the patency is confirmed with isosulfan blue and ICG.

Vascularized lymph node transfer

Another approach to treating lymphedema is to replenish the missing lymph nodes of the affected extremity by harvesting healthy lymph nodes from one area of the body and transplanting them to either the affected basin or a non-anatomic area on the affected limb. This was first reported in humans by Clodius in 1982 for treatment of lower extremity lymphedema in two patients. In the first patient, a pedicled groin flap including the inguinal lymph nodes was transferred to the contralateral inguinal region of the affected lower extremity resulting in a stable volume reduction. In the second patient, a free groin flap was transferred to the medial knee to bridge a lymphatic defect caused by trauma. This patient initially experienced limb volume reduction, but his lymphedema recurred within 6 months postoperatively.[17] Since then, many surgeons have worked at perfecting the technique. In 2006, Becker reported favorable long-term outcomes in 24 patients who underwent free transfer of nodes from the groin to either the axilla or elbow of the affected upper extremity, including objective evidence of functioning transplanted lymph nodes with lymphoscintigraphy in 30% of the patients.[18] Saaristo combined vascularized lymph node transfer with autologous breast reconstruction and also reported favorable outcomes, with one-third of patients no longer needing compression therapy and evidence of improved lymphatic flow on lymphoscintigraphy in five of six cases.[19] The mechanism by which vascularized lymph node transfer works is unclear, either the lymph nodes act as a sponge to absorb lymphatic fluid or they induce lymphangiogenesis.[20] It does seem however, that preserving the vascular supply is necessary and results in greater improvement.[21] Therefore rather than just grafting the lymph nodes, they are harvested with a vascular pedicle, transferred, and anastomosed to the recipient artery and vein, however it is thought that it is unnecessary to reconnect the actual lymphatics.

There are many options for potential donor sites for this surgery. The groin is the most common, but thoracic, submental, and supraclavicular nodes as well as the omentum have been used as well. The other consideration when performing this surgery is where to place the transplanted tissue in the affected limb: anatomic versus non-anatomic. The theory behind placement in non-anatomic sites is that they work as a "lymphatic pump". Pulsations from the arterial anastomosis act as a pump providing a strong hydrostatic force into the flap and then the low-pressure flap vein acts as suction. Since lymph has lower colloid osmotic pressure than blood, lymphatic fluid is drawn into the capillaries. It is also theorized that a "catchment" effect is at play with non-anatomic placement as well. Distal flap placement allows gravitational drainage of the limb, and as interstitial pressures normalize old lymphatic channels may open allowing improved lymphatic drainage. Proponents of non-anatomic placement also believe it is better to avoid the scarred bed present in anatomic placement. A disadvantage to non-anatomic placement is the presence of a visible, bulky flap on the extremity. It also is commonly difficulty to primarily close the recipient site due to compression on the pedicle and skin grafts are often needed. The advantages of anatomic placement are excision of scar tissue, which is likely contributing to the lymphedema and placement of healthy vascularized lymph nodes to promote lymphangiogenesis where lymphatics are known to be deficient. Additionally there is abundant surrounding soft tissue to allow easy closure and the scar is usually well-hidden. In the upper extremity, vascularized lymph nodes have been placed in the axilla, elbow, or wrist. In the lower extremity, vascularized lymph nodes have been placed in the ankle, knee, or groin.[22]

A recent meta-analysis looked at 5 quantitative studies reporting outcomes with vascularized lymph node transfer. One of these studies provided level III evidence and the remaining were level IV. 100% of patients reported subjective improvement, 91%

had a quantitative improvement, and 78% were able to discontinue compression therapy. Complications included infection (8%), lymphorrhea (15%), re-exploration (3%), and need for additional procedures (36%).[16] As mentioned previously, although helpful in summarizing outcomes, these results should be interpreted with scrutiny given the great amount of heterogeneity between the studies. The largest series included in the meta-analysis was from Becker who reported experience with 24 patients.[18] Since then, that group has reported operating on 1500 patients with an average 3-year follow-up, and they have briefly commented on their outcomes, although they have not published detailed results. They reported 98% of patients have some degree of improvement, with 40% of clinical stage 1 or 2 patients experiencing normalization of their affected extremity.[23] Indications for vascularized lymph node transfer include fibrosis that precludes performing lymphovenous bypass, evidence of total occlusion on lymphoscintigraphy or clinical stage 2 lymphedema with a history of repeated episodes of cellulitis.

For isolated extremity lymphedema, the senior author tends to harvest the supraclavicular nodes and place the tissue in the anatomic location. It is important to excise all scar in the recipient site as it hinders lymphatic flow and inhibits lymphangiogenesis. If it is difficult to access or remove scar in the anatomic location, the author's preference is to place the vascularized lymph nodes just distal on the limb to the site of lymphatic obstruction. For example in a patient who had removal of pelvic lymph nodes via laparotomy, the flap would be placed in the proximal thigh along the femoral artery and saphenous vein. Additionally if a patient has no definitive site of injury or primary lymphedema with edema localized to the distal limb, the author prefers to place lymph nodes at the medial portion of the leg along the posterior tibial vessels as opposed to the dorsum of the ankle. This results in a less bulky flap and allows better ease in wearing shoes. The supraclavicular nodes are based off the transverse cervical artery located at the midpoint between the acromial-clavicular joint and the sternal notch (Figure 37-4). The external jugular vein can be harvested with the nodes as well if adequate vena comitantes are not present with the artery. Dissection of this flap can be tedious, and care must be taken to avoid injury to the lymphatic ducts. Additionally, a skin paddle is usually not included in the flap design as it is not reliable.[24]

If a large skin paddle is required or the patient has had a previous mastectomy and desires breast reconstruction in addition to vascularized lymph node transfer for upper extremity lymphedema, the author will harvest the superficial lateral groin lymph nodes based off the superficial circumflex iliac vessels. The lateral, superficial groin lymph nodes are harvested for transfer leaving behind the deeper lymph nodes that drain the leg. The desired nodes are usually located deep to Scarpa's fascia within a 3 cm radius of a point 3 cm inferior and perpendicular to a point 1/3 the distance from the pubic tubercle to the anterior superior iliac spine, clustered at the junction of the superior inferior epigastric and superficial

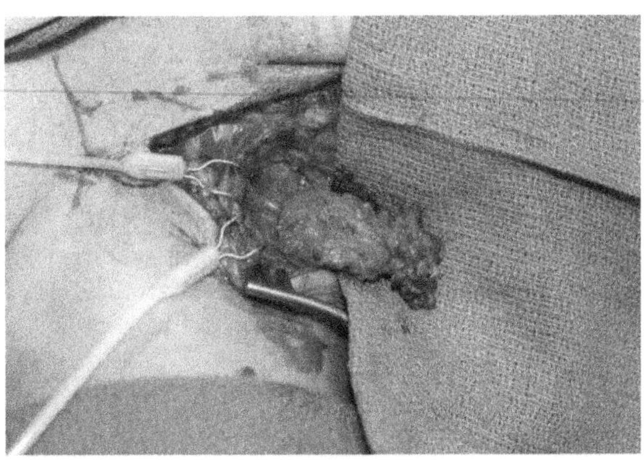

Figure 37-4. Supraclavicular nodes are a good source for vascularized lymph nodes.

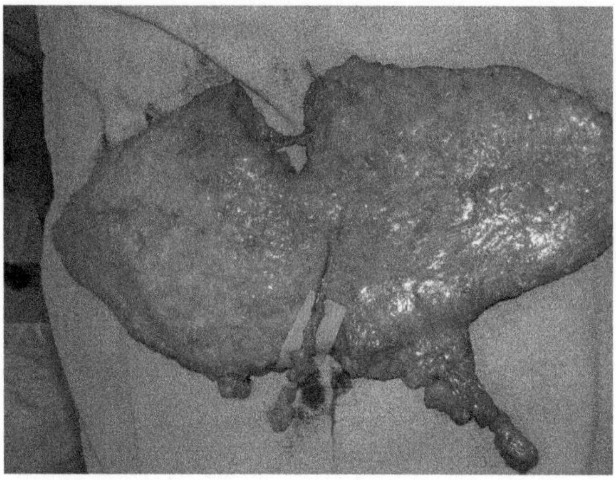

Figure 37-5. Lymph nodes adjacent to superficial cirmflex iliac vessels can be harvested together with free abdominal flap for combined breast reconstruction and lymph node transfer.

circumflex iliac veins (Figure 37-5). Reverse lymphatic mapping with Technetium and indocyanine green is performed to decrease the risk of causing donor site lymphedema. In combined breast reconstruction cases, this tissue is taken as an extension of the abdominal tissue based on the deep inferior epigastric system used to reconstruct the breast. In these cases, the superficial circumflex iliac vein is anastomosed in the axilla in addition to the arterial and venous anastomosis of the deep inferior epigastric vessels to the internal mammary vessels for the breast reconstruction.[22]

PROPHYLACTIC SURGERY

As we have gained more experience with lymphatic surgery, the idea of prophylactic surgery has been proposed. Boccardo et al. have proposed a procedure named LYMPHA (lymphatic microsurgical preventing healing approach). This involves anastomosing arm lymphatics to a collateral branch of the axillary vein at the time of nodal dissection to prevent lymphedema. They have reported 4-year outcomes in 74 patients undergoing this procedure and only 3 patients have developed lymphedema determined by volumetry and lymphoscintigraphy.[25] This 4% risk of lymphedema compares favorably to the 13% 65% incidence of lymphedema in women undergoing axillary lymph node dissection. Although these results are intriguing, further study needs to be performed before this can truly be determine to be efficacious or oncological safe.

CONCLUSIONS

Lymphedema is a debilitating disease that to date has been very difficult to successfully treat. New surgical techniques including lymphovenous bypass and vascularized lymph node transfer offer great promise in helping control disease and free patients from labor intensive compression treatment. To better understand the effects and potential benefits of these procedures we need to report standardized grading and outcomes. Although these techniques show promise, they are best utilized before extensive fibrosis sets in. There is still a role for older excisional techniques in late-stage lymphedema. Table 37-1 summarizes the indications and outcomes of surgical options for lymphedema.

TABLE 37-1. RECOMMENDED INDICATIONS AND OUTCOMES FOR LYMPHEDEMA SURGERY

Surgery	Recommended Indication	Outcomes
Excision and skin graft	Severe end-stage lymphedema	Resolution of lymphedema Significant blood loss and fluid shifts Poor cosmesis
Liposuction	Later clinical stage (II-III) lymphedema that has failed conservative management Patient willing to comply to continued compression garments Best in upper extremity	Decreased cellulitis significant volume reduction Must wear compression postoperatively
Lymphovenous bypass	Mild upper extremity lymphedema with moderate amount of functioning lymphatics and minimal fibrosis (ICG stage 2)	Decreased cellulitis variable subjective improvement variable quantitative improvement variable volume reduction
Vascularized lymph node transfer	Fibrosis which precludes performing lymphovenous bypass Evidence of total occlusion on lymphoscintigraphy Advanced lymphedema with a history of repeated episodes of cellulitis	variable subjective improvement variable quantitative improvement variable volume reduction

REFERENCES

1. Chang DW, Suami H, Skoracki R. A prospective analysis of 100 consecutive lymphovenous bypass cases for treatment of extremity lymphedema. *Plast Reconstr Surg*. 2013;132:1305–14.
2. Dumanian GA, Futrell JW. The Charles procedure: misquoted and misunderstood since 1950. *Plast Reconstr Surg*. 1996;98:1258–63.
3. O'Brien BM, Khazanchi RK, Kumar PA, et al. Liposuction in the treatment of lymphoedema; a preliminary report. *Br J Plast Surg*. 1989;42:530–3.
4. Brorson H, Svensson H. Liposuction combined with controlled compression therapy reduces arm lymphedema more effectively than controlled compression therapy alone. *Plast Reconstr Surg*. 1998;102:1058–67. discussion 68.
5. Frick A, Hoffmann JN, Baumeister RG, et al. Liposuction technique and lymphatic lesions in lower legs: anatomic study to reduce risks. *Plast Reconstr Surg*. 1999;103:1868–73. discussion 74–5.
6. Sistrunk WE. Contribution to Plastic Surgery: removal of scars by stages; an open operation for extensive laceration of the anal sphincter; the Kondoleon operation for elephantiasis. *Ann Surg*. 1927;85:185–93.
7. Thompson N. Buried dermal flap operation for chronic lymphedema of the extremities. Ten-year survey of results in 79 cases. *Plast Reconstr Surg*. 1970;45:541–8.
8. Gilles H. The lymphatic wick. *Proc R Soc Med*. 1950;43:1054-56.
9. Goldsmith HS. Long term evaluation of omental transposition for chronic lymphedema. *Ann Surg*. 1974;180:847–49.
10. Jacobson JH, Suarez EL. Microvascular Surgery. *Dis of Chest*. 1962;41:220–4.
11. Sedlacek J. Lymphovenous shunt as supplementary treatment of elephantiasis of lower limbs. *Acta Chir Plast*. 1969;11:157–62.
12. Yamada Y. Studies on lymphatic venous anastomosis in lymphedema. *Nagoya J Med Sci*. 1969;32:1–21.

13. Ho LC, Lai MF, Kennedy PJ. Micro-lymphatic bypass in the treatment of obstructive lymphoedema of the arm: case report of a new technique. *Br J Plast Surg.* 1983;36:350–7.
14. Baumeister RG, Siuda S. Treatment of lymphedemas by microsurgical lymphatic grafting: what is proved? *Plast Reconstr Surg.* 1990;85:64–74.
15. Campisi C. Use of autologous interposition vein graft in management of lymphedema: preliminary experimental and clinical observations. *Lymphology.* 1991;24:71–6.
16. Basta MN, Gao LL, Wu L. Operative Treatment of peripheral lymphedema: Aa systematic meta-analysis of the efficacy and safety of lymphovenous microsurgery and tissue transplantation. *Plast Reconstr Surg.* 2014;133:905–13.
17. Clodius L, Smith PJ, Bruna J, et al. The lymphatics of the groin flap. *Ann Plast Surg.* 1982;9:447–58.
18. Becker C, Assouad J, Riquet M, et al. Postmastectomy lymphedema: Long-term results following microsurgical lymph node transplantation. *Ann Surg.* 2006;243:313–5.
19. Saaristo AM, Niemi TS, Viitanen TP, et al. Microvascular breast reconstruction and lymph node transfer for postmastectomy lymphedema patients. *Ann Surg.* 2012;255:468–73.
20. Cheng MH, Huang JJ, Wu CW, et al. The Mechanism of Vascularized Lymph Node Transfer for Lymphedema: Natural Lymphaticovenous Drainage. *Plast Reconstr Surg.* 2014;133:192e–8e.
21. Tobbia D, Semple J, Baker A, et al. Experimental assessment of autologous lymph node transplantation as treatment of postsurgical lymphedema. *Plast Reconstr Surg.* 2009;124:777–86.
22. Raju A, Chang DW. Vascularized Lymph Node Transfer for Treatment of Lymphedema A Comprehensive Literature Review. *Ann Surg.* 2015;261:1013–23.
23. Becker C, Vasile JV, Levine JL, et al. Microlymphatic surgery for the treatment of iatrogenic lymphedema. *Clin Plast Surg.* 2012;39:385–98.
24. Althubaiti GA, Crosby MA, Chang DW. Vascularized supraclavicular lymph node transfer for lower extremity lymphedema treatment. *Plast Reconstr Surg.* 2013;131:133e–5e.
25. Boccardo F, Casabona F, DeCian F, et al. Lymphatic microsurgical preventing healing approach (LYMPHA) for primary surgical prevention of breast cancer-related lymphedema: over 4 years follow-up. *Microsurgery.* 2014;34:421–4.

38

Catheter-Directed Thrombolysis for Acute Finger Ischemia

Matthew A. Corriere MD, MS

Acute finger ischemia (AFI) is a relatively uncommon clinical presentation with specific considerations for diagnosis and management. In contrast to acute upper extremity ischemia, which presents with signs and symptoms (such as pain, pallor, paralysis, paresthesias, pulselessness, and poikilothermia) that involve and potentially threaten the limb,[1] AFI is distinguished by more focal symptoms involving one or more fingers but not the entire arm or hand. In fact, patients with AFI frequently (but not always) present palpable radial and/or ulnar pulses. The designation *acute* refers to symptoms and signs that are new-onset and have been present ≤ 30 days; although this time interval is somewhat arbitrary, it is meant to distinguish AFI from more chronic presentations where the time frame for diagnosis and treatment may be less urgent. AFI therefore does not include ischemic finger symptoms that are intermittent in nature or chronically wax and wane (as commonly seen with many rheumatologic disorders such as Raynaud's disease).

Within the limits of this relatively precise definition, diagnosis and treatment of AFI differs in several ways from more proximal upper extremity arterial occlusive disease. This chapter will review the epidemiology, diagnosis, and management of AFI with a focus on the role of catheter-directed thrombolysis. Because AFI resulting from penetrating trauma or known iatrogenic causes (such as an ipsilateral arterial catheter or arteriovenous hemodialysis access) involves distinct diagnostic and treatment considerations reviewed elsewhere, these presentations are more appropriately considered separately from *de novo* AFI and therefore will not be discussed.

EPIDEMIOLOGY

Although the epidemiology of AFI is poorly understood, limited data suggests several characteristics that distinguish these patients from those with lower extremity peripheral arterial disease (PAD): patients presenting with AFI are relatively younger and have a higher prevalence of both connective tissue disease. In a single center review of 35 patients treated with catheter-directed thrombolysis for AFI, Islam et al. noted a mean age of 48 years with a 31% prevalence of connective tissue disease.[2] Current or previous history of smoking was present in 65% of patients in this cohort, while 29% had a history of ipsilateral repetitive motion or minor blunt trauma, and 14% had a hypercoagulable disorder.

ANATOMIC CONSIDERATIONS

The upper extremity arteries are superficial, small in diameter (relative to the lower extremity arteries), and sensitive to temperature and mechanical stimuli.[3] The arterial circulation of the hand and fingers is highly variable, and the clinical manifestations of AFI usually depend on the amount of collateral flow between the radial, ulnar, and proper digital arteries. The normal arterial anatomy of the hand involves duplicated systems between the radial and ulnar arteries which communicate through the superficial and deep palmar arches. This rich collateral network makes it possible for acute occlusion of either the radial or ulnar arteries to occur without clinically apparent signs, symptoms, or severe alterations of either nutritional blood flow or thermoregulatory function.[4] An incomplete palmar arterial arch, however, has been reported in up to 65% of patients with AFI and may predispose patients to develop relatively severe ischemia from disease that otherwise might be tolerated in the setting of intact collateral flow.[2] AFI presenting with severe signs and symptoms therefore should prompt suspicion of atypical arterial anatomy as a potential predisposing factor.

Anatomic assessment and classification of AFI requires consideration of the level of the occlusive lesion(s) and the adequacy of collateral flow (Figure 38-1).[4] AFI is characterized by a high prevalence of both distal lesions and multi-level disease. Lesions distal to the level of the wrist have been reported based on angiography in over 90% of patients presenting with AFI,[2] while approximately 75% of patients with upper extremity ischemia have lesions of the forearm or hand.[4, 5] Ruch et al. reported multi-level occlusive disease in 76% of patients with upper extremity ischemia based on angiography, with lesions the distal forearm or Guyon's canal in combination with a second distal occlusion of one or more proper digital arteries as the most common combinations of occlusive disease levels.[4] Islam et al. reported disease involving the contralateral upper extremity among 32% of patients with AFI who were studied with bilateral upper extremity arteriography, although only 6% of patients presented with bilateral symptoms.[2] Other anatomic findings of interest reported from this study included a 23% prevalence of radial and/or ulnar artery aneurysms and a 20% prevalence of a proximally located (upper arm) brachial artery bifurcation.

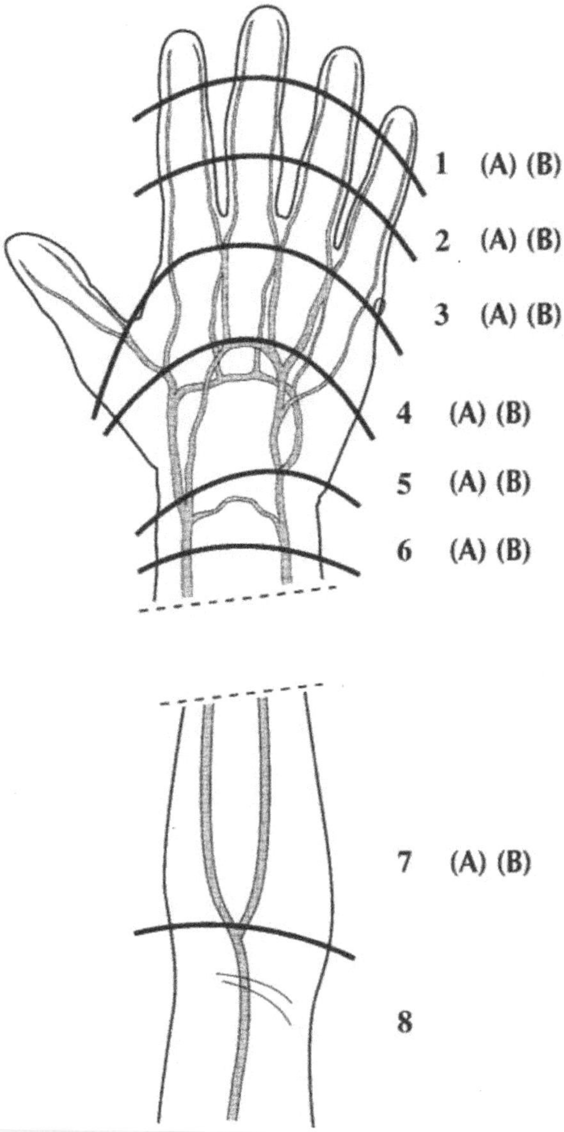

Figure 38-1. Classification system for describing arterial occlusive disease associated with acute finger ischemia. Numbers 1-8 indicate level of occlusion, while letters refer to whether occlusion of either the radial or ulnar (A) versus both the radial and ulnar sources of inflow (B) at the given level. (Figure originally published but Ruch et al, and used with permission from the publisher.[4])

CLINICAL PRESENTATION OF ACUTE FINGER ISCHEMIA

AFI usually presents with finger pain, numbness, and/or paresthesias; motor deficits are much less common. In more severe cases, patients may also present with digital ulcers or focal gangrene. Skin discoloration (including mottling or pallor) may also be seen with AFI but is more consistently associated with diseases characterized by intermittent vasospasm (such as Raynaud's), although AFI may also occur without visible skin changes. Patients with AFI often delay seeking medical evaluation for several days or weeks after onset, sometimes mistakenly attributing their initial symptoms to minor blunt trauma or other causes.[2] Symptoms may be vague and have multiple similarities to other conditions such as compressive neuropathy (Table 38-1).[4] AFI is seldom associated with significant finger or hand edema, so these symptoms should prompt consideration of alternative etiologies such as venous or lymphatic disease, local traumatic injury (including insect bites or stings), or focal allergic reactions (such as contact dermatitis).

DIAGNOSTIC EVALUATION AND TESTING

History and physical examination

When AFI is suspected, the history and physical examination can provide valuable information that helps to narrow the differential diagnosis and to focus subsequent diagnostic testing. The history of present illness interview should include focused questions exploring precipitating factors (such as cold exposure, positional changes,

TABLE 38-1. DIFFERENTIAL DIAGNOSIS FOR ACUTE FINGER ISCHEMIA

Embolism from proximal source	Aortic aneurysm
	Cardiac mural thrombus
	Patent foramen ovale
	Valvular heart disease/endocarditis
Embolism from ipsilateral arm	Subclavian artery aneurysm/psuedoaneursm
	Radial or ulnar artery aneurysm
Atherosclerotic disease	Subclavian steal syndrome
Non-atherosclerotic vascular disease	Buerger's disease
	Takayasu arteritis
	Giant cell arteritis
	Kawasaki disease
	Arterial dissection (aortic, subclavian)
	Collagen vascular disease
Vasospasm	Temperature-induced (e.g., Raynaud's syndrome)
	Drug-induced (e.g., cocaine, methamphetamine)
	Systemic shock
Neurologic	Compressive neuropathy (e.g., carpal tunnel syndrome)
	Cerebrovascular accident
	Complex regional pain syndrome
Steal syndrome	Proximal arteriovenous fistula
	Subclavian stenosis
	Hypothenar hand syndrome
Traumatic	Pectoralis minor syndrome
	Iatrogenic (arterial catheterization)
	Brachial artery injection
Other	Hypocalcemia
	Hypersensitivity

repetitive motion or blunt force, or other physical activities) or associated symptoms (including palpitations, transient ischemic attacks or other cerebrovascular manifestations, or hyperventilation) that might establish suspicion of a likely cause or alternative diagnosis. Physical examination should include a thorough pulse examination of all extremities, chest auscultation, and visual inspection of the symptomatic extremity with direct comparison to the contralateral arm and hand. Finger inspection should include examination of the nail beds for evidence of micro-embolization.[6] Ulcers or focal gangrene should be documented if present and may be identified in up to 20% of patients at the time of initial evaluation.[2] Visual inspection of the ipsilateral arm should also be performed to screen for ecchymosis, skin lesions, needle tracks, or other signs that may indicate a likely etiology. Photographs of both hands are useful to obtain at the time of presentation, particularly if these images can be added to the electronic medical record for longitudinal comparisons to assess wound healing and/or response to revascularization. The Allen test can assess the relative contributions from the radial and ulnar arteries to hand blood flow, but is less useful for AFI than for chronic disease.[6] Continuous wave Doppler evaluation of the palmar arch, proper digital arteries, and both the radial and ulnar arteries allows bedside assessment of these vessels but is inadequate for confirming the diagnosis or developing a treatment plan.[6] Nonetheless, abnormal continuous wave Doppler findings may establish increased suspicion for AFI, while normal signals may help lower AFI on the differential diagnosis and direct the subsequent workup toward other diagnoses if plausible alternative explanations exist.

Laboratory Testing

Laboratory testing for patients with AFI can inform both short-term and long-term management. Screening for thrombophilia should be considered at the time of presentation before initiating therapeutic anticoagulation, which can affect the results of several of these tests (including proteins C and S), making it difficult to interpret the results and sometimes necessary to obtain repeat testing. Assessment of coagulation parameters is also important for evaluating patients as candidates for thrombolysis; patients with severe coagulopathy (such as a profoundly elevated INR or low fibrinogen) may not be appropriate candidates due to increased risk of hemorrhagic complications. Longer-term considerations include testing for vasculitis, rheumatologic, or other inflammatory conditions that may not be critical to management during the acute presentation but may identify opportunities to decrease risk for disease progression or relapses through pharmacotherapy for systemic disease. From a practical perspective, it is also worth obtaining a serum creatinine for glomerular filtration rate estimation to determine risk of contrast-induced nephropathy. When contrast imaging is necessary in a patient with kidney disease, it is prudent to consider catheter arteriography as the primary modality to minimize the volume of iodinated contrast. Prophylactic hydration and medications should also be considered in patients with severe kidney disease. Although evidence supporting pharmacotherapy for prevention of contrast-induced nephrotoxicity is not robust, these medications are safe and inexpensive. We routinely administer prophylactic intravenous hydration for patients with an estimated glomerular filtration rate (eGFR) <60 ml/min/m^2 and add pharmacologic prophylaxis with oral N-acetylcysteine and vitamin C for those with an eGFR <30 ml/min/m.[2] Obtaining a serum pregnancy test in women at risk will maximize safety while avoiding subsequent delays if imaging requiring radiation exposure and/or thrombolysis are pursued. Table 38-2 summarizes laboratory tests worthy of consideration during initial evaluation of AFI; this list is not all-inclusive, and the tests ordered should be individualized based on the history, patient gender, and clinical suspicion.

Physiologic Testing

Digital brachial index assessment, digital plethysmography, and laser Doppler may be useful for confirming the symptom etiology and quantifying the severity of ischemia; these tests can also provide an assessment of the microcirculation (and related likelihood of wound healing with conservative management) that cannot be obtained through routine anatomic imaging tests.[4] A digital pressure <30 mm Hg or digital brachial index <0.5 indicates likely finger ischemia, while a digital brachial index <0.3 has been suggested as consistent with imminent digital gangrene.[6,7] Laser Doppler may

TABLE 38-2. USEFUL LABORATORY TESTS DURING INITIAL EVALUATION OF ACUTE FINGER ISCHEMIA

Category	Test(s)
Renal function and acid-base status	Electrolytes
	Serum creatinine (with estimated glomerular filtration rate)
	Serum creatine phosphokinase
Bleeding risk	Complete blood count (with platelet count)
	Prothrombin time with International Normalized Ratio
	Partial thromboplastin time
	D-dimer
	Type and screen
Thrombophilia	Protein C
	Protein S
	Plasminogen
	Antithrombin III
	Antiphospholipid antibodies (lupus anticoagulant, anti-cardiolipin, anti-beta-2 glycoprotein)
	Factor V Leiden
	Prothrombiin (Factor II) 20210 mutation
Connective tissue disorders, vasculitis	Antinuclear antibody
	Anti-neutrophil cytoplasmic antibody
	Erythrocyte sedimentation rate
	Serum complement
Miscellaneous	Ionized calcium
	Serum/urine pregnancy
	Drug screen

Note: Testing should be individualized based on the history, patient gender, and clinical suspicion, and list is not all-inclusive.

provide additional information related to cutaneous finger perfusion, although poor correlation has been reported between laser Doppler and arteriogram findings in the setting of finger ischemia.[4] Non-invasive physiologic testing can also sometimes provide useful information when attempting to rule out a non-vascular etiology, but may be less useful in the setting of bilateral disease, poorly tolerated in patients with severe finger pain, or inadequate if gangrene and/or ulcers warrant proceeding directly to a more definitive anatomic assessment. In contrast to evaluation of chronic symptoms, cold/warm stress testing and digital temperature evaluation are less useful for AFI.

Anatomic Imaging

Diagnostic imaging selection or AFI should be guided by the clinical presentation, pulse examination, and suspected anatomic location of the causative pathology. When a proximal brachial artery occlusion is suspected based on the clinical presentation, it may be most efficient to forego extensive imaging and proceed with immediate surgical exploration; one example of such a situation would be a patient who has chronic history of atrial fibrillation, is not therapeutically anticoagulated, and presents with numbness and weakness involving the arm and hand ipsilateral to an absent brachial pulse. When the clinical presentation does not clearly point to a likely etiology, however, anatomic imaging can provide useful information for both making the diagnosis and developing an appropriate treatment plan based on the findings.

Duplex ultrasound (DUS) is often helpful for assessing flow in the brachial and axillary arteries and can provide confirmation of suspected proximal disease (such as a brachial artery thrombus) sufficient for proceeding with exploration without need for contrast imaging. DUS may also serve as a non-invasive screening test that informs subsequent imaging selection; Barbiero et al. described using DUS confirmation of distal arterial ischemia as a criterion for proceeding with catheter angiography, while patients with non-diagnostic or equivocal DUS findings were instead studied with cross-sectional imaging.[3]

Cross-sectional contrast imaging (including both computed tomography angiography [CTA] and magnetic resonance angiography [MRA]) can provide useful information related to proximal sources of embolism (such as aneurysmal disease) or non-vascular anatomic findings relevant to both etiology and treatment (such as a cervical rib). Cross sectional imaging can also be used for imaging more distal arterial pathology involving the small vessels of the hand and fingers, although issues such as motion artifact, vascular calcification, and timing of image acquisition relative to contrast infusion (particularly for patients with multilevel occlusive disease) can sometimes result in an inadequate study. Cross sectional imaging systems may require patients to assume non-anatomic positions such as abducting the symptomatic extremity above their head while lying supine or extending their hand while prone in the "Superman" position so that the hand enters the imaging field first.[6,8] Because these maneuvers can sometimes reduce blood flow in asymptomatic patients without known arterial pathology, catheter angiography may be necessary when studies performed in this position suggest abnormal distal flow without a clear proximal lesion. MRA may also be limited by length of coverage or overlap between arteries and veins in the hand, and is contraindicated for patients with implanted devices that are not magnetic resonance compatible.[6] Given these considerations, cross-sectional imaging may be most useful for evaluating the aortic arch and subclavian vessels, particularly when clinical suspicion for AFI is low or there is reason to suspect proximal disease.

Catheter angiography is considered the gold standard for anatomic imaging of upper extremity arterial occlusive disease,[6, 9] and plays an even more prominent role in the diagnosis and treatment of AFI. Because AFI often results from occlusive disease affecting the more distal arterial circulation (including the radial, ulnar, palmar arch, and/or proper digital vessels), angiography can often provide the most definitive evaluation of the distal vasculature by avoiding issues related to motion artifact and timing of image acquisition relative to contrast infusion. This advantage is especially important in the setting of multi-level disease (as may be seen in the setting of an embolizing proximal lesion) (Figure 38-2). Catheter angiography also allows immediate initiation of endovascular treatment if anatomically suitable pathology is identified, resulting in greater efficiency while avoiding the additional time, contrast volume, and/or radiation exposure from an initial cross-sectional study if endovascular treatment is selected based on the findings. Catheter angiography also provides real-time evaluation of flow (including both direction and rate) that is not available with cross sectional imaging.[8] When distal vasospasm is suspected, intra-arterial

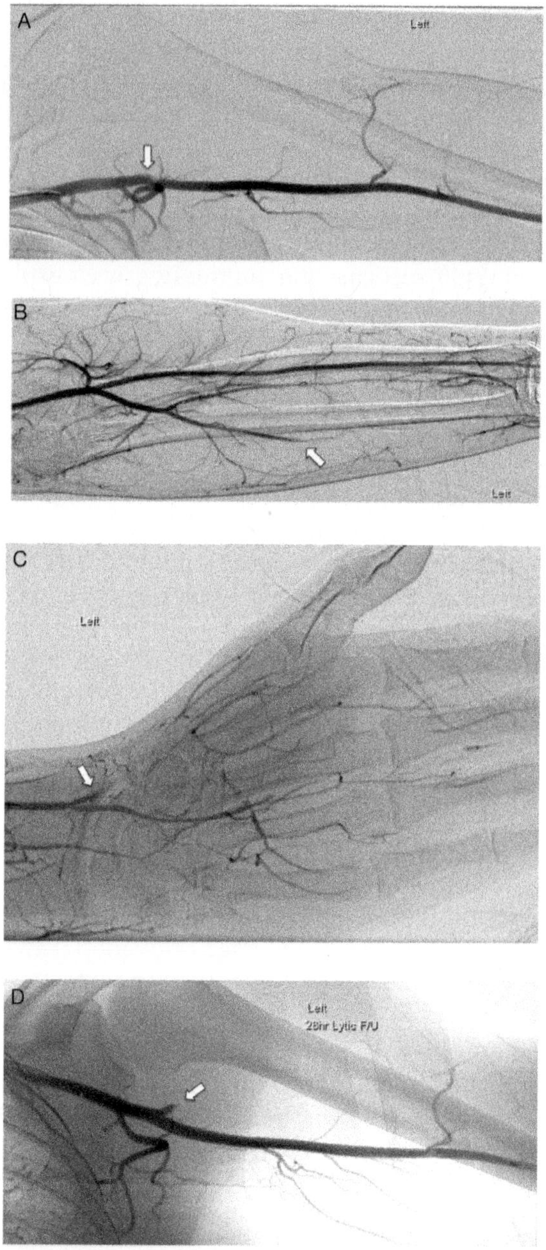

Figure 38-2. Proximal upper extremity arterial lesion with distal embolization to radial and ulnar arteries. The patient was a baseball pitcher who presented with acute finger ischemia. (**A**) Catheter angiogram demonstrates focal filling defect with intraluminal thrombus at junction between third portion of the left axillary artery and the brachial artery (arrow). (**B**) Forearm arteriogram performed using axillary artery injection demonstrates occlusion of the ulnar artery (arrow), with patent radial and interosseus arteries. (**C**) Distal catheter arteriogram performed using same injection indicates occlusion of the princeps pollicis artery (arrow) with absent deep and superficial palmar arches and pruning of the proper digital vessels. (**D**) Repeat catheter angiography after 28 hours if catheter-directed thrombolysis with alteplase (infused through an end-hole catheter positioned with its tip in the axillary artery) demonstrates thrombosed, aneurysmal subscapular artery as source of embolizing lesion. Patient was treated with ligation of the aneurysmal branch, axillary artery repair, and pectoralis minor tendon lengthening after a two week period of temporary anticoagulation.

administration of vasodilator medications (400 μg boluses of nitroglycerine can be administered every 3–5 minutes with minimal effects on systemic blood pressure) will sometimes reduce vasoconstriction adequately to allow angiographic characterization of distal small vessels (such as the metacarpal and proper digital arteries) that were not previously visible.

An additional advantage of contrast arteriography for diagnostic imaging of AFI is the ability to immediately initiate catheter-directed thrombolysis if anatomically suitable findings are identified. In contrast to arteriography for lower extremity ischemia, where it is common to identify lesions that are treatable with other endovascular techniques such as angioplasty, stenting, and/or atherectomy, these treatments are utilized less often for AFI for several reasons. Non-atherosclerotic pathology that is less often amenable to endovascular treatment (such as radial or ulnar artery aneurysm) is commonly identified during arteriography for AFI, and longer working lengths between the lesion and femoral artery access can create issues with reaching the lesion or delivering a device to its intended location.

Other Diagnostic Testing

An electrocardiogram should be obtained at the time of initial evaluation for AFI to rule out arrhythmia, particularly if the patient is tachycardic (as is often the case in the setting of significant pain or anxiety due to symptoms) and the ability to distinguish an irregular heart rhythm therefore may be limited based on physical examination alone. Additional evaluation with echocardiography and/or three-dimensional cardiac imaging should also be obtained when an arrhythmia is identified or physical exam findings (such as a murmur) suggest valvular or structural heart disease. Echocardiography with saline injection may also be useful for excluding paradoxical embolism associated with a septal defect (such as a patent foramen ovale) if the presentation is consistent with embolism and a proximal arterial source is not identified.

CATHETER ANGIOGRAPHY FOR ACUTE FINGER ISCHEMIA

Careful pre-procedure planning with anticipation of the necessary wires, catheters, and other equipment is therefore important for successful angiography. Anticipating challenges, carefully planning the approach, and minimizing potential for adverse circumstances related to equipment or technique can optimize imaging success. With the possible exception of trans-radial access for lower extremity angiography, catheter access of the brachial artery or more distal arm vessels from a femoral approach generally involves one of the longest distances between the access and target vessels routinely encountered, particularly for patients who are tall or lanky. Accordingly, it is wise to confirm availability of adequate length catheters and wires to avoid technical limitations during angiography. Providers who routinely perform carotid stenting will find many of the catheters used for this purpose (including vertebral, headhunter, and VTK catheters) also useful for selective innominate and/or subclavian artery access during upper extremity angiography. Although long (90 cm) sheaths and/or guide catheters are useful for treating disease of the proximal innominate or subclavian arteries, these devices are often impractical for dealing with more distal upper extremity pathology due to flow limitations, tendency to induce vasospasm, and (for right upper extremity disease) the disadvantage of leaving a larger diameter device positioned across the remaining arch vessels if catheter-directed thrombolysis is utilized. It is also helpful to anticipate what medications will likely be needed on the field for trans-arterial administration so that they can be prepared and immediately available during the procedure.

The patient is positioned supine on a radiolucent imaging table with one or both arms abducted depending on whether unilateral versus bilateral imaging is planned. To minimize potential for vasospasm, the room should be warmed and local warming of the affected hand should be arranged using forced heated air and/or a warmed intravenous fluid bag placed over the patient's hand. The hand should be taped to a radiolucent arm board to minimize motion artifact during angiography. At the time of positioning, it is useful to ensure that external devices with potential to obscure important anatomy or create imaging artifacts (such as ECG leads) are positioned outside the anticipated fields of view. If thrombolysis is being considered, it is wise to establish all invasive access and monitoring devices that will likely be needed prior to angiography to avoid bleeding complications resulting from invasive procedures performed during thrombolytic medication infusion. Relatively minor procedures (such as insertion of nasogastric tubes, urethral catheters, or intravenous lines) during catheter-directed thrombolysis can provoke significant bleeding during thrombolytic infusion, so it is better to perform these procedures beforehand to minimize risk of major complications or need to discontinue the infusion prematurely.

Although the additional diagnostic yield or therapeutic benefit gained from bilateral upper extremity imaging in the setting of unilateral AFI has not been definitively evaluated or proven, some providers advocate routine bilateral imaging to avoid the need for subsequent evaluation of the contralateral extremity with a separate procedure. This approach may be particularly wise when a systemic disease process is suspected as the most likely etiology for AFI, as information related to the contralateral upper extremity may be useful in confirming the diagnosis or potentially provide useful anatomic information if contralateral symptoms occur in the future. Contralateral imaging may also identify pathology warranting pre-emptive intervention under elective circumstances in the future (such as asymptomatic aneurysms of the radial or ulnar arteries). Conversely, bilateral imaging may have less benefit when the history or presenting signs and symptoms suggest a cause that is more likely to be unilateral (such as AFI involving the dominant hand in a throwing athlete or a history of repetitive hand trauma affecting one hand but not the other).

A large proportion of procedure-related adverse events related to upper extremity arteriography and thrombolysis are access-related,[2] and use of ultrasound guidance can minimize risk of iatrogenic complications resulting from repeated access attempts in multiple locations. If femoral access is utilized, the femoral head should be localized with fluoroscopy, and percutaneous access of the common femoral artery at this location should then be attempted after confirming that this site is free of dense plaque or calcification and proximal to the origin of the deep femoral artery. Antegrade brachial access has also been described for upper extremity arteriography and/o thrombolysis, but this approach does not permit imaging or treatment of more proximal disease and has a higher rate of access-related complications.[3,5,7,10] After infiltrating the overlying skin with local anesthetic and establishing access with a 4 French micro-catheter over an 0.014 "wire, an 0.035" wire can then be advanced and used to insert a short sheath. A 6 French sheath may be preferred due to easier infusion and blood sampling through the side port during thrombolysis, which is associated with greater resistance when performed around an infusion catheter through a smaller 5 French sheath. After establishing percutaneous access, the patient should be anticoagulated (unless anticoagulation was initiated preoperatively) with a bolus of unfractionated heparin prior to advancing a guide wire retrograde into the aortic arch. An activated clotting time (ACT) obtained 3–5 minutes following heparin administration allows confirmation of adequate anticoagulation before proceeding with selective catheterization. To minimize risk of cerebrovascular embolization during angiography and catheter manipulation, an ACT can be assessed every 30–45 minutes during the procedure with a target of >280 seconds as the criterion for repeat heparin administration.

Arch aortography is useful for identifying the location of the targeted access vessels and evaluating them for ostial disease, but is not always necessary. Aortography may be omitted if preoperative cross sectional imaging has been obtained and provides adequate information for procedure planning (including catheter selection), particularly if there is no proximal arch vessel disease. Arch angiography should be performed if cross-sectional contrast imaging has not been obtained, however, and may be preferred for patients with impaired renal function in order to minimize contrast volume. A reasonable arch aortogram can be obtained with a single dose of half-strength contrast while still managing to keep the total contrast volume for the procedure well below the volume needed for a routine CTA. Arch angiography should utilize a left anterior oblique (LAO) projection of 25°–30°, and the ideal projection can be identified by rotating the C-arm during live fluoroscopy until the maximum AP distance between the guidewire in the ascending versus descending thoracic aorta. Selective access to the targeted arch vessel is then established using a configured catheter in combination with an angled hydrophilic guide wire. Difficulty of arch access and catheterization may be anticipated using one of several scoring systems, such as that described by Schneider et al.[11] Left subclavian access is usually the least difficult and can often be accomplished using a catheter with a single angle such as a vertebral artery, Berenstein, or MP catheter. More difficult access in the setting of a severely angulated or diseased aortic arch may require more advanced catheter configurations such as a Simmons, Headhunter, or VTK catheter. Once selective access is established, the more distal subclavian artery can then be imaged using serial hand injections of dilute contrast with digital subtraction.

If proximal arch vessel disease suitable for endovascular treatment is identified, it is usually prudent to proceed with intervention prior to obtaining more distal imaging. Proximal disease is identified in only a minority of patients presenting with AFI, however, and is seldom the sole cause for symptoms other than arm claudication in the absence of distal embolization. If no proximal arch disease is identified, a 5 French angled diagnostic catheter is then advanced into the proximal axillary artery and used to image the distal axillary and brachial vessels. If appears satisfactory arteriograms of the brachial, radial, and ulnar arteries are obtained with the catheter tip positioned in the distal axillary artery, it may be worthwhile to also perform arteriography of the distal forearm and hand injecting from this same location. Alternatively, a catheter can advanced more distally into the brachial artery for more selective contrast injection but this approach risks provoking vasospasm which can be severe enough to result in arterial occlusion, may jeopardize both imaging and catheter-based therapy, and may be resistant to intra-arterial vasodilators.[3] For this reason, selective catheterization of the brachial, radial or ulnar arteries should be performed with an 0.018 "or 0.014" guide wire and a smaller diameter catheter (such as a 4 French catheter or microcatheter), although rapid injection may be more challenging due to increased resistance with the latter.

CATHETER-DIRECTED THROMBOLYSIS FOR ACUTE FINGER ISCHEMIA

Patient selection

Arteriography should guide selection of the most appropriate treatment strategy based on the anatomic findings and suspected disease etiology. A management algorithm proposed for imaging and use of thrombectomy versus catheter-directed thrombolysis for AFI is shown in Figure 38-3.[2] Catheter-directed thrombolysis should be considered for one or more of the following findings: pruning of the distal small

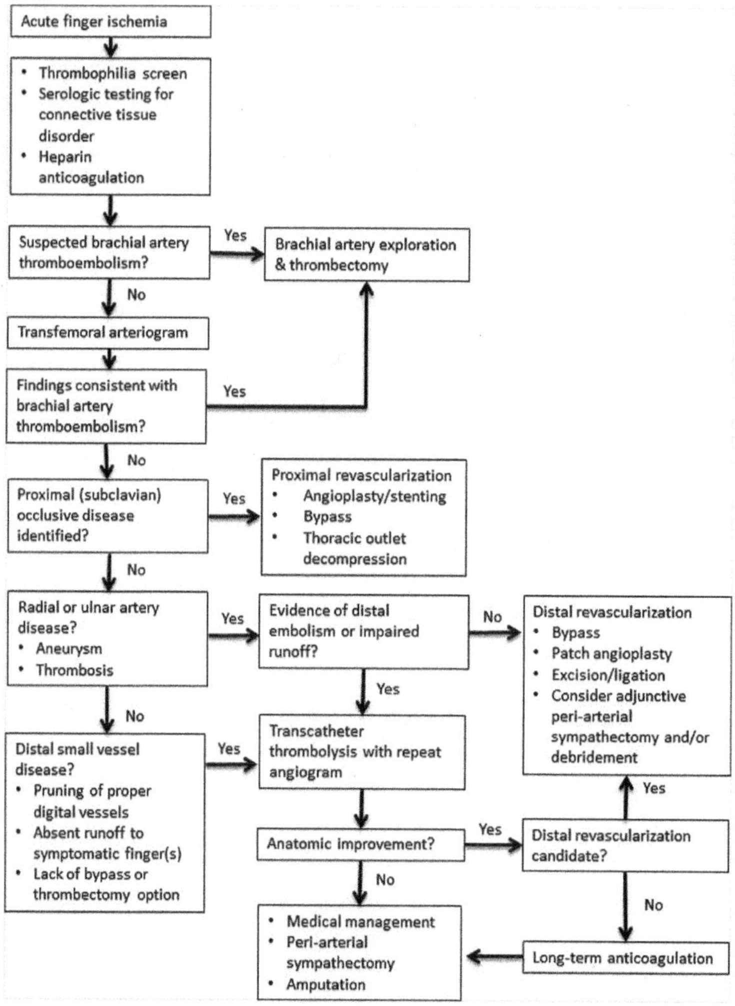

Figure 38-3. Proposed management algorithm for patients with acute finger ischemia. (Figure originally published by Islam et al. and used with permission from publisher.[2])

vessels consistent with proper digital vessel thrombosis and/or embolism, radial or ulnar artery aneurysm with thrombosis or distal embolization, or absent distal outflow to the fingers with lack of alternative revascularization options.[2] Digital emboli are present in the most patients with AFI resulting from radial or ulnar artery aneurysms[9]; because these small diameter vessels are poorly suited to thrombectomy, there are limited alternatives apart from catheter-directed thrombolysis for re-establishing their patency. Alternatively, when arteriography demonstrates more proximal large vessel thrombosis involving the brachial, radial, and/or ulnar arteries with patent palmar and digital vessels, exploration with thrombectomy should be considered as primary therapy rather than thrombolysis, as this treatment will allow more rapid and definitive restoration of arterial perfusion.[3,12] Thrombectomy and/or bypass should also be considered for patients who present with severe acute neurologic deficits, as the interval of time required for catheter-directed thrombolysis to achieve a clinically apparent effect may not be rapid enough to salvage function or prevent permanent neurologic symptoms. Patients with small diameter brachial arteries or those who develop significant arterial spasm during angiography are also suboptimal candidates for catheter directed thrombolysis. Patients with these symptoms who have limited alternatives for treatment may require intra-arterial vasodilator medications and/or withdrawal of the catheter tip to a more proximal location for contrast injection and/or thrombolytic infusion.

Prior to proceeding with angiography, it is critical to review the patient's history and ask specific questions to confirm that there are no contraindications to thrombolytic administration. Because many contraindications to thrombolysis cannot be identified based on physical examination alone (Table 38-3),[5,13–18] a detailed and accurate history is critical for minimizing risk of bleeding complications and may require confirmatory imaging (such as brain imaging) to ensure safety when details are unclear.

TABLE 38-3. CONTRAINDICATIONS TO CATHETER-DIRECTED THROMBOLYSIS

Contraindications to catheter-directed thrombolysis
Intracranial tumor
History of intracranial bleeding
Known peptic ulcer or history of gastrointestinal bleeding
Recent major surgery or trauma
Stroke within past 2 months
Thrombocytopenia
Coagulation disorder
Severe uncontrolled hypertension
Irreversible ischemia (i.e., severe motor deficit or rigor)
Sensory/motor deficit (inability to tolerate ≤24 additional hours of ischemia)
Infected bypass graft
Infective endocarditis
Pregnancy
Cardiopulmonary resuscitation

Approach and technical considerations

Tissue plasminogen activator (t-PA) (alteplase) is a naturally occurring serine protease that activates fibrin-bound plasminogen several hundred times more rapidly than circulating plasminogen.[18] t-PA is secreted naturally by vascular endothelial cells, plays an important role in normal endogenous fibrinolysis, and is primarily cleared by hepatic metabolism with a half-life of approximately 5 minutes.[13] Other recombinant variants of t-PA (sometimes alternatively abbreviated as rt-PA to specifically designate them as such, including reteplase and tenecteplase) have longer half-lives than native t-PA but are similar in terms of both efficacy and toxicity.[13,18] Catheter-directed thrombolysis using streptokinase and urokinase for upper extremity ischemia has also been described.[3,19,20] Limited evidence suggests that intra-arterial t-PA is more effective than either intra-arterial streptokinase or intravenous t-PA for improving vessel patency in people with peripheral arterial occlusion.[21] Recombinant t-PA is packaged in vials as a lyophilized powder that requires reconstitution prior to infusion.[13] When using alteplase for catheter-directed thrombolysis, a bolus dose of 6–10 mg is often administered prior to initiating an infusion at 1–2 mg/hr. When preparing the infusion, the alteplase should be reconstituted and diluted in an adequate volume. A practically useful concentration can be obtained by reconstituting 10 mg alteplase in 250 mL of saline, which yields a concentration of 0.04 mg/mL; this concentration permits easy dose adjustment for infusion at 1 mg (25 mL) or 2 mg (50 mL) per hour, allows easy bedside dose identification based on the infusion rate during rounds, and minimizes potential for accidental administration of large doses of atleplase as the result of line flushes (which may happen with more concentrated doses, although line flushes through the infusion catheter should be avoided if at all possible).

Once catheter angiography is complete and the decision has been made to proceed with catheter-directed thrombolysis, a bolus of thrombolytic agent can be administered through the catheter while the infusion is being prepared. An end-hole catheter positioned in the distal axillary or proximal brachial artery is well suited for both infusion and repeat arteriography to assess the treatment response. A proximally positioned catheter may also result in wider thrombolytic distribution through the radial, ulnar, and interosseus arteries.[7] Alternatively, infusion through a multiple side-hole catheter placed within the thrombus (as commonly performed for lower extremity arterial or venous thrombosis) has been described for upper extremity arterial thrombolysis,[3,7] but may be impractical due to relatively smaller arterial diameters, access length, and tendency to induce vasospasm. If arterial spasm is a problem but thrombolysis is necessary, a smaller diameter microcatheter or infusion wire can be used for thrombolytic infusion but usually requires exchange for a larger catheter to obtain adequate images during follow-up arteriography.

Once the thrombolytic infusion has been initiated, the catheter and sheath should be secured to one another and to the patient to avoid inadvertent withdrawal or repositioning during port manipulation or transportation. The infusion catheter can be secured to the sheath using adhesive strips wound in a spiral fashion, and the sheath then sutured to the skin before covering the entire apparatus with an adhesive barrier drape. When attached in this fashion, traction on the infusion catheter will transfer tension to the patient's skin without resulting in catheter withdrawal. Peri-catheter thrombosis has been reported as a complication of catheter-directed thrombolysis,[19,22] and a low-dose heparin infusion (500 units/hr) should therefore be administered through the side port of the sheath to minimize risk of local thrombus accumulation. The heparin dose should not be adjusted or titrated based on the pTT. To maximize safety and reduce risk of errors, it is wise to clearly label both the catheter and sheath in a manner consistent with the infusion orders (such as "catheter-TPA" and "sheath-heparin"), particularly if the patient will be cared for or observed (even temporarily) in a unit where experience with catheter-directed thrombolysis is limited. For this reason, it is worthwhile to routinely transport patients receiving thrombolytic infusions directly to the intensive care unit and personally review the orders, labeling, and intended infusion doses directly with the receiving nurse and other team members.

PATIENT CARE AND MONITORING

Patients treated with catheter-directed thrombolysis should be monitored in a unit staffed appropriately for high-acuity patients, preferably by a nursing and pharmacy team experienced with their specific care and monitoring needs. If circumstances require the patient to temporarily reside in a location other than the definitive care unit (such as a postoperative anesthesia care unit or imaging department), it is important that all personnel involved with medication administration, phlebotomy, and management of intravenous fluids are aware that the patient is receiving a thrombolytic infusion so that appropriate safety precautions can be followed. Patients should be closely monitored with a heightened sense of awareness for potential bleeding complications related to thrombolysis. Accordingly, any new symptoms that are potentially attributable to bleeding (including acute headache or back pain) must be pursued immediately with appropriate diagnostic imaging while the thrombolytic infusion is temporarily held until bleeding has been ruled out. As previously mentioned, any invasive procedures (including arterial or intravenous lines, Foley catheters, nasogastric tubes, or even suppositories) should be avoided during infusion if at all possible. In order to avoid needle phlebotomy during thrombolytic infusion (and associated bleeding risk), blood samples can be obtained from the side port of the access sheath provided that it is flushed with non-heparinized saline and an adequate amount of blood is temporarily aspirated to clear the sheath before obtaining the sample. Radial artery catheters and other upper extremity arterial lines, which are sometimes used for blood sampling in intensive care unit settings, should be avoided in patients with AFI (including in the contralateral arm).

During catheter-directed thrombolysis, patients should be re-evaluated after 8–24 hours of infusion with repeat angiography to determine whether treatment has resulted in anatomic improvement (i.e., partial or complete resolution of previously identified occlusive disease) and decide whether the infusion should be resumed or discontinued (Figure 38-4). Angiography can be performed through the infusion catheter without need for removal of the securing adhesive attachments if adequate rates of injection are possible. When anatomic improvement is observed but is incomplete (such as re-established radial artery patency with persistent proper digital artery occlusion), continued thrombolysis has potential to yield further improvement and should be considered. Conversely, catheter-directed thrombolysis should be discontinued in the absence of anatomic improvement, particularly if the total duration of the

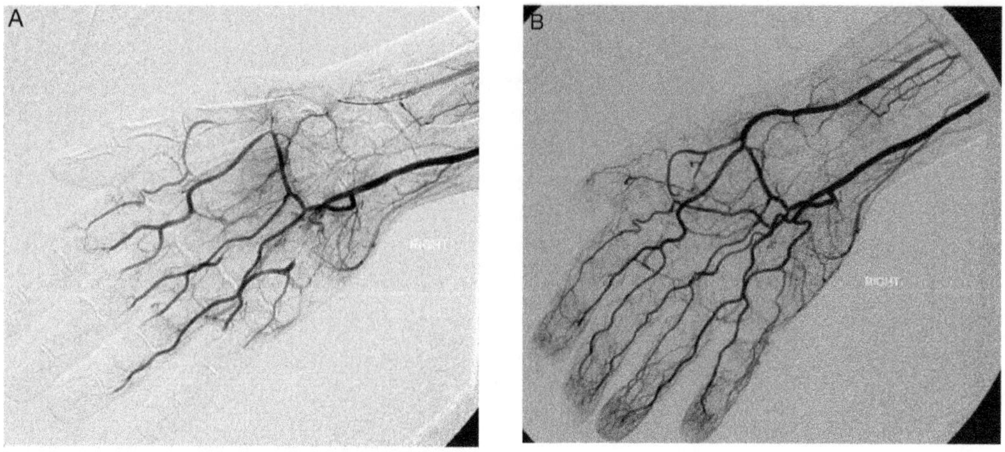

Figure 38-4. Interval anatomic improvement based on angiography following catheter-directed thrombolysis. (**A**) Catheter angiogram demonstrates occluded right radial artery, occluded superficial palmar arch, incomplete deep palmar arch with occlusion of multiple metacarpal arteries and pruning of the proper digital arteries. (**B**) Repeat angiogram following catheter-directed thrombolysis for 24 hours demonstrates re-established patency of previously occluded superficial palmar arch, metacarpal, and proper digital arteries.

infusion is approaching 48 hours, the total dose of alteplase has exceeded 20–25 mg, or severe and persistent vasospasm is observed.

Risk of bleeding during catheter-directed thrombolysis is related to both the dose and duration of infusion.[13,15] Use of weight-based dosing or a maximum total dose (such as 20 mg of alteplase) has been described by some and may limit the risk of bleeding complications.[1,20] During catheter-directed thrombolysis, patients should be monitored regularly (i.e., every 4–8 hours) with surveillance laboratory testing that includes fibrinogen, pTT, platelet count, and hemoglobin. A significant decrease in the hemoglobin, platelet count, or fibrinogen, or a fibrinogen level <100 mg/dL, should prompt an immediate patient assessment and consideration of either decreasing or discontinuing the infusion to avoid bleeding. Other reasons to discontinue the thrombolytic infusion include lack of improvement during the previous infusion interval (which may be assessed based on symptoms, physical examination, or arteriogram findings), restoration of flow without an identifiable need for continuation of thrombolysis, or infusion for a period >48 hours. When the infusion is discontinued, the catheter should be removed to avoid adjacent thrombus accumulation and associated risk of arterial thrombosis or embolization (unless repeat arteriography to assess the anatomy at the conclusion of thrombolysis is immediately pending). Sheath removal should be deferred for 2–4 hours following cessation of both the thrombolytic and heparin infusions to allow these medications to dissipate, and a repeat ACT should be obtained if the previous value was >200 seconds.

ADJUNCTIVE TREATMENTS

Several adjunctive treatments have been described in combination (either simultaneously or in a staged fashion) with catheter-directed thrombolysis for AFI.

Thromboaspiration in combination with thrombolysis has been described for endovascular management of organized thrombus embolizing from a proximal anatomic location.[20] Because aspiration catheters are seldom long enough to reach the distal arm from the femoral artery, this technique requires retrograde access from a patent distal arterial segment and often requires multiple aspiration sessions with a 6 French catheter. Use of pulse-spray thrombolytic infusion for acute upper extremity ischemia has also been described.[20]

Although use of ultrasound-accelerated thrombolysis has been associated with reduced thrombolysis time for acute lower extremity ischemia, this adjunctive treatment was not associated with a patency advantage has not been described extensively for upper extremity ischemia.[14] Proposed mechanisms of action for ultrasound-accelerated thrombolysis include increased thrombus permeability resulting from loosening of fibrin strands, increased exposure of plasminogen receptors, and acoustic cavitation.

OUTCOMES

Adverse procedure-related events occur in in 11%–12% of patients treated with catheter-directed thrombolysis for upper extremity disease, with access-related bleeding complications being the most common.[2] Rates of major bleeding reported from larger series of patients undergoing catheter-directed thrombolysis for lower extremity arterial disease range from 6%–13% with a 2%–3% rate of intracranial bleeding,[23–26] while a meta-analysis identifying a 9% rate of major bleeding within 30 days.[17] Bleeding risk is related to both the duration of the infusion and the total dose of the thrombolytic agent.[13] Other reported procedure-related adverse events include access site pseudoaneurysm, guide wire perforation of branch arteries, stroke or transient ischemic attack, and upper extremity compartment syndrome.[2,7,19,20,27] Compartment syndrome of the hand during catheter-directed thrombolysis is associated with instrumentation of the affected extremity;[27] avoiding ipsilateral antegrade brachial access may therefore be wise, particularly among patients with neurologic symptoms at the time of presentation (which may make clinical diagnosis of compartment syndrome challenging).

Rates of angiography-based anatomic improvement reported with catheter-directed thrombolysis for upper extremity arterial disease are between 33%–50%.[2,5] Finger amputation is necessary 5%–6% of patients and is usually performed within 60 days of initial evaluation; the majority of these patients present with ulcers or gangrene.[2] Surgical revascularization (including aneurysm resection, ligation, or bypass) was performed in approximately 12% of patients following angiography with or without catheter directed thrombolysis for AFI,[2] with a bypass patency of 77% reported at 2 years.[28]

Although one year amputation-free survival following presentation with AFI is 70%–80% overall, nearly half of patient report continued long-term symptoms.[2] Amputation-free survival appears similar between patients treated with versus without catheter-directed thrombolysis, limited data suggests a possible benefit associated with thrombolysis among those patients without ulcers or gangrene at the time of initial presentation (Figure 38-5).[2]

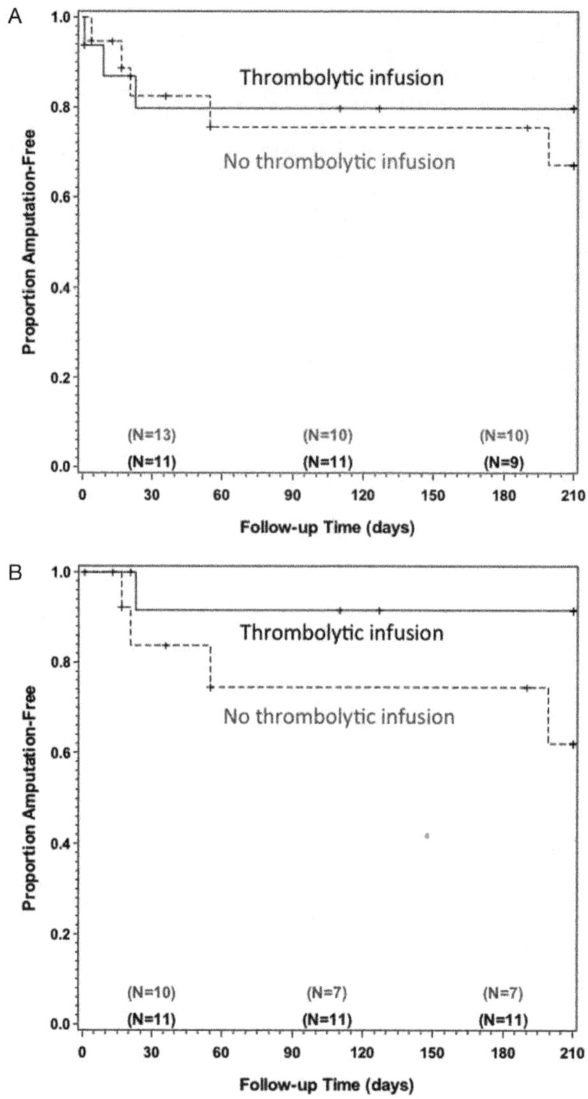

Figure 38-5. Estimated amputation-free survival following presentation with acute finger ischemia stratified by use of catheter directed thrombolysis. Figures represent overall cohort of 35 patients (**A**) versus subgroup without tissue loss or gangrene at time of initial evaluation (**B**). Solid line indicates group treated with catheter-directed thrombolysis, while interrupted line indicates those treated without catheter-directed thrombolysis.

REFERENCES

1. Schernthaner MB, Samuels S, Biegler P, et al. Ultrasound-accelerated versus standard catheter-directed thrombolysis in 102 patients with acute and subacute limb ischemia. *J Vasc Interv Radiol.* 2014;25(8):1149–56; quiz 1157.
2. Islam A, Edgerton C, Stafford JM, et al. Anatomic findings and outcomes associated with upper extremity arteriography and selective thrombolysis for acute finger ischemia. *J Vasc Surg*. 2014;60(2):410–7.

3. Barbiero G, Cognolato D, Casarin A, et al. Intra-arterial thrombolysis of acute hand ischaemia with or without microcatheter: preliminary experience and comparison with the literature. *Radiol Med.* 2011;116(6):919–31.
4. Ruch DS, Smith TL, Smith B,P et al. Anatomic and physiologic evaluation of upper extremity ischemia. *Microsurgery.* 1999;19(4):181–8.
5. Cejna M, Salomonowitz E, Wohlschlager H, et al. rt-PA thrombolysis in acute thromboembolic upper-extremity arterial occlusion. *Cardiovasc Intervent Radiol.* 2001;24(4):218–23.
6. Grasu BL, Jones CM, Murphy MS. Use of diagnostic modalities for assessing upper extremity vascular pathology. *Hand Clin.* 2015;31(1):1–12.
7. Breguet R, Terraz S, Righini M, et al. Acute hand ischemia after unintentional intraarterial injection of drugs: is catheter-directed thrombolysis useful. *J Vasc Interv Radiol.* 2014;25(6):963–8.
8. Friedrich KM, Frühwald-Pallamar J, Stadlbauer A, et al. Hypothenar hammer syndrome: long-term follow-up of selective thrombolysis by 3.0-T MR angiography. *Eur J Radiol.* 2010;75(2):e27–e31.
9. Vayssairat M, Debure C, Cormier JM, et al. Hypothenar hammer syndrome: seventeen cases with long-term follow-up. *J Vasc Surg.* 1987;5(6):838–43.
10. De Martino RR, Moran SL. The role of thrombolytics in acute and chronic occlusion of the hand. *Hand Clin.* 2015;31(1):13–21.
11. Schneider PA, Bohannon WT, Silva MB. *Carotid interventions.* Boca Raton, FL: Marcel Dekker; 2005.
12. Andersen LV, Mortensen LS, Lindholt JS, et al. Upper-limb thrombo-embolectomy: national cohort study in Denmark. *Eur J Vasc Endovasc Surg.* 2010;40(5):628–34.
13. Semba CP, Sugimoto K, Razavi MK, et al. Alteplase and tenecteplase: applications in the peripheral circulation. *Tech Vasc Interv Radiol.* 2001;4(2):99–106.
14. Schrijver AM, van Leersum M, Fioole B, et al. Dutch randomized trial comparing standard catheter-directed thrombolysis and ultrasound-accelerated thrombolysis for arterial thromboembolic infrainguinal disease (DUET). *J Endovasc Ther.* 2015;22(1):87–95.
15. Ebben HP, Nederhoed JH, Lely RJ, et al. Low-dose thrombolysis for thromboembolic lower extremity arterial occlusions is effective without major hemorrhagic complications. *Eur J Vasc Endovasc Surg.* 2014;48(5):551–8.
16. Yusuf SW, Whitaker SC, Gregson RH, et al. Prospective randomised comparative study of pulse spray and conventional local thrombolysis. *Eur J Vasc Endovasc Surg.* 1995;10(2):136–41.
17. Berridge DC, Kessel DO, Robertson I. Surgery versus thrombolysis for initial management of acute limb ischaemia. *Cochrane Database Syst Rev.* 2013;6 CD002784.
18. Weitz JI. Chapter 30. Blood Coagulation and Anticoagulant, Fibrinolytic, and Antiplatelet Drugs. In: Goodman LS, Brunton LL, Chabner B, et al. *Goodman & Gilman's Pharmacological Basis of Therapeutics.* 12th ed. ed. New York: McGraw-Hill; 2011.
19. Coulon M, Goffette P, Dondelinger RF. Local thrombolytic infusion in arterial ischemia of the upper limb: mid-term results. *Cardiovasc Intervent Radiol.* 1994;17(2):81–6.
20. Miyayama S, Yamashiro M, Shibata Y, et al. Thrombolysis and thromboaspiration for acute thromboembolic occlusion in the upper extremity. *Jpn J Radiol.* 2012;30(2):180–4.
21. Robertson I, Kessel DO, Berridge DC. Fibrinolytic agents for peripheral arterial occlusion. *Cochrane Database Syst Rev.* 2013;12 CD001099.
22. Wheatley MJ, Marx MV. The use of intra-arterial urokinase in the management of hand ischemia secondary to palmar and digital arterial occlusion. *Ann Plast Surg.* 1996;37(4):356–62; discussion 362.
23. Results of a prospective randomized trial evaluating surgery versus thrombolysis for ischemia of the lower extremity. The STILE trial. *Ann Surg.* 1994;220(3):251–66; discussion 266.
24. Cragg AH, Smith TP, Corson JD, et al. Two urokinase dose regimens in native arterial and graft occlusions: initial results of a prospective, randomized clinical trial. *Radiology.* 1991;178(3):681–6.

25. Duda SH, Tepe G, Luz O, et al. Peripheral artery occlusion: treatment with abciximab plus urokinase versus with urokinase alone–a randomized pilot trial (the PROMPT Study). Platelet Receptor Antibodies in Order to Manage Peripheral Artery Thrombosis. *Radiology.* 2001;221(3):689–96.
26. Ouriel K, Veith FJ, Sasahara AA. A comparison of recombinant urokinase with vascular surgery as initial treatment for acute arterial occlusion of the legs. Thrombolysis or Peripheral Arterial Surgery (TOPAS) Investigators. *N Engl J Med.* 1998;338(16):1105–11.
27. Freyer M, Vachalova I, Zirngibl B, et al. Compartment syndrome following thrombolysis: clinical features and associated conditions. *J Thromb Thrombolysis.* 2014;38(2):201–7.
28. Chloros GD, Lucas RM, Li Z, et al. Post-traumatic ulnar artery thrombosis: outcome of arterial reconstruction using reverse interpositional vein grafting at 2 years minimum follow-up. *J Hand Surg Am.* 2008;33(6):932–40.

39

Soft Tissue Coverage of the Open Groin Wound with Emphasis on the Gracilis Flap

Lauren Mioton, MD and Gregory Dumanian, MD

Groin wounds are a common problem following vascular surgery. Patient factors such as diabetes, poor nutrition, and tobacco use, along with local fluid collections and infection, prevent proper healing. Even the basic movements of hip flexion and extension place undo pressure on groin incisions and predispose them to breakdown. These wounds present a challenge as they can lead to graft infection, pseudoaneurysm, sepsis, graft blow-out, and additional procedures. Soft tissue flap coverage of groin wounds is often necessary to protect underlying vascular bypasses and expedite healing.

This chapter will provide an overview of the decision-making process for determining soft tissue coverage in patients with groin wounds after vascular surgery. A brief overview of various muscle flap options will be detailed with a specific focus on the gracilis muscle flap.

DECISION-MAKING PROCESS

Effective evaluation and treatment of groin wounds must account for a patient's individual risk factors for wound breakdown, the location of vascular bypass grafts, and the chronicity and severity of the wound. The confluence of local elements such as seroma, hematoma, lymphocele, and infection combined with intrinsic patient risk factors often hinders healing and facilitates tissue breakdown. Fluid collections create planes between adjacent structures and prevent tissues from falling into their natural position after dissection. Infection can cause local inflammation and cell death that places incisions at risk of breakdown. Bacteria-laden prosthetic grafts with surface biofilm are difficult for the body to incorporate. The groin is prone to moisture accumulation that predisposes patients to infection in the setting of poor hygiene. The location of femoral access incisions in the groin crease also makes it hard to provide adequate compression with dressings and allows for swelling to build up, in turn placing stress on the suture line. The vascular surgery patient population is often more medically complex than other surgical populations with diabetes, obesity, poor diet, and tobacco use being known contributors to vascular disease and deterrents of wound healing. Prior surgery through the groin leaves surgeons sewing scar to scar during subsequent operations.

Groin wounds, as defined by missing soft tissue over the inguinal area, encompass a wide spectrum of presentations. Some patients suffer from superficial wound infections with surrounding cellulitis and minimal if any incisional breakdown, while others may have a noninfected hematoma or seroma that can lead to graft exposure. In extreme situations, patients can have deep wound infections that threaten vascular bypasses or already have exposed graft material with palpable vessels at the base of their wounds. The later cases definitively need coverage to protect exposed critical structures.

It is important to be aware of prior vascular procedures and the location of current bypass grafts before elevating flaps for soft tissue coverage. A large percentage of patients undergo multiple bypass procedures for occlusive arterial disease; for this reason, the arterial supply to various muscles and muscle groups may be precarious following aorto-femoral grafting. Additionally, aorto-bifemoral bypass grafts, femoro-femoral bypass grafts, and iliofemoral bypass grafts can present with relatively cephalad wounds located above the inguinal ligament. These cases are more demanding to achieve soft tissue coverage with leg flaps than for wounds developing after infrainguinal bypass grafts.

The chronology of the wound is also an important factor since chronic wounds are more difficult to heal. By definition, chronic wounds have failed to proceed through the normal healing cycle in a timely manner and can be plagued with prolonged inflammation, local ischemia, biofilm, and cellulitis. While there is no definitive time at which a wound transitions from being acute to chronic, certain clinical signs can help determine the age of the problem. Specifically, a mildly erythematous incision leaking serous or lymphatic fluid within one week of surgery is an acute wound. Chronic wounds have well-developed bursa-lined walls, thick surrounding scar, small areas of exposed bypass grafts in the midst of an otherwise well incorporated graft, and often have a history of suppressive antibiotics having been given. Chronically exposed vascular bypass material are at higher risk of infection and may require explantation of graft material—early treatment of acute wounds in order to avoid these chronic situations is preferable. The success of the procedure and likelihood of obtaining healed wounds is dependent on the chronicity of the wound.

SOFT TISSUE FLAPS

The abdomen and legs serve as the primary sources of tissue for local flap coverage of problematic groin wounds. Abdominal flap options are based off of branches from the external iliac artery and include rectus abdominis and internal oblique muscle flaps. These flaps have an arc of rotation that allows for coverage of wounds both above and below the inguinal ligament. Long abdominal flaps such as the oblique rectus abdominis myocutaneous flap permit the coverage of a groin wound using contralateral tissue.[1] However, they carry high donor site morbidity rates, with abdominal hernia and abdominal wounds that require further treatment being frequent complications. Leg flaps, which receive blood supply from the femoral artery system, are distinctly advantageous for groin wound coverage given their lower donor site morbidity rates and ability to keep the surgical site localized near the wound. Flaps originating from the leg include the sartorius, rectus femoris, anterolateral thigh, and gracilis muscle flaps. As long as leg flaps of the appropriate size are available with patent vessels, they are the preferred option for soft tissue coverage of the groin following vascular surgery.

The sartorius muscle flap has been a longstanding option for coverage of certain groin wounds.[2,3] One of the earliest descriptions of its use stems from a discussion on flap coverage after lymph node dissection in 1948. The muscle is often detached from its origin at the anterior superior iliac spine and transposed medially to cover any exposed vasculature. However, the superficial femoral artery, which provides the segmental arterial supply to the muscle, is often occluded in the vascular surgery population. If by chance it is patent, the trauma from dissection around the proximal portion of the muscle can compromise the blood supply to the end of the muscle and cause ischemia. Another inherent disadvantage to using this flap is that dissection of the flap off of the iliac spine for medialization of the muscle can lead to injury of the lateral femoral cutaneous nerve. Additionally, the limited width of the muscle allows for coverage of the femoral artery and vein but little else in larger wounds. The flap works best for coverage of the bifurcation of the common femoral artery into superficial and profunda femoral branches. Trying to preserve all of the pedicles from the segmental blood supply can keep the muscle tethered and limit its arc of rotation. However, anatomic studies have shown that the first vascular pedicle is vital for sartorius muscle survival, and it is reliably located 6.6 cm away from the anterior superior iliac spine. Therefore, the muscle can be detached from the anterior superior iliac spine and elevated judiciously until the first vascular pedicle is encountered in the proximal portion. The muscle can then be turned over to fill the defect with the tendinous portion anchored to the inguinal ligament.[1,4]

The rectus femoris muscle flap is another option for groin wound coverage. It is bulky, long and has a wide arc of rotation to cover wounds both above and below the inguinal ligament. Compared to the segmental arterial supply of the sartorius, the rectus femoris muscle derives its blood supply from the profunda femoris artery; the vessel arises off the lateral circumflex artery in seventy percent of cases and directly off the profunda femoris artery in the remaining cases. Mobilization of the muscle requires elevation from distal to proximal in order for the proximal arterial inflow to be preserved. The muscle contributes to terminal knee extension and a desire to retain this function has deterred surgeons from using this flap as a first line option. However, studies have shown that the lower peak torque values seen during isometric knee extension in the donor leg when compared to the non-operative (or dominant) leg is of equal deficit when thigh strength was evaluated in matched control cohorts.[5] Thus, sacrificing the rectus femoris for groin wound coverage may not negatively impact knee extension to the extent it was previously thought. One must be certain before elevation of this flap that the tunneled bypass graft does not run anywhere in the vicinity, because donor site healing is not always routine and one must not cause a graft exposure in a second location. A final less important drawback to the use of this flap is the need to divide the sartorius muscle for proper inset. Having discussed these issues, it should be noted that these are all relative issues, and the rectus femoris flap is a viable surgical option and the preferred flap of many reconstructive surgeons.[6]

When faced with medium to large groin wounds, the pedicled anterolateral thigh flap is a safe and reliable flap for soft tissue reconstruction. This fasciocutaneous flap is appealing due to the relative ease of dissection, long vascular pedicle, and adequately sized vessels that emerge off of the profunda femoris.[7] The longitudinal axis of the flap is marked on a line extending between the anterior superior iliac spine and the lateral border of the patella. The anterolateral thigh flap shares the same vascular pedicle as the rectus femoris muscle flap, yet it does not share the same potential negative impact on knee extension. The anterolateral thigh flap also has the advantage of low donor site morbidity, with a majority of wounds closed in a cosmetically acceptable linear scar. However, there is some animal data demonstrating improved soft tissue coverage with muscle flaps as compared to fasciocutaneous flaps due to improved filling of dead spaces and more rapid bacterial clearance.[8] The debate between fasciocutaneous flaps and muscle flaps for coverage of important defects is currently unsettled, and both flap options are reasonable alternatives.

Our preferred flap for groin wound coverage following vascular surgery is the gracilis muscle flap.[9,10] Like the rectus femoris and anterolateral thigh flaps, the gracilis muscle flap depends on the profunda femoris for its blood supply. This dominant pedicle often enters the muscle 5 to 10 cm distal to the pubic tubercle as it passes superficial to the adductor magnus muscle and underneath the adductor longus. The intramuscular neurovascular anatomy, specifically the three neural branches supplying the anterior, mid, and posterior muscle segments, allow for muscle debulking if necessary. The muscle is often unscarred even in the setting of prior surgeries and bypass grafts rarely travel in this area, reducing the risk of bypass exposure during flap elevation and in the event of donor site breakdown. Moreover, elevating the muscle does not result in *any* functional loss to the leg.

SURGICAL ANATOMY AND TECHNIQUE

The gracilis muscle is approached through a standard 10-cm longitudinal medial thigh incision (Figure 39-1). This incision is typically placed slightly posterior to an incision for saphenous vein harvesting; a recent vein incision may even be reopened to locate and mobilize the gracilis muscle. The access incision is often not connected with the groin incision to help preserve skin vascularity (Figure 39-2).

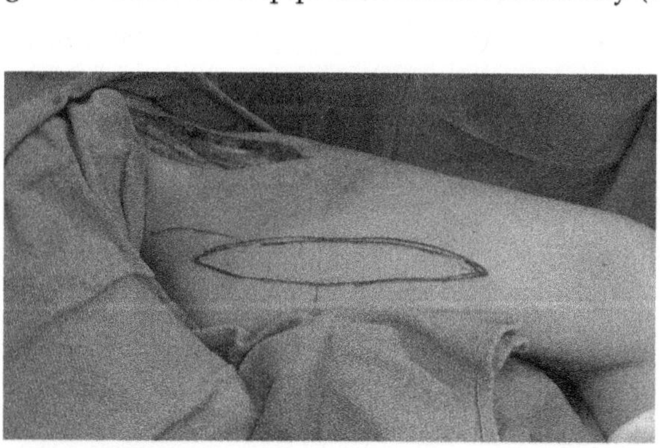

Figure 39-1. Large radiated tumor defect in the proximal left thigh. Gracilis muscle markings are shown on the medial thigh prior to flap dissection.

There are three aids to identify the gracilis during dissection. First, no superficial sensory or motor nerves are encountered during the dissection. Second, the muscle is triangular in shape due to its taper distally as it becomes tendinous two thirds of the way down the thigh; surrounding muscles are rectangular. Third, the muscle can easily be freed along the superficial and deep surfaces.

The investing fascia is opened, and the medial and lateral aspects of the gracilis muscle are thoroughly exposed. Upon incising the fascia along the proximal one-third of the muscle, a consistent skin perforator should be noted. This perforator is the distal continuation of the major vascular vessel after it travels through the muscle. The muscle is detached distally at the level at which the gracilis transitions into tendinous fibers. Dissection of the deep surface of the muscle then begins and all minor segmental pedicles are identified and ligated. The major pedicle enters the muscle on the deep medial surface, 10 cm distal from the pubic symphysis (Figure 39-3). An essential step to properly visualizing the vascular pedicle is wide elevation of the adductor longus muscle off of the gracilis. The origin of the gracilis at the pubic tubercle is then transected.

The major vascular pedicle is traced medially as it travels underneath the adductor longus, and intramuscular branches from the vascular pedicle to the adductor longus should be ligated (Figure 39-4). The space between the adductor longus and sartorius is opened bluntly to reach the proximal aspect of the gracilis vascular pedicle as it just comes off the profunda. Any final attachments connecting the gracilis or its pedicle are freed, allowing the flap to be passed under the adductor into the space in between the sartorius and adductor and within the femoral triangle (Figures 39-5 and 39-6). With the new position of the gracilis, the final dissection of the proximal pedicle at the junction with the profunda femoris is easily accomplished. Rotating the pedicle 180 degrees for placement does not appear to affect the patency of the vessels, and blood flow is confirmed by Doppler. Drains are left in the donor site and underneath the muscle flap. The skin is closed over the flap, typically leaving a small postage stamp size area open to visualize the muscle in the postoperative period. This tends to simply contract and epithelialize closed with

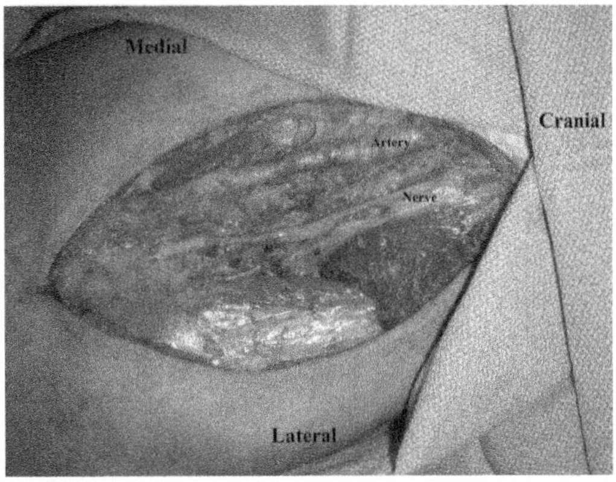

Figure 39-2. Enlarged view of the radiated tumor defect with exposed femoral nerve and artery identified at the base. The incision to access the gracilis muscle is not connected with the defect.

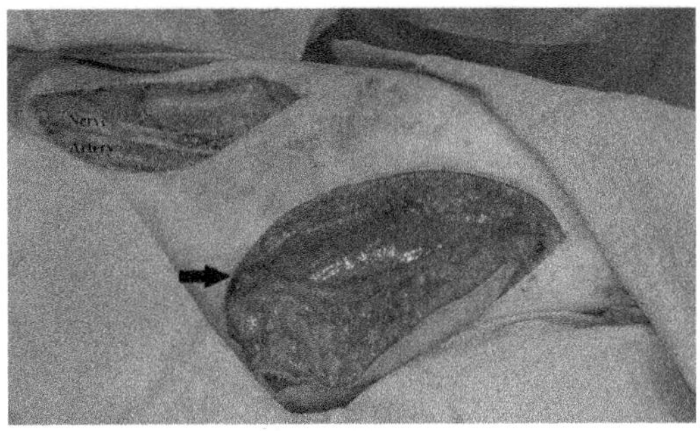

Figure 39-3. Illustration of the gracilis muscle in relation to the proximal thigh defect. The gracilis muscle has been dissected out through a medial thigh incision. The large arrow indicates the proximal vascular pedicle to the gracilis muscle flap, traveling underneath the adductor longus muscle.

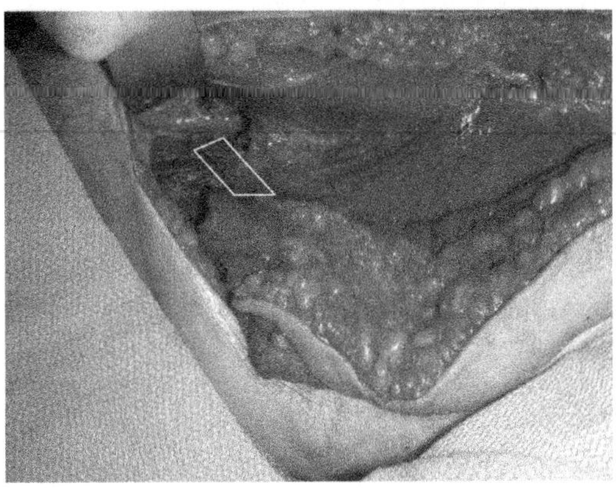

Figure 39-4. The vascular pedicle to the gracilis muscle is highlighted as it passes underneath the retracted adductor longus muscle. A skin paddle was taken with the gracilis muscle due to the large size of the radiated tumor defect with exposed vessels.

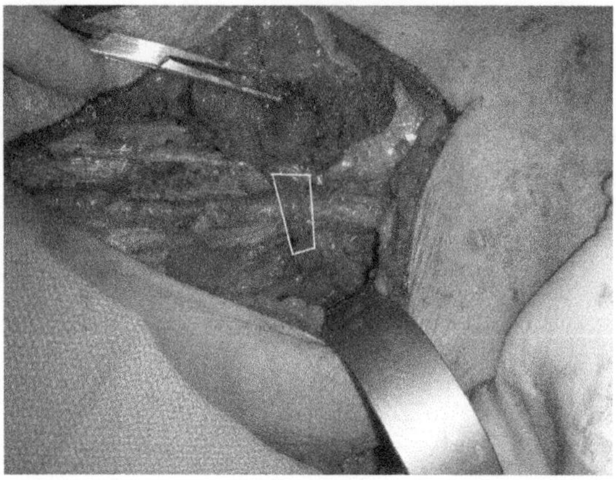

Figure 39-5. Gracilis flap has been passed underneath the adductor longus and transposed into the femoral triangle. The vascular pedicle to the flap is shown overlying the femoral vessels.

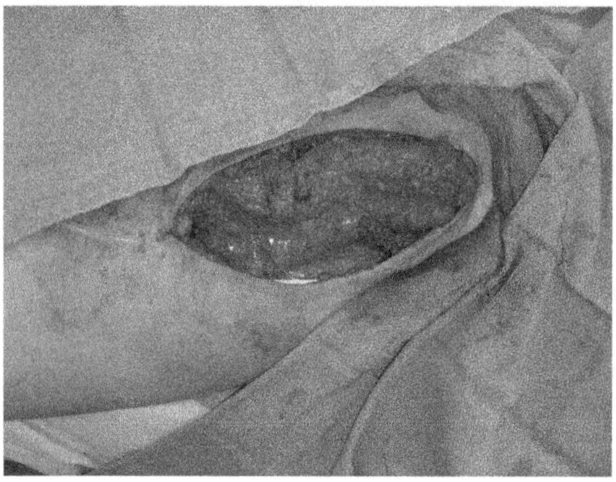

Figure 39-6. Gracilis flap in place for coverage of femoral artery and nerve. In the majority of cases, skin is present to close over the flap (not so in this tumor case).

local wound care over time. For the donor site, any excess skin is excised to reduce the potential for fluid to collect in potential dead spaces.

DISCUSSION

Groin complications after vascular surgery can lead to devastating outcomes and be a significant healthcare burden with prolonged hospital stays and higher medical bills. Early soft tissue coverage is the standard of care for non-healing groin wounds to expedite wound healing and salvage limbs. Our results of the use of the gracilis flap at Northwestern Memorial Hospital were detailed over a decade ago, showing successful wound healing with gracilis muscle flap coverage.[9] The gracilis flap remains our flap of choice to achieve wound closure as it offers a long vascular pedicle with coverage both above and below the inguinal ligament, a large enough surface area for coverage, a donor site without functional loss, and a reliable blood supply off of the profunda femoris.[9] It carries a low donor site morbidity rate and avoids exposure of vital structures if incisional breakdown were to occur.

In an effort to circumvent the aforementioned catastrophic complications associated with groin wounds, the use of prophylactic flaps has been advocated in certain patient populations. Some institutions have gone so far as to employ risk stratification models in an attempt to determine the high risk patients who might benefit the most from prophylactic flaps.[11,12] Along this line, models have shown that patients with risk factors such as obesity and tobacco use, as well as patients deemed to have complex surgical cases that include prosthetic graft and redo operations, are high risk. Even with such criteria, it is not clear-cut as to who warrants prophylactic flap placement. Our own recommendations for prophylactic flaps have both similarities and variances with such stratification systems. We agree that patients who have undergone multiple groin operations and individuals undergoing "re-do" prosthetic reconstructions potentially have the most to benefit from prophylactic flap coverage. We also contend that patients with a history of radiation to the groin, those with pseudoaneurysms, and patients with prior infection in the immediate area of surgery warrant prophylactic flaps. Utilization of prophylactic gracilis flap coverage in such cases can cause a marked decrease in groin incision breakdown, thereby reducing lengths of hospital stay and medical bills.

REFERENCES

1. Lee MJ, Dumanian GA. The oblique rectus abdominis musculocutaneous flap. Revisited clinical applications. *Plast Reconstr Surg.* 2004;114:367–73.
2. Maser B, Vedder N, Rodriguez D, Johansen K. Sartorius myoplasty for infected vascular grafts in the groin: Safe, durable, and effective. *Arch Surg.* 1997;132(5):522–5.
3. Petrasek PF, Kalman PG, Martin RD. Sartorius myoplasty for deep groin wounds following vascular reconstruction. *Am J Surg.* 1990;160(2):175–8.
4. Wu LC, Djohan RS, Liu TS, et al. Proximal vascular pedicle preservation for sartorius muscle flap transposition. *Plast Reconstr Surg.* 2006;117(1):253–8.
5. Sbitany H, Koltz PF, Girotto JA, et al. Assessment of donor-site morbidity following rectus femoris harvest for infrainguinal reconstruction. *Plast Reconstr Surg.* 2010;126(3):933–40.
6. Nelson JA, Fischer JP, Mackay DJ, et al. The limited incision harvest of the rectus femoris flap for complex groin wound management. *Ann Plast Surg.* 2014;73 Suppl 2:S161–4.
7. Ng RW, Chan JY, Mok V, Li GK. Clinical use of a pedicled anterolateral thigh flap. *J Plast Reconst Aesthet Surg.* 2008;61(2):158–64.
8. Gosain A, Chang N, Mathes S, et al. A study of the relationship between blood flow and bacterial inoculation in musculocutaneous and fasciocutaneous flaps. *Plast Reconst Surg.* 1989;86(6):1152–62.
9. Morasch MD, Sam AD 2nd, Kibbe MR, et al. Early results with use of gracilis muscle flap coverage of infected groin wounds after vascular surgery. *J Vasc Surg.* 2004;39(6):1277–83.
10. Hasen KV, Gallegos ML, Dumanian GA. Extended approach to the vascular pedicle of the gracilis muscle flap: anatomical and clinical study. *Plast Reconst Surg.* 2003;111(7):2203–8.
11. Fischer JP, Nelson JA, Mirzabeigi MN, et al. Prophylactic muscle flaps in vascular surgery. *J Vasc Surg.* 2012;55(4):1081–6.
12. Fischer JP, Nelson JA, Rohrbach JI, et al. Prophylactic groin flaps in vascular surgery: the Penn Groin Assessment Scale. *Plast Reconst Surg.* 2012;129(6):940e–9e.

40

Upper Extremity Trauma and the Advanced Surgical Skills Exposures for Trauma (ASSET) Course

Col. (ret.) Mark W. Bowyer, MD, FACS, DMCC

Vascular trauma is a leading cause of morbidity and mortality worldwide, and rapid identification and control of hemorrhage is essential to survival. It is imperative that surgical trainees be proficient in the management of traumatically injured patients to include operative exposure and control of bleeding. Surgical training and vascular surgery training in particular face a number of significant current and future challenges. The introduction of work hour restrictions in the United States, the United Kingdom, and the European Union has led to dramatically decreased opportunities for exposure to clinical material.[1–8] The full impact of work hour restrictions has yet to be fully assessed. However, a recent study by the Royal College of Surgeons of England suggests that the quality of patient care has sharply declined because of the lack of continuity of care and further suggests that operative exposure is insufficient to ensure competency in a range of adequate procedures for independent practice.[9] The introduction of increasing complex procedures to include endovascular techniques has placed additional strain on the ability to ensure that competence and proficiency are achieved during the course of a residency or fellowship program.

In addition to the above, there has also been an increasing trend towards nonoperative management of trauma patients which has resulted in significant decrease in exposure by trainees to surgical experience with trauma.[10–13] The increasing specialization of vascular surgeons and their training has also diluted the available training cases for general surgery residents with the majority of open vascular cases being done by vascular surgeons and vascular residents/fellows to the detriment of general surgery trainees.[14–16] In spite of vascular surgery still being considered an integral part of general surgery training there has been a decreasing experience with vascular trauma among graduating residents. Over the last ten years the average number of major vascular repairs for trauma (includes repair of thoracic aorta, innominate, subclavian, neck vessels, abdominal aorta, peripheral and other vascular injuries) reported by graduating chief residents to the American Board of Surgery decreased from 4.7 in 2003–2004 to 2.3 in 2013–2014 over the course of a residency in general surgery (see Table 40-1).[17] It is important to bear in mind that the numbers reported are averages and as such there are significant numbers of trainees who have zero experience with caring for major vascular trauma. The exposure to vessels to the upper extremity either electively or in the management of trauma is likewise very limited. The Accredited Council of Graduate Medical Education (ACGME) case logs do not specifically report axillary artery exposures, but do list axillary-peripheral bypass which is an adequate surrogate for axillary artery exposure.[17] As seen in Table 40-1, axillary-femoral and other axillary-peripheral bypass procedures done by surgical residents over a residency have averaged between 0.6 and 0.9 with a trend towards decreasing performance. Brachial artery exposures for trauma were not tracked by the ACGME until the 2009–2010 reporting period and have averaged a dismal 0.0 to 0.1 since that time (Table 40-1). Experience with elective exposure of the brachial artery may be postulated from the tracked entry "Upper Extremity Bypass, Endarterectomy, or Repair"; which has an average over the last 10 years of 0.6 to 0.9 (Table 40-1). Additional experience with exposure of the vessels of the upper arm (brachial, radial, and ulnar arteries) can be postulated from the ACGME tracked entry "Vascular Access: Arterio-Venous fistulas and grafts," which averaged between 33.7 and 38.4 over the last decade (Table 40-1). Though only recently added to the case logs, reported experience with fasciotomy by graduating residents was similarly scant with a reported average of 1.5 in 2009–2010, with a decrease each subsequent year to 0.8 in 2013–2014 (Table 40-1).[17] This category does not describe which extremity the fasciotomy was done on, and it is likely that the average experience with fasciotomy of the upper extremity is closer to 0.0.

TABLE 40-1. AVERAGE NUMBER OF SELECTED CASES OVER DURATION OF TRAINING REPORTED BY GRADUATING SURGICAL CHIEF RESIDENTS SUPPLIED AS PART OF CASE LOGS SUBMITTED TO THE AMERICAN BOARD OF SURGERY FROM 2004 TO 2014

Report Year	04–05	05–06	06–07	07–08	08–09	09–10	10–11	11–12	12–13	13–14
Major Vascular Cases (trauma)	4.7	4.6	4.7	4.4	4.7	3.2	2.1	2.9	2.4	2.3
Ax-Fem, Axillary Peripheral Bypass	0.9	0.9	0.9	0.9	0.8	0.7	0.6	0.6	0.6	0.6
Brachial Artery Exposure	X	X	X	X	X	0.1	0.0	0.1	0.1	0.1
UE Bypass, Endarterectomy or repair	0.7	0.8	0.8	0.8	0.8	0.9	0.8	0.7	0.6	0.6
Vascular Access: AV fistulas/ grafts	36.4	38.4	37.9	36.3	36.3	36.2	35.2	36.3	34.2	33.7
Fasciotomy for Injury	X	X	X	X	X	1.5	1.2	1.0	0.8	0.8

Note: Numbers represent the mean for each procedure, and if missing (X), that procedure was not requested during that particular data collection year. Data collated from http://www.acgme.org/acgmeweb/tabid/274/DataCollectionSystems/ResidentCaseLogSystem/CaseLogsStatisticalReports.aspx.

Abbreviations: Ax-Fem = Axillo-Femoral; UE= Upper Extremity; AV = Arterio-Venous.

On the basis of the numbers presented, it is clear that general surgery residents in the United States have, on average, a suboptimal experience with the surgical management of vascular trauma, in spite of it being an integral part of general surgery training. In Canada, vascular surgery has been removed from the Canadian general surgery training objectives. In a recent survey of 29 Canadian surgical residents, 90% reported an intention to perform vascular procedures after training though they reported being inadequately trained in 10 of 13 procedures surveyed.[18] The authors of this study concluded that current trainees may lack the skills and abilities to deal with vascular emergencies. In spite of the growing prevalence of specialist trained vascular surgeons, there are still many areas in the world (developed and developing) where the primary surgeon may not always be a vascular surgical specialist. He or she may have had limited previous exposure to vascular surgery (which is becoming more limited with the specialization of training) and not be practicing the skills set regularly.

While it may be argued that the solution to this is to ensure that a fully trained vascular surgical specialist is available for every trauma case, this is not practical at the present time in many situations outside major centers and certainly in most areas of military and humanitarian surgical practice. Thus the need to train competent practitioners who can handle vascular trauma is universal.[19–21]

In the developed world, vascular trauma is being managed to a greater extent by trauma surgeons and vascular specialists than it has in the past.[20] In spite of this concentration, outside of major urban trauma centers with high percentages of penetrating trauma the experience in vascular trauma is also surprisingly limited for this group as well. As can be seen in Table 40-2, the numbers of major vascular repairs for trauma (thoracic, neck, abdomen, and peripheral vessels) reported to the ABS by vascular surgery fellows though significantly greater than reported by graduates of general surgery residencies, is limited with an average number of cases in the last decade reported between 8.7 and 12.5 during a vascular fellowship.[17] The experience with repair of peripheral vessels (included in the major vascular repairs cited above) averaged 7.2 to 9.0, and exposure of the axillary artery (Axillary-distal bypass) had an average range of 3.4 to 4.4 over the same period (Table 40-2). Experience with brachial

TABLE 40-2. AVERAGE NUMBER OF SELECTED CASES OVER DURATION OF TRAINING REPORTED BY VASCULAR FELLOWS DURING FELLOWSHIP SUPPLIED AS PART OF CASE LOG SUBMITTED TO THE AMERICAN BOARD OF SURGERY FROM 2004 TO 2014

	04–05	05–06	06–07	07–08	08–09	09–10	10–11	11–12	12–13	13–14
Major Vascular Cases (trauma)	8.7	10.9	10.6	10.9	12.5	11.3	10.8	10.7	11.2	12.2
Repair Peripheral Vessels	7.8	8.0	8.2	8.4	9.0	8.3	7.6	7.4	7.2	8.2
Ax-Fem, Axillary Peripheral Bypass	3.5	3.3	3.5	3.4	3.9	3.7	3.9	4.0	3.9	4.4
Brachial Artery Exposure	X	X	X	0.1	0.1	0.3	0.3	0.2	0.4	0.3
Vascular Access: AV fistulas/ grafts	16.6	20.0	21.6	22.2	25.5	28.1	31.1	34.7	34.6	38.7
Fasciotomy for Injury	1.2	1.0	1.2	1.0	1.4	1.4	1.4	2.0	2.0	2.3

Note: Numbers represent the mean for each procedure, and if missing (X), that procedure was not requested during that particular data collection year. Data collated from http://www.acgme.org/acgmeweb/tabid/274/DataCollectionSystems/ResidentCaseLogSystem/CaseLogsStatisticalReports.aspx.

Abbreviations: Ax-Fem = Axillo-Femoral; UE= Upper Extremity; AV = Arterio-Venous.

artery exposure (average 0.1 to 0.4) and fasciotomy, not specified by extremity (1.0 to 2.3) was also remarkably low, and the experience with AV fistulas and grafts (surrogate of elective exposure to brachial, radial, and ulnar arteries was similar if not somewhat less than surgical residents averaging between 16.6 and 38.7 (Table 40-2).[17]

When looking at the practice of specialist vascular surgeons in the United States who recertify in vascular surgery, the number of cases of vascular trauma experience is also quite low. Only 46% of vascular surgeons reported a vascular trauma experience (a one-year experience prior to taking the recertification exam) of greater than zero with a mean average of 4.0 for the remainder in 2003, and in 2009 only 23% reported a vascular trauma experience of greater than zero with a mean of 4.0 for the remainder.[22]

Though it is difficult to judge proficiency and competence by numbers alone, it is clear that the experience of trainees is anything but uniform and that we are graduating specialists with a surprisingly wide spectrum of abilities who when called upon to care for vascular trauma may or may not have the requisite skill set to ensure optimal outcomes. Likewise, a minority of practicing vascular surgeons report having the management of vascular trauma as even a small part of their clinical practice. As such there is a critical need to improve the way we train and maintain the skills of the surgeon caring for vascular trauma in the future.

THE ASSET COURSE

In recognition of these significant training gaps, the American College of Surgeons (ACS) Committee on Trauma (COT) leadership established a Surgical Skills Committee in 2005. This committee was charged with developing a standardized, skills-based cadaver course designed to teach surgical exposure of vital structures that are most likely to pose an immediate threat to life or limb when injured.[23,24] The result of this effort was the development of the Advanced Surgical Skills for Exposure in Trauma (ASSET) course.

The ASSET course is a one-day, case-based, scenario-driven dissection course using unpreserved (fresh) human cadavers, emphasizing surgical exposure of extremity, neck, chest, abdomen, and pelvic vasculature, with additional instruction in fasciotomies and pelvic packing. The target audience of this course is senior surgical residents, trauma fellows, and practicing surgeons who care for victims of trauma. The course is done entirely in the lab with a student to faculty ratio of 4:1. The skills included in the course were culled from a comprehensive list of all possible exposures needed for trauma and a modified Delphi approach was utilized to choose 59 separate skills deemed relevant to the management of trauma for inclusion in the course.[23,24] The committee subsequently developed a course manual, narrated videos of selected procedures, faculty manual, lab slides, and assessment tools, all of which were subjected to review by subject matter and educational experts. A demonstration course was conducted at the Uniformed Services University of the Health Sciences in March of 2008, followed by three additional beta courses, during which the course was further refined prior to final approval and released of the course as an ACS-branded continuing medical education course in March of 2010.[23,24] Since that time the course has been widely adopted, and there are now over 80 approved sites throughout the United States and Canada,[25] as well as sites in Thailand, the United Kingdom, Norway, France, Germany, and Sweden that have conducted more than 300 courses to date.

Additionally, the ASSET course has become the de facto cadaver training course for predeployment training of U.S. military surgeons.

The skills taught in the ASSET course relevant to the upper extremity (UE) include exposure of the axillary artery, the brachial artery, and the ulnar and radial arteries in the forearm. Additionally, fasciotomy of the forearm and hand is taught in the course as well. The course is accompanied by a richly illustrated manual that describes the detailed steps of the exposures in a bullet point format. Examples of the photos used in the text (shot by the author but not included in the ASSET manual) can be found in Figures 40-1 and 40-2.

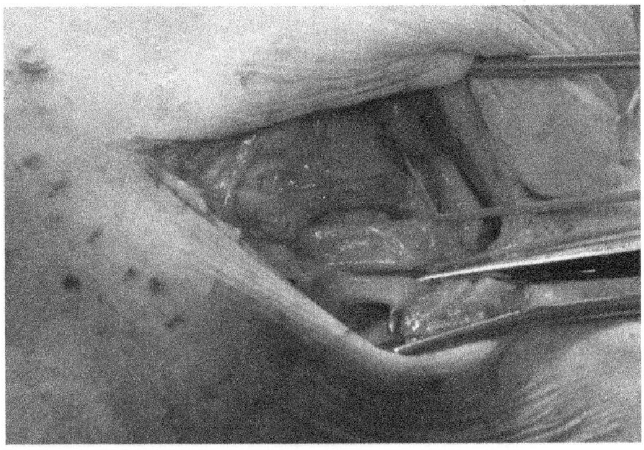

Figure 40-1. Representative photo of the step by step exposure of the axillary artery taught in the ASSET course. The photo is oriented with the right neck to the left lower corner. An infra-clavicular incision has been made, the pectoralis major muscle split, and the pectoralis minor muscle divided to demonstrate (from top to bottom) the axillary vein, axillary artery (with red vessel loop), and the brachial plexus (retracted upwards by right-angle clamp)

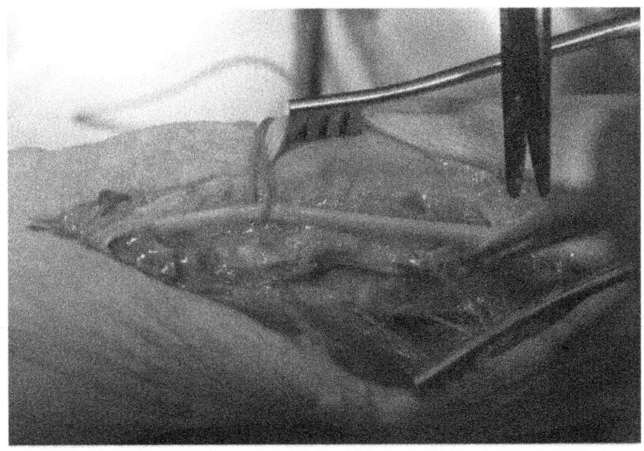

Figure 40-2. Representative photo of the step-by-step exposure of the brachial artery taught in the ASSET course. The photo depicts the right arm of a fresh cadaver with the radial aspect of the arm superior and the wrist to the left of the photo. The median nerve is tagged with a red vessel loop, and the brachial artery is seen immediately inferior to the nerve.

The course has been well received and prior reviews of the course effect have shown significant improvements over base line for both surgical trainees and practicing surgeons for all of the procedures taught in the course. In a review of the first 25 courses, Bowyer et al. found that for 214 participants, significant improvements over baseline self-reported efficacy or comfort level (on a 5-point Likert scale) for exposure of the axillay artery (2.95 vs. 4.19; $P < 4.2 \times 10^{-37}$); exposure of the brachial artery (3.35 vs. 4.27; $P < 1.7 \times 10^{-27}$); and for the performance of forearm fasciotomy (2.76 vs. 4.05; $P < 2.7 \times 10^{-32}$).[15] The ASSET course is currently undergoing a validation study in which surgical trainees who have not taken the course (novices) are asked to perform both axillary and brachial artery exposures (among others) in a fresh cadaver without coaching, while being scored with rigidly developed metrics both in real time and by blinded experts reviewing videos of their performance. In this ongoing validation study, senior surgical trainees were noted in this study to have significantly more confidence in their both the ability to expose the axillary and brachial arteries and their knowledge of anatomy required to perform these exposures than did expert evaluators.[27] This study highlighted significant gaps in anatomical knowledge and the preparation of surgical trainees to care for vascular injuries to the upper extremity, and should serve as a wake-up call for surgical educators.

CONCLUSIONS

Current graduates of general surgical residencies and vascular fellowships are in general ill-prepared to care for vascular injuries to the upper extremities. The reasons behind this are multi-factorial as outlined above, and the solution will need to be multi-modality as well. Increased emphasis on anatomy and broad operative experience with exposure and repair of blood vessels is needed and will require augmentation with specifically designed curricula such as the ASSET course to fill the gaps.

DISCLAIMER

The views, opinions and/or findings contained in this publication are those of the author and do not necessarily reflect the views of the Department of Defense and should not be construed as an official DoD/Army/Air Force position, policy, or decision unless so designated by other documentation. No official endorsement should be made.

REFERENCES

1. Lamont PM, Scott DJ. The impact of shortened training times on the discipline of vascular surgery in the United Kingdom. *Am J Surg.* 2005;190:269–72.
2. Pellegrini CA, Warshaw AL, Debas HT. Residency training in surgery in the 21st century: a new paradigm. *Surgery.* 2004;136:953–65.
3. Bell RH Jr, Banker MB, Rhodes RS, Biester TW, Lewis FR. Graduate medical education in surgery in the United States. *Surg Clin North Am.* 2007;87:811–23.
4. Ferguson C, Kellog K, Hutter M, Warshaw A. Effect of work-hour reforms on operative case volume of surgical residents. *Curr Surg.* 2005;62:535–8.
5. De Martino RR, Brewster LP, Kokkosis AA, et al. The perspective of the vascular surgery trainee on new ACGME regulations, fatigue, resident training and patient safety. *Vasc Endovascular Surg.* 2011;45:697–702.
6. Sadababa JR, Urso S. Does the introduction of duty-hour restrictions in the United States negatively affect the operative volume of surgical trainees? *Interact Cardiovasc Thorac Surg.* 2011;13:316–319.
7. Damadi A, Davis AT, Saxe A, Apelgren K. ACME duty-hour restrictions decrease resident operative volume: a 5-year comparison at an ACGME-accredited university general surgery residency. *J Surg Educ.* 2007;64:256–9.
8. Drake FT, Van Eaton EG, Huntington CR, et al. ACGME case logs: Surgery resident experience in operative trauma for two decades. *J Trauma Acute Care Surg.* 2012;73:1500–6.
9. Thomas RL, Karanja N. Comparison of SHO surgical log books a generation apart. *Ann R Coll Surg Eng.* 2009;9(suppl):356–9.
10. Bulinski P, Bachulis B, Naylor DF, et al. The changing face of trauma management and its impact on surgical resident training. *J Trauma.* 2003;54:161–3.
11. Bittner JG 4th, Hawkins ML, Medeioros RS, et al. Nonoperative management of solid organ injury diminishes surgical resident operative experience: is it time for simulation training? *J Surg Res.* 2010;163:179–85.
12. Brigham RA, Salander JM. Lack of a significant exposure to trauma by residents. *Mil Med.* 1989 Nov;154(11):581.
13. Gaarder C, Skaga NO, Eken T, et al. The impact of patient volume on surgical trauma training in a Scandinavian trauma centre. *Injury.* 2005;36:1288–92.

14. Joels CS, Langan EM 3rd, Cull DL, Kalbaugh CA, Taylor SM. Effects of increased vascular surgical specialization on general surgery trainees, practicing surgeons, and the provision of vascular surgical care. *J Am Coll Surg.* 2009 May;208(5):692–7.
15. Grabo DJ, DiMuzio PJ, Kairys JC, et al. Have endovascular procedures negatively impacted general surgery training? *Ann Surg.* 2007;246:472–7.
16. Cronenwett JL. Vascular surgery training: is there enough case material? *Semin Vasc Surg.* 2006;19:187–90.
17. Accreditation Council for Graduate Medical Education. http://www.acgme.org/acgmeweb/tabid/274/DataCollectionSystems/ResidentCaseLogSystem/CaseLogsStatisticalReports.aspx. Accessed June 5, 2015.
18. Boutros J, Sekhon M, Webber E, et al. Vascular surgery training, exposure, and knowledge during general surgery residency: implications for the future. *Am J Surg.* 2007;193:561–6.
19. van Bockel JH, Bergqvist D, Cairols M, et al. European Section and Board of Vascular Surgery of the European Union of Medical Specialists. Education in vascular surgery: critical issues around the globe-training and qualification in vascular surgery in Europe. *J Vasc Surg.* 2008 Dec;48(6 Suppl):69S–75S.
20. Burkhardt GE, Rasmussen TE, Propper BW, et al. A national survey of evolving management patterns for vascular injury. *J Surg Educ.* 2009 Sep-Oct;66(5):239–47.
21. Eckert M, Cuadrado D, Steele S, et al. The changing face of the general surgeon: national and local trends in resident operative experience. *Am J Surg.* 2010 May;199(5):652–6.
22. Eidt JF, Mills J, Rhodes RS, et al. Comparison of surgical operative experience of trainees and practicing vascular surgeons: a report from the Vascular Surgery Board of the American Board of Surgery. *J Vasc Surg.* 2011 Apr;53(4):1130–9.
23. Kuhls DA, Risucci DA, Bowyer MW, Luchette FA. Advanced surgical skills for exposure in trauma: A new surgical cadaver course for residents and fellows. *J Trauma Acute Care Surg.* 2013;74:664–70.
24. Kuhls DA, Risucci DA, Bowyer MW, Luchette FA. ASSET: An effective educational experience for practicing surgeons. *Bull Am Coll Surg.* 2012;97:31–5.
25. Ali J, Sorvari A, Haskin D, Luchette F, Bowyer M. Potential role of the Advanced Surgical Skills for Exposure in Trauma (ASSET) course in Canada. *J Trauma.* 2011;71:1491–3.
26. Bowyer MW, Kuhls DA, Haskin D, et al. Advanced Surgical Skills for Exposure in Trauma (ASSET): the first 25 courses. *J Surg Res.* 2013;183:553–8.
27. Bowyer MW, Shackelford SA, Garofalo E, Pugh K, Mackenzie CF. Perception does not equal reality for resident vascular trauma skills. *J Surg Res.* 2015 Apr 1. pii: S0022-4804(15)00347-9. doi: 10.1016/j.jss.2015.03.082. [Epub ahead of print]

41

Outcomes after Interfacility Transfer for Ruptured Aneurysms

Matthew Mell, MD, MS

Ruptured abdominal aortic aneurysm continues to be a common and challenging surgical illness in the United States, with an estimated 8,000 to 10,000 deaths per year.[1] Including those for whom death is immediate, overall mortality may be as high as 75%.[2] For patients who survive the immediate rupture event ruptured abdominal aortic aneurysm remains a highly time-sensitive condition: if untreated 25% die within 2–4 hours[3] (Figure 41-1). Conversely, many patients remain clinically stable for a short time after rupture thereby creating a window of opportunity for successful definitive treatment for this otherwise fatal event. As such, it is imperative for patients with ruptured abdominal aortic aneurysm to receive definitive diagnosis and therapy as quickly as possible.

Population studies of patients treated for ruptured abdominal aortic aneurysm have shown modest improvement in operative survival after ruptured abdominal aortic aneurysm over the past decade, thought to be related to technical advances in care as well as improved management of blood loss, hypotension, and metabolic derangements.[4] Contemporary single center studies have shown even better success in treating ruptured abdominal aortic aneurysm.[5–7] These improvements have been attributed to a standardization of care and immediate availability of appropriate personnel, physical resources, and endovascular technology and device inventory. These exemplary studies show that excellent outcomes are possible after treating ruptured abdominal aortic aneurysm, supporting the concept of an unrealized potential for improving survival at a population level.

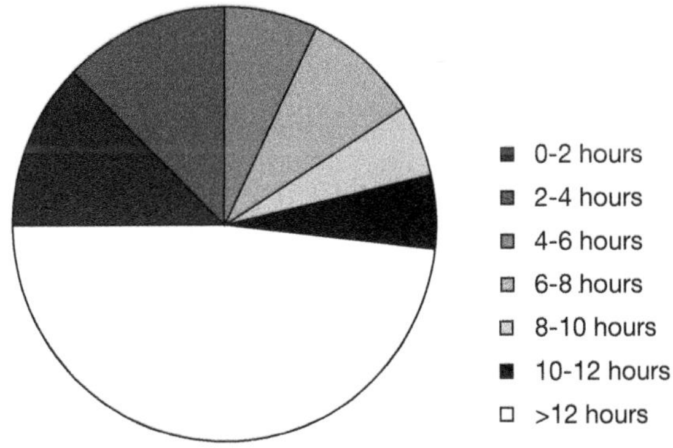

Figures 41-1. Time from admission to death for untreated ruptured abdominal aortic aneurysms.

When confronted with a patient with a suspected ruptured abdominal aortic aneurysm, a health care provider must act quickly to secure the diagnosis and treatment. For patients presenting to a hospital replete with vascular expertise and resources, the episode of care is likely to be seamless from diagnosis to treatment. For patients presenting to a facility without such resources, the pathway for care immediately becomes more complex. Many questions must be answered in a short span of time to expedite care and optimize the opportunity for a good outcome. Is the patient a suitable candidate for treatment? Which diagnostic tests are necessary? Is there a nearby facility that is able to accept a transfer? What is the best mode of transportation? What is the most appropriate management to maintain a clinically stable patient during the transfer? As many sending or receiving hospitals do not have systems in place and no standards exist to address these clinically relevant questions, care may be disorganized with negative impact on outcomes.

CURRENT STATE

Emergency Department Deaths for Ruptured Abdominal Aortic Aneurysm

A potential consequence of poorly organized systems of care for ruptured abdominal aortic aneurysm when local treatment is unavailable is a high Emergency Department (ED) death rate. ED deaths may reflect both those who arrive in extremis as well as those who deteriorate while awaiting definitive care.[8] Using the Nationwide Emergency Department Sample (NEDS) data, we found that 7% of those who present to an ED with ruptured abdominal aortic aneurysm die in the ED, and another 6% die without receiving treatment. ED death for ruptured abdominal aortic aneurysm was independently associated with increasing age, female sex, and initial presentation in non-metropolitan hospitals (Table 41-1). Non-metropolitan hospitals not surprisingly were also most likely to transfer patients for definitive care. This

TABLE 41-1. PREDICTORS OF ED DEATH FOR RUPTURED ABDOMINAL AORTIC ANEURYSM

Factor		Adjusted OR*	95% CI	p-value
Rural vs. Urban teaching hospital		1.9	1.2 – 2.9	0.001
Rural vs. Urban non-teaching hospital		1.4	0.9 – 2.1	0.12
Low-volume ED		1.3	0.8 – 2.2	0.25
Moderate-volume ED		1.0	0.7 – 1.4	0.92
High-volume ED		1.0	Referent	
Region	East	0.5	0.3 – 0.8	0.008
	South	0.4	0.3 – 0.7	0.001
	Midwest	0.6	0.4 – 0.9	0.02
	West	1.0	Referent	
Trauma designation		0.9	0.5 – 1.4	0.54
Age (per decade)		1.9	1.6 – 2.2	<0.0001
Male gender		0.7	0.5 – 0.9	0.008

*Adjusted for co-morbidity and insurance status.

pattern of high ED death rate and high transfer rate suggests that these facilities were not able to provide local care but were also without a rapid and reliable transfer process to move patients for definitive care during a window of hemodynamic stability. Some of these deaths may therefore have been preventable with better systems of care.

We also identified differences in ED death by region, with the West having roughly double the ED death rate even after adjusting for demographic and hospital factors. This region was also less likely to transfer patients. As the Western region of the United States has approximately 25% of the US population but 50% of the land mass, our findings suggest that patients who have greater travel distances and travel times to the initial ED may be more likely to become clinically unstable upon arrival or before transfer can be arranged.

Transfer for Treatment of Ruptured Abdominal Aortic Aneurysm

Single-institution experiences have reported equivalent outcomes for treatment of ruptured abdominal aortic aneurysm after transfer.[6,7,9–11] These studies were limited in that they focused only on patients receiving treatment, excluding those transferred who did not undergo treatment or who died prior to reaching the receiving hospital. Reported outcomes may therefore have been subject to survivor bias as only patients stable enough to receive treatment were included, and those stable after transfer may have self-selected for increased likelihood of survival. As an intent-to-treat analysis, we linked State Inpatient Databases and Emergency Department Databases for New York, California, and Florida to compare outcomes for ruptured abdominal aortic aneurysm for those transferred for care with those treated at the presenting institution.[12] Our goal was to determine the utilization of transfer for ruptured abdominal aortic aneurysm care, and to determine the outcomes over the entire episode of care.

We found that nearly 20% of patients who presented with ruptured abdominal aortic aneurysm were transferred for definitive care. Median travel distance was 27 miles with travel distance of >100 miles for less than 8% of those transferred. Transfer was more commonly used in each subsequent year of the study, from 15% in 2005 to 24% in 2010. Transfer was more likely on weekends, suggesting that at some facilities the resources for local treatment are inconsistently present. Transferred patients had fewer co-morbid medical conditions, and were more likely to present in a smaller nonteaching hospital with fewer nursing resources.

Of those transferred, 17% died without receiving treatment. Overall mortality of transferred (45%) patients was no different than those treated without transfer (43%). When analyzing only those who received treatment, inter-facility transfer was associated with lower mortality, but when including those who died without treatment inter-facility transfer was associated with *increased* mortality (Table 41-2). Mortality was not associated with travel distance or weekend presentation. Our findings support the hypothesis that those surviving the transfer process stable enough to receive an operation are more likely to survive. They also indicate, however, that in the current state the benefits of transfer for operative repair are overshadowed by the mortality of the transfer process. Improving initial patient selection for repair and improving the transfer process should improve the likelihood of clinical stability during transfer and consequently improve overall survival.[13]

TABLE 41-2. INTER-FACILITY TRANSFER AND RUPTURED ABDOMINAL AORTIC ANEURYSM MORTALITY

	Adjusted Odds Ratio*	95% CI	P-value
Non-operative deaths excluded	0.81	0.68–0.97	0.02
Non-operative deaths included	1.30	1.05–1.60	0.01

*Adjusted for age, gender, weekend presentation, admission year, state, comorbidity and insurance status.

PATIENT SELECTION

The cohort of transferred ruptured abdominal aortic aneurysm patients who die without repair comprises two general categories of patients: those who are not suitable for repair, and those who are suitable for repair but deteriorate or die before repair can be performed. Some patients with known AAA have previously declined elective repair and continue to decline emergent repair; however, it is not uncommon for patients who had declined elective repair to request emergent ruptured abdominal aortic aneurysm repair when the alternative is certain death. This scenario provides a challenge for the physician, as these patients frequently have other significant co-morbidities that factored into the decision to forego elective repair yet make survival after ruptured abdominal aortic aneurysm repair more challenging.

No standards exist for selecting the ruptured abdominal aortic aneurysm patient suitable for repair, especially when inter-facility transfer is required for evaluation and repair. Clinical algorithms[14–19] for predicting death have been reported but have not proven to be clinically useful. A recent survey concluded that surgeons in the Western United States most vascular surgeons had few if any exclusion criteria for accepting transfers for ruptured abdominal aortic aneurysm.[20] Specifically, age was not a criterion for suitability, with 7% reporting age greater than 90 years a contraindication to transfer. Similarly, 19% did not consider transfer for those with severe underlying systemic disease and 34% for those unable to perform activities of daily living. These finding contrast results from a similar United Kingdom survey showing that underlying health and lifestyle were far more important the decision-making process.[21] Conversely, both groups reached consensus that hypotension requiring inotropic support did not preclude consideration for transfer, but cardiac arrest requiring CPR generally did.

In the absence of reliable data for determining if a patient is suitable for transfer, the decision to transfer is generally made on a case-by-case basis. As such, requested information to make such a determination varies widely by both institution and physician, which may lead to avoidable delays in transfer. Requests for clinical evaluation, diagnostic laboratory tests or radiographic imaging may be extensive, time-intensive and ultimately unnecessary. For example, respondents in the US study were far more likely to require evaluation by a surgeon or a CT scan prior to transfer compared with UK respondents, perhaps in part explained by the possibility that UK surgeons are more comfortable with an ED diagnosis of ruptured abdominal aortic aneurysm because abdominal ultrasound skills for detecting ruptured abdominal aortic aneurysm are a core competency of ED physician training and are integral to routine ED practice in the United Kingdom.

IMPROVING OUTCOMES AFTER TRANSFER FOR RUPTURED ABDOMINAL AORTIC ANEURYSM

Once a patient with ruptured abdominal aortic aneurysm is determined to benefit from transfer and attempted repair, the prime objective is to rapidly and efficiently provide transport with only necessary diagnostic information and with minimal delay. Previous research has demonstrated that with an organized regional system of care operative repair can be performed in over 95% transferred ruptured abdominal aortic aneurysm patients, with 67% survival.[22] Transfer is most seamless when organized at the sending facility, at the receiving facility, and between the two facilities (Table 41-3). Regional care may be better organized with either a hub-and-spokes or network model.

Key components of an efficient transfer process for the sending hospital include rapid diagnosis, pre-determined receiving hospital(s) and vascular surgeons, simple method of communication with the receiving hospital, rapid and reliable access to appropriate transport (ground or air), and infrastructure to provide the receiving hospital with all pertinent information. Reliable means of transferring CT images when performed, either by disc or sent electronically, should be available.

For the receiving hospital, key components for effective transfer include rapid connectivity between the referring and receiving physicians, a standard approach to patient management during the transport, and an organized approach to operative repair. Rapid connectivity with a simple access phone number is important so that a receiving treating surgeon can be contacted without delay to discuss the transfer, obtain necessary diagnostic information, and determine if treatment is appropriate. Additionally, a transfer center or hospital administrator should participate in the phone call to approve the transfer based on required available operating room, catheterization lab, and hospital bed resources. Ideally, the receiving hospital may have a "no denial" policy to avoid the need for referring facilities to simultaneously call multiple hospitals in order to identify one that is able to accept the transfer. When such a policy is not possible, pre-determined required resources should be known so a denial when necessary it is done so quickly if such resources are not available.

Data are limited as to the optimal approach to management during transport. Most would agree that intravenous access should be obtained but fluid resuscitation should

TABLE 41-3. KEY COMPONENTS FOR AN EFFICIENT RUPTURED ABDOMINAL AORTIC ANEURYSM TRANSFER SYSTEM

Sending facility	Receiving facility	Inter-facility
• Rapid diagnosis	• Easily accessible vascular surgeons	• Rapid and reliable communication
• Avoidance of unnecessary diagnostic work-up	• Pre-determined minimal criteria for accepting transfer	• Electronic means of transferring images
• Pre-determined receiving hospital(s)	• Standard resuscitation protocol for transport	
• Simple method of reaching receiving physician	• Rapid decision-making for acceptance of transfer based on available hospital resources	
• Rapid access to transport	• Organized system of care for ruptured abdominal aortic aneurysm	

be minimal, allowing for permissive hypotension with systolic blood pressure between 70 mmHg to 100 mmHg. Although hypotension is best treated with blood products, obtaining blood for transport generally is not recommended if it will delay the transfer. Pain should be managed with small doses of narcotic pain medication. Sustained hypertension must be avoided as it may lead to frank rupture, and should be treatment with intravenous nitroglycerin, esmolol, or sodium nitroprusside in additional to pain medication. The mode of transportation that provides the most rapid transport should be utilized, which may depend on distance, traffic, weather, and availability.

An organized treatment algorithm for ruptured abdominal aortic aneurysm has led to improved operative survival, approaching 75% in some single-institution studies.[5–7] In addition to the elements previously discussed, such an approach should include trained physicians, operating room, and radiology personnel; immediate availability of blood products and a standard resuscitation protocol; rapid access to endovascular inventory; and a predefined treatment algorithm including guidelines for converting endovascular to open repairs. Resuscitation with trauma-based massive transfusion protocols may provide a survival benefit[6]. The costly and extensive nature of the required resources to optimize outcomes after ruptured abdominal aortic aneurysm may preclude many hospitals from providing such services and thereby supporting the ongoing need for efficient transfer for care. Providing ubiquitous ruptured abdominal aortic aneurysm care at all facilities in fact may not be practical or necessary.

The utilization of transfer for the patient with ruptured abdominal aortic aneurysm has increased yearly since 2005, as has the utilization of transfer for rural patients with ruptured abdominal aortic aneurysm.[12,23] These trends are likely to continue and underscore the need for developing organized systems of care. As specialized centers for treatment of acute aortic conditions improve expand, they may siphon case volume and diminish expertise of local facilities[24], thereby increasing the future need for transfer. This pattern of care may be accentuated by the increasing cost of providing a complete vascular device inventory, as well as the changing patterns of providing vascular care. As community general surgeons who provide vascular coverage leave the work force and are replaced by current-generation general surgeons who are not trained to offer contemporary vascular treatment options. These facilities may not have the resources or case volume to support a vascular surgeon and must therefore refer vascular conditions including ruptured abdominal aortic aneurysm.

THE POTENTIAL ROLE FOR BEST-PRACTICE GUIDELINES

Even with mounting evidence that an organized, systematic approach to ruptured abdominal aortic aneurysm improves outcomes, adoption of such a strategy has been inconsistent: in the Western region of the US 60% of physicians who accept ruptured abdominal aortic aneurysm transfers do not have a formal protocol for treatment, and 70% do not use a transfer protocol or clinical guidelines[20]. Absence of evidence has likely contributed to the range of opinion and approaches regarding essential clinical characteristics, criteria, patient management, and transfer conditions in considering transfer for patients with ruptured abdominal aortic aneurysm.

In the absence of data, the development of best-practice guidelines may provide a framework to address key components of an effective transfer process. For example, eliminating unnecessary diagnostic tests, instituting a pre-defined resuscitation strategy, or more efficiently identify an accepting hospital and physician should reduce variation and improve efficiency of the transfer. Significant time delays from diagnosis at the sending hospital to arrival at the receiving hospital can be reduced, thereby increasing the likelihood that the patient will arrive clinically stable and remain suitable for repair. Improving the proportion of transferred patients who arrive in condition to receive AAA repair will increase the overall ruptured abdominal aortic aneurysm survival.[13] No best practice guidelines exist in the United States. Guidelines have been developed in the United Kingdom and are jointly endorsed by the Vascular Society of Great Britain & Ireland, The College of Emergency Medicine, and the Royal College of Radiologists[25] (Table 41-4). The acceptance of these guidelines and their effect on reducing variation in care, increasing the utilization of operative repair, or improving survival has not been reported.

TABLE 41-4. BEST PRACTICE GUIDELINES FOR THE MANAGEMENT AND TRANSFER OF PATIENTS WITH A DIAGNOSIS OF RUPTURED ABDOMINAL AORTIC ANEURYSM TO A SPECIALIST VASCULAR CENTRE[25]

1. A clinical diagnosis of ruptured abdominal aortic aneurysm (ruptured abdominal aortic aneurysm) should be considered:
   - In patients over the age of 50 years presenting with abdominal/back pain AND hypotension
   - In patients with a known AAA and symptoms of either abdominal/back pain OR hypotension/collapse
   - In patients where an alternative diagnosis is considered more likely on clinical grounds, ruptured abdominal aortic aneurysm still must be excluded, with radiological confirmation made prior to referral. *Level 3, strong recommendation*
2. Permissive hypotension is advocated for patients with a clinical diagnosis of ruptured abdominal aortic aneurysm to maintain an alert patient and systolic blood pressure >70 mm Hg is acceptable. *Level 4, strong*
3. If a specialist vascular service cannot be provided on-site the patient requires transfer to a center with appropriate facilities and expertise. Transfer agreements with the local ambulance service should be in place. *Level 4, strong recommendation*
4. Rapid and coordinated transfer can reduce delays in the patient journey and improve outcome. *Level 3, strong.* To expedite transfer the most senior doctor available should lead and be actively involved the care of any patient with suspected ruptured abdominal aortic aneurysm. Outgoing referrals should go to a senior vascular trainee or consultant.
   Items 5–18 below are all Level 5, with strong recommendation
5. All patients with a clinical or radiological diagnosis of ruptured abdominal aortic aneurysm should be assessed as to their current clinical state AND premorbid level of function to determine suitability for transfer.
6. Patients aged <85 with no/mild/moderate systemic disease should be referred to the receiving hospital's on-call vascular service without delay.
7. Patients age >85 or with severe systemic disease will benefit from a consultant*–consultant discussion prior to transfer to a vascular unit.
8. Impaired mental capacity is not a contraindication to assessment and transfer.
9. Patients who have been previously turned down for elective surgery should still be discussed via a consultant–consultant referral.
10. Contraindications to transfer are restricted to those with cardiac arrest in the current admission and intubated patients. Such patients are unlikely to survive transfer and surgery.
11. There are no ESSENTIAL investigations required prior to transfer. However, a blood gas and an emergency department ultrasound are considered useful, if these incur no delay.
12. Investigations including FBC, U&E, amylase, X-match, CT scans MUST not delay transfer to a center that can provide definitive care. If an alternative diagnosis is more likely, or the investigation can be performed without causing delay, it is reasonable to perform these investigations before transfer.

(Continued)

TABLE 41-4. ***(Continued)***

13. Patients should be treated, if necessary, with both analgesia (according to the College of Emergency Medicine [CEM] guidelines) and fluids before and during transfer. Blood products and inotropes may be required, their use should be supervised by a ST4 or above, trainee or equivalent or consultant.
14. A time-critical transfer in a 999 ambulance, preferably with a paramedic crew is required, although this is not essential.
15. Patients requiring inotropic support will need a suitably experienced and trained medical escort for transfer.
16. The facility to transfer CT images electronically must be in place to ensure all images are transferred to the receiving hospital. If electronic transfer is not possible, a CD or DVD of DICOM files must accompany the patient.
17. Patients should not travel with blood products, unless transfusion already commenced.
18. Patients who remain cardiovascularly stable should be transferred to either an emergency department resuscitation bed or local equivalent. Patients who are unstable may need rapid transfer to theatres.
19. Transfer to a specialist vascular center should occur within 30 minutes of diagnosis.

FUTURE DIRECTIONS

Accepted guidelines may reduce variation in contemporary ruptured abdominal aortic aneurysm diagnosis and treatment. Even with established guidelines based on current evidence, many knowledge gaps can be bridged to optimize the care for the patient with ruptured abdominal aortic aneurysm who requires inter-facility transfer for definitive care. Yet-to-be-determined factors those that better determine suitability for transfer based on likelihood of meaningful survival, most rapidly establish ruptured abdominal aortic aneurysm with the minimal required diagnostic evaluation, and most effectively support a successful regional organization. Furthermore, additional research can improve the transport process including resuscitation efforts during transport as well as communication between facilities to assure accurate sharing of data and information with avoidance of redundant or unnecessary information and preventable delays. Finally, efforts could be made to improve triage in the field. If for example paramedics or emergency medical technicians were able make the diagnosis of ruptured abdominal aortic aneurysm in the field, patients could be triaged to hospitals equipped with the capability to diagnose and treat ruptured abdominal aortic aneurysms thereby avoiding detours to facilities without them. With these and other advances, it is possible to translate the exemplary results of single centers to improved population-level outcomes.

REFERENCES

1. http://hcupnet.ahrq.gov/HCUPnet (accessed June 11, 2015).
2. Heikkinen M, Salenius JP, Auvinen O. Ruptured abdominal aortic aneurysm in a well-defined geographic area. *J Vasc Surg*. 2002;36(2):291–296.
3. Lloyd GM, Bown MJ, Norwood MG, et al. Feasibility of preoperative computer tomography in patients with ruptured abdominal aortic aneurysm: a time-to-death study in patients without operation. *J Vasc Surg*. 2004;39(4):788–791.

4. Mureebe L, Egorova N, Giacovelli JK, et al. National trends in the repair of ruptured abdominal aortic aneurysms. *J Vasc Surg.* 2008;48(5):1101–1107.
5. Mehta M, Taggert J, Darling RC, 3rd, et al. Establishing a protocol for endovascular treatment of ruptured abdominal aortic aneurysms: outcomes of a prospective analysis. *J Vasc Surg.* 2006;44(1):1–8; discussion 8.
6. Mell MW, O'Neil AS, Callcut RA, et al. Effect of early plasma transfusion on mortality in patients with ruptured abdominal aortic aneurysm. *Surgery.* 2010;148(5):955–962.
7. Starnes BW, Quiroga E, Hutter C, et al. Management of ruptured abdominal aortic aneurysm in the endovascular era. *J Vasc Surg.* 2010;51(1):9–17; discussion 17–18.
8. Mell MW, Callcut RA, Bech F, et al. Predictors of emergency department death for patients presenting with ruptured abdominal aortic aneurysms. *J Vasc Surg.* 2012;56(3):651–655.
9. Vogel TR, Nackman GB, Brevetti LS, et al. Resource utilization and outcomes: effect of transfer on patients with ruptured abdominal aortic aneurysms. *Ann Vasc Surg.* 2005;19(2):149–153.
10. Hames H, Forbes TL, Harris JR, et al. The effect of patient transfer on outcomes after rupture of an abdominal aortic aneurysm. *Can J Surg.* 2007;50(1):43–47.
11. Azizzadeh A, Miller CC 3rd, Villa MA, et al. Effect of patient transfer on outcomes after open repair of ruptured abdominal aortic aneurysms. *Vascular.* 2009;17(1):9–14.
12. Mell MW, Wang NE, Morrison DE, Hernandez-Boussard T. Interfacility transfer and mortality for patients with ruptured abdominal aortic aneurysm. *J Vasc Surg.* 2014;60(3):553–557.
13. Karthikesalingam A, Holt PJ, Vidal-Diez A, et al. Mortality from ruptured abdominal aortic aneurysms: clinical lessons from a comparison of outcomes in England and the USA. *Lancet.* 2014;383(9921):963–969.
14. Antonello M, Frigatti P, Maturi C, et al. Open repair for ruptured abdominal aortic aneurysm: is it possible to predict survival? *Ann Vasc Surg.* 2009;23(2):159–166.
15. Chen JC, Hildebrand HD, Salvian AJ, et al. Predictors of death in nonruptured and ruptured abdominal aortic aneurysms. *J Vasc Surg.* 1996;24(4):614–620; discussion 621–613.
16. Hardman DT, Fisher CM, Patel MI, et al. Ruptured abdominal aortic aneurysms: who should be offered surgery? *J Vasc Surg.* 1996;23(1):123–129.
17. Samy AK, Murray G, MacBain G. Glasgow aneurysm score. *Cardiovasc Surg.* 1994;2(1):41–44.
18. Samy AK, Murray G, MacBain G. Prospective evaluation of the Glasgow Aneurysm Score. *J R Coll Surg Edinb.* 1996;41(2):105–107.
19. Tambyraja A, Murie J, Chalmers R. Predictors of outcome after abdominal aortic aneurysm rupture: Edinburgh Ruptured Aneurysm Score. *World J Surg.* 2007;31(11):2243–2247.
20. Mell MW, Schneider PA, Starnes BW. Variability in transfer criteria for patients with ruptured abdominal aortic aneurysm in the western United States. *J Vasc Surg.* 2015.
21. Hinchliffe RJ, Ribbons T, Ulug P, Powell JT. Transfer of patients with ruptured abdominal aortic aneurysm from general hospitals to specialist vascular centres: results of a Delphi consensus study. *Emerg Med J.* 2013;30(6):483–486.
22. Haveman JW, Karliczek A, Verhoeven EL, et al. Results of streamlined regional ambulance transport and subsequent treatment of acute abdominal aortic aneurysms. *Emerg Med J.* 2006;23(10):807–810.
23. Maybury RS, Chang DC, Freischlag JA. Rural hospitals face a higher burden of ruptured abdominal aortic aneurysm and are more likely to transfer patients for emergent repair. *J Am Coll Surg.* 2011;212(6):1061–1067.
24. Davies MG, Younes HK, Harris PW, et al. Outcomes before and after initiation of an acute aortic treatment center. *J Vasc Surg.* 2010;52(6):1478–1485.
25. Vascular Society, College of Emergency Medicine, Royal College of Radiologists. Best Practice Guidelines for the Management and Transfer of Patients with a Diagnosis of Ruptured Abdominal Aortic Aneurysm to a Specialist Vascular Centre. London: VSGBI, CEM, RCR; 2012. http://www.collemergencymed.ac.uk/Shop-Floor/Clinical%20Guidelines/default.asp. [Cited June 2015].

42

Aortic Aneurysms in Abdominal Organ Transplant Recipients

David C. Cron, BS and Michael J. Englesbe, MD

Solid-organ transplantation is the only cure for end-stage organ failure. Post-transplant survival has been improving for abdominal organ transplant recipients. Five-year graft survival is currently around 82% for kidney transplant recipients and 71% for liver transplant recipients.[1,2] As a result, the number of patients living with a transplanted organ continues to rise. In 2013, nearly 200,000 patients were living with a functioning kidney graft, and 70,000 were living with a functioning liver graft.[1,2]

Organ demand continues to outweigh supply, and surgeons are transplanting older and higher-risk organs into older patients with more medical comorbidities.[3] These patients are at increased risk for developing aneurysms, and therefore, vascular surgeons will begin to see more transplant recipients presenting for management of aortic aneurysms. Aneurysms are believed to be more aggressive in transplant patients, and clinical management of aneurysms in these patients is challenging.[4,5] Careful consideration must be given to perioperative management of immunosuppression and repair of aortic aneurysms in the transplant population.

With this chapter, we discuss aortic aneurysms in abdominal transplant recipients, with a focus on abdominal aortic aneurysms (AAA). This chapter has the following goals:

1. Review the natural history of aneurysms in transplant patients.
2. Explain the pathophysiology of aneurysmal disease in transplant patients compared to non-transplant patients.
3. Explain the key concepts behind immunosuppression management in these patients.
4. Identify specific technical issues relevant to the management of aortic aneurysms in liver and kidney transplant patients.

WHAT DO WE KNOW ABOUT ANEURYSMS IN TRANSPLANT PATIENTS?

Natural history

Aneurysms are believed to have a more aggressive course following solid-organ transplantation.[4–9] Unfortunately, the literature on this topic is limited to single-center retrospective studies and case reports. Despite this, there is a general consensus that AAA have higher rates of expansion and rupture in solid-organ transplant recipients.[4,5] Post-transplant, AAA expansion rates are high, ranging from 0.58 to 1.2 cm/yr.[4,5,7,8,10] Average age at aneurysm diagnosis ranges from 55 to 60.[4,5,7,8] Heart transplant patients and abdominal transplant patients both seem to suffer from aggressive expansion and younger age of onset. Most studies focus on AAA, and less is known about the nature of thoracic aortic aneurysms.

Prevalence

The prevalence of aortic aneurysms in transplant patients is poorly defined due to lack of screening studies. One single-center study followed 394 kidney transplant recipients and identified a AAA prevalence of 1.0% in this group.[6] Other retrospective studies identified overall AAA prevalence ranging from 0.2% to 1.4% in kidney transplant patients and 0.3% to 0.7% in liver transplant patients.[4,5] The prevalence of AAA in the general population depends on age and ranges from 1.3% to 8.9% in men and 1.0% to 2.2% in women.[11] It is likely that the true prevalence of AAA in abdominal transplant patients is higher than stated by these retrospective studies, but in the absence of proper screening studies, it is uncertain whether aneurysms are more common in liver and kidney transplant patients compared to other populations.

Importantly, visceral artery aneurysms (most commonly splenic and hepatic artery) are particularly common in liver transplant recipients[5].

WHAT IS UNIQUE ABOUT ANEURYSMS IN TRANSPLANT RECIPIENTS?

It is hypothesized that immunosuppression promotes the progression of atherosclerosis and aneurysmal disease in transplant patients. This hypothesis is not supported by animal studies of immunosuppression and aneurysm growth, and thus the mechanistic relationship between immunosuppression and aortic wall integrity in transplant patients remains unclear. Clinically, new-onset diabetes, hyperlipidemia, and hypertension are common post-transplant due to immunosuppression therapy. These new-onset atherogenic risk factors and altered hemodynamics may contribute to the aggressive nature of aneurysm expansion observed in transplant patients. The influence of immunosuppression medications on the aortic wall is likely a combination of protective factors (anti-inflammatory effects) and risk factors (new-onset cardiovascular risk factors); the balance between these domains may be shifted to favor atherogenesis and aneurysmal growth (Figure 42-1).

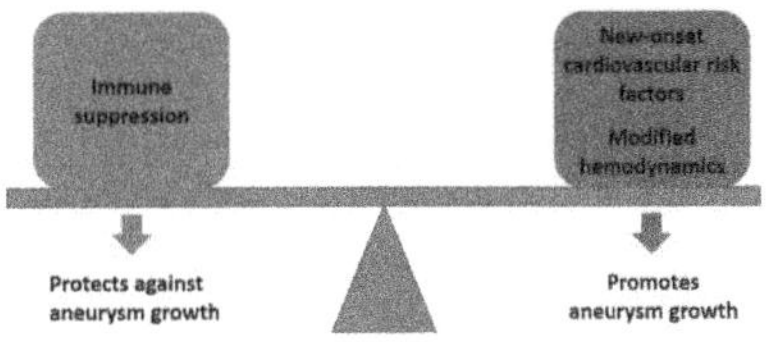

Figure 42-1. This figure depicts the complex, hypothetical relationship between immunosuppressive medication and aortic wall integrity. The relationship is a balance between: (A) the protective immune suppression and anti-inflammatory effects; and (B) the new-onset cardiovascular risk factors and modified hemodynamics associated with immunosuppressive medications.

Immunosuppression: overview

Most transplant recipients receive a calcineurin inhibitor, an antimetabolite, and corticosteroids. Further, a subset of patients receive induction immunosuppression (usually a T-cell depleting biological agent). In the immediate post-operative period, transplant patients are profoundly immunosuppressed, and all discretionary care should be delayed until at least 3 months following the transplant event. Immunosuppression medications are slowly weaned depending on the specific organ, risk of rejection, and clinical course of the patient. The degree of immunosuppression ranges widely; early post-heart or kidney recipients are the most immunosuppressed, whereas long-term liver transplant recipient are minimally immunosuppressed.

Immunosuppression: aortic wall integrity

AAA growth is characterized by atherosclerotic degeneration of the aortic wall, which is in part a cellular immune response. Immunosuppression targets cell-mediated immunity by inhibiting T-cell proliferation and blocking T-cell promoting cytokines such as IL-2. It is therefore intuitive that immunosuppression may inhibit aneurysm growth. Experimental aneurysm models in animals support this hypothesis. Calcineurin inhibitors and mTOR inhibitors have been shown to stabilize atherosclerotic lesions and inhibit aneurysm expansion in animal models[12–14]. There are ongoing clinical trials investigating the utility of anti-inflammatory agents in the prevention of adverse cardiovascular events[15]. Though the experimental biology supports a link between immunosuppression and aortic wall stability, the opposite effect has been seen clinically in transplant patients, as aneurysm expansion is reportedly more rapid. However, these clinical observations are based on limited data, and more investigation is needed.

Immunosuppression: hemodynamics and cardiovascular risk

The more virulent course of AAA in transplant patients is possibly related to changes in hemodynamics following transplant. Hypotension is common in patients with end stage liver and heart disease. Following transplantation, hypertension is common. These hemodynamic changes affect aortic wall stress and potentially the natural history of AAA.

Additional cardiovascular risk factors that commonly develop following transplantation include diabetes and hyperlipidemia. Further, many transplant recipients develop end-organ failure related to cardiovascular disease, especially renal and cardiac failure. This exacerbation of cardiovascular risk likely affects the rate of AAA progression in these patients. Aggressive management of cardiovascular risk factors is key for all transplant patients, as death related to cardiovascular disease is the most common cause of mortality in these patients.[16]

CLINICAL MANAGEMENT OF ANEURYSMS IN TRANSPLANT PATIENTS

Aneurysm screening

As discussed above, there is no conclusive evidence suggesting that the prevalence of AAA is higher in transplant patients. As such, we do not recommend that all patients be screened for aneurysm prior to transplantation. Patients with a clinical suspicion or strong family history need to be screened for AAA prior to transplantation. In practice, many transplant patients have available pre-transplant imaging that can be used to screen for aneurysm. At our institution, standard pre-transplant workup includes an abdominal ultrasound and likely MRI for liver transplant recipients and a non-contrast CT scan of the abdomen for renal transplant recipients with significant cardiovascular risk factors. The CT scan of the abdomen is for operative planning; circumferential calcification of the external iliac vessels may preclude transplantation in marginal renal transplant candidates.

Given the data suggesting rapid AAA expansion and increased rate of rupture in post-transplant patients, any patients with known aneurysm prior to transplantation should be followed closely with a low threshold for repair.

Timing of repair

Transplant recipient selection considers a broad range of physiologic, anatomic, and psychosocial factors. Transplant teams lack expertise in AAA management. Close collaboration between vascular surgeons and the transplant team is necessary to assure these complex patients get appropriate care. Vascular surgeons should consult with transplant surgeons regarding a patient's ability to tolerate major surgery.

When an aneurysm is detected prior to transplantation, timing of elective AAA repair must be carefully considered. Kidney transplant candidates presenting with AAA should have their aneurysm repaired prior to transplantation since the risk of renal complications following aneurysm repair puts the allograft at risk. These patients are generally stable enough to tolerate the operation by endovascular or open approach. When pre-transplant AAA repair is not possible, repair can be deferred until after transplantation. Methods of perioperative renal allograft protection are discussed below.

Elective AAA repair on patients with significant liver disease is risky. Any signs of hepatic decompensation such as muscle wasting, ascites, platelet count less than 50, or encephalopathy are contraindications to elective repair. If a well-compensated cirrhotic patient requires repair, endovascular AAA repair is preferable.

When a post-transplant patient presents with a de novo AAA, the decision to repair is less complicated. Transplant patients recovering from an infection or rejection are unstable, and aneurysm repair should be deferred until the patient fully recovers. When stable, transplant patients tolerate AAA repair well.[4,17–19] Aortic aneurysms are reported to rupture at smaller sizes in transplant patients, and therefore, repair should be offered once the AAA is 5 cm.[4,6]

Perioperative management of immunosuppression

Transplant patients are all maintained on immunosuppressive medications to prevent graft rejection, and it is imperative that they remain on these medications. Most immunosuppressive medication are oral, and they should be kept on these medications even if they are taking no oral food or drink. Intravenous immunosuppressive medications should not be used, as they are difficult to administer and can have serious adverse effects.

If a transplant patient has a prolonged hospital stay following aneurysm repair, monitoring of drug levels should occur to assure proper levels of immunosuppression. If a transplant patient has a complicated postoperative course following aneurysm repair, immunosuppression doses may need to be lowered. This is due to the natural immunosuppression associated with a critically ill state. Transplant physicians should always be contacted in these scenarios prior to modifying immunosuppression regimens.

Wound complications are common in transplant patients. It is unclear if this is due to immunosuppression or their underlying disease processes. It is well recognized among surgeons that patients on chronic steroid maintenance have altered tissue integrity. Despite this, immunosuppression medications should not be altered, with the exception of Rapamycin. This drug works by inhibiting the mammalian target of Rapamycin (mTOR) pathway, and it is known to impair wound healing by suppressing smooth muscle cell growth and fibroblast migration. In the authors experience as well as others, wound complications rates are high after major surgery in the vast majority of patients maintained on Rapamycin.[20,21] In patients undergoing open AAA repair, Rapamycin should be replaced with another immunosuppressive medication for the duration of the perioperative period. It is not necessary to discontinue Rapamycin for endovascular aneurysm repair, but wound complications from a femoral incision can still be expected. Table 42-1 provides a

TABLE 42-1. PERIOPERATIVE RECOMMENDATIONS FOR MANAGEMENT OF TRANSPLANT IMMUNOSUPPRESSION IN ANEURYSM PATIENTS

Medication	Recommendations
Calcineurin inhibitors (cyclosporine, tacrolimus)	• Maintain oral medication throughout perioperative period • May need to adjust dose if postoperative course is complicated or if prolonged NPO status • Acute nephrotoxicity if serum levels elevated
Corticosteroids	• Perioperative stress dose steroids typically unnecessary • In case of life-threatening infection, corticosteroids should be aggressively weaned
Antimetabolites (mycophenolic acid, azathioprine)	• In case of life-threatening infection, consider decreasing dose or discontinuing
mTOR Inhibitors	• High rates of wound complications due to inhibition of smooth muscle cells and fibroblasts • Consider replacing with a different medication prior to open repair • Can be maintained though endovascular repair, but expect wound complications
Monoclonal and polyclonal antibodies Intravenous immunoglobulins	• In patients who have recently received these, elective surgery should be deferred until patient is more stable
Plasmapheresis	• Avoid in perioperative period due to profound immunosuppression • Post-plasmapheresis coagulopathy is possible

summary of recommendations for management of the various classes of immunosuppressive medications. A transplant physician should be involved with immunosuppression management.

Technical considerations for aneurysm repair

Transplantation is associated with increased risk of renal failure. The overall incidence of chronic renal failure ranges from 7% to 21% following nonrenal organ transplantation.[22] The cause is in large part related to the nephrotoxic side effects of calcineurin inhibitors—a mainstay of immunosuppression for most transplant patients. Additionally, the same factors that predispose transplant patients to aneurysm—modified hemodynamics, diabetes, hypertension—also contribute to renal dysfunction. Outcomes are poor for transplant patients who develop renal failure.[22] Renal impairment can go undetected in patients with seemingly normal renal function. It is therefore imperative to implement kidney protective measures when caring for all transplant recipients. Intravenous contrast should be minimized to the extent possible during imaging or endovascular repair in all patients. When contrast is used, patients should be hydrated to protect kidney function.

As an additional consideration for abdominal organ transplant patients, if an aneurysm is recognized near the anastomosis, it is likely an anastomotic pseudoaneurysm. Endovascular management of this problem is preferred. In kidney patients in particular, surgical management of these pseudoaneurysms typically results in transplant nephrectomy.

Kidney recipients

Kidney recipients presenting with aortic aneurysm will be encountered more frequently than other groups of organ recipients. It is critical to maintain function of the transplanted kidney, as mortality is high in these patients following graft loss.[23] Endovascular repair is preferred whenever possible. Prior to repair, imaging of the aorta from aneurysm to kidney allograft is mandatory. The renal graft is most often sewn to the external iliac artery, 3 to 10 cm from the bifurcation of the external and internal iliac. For this reason, repair is challenging when aneurysmal disease includes the iliac artery. Though the external iliac is less commonly affected by aneurysmal dilatation, stenting an iliac aneurysm will still often compromise inflow to the transplanted kidney. When this cannot be avoided by endovascular approach, open repair must be considered. In an open approach, the transplanted kidney does not need to be mobilized. If mobilization is necessary, be aware that doing so will be difficult, as there will be significant adhesions between the graft and the retroperitoneal structures. Injury to the transplant ureter may lead to graft loss and vascular graft infectious complications.

There are various surgical techniques to preserve renal function in open AAA repair in renal transplant recipients. The literature describing the techniques is limited to small case reports.[18,19] The most commonly reported technique involves axillofemoral bypass. By this method, the transplant kidney receives retrograde perfusion while the aorta and or iliac are clamped during aneurysm repair. Similarly, an aortofemoral shunt can be used to provide temporary perfusion of the allograft. An extracorporeal circuit can be used to provide perfusion to the transplant kidney via cannulation of the femoral artery and vein, but this technique requires significant experience and resources to manage the extracorporeal membrane oxygenation. Cold perfusion with Ringer's lactate or topical cooling can also be used to extend aortic cross-clamp time. In the author's experience, though these methods improve perfusion and may reduce ischemia, they are largely unnecessary. Though limited to case reports and subject to positive outcome bias, critical reviews of the literature suggest no difference in renal function or outcomes when using the above methods compared to a "clamp-and-go" approach.[18,19] In general, surgical outcomes are favorable for renal transplant patients following AAA repair by both endovascular and open approach.[4,17–19] We advise against these aggressive renal protection techniques in patients with low creatinine as these techniques are not without their own risk of complications. However, these techniques are appropriate in patients with marginal or impaired renal function.

Liver recipients

When a liver transplant recipient presents with AAA needing repair, there are a few important technical considerations. Assuming a patent portal vein and functioning graft, these patients are cured of portal hypertension. However, liver transplant recipients often still have considerable splenomegaly. Importantly, about 5% of these patients have an aortic conduit from either the supraceliac or infrarenal aorta to the hepatic artery. It is important to consider the location of this conduit prior to aneurysm repair. For these reasons, preoperative imaging of the aneurysm and transplant liver is essential for operative planning. Except for the right upper quadrant, a liver transplant abdomen is relatively free of abdominal adhesions in most patients. Endovascular repair is preferred if technically and anatomically feasible, but in general, open repair can be tolerated in a stable liver transplant recipient.

Pancreas recipients

Pancreas transplants are less commonly performed compared to kidney and liver. Therefore, pancreas transplant recipients with aneurysms will be seen less frequently. Most pancreas transplants are performed as a simultaneous kidney-pancreas transplant. In this case, it will be important to consider the renal-specific recommendations provided above.

Aneurysm repair in a pancreas transplant recipient is easiest to manage by endovascular approach. If an open approach is taken, it may be difficult to access the aorta or iliac arteries without jeopardizing the transplant. The pancreas allograft is usually anastomosed to the right common iliac. Occasionally, it is sewn instead to the external iliac or the aorta. Mobilization is hazardous due to the delicacy of the pancreas parenchyma. Further, the pancreas is usually attached to its loop of small bowel, and it is therefore often necessary to detach this bowel anastomosis to expose the aorta or iliac vessels. Reconstruction of this anastomosis is often difficult.

If integrity and or perfusion of the pancreas allograft cannot be maintained during repair of a life-threatening aneurysm, priority is given to the aneurysm repair. Unlike other organs, a pancreas transplant does not confer a survival benefit. If the aortoiliac stent must be deployed across the pancreas anastomosis, management of the compromised allograft will depend on the preoperative status of the transplant pancreas. If the pancreas allograft was not functioning and did not take up contrast on imaging at the time of aneurysm repair, then the graft can be left in place. However, if the graft was functioning at the time of aneurysm repair but inflow was compromised by stent placement, then the graft should be removed in the immediate postoperative period.

SUMMARY

Post-transplant patients suffer a more virulent course of AAA. Endovascular repair is preferable to open aneurysmectomy in the majority of cases. Careful titration of immunosuppression should be done in close collaboration with transplant physicians. Specific technical considerations are important in transplant patients related to location of and inflow to the allograft.

REFERENCES

1. Matas AJ, Smith JM, Skeans MA, et al. Optn/srtr 2013 annual data report: Kidney. *Am J Transplant.* 2015;15 Suppl 2:1–34.
2. Kim WR, Lake JR, Smith JM, et al. Optn/srtr 2013 annual data report: Liver. *Am J Transplant.* 2015;15 Suppl 2:1–28.
3. Abecassis M, Bridges ND, Clancy CJ, et al. Solid-organ transplantation in older adults: Current status and future research. *Am J Transplant.* 2012;12(10):2608–22.
4. Englesbe MJ, Wu AH, Clowes AW, Zierler RE. The prevalence and natural history of aortic aneurysms in heart and abdominal organ transplant patients. *J Vasc Surg.* 2003;37(1):27–30.
5. Cron DC, Coleman DM, Sheetz KH, et al. Aneurysms in abdominal organ transplant recipients. *J Vasc Surg.* 2014;59(3):594–8.
6. Favi E, Citterio F, Tondolo V, et al. Abdominal aortic aneurysm in renal transplant recipients. *Transplant Proc.* 2005;37(6):2488–90.
7. Fazel S, Lawlor DK, Forbes TL. Abdominal aortic aneurysms following orthotopic heart transplantation. *Vasc Endovascular Surg.* 2004;38(2):149–55.
8. Piotrowski JJ, McIntyre KE, Hunter GC, et al. Abdominal aortic-aneurysm in the patient undergoing cardiac transplantation. *J Vasc Surg.* 1991;14(4):460–7.
9. Vantrimpont P, van Dalen BM, van Riemsdijk, et al. Abdominal aortic aneurysms after heart transplantation. *J Heart Lung Transplant.* 2004;23(2):171–7.
10. Ballotta E, Merenda R, Mion E, Da Giau G. Abdominal aortic aneurysm in liver transplant recipients. *Langenbecks Arch Surg.* 2001;386(6):426–9.
11. Sakalihasan N, Limet R, Defawe OD. Abdominal aortic aneurysm. *Lancet.* 2005; 365(9470):1577–89.
12. Dai J, Michineau S, Franck G, et al. Long term stabilization of expanding aortic aneurysms by a short course of cyclosporine a through transforming growth factor-beta induction. *PLoS One.* 2011;6(12):e28903.
13. Yamaguchi T, Yokokawa M, Suzuki M, et al. The effect of immunosuppression on aortic dilatation in a rat aneurysm model. *Surg Today.* 2000;30(12):1093–9.
14. Rouer M, Xu BH, Xuan HJ, et al. Rapamycin limits the growth of established experimental abdominal aortic aneurysms. *Eur J Vasc Endovasc Surg.* 2014;47(5):493–500.
15. Everett BM, Pradhan AD, Solomon DH, et al. Rationale and design of the cardiovascular inflammation reduction trial: A test of the inflammatory hypothesis of atherothrombosis. *Am Heart J.* 2013;166(2):199–207 e115.

16. Lentine KL, Costa SP, Weir MR, et al. Cardiac disease evaluation and management among kidney and liver transplantation candidates: A scientific statement from the american heart association and the american college of cardiology foundation: Endorsed by the american society of transplant surgeons, american society of transplantation, and national kidney foundation. *Circulation.* 2012;126(5):617–63.
17. Gallagher KA, Ravin RA, Schweitzer E, et al. Outcomes and timing of aortic surgery in renal transplant patients. *Ann Vasc Surg.* 2011;25(4):448–53.
18. Leon LR, Jr., Glazer ES, Hughes JD, Bui TD, Psalms SB, Goshima KR. Aortoiliac aneurysm repair in kidney transplant recipients. *Vasc Endovascular Surg.* 2009;43(1):30–45.
19. Sadat U, Huguet EL, Varty K. Abdominal aortic aneurysm surgery in renal, cardiac and hepatic transplant recipients. *Eur J Vasc Endovasc Surg.* 2010;40(4):443–9.
20. Burgos FJ, Pascual J, Quicios C, et al. Post-kidney transplant surgical complications under new immunosuppressive regimens. *Transplant Proc.* 2006;38(8):2445–47.
21. Kuppahally S, Al-Khaldi A, Weisshaar D, et al. Wound healing complications with de novo sirolimus versus mycophenolate mofetil-based regimen in cardiac transplant recipients. *Am J Transplant.* 2006;6(5):986–92.
22. Ojo AO, Held PJ, Port FK, et al. Chronic renal failure after transplantation of a nonrenal organ. *N Engl J Med.* 2003;349(10):931–40.
23. Merion RM, Ashby VB, Wolfe RA, et al. Deceased-donor characteristics and the survival benefit of kidney transplantation. *JAMA.* 2005;294(21):2726–33.

43

Complications of Indwelling Retrievable versus Permanent IVC Filters

Benjamin B. Lind, MD and Tina R. Desai, MD

Interruption of the inferior vena cava has become increasingly popular as a treatment modality for venous thromboembolism (VTE). The first vena cava interruption procedure to prevent pulmonary embolization of deep venous thrombosis was described by Armand Trousseau in 1865.[1] Initial reported morbidity and mortality were high, and the technique was modified to allow some blood flow through the cava, such as the DeWeese clip. However, these techniques did not gain widespread acceptance until the introduction of percutaneous devices was made possible by the introduction of the Seldinger technique. The Greenfield filter, introduced by Lazar Greenfield in 1973,[2] represented the first use of a modern conical design inspired by discussion with an engineer who worked on oil pipelines, which are prone to sludge collection. The conical design allowed sludge collection towards the apex of the structure while flow was maintained at the periphery. The introduction of this concept to the inferior vena cava (IVC) filter facilitated percutaneous insertion and improved patency compared to the disc shaped Mobin-Uddin Umbrella that preceded it.[3]

Following the introduction of the Greenfield filter and the development of several other percutaneous devices, there was an exponential rise of 2000% in IVC filter use between 1979 and 1999.[4] Although anticoagulation remains the primary treatment modality for VTE, there has been a liberalization of IVC filter use with expanding indications, which continued with the introduction of retrievable filters in 2003. Retrievable filters, with the theoretical option of retrieval when no longer necessary, represented the next phase in the development of IVC filters. Introduction of retrievable filters led to a continued expansion of the indications for filter placement. In fact, a number of studies of retrievable filters now report that 14%–58% of filters are placed prophylactically in patients who do not have a diagnosis of acute venous thromboembolism.[5–8] Consideration of the complications associated with IVC filters is essential in defining appropriate use of these devices.

There are a number of different filters on the market, which can be classified as either "permanent," "retrievable," "temporary," or "convertible." Retrievable filters are defined as devices designed for image-guided percutaneous removal during device-specific time windows of retrievability with the use of catheter-based technologies. All commercially available retrievable filters in the US are FDA-approved for permanent placement but have the theoretical benefit of being able to be retrieved when the risk of pulmonary embolism is no longer significant. The design of retrievable filters differs from that of most permanent filters and their natural history, if left in the IVC indefinitely, is not known. With regards to retrievable filters, they are designed to be collapsed like an umbrella and withdrawn through a vascular sheath. It is felt that this structural modification, in comparison to permanent filter designs, is an engineering trade-off balancing long-term design integrity and retrievability. Convertible filters are those devices engineered to allow the filter to be structurally modified within a time window after placement, allowing the filter to collapse against the IVC wall thereby no longer providing caval filtration.[5,9] The majority of filters in use today are either permanent or retrievable. Each of these filter types may have common and unique complications associated with them.

It is important to consider that most retrievable filters, whether placed therapeutically or prophylactically, are not retrieved. The majority are left in place permanently, with retrieval rates ranging from 4 to 50%.[6,8,10–15] Little is known about the long-term consequences of leaving retrievable filters in place indefinitely. The complications associated with retrievable filters must be considered in the context of these filters being left in place permanently.

Complications of IVC filter placement can be categorized into implantation complications related to percutaneous access (such as puncture site hematoma, puncture site DVT, AV fistula, pneumothorax); complications unique to IVC filter implantation (such as filter misplacement or tilt, IVC perforation); and complications unique to long term indwelling IVC filters (such as strut perforation, device fracture, filter thrombosis, and filter migration) which will be the primary focus of this chapter.

Implantation-related complications such as filter misplacement are relatively unusual with the availability of modern imaging technology but filter placement in the gonadal veins (Figure 43-1), iliac veins or suprarenal vena cava can occur. IVC

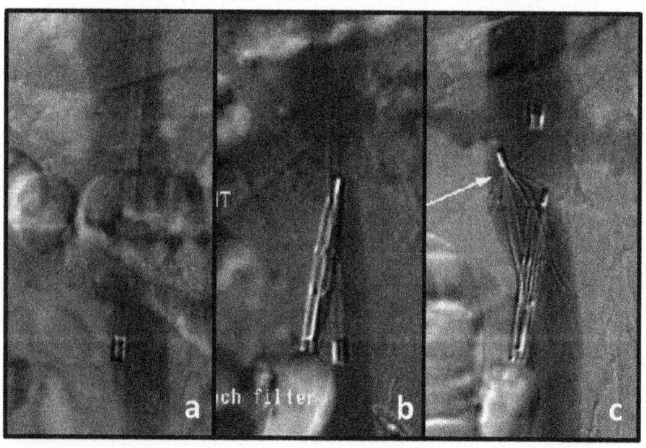

Figure 43-1. Filter malposition: (**a**) Venogram prior to filter position with sheath tip inadvertently positioned into right gonadal vein; (**b**) filter placement into right gonadal vein with incomplete deployment; (**c**) second filter placement in IVC above initial malpositioned filter.

perforation was a concern with the original Greenfield filters but is a rare occurrence with modern retrievable and permanent IVC filters and not clinically significant when it does occur. Technical success rates of 97%–100% are reported with IVC filter placement in most centers.

Specific complications of indwelling filters (permanent or retrievable filters) include thrombotic and device-related complications. Thrombotic complications of filters include recurrent deep vein thrombosis, IVC thrombosis, and pulmonary embolism after filter placement. Reported rates of recurrent thromboembolism after IVC filter placement vary depending on type of filter and type and length of follow-up, and range from 4 to 36%. Notably, routine follow-up evaluation for lower extremity deep vein thrombosis is extremely variable in these studies and the continued use of anticoagulation after filter placement is not well documented. IVC thrombosis, which was more common with earlier types of caval interruption, now occurs uncommonly after filter placement (0.5%–3%) but can result in significant morbidity if it occurs (Figure 43-2). Some reports of IVC "stenosis" after filter placement may also represent caval thrombosis in its chronic state. Finally, protection from pulmonary embolism (PE) is greatest in the early period after filter placement and the rate of PE can increase to 6.2% at 8 year follow-up, according to a long-term prospective study by Decouses and colleagues.[16]

Device-related complications of IVC filters have been reported with both permanent and retrievable filters and include strut perforation, strut fracture, and filter migration. Strut perforation is commonly seen after retrievable IVC filter placement and is a result of the design of these filters that facilitates retrieval. One review found that 86% of Gunther Tulip and Celect filters showed evidence of perforation on imaging between 1 and 880 days after placement.[17] Other studies have shown filter penetration of the IVC ranging from 10 to 56%.[15,18,19] Given the large number of retrievable filters left in place, it is likely that most perforations are asymptomatic. However, a subset of these patients will present with symptomatic perforation. Any structure adjacent the IVC may be affected, and perforations are seen into the duodenum, mesocolon, aorta, and lumbar vertebral body (Figure 43-3). Fracture of filter struts may be associated with penetration through the wall of the IVC and has the additional risk of embolization to vital structures such as the heart (Figure 43-4 and 43-5). Filter fracture is most commonly

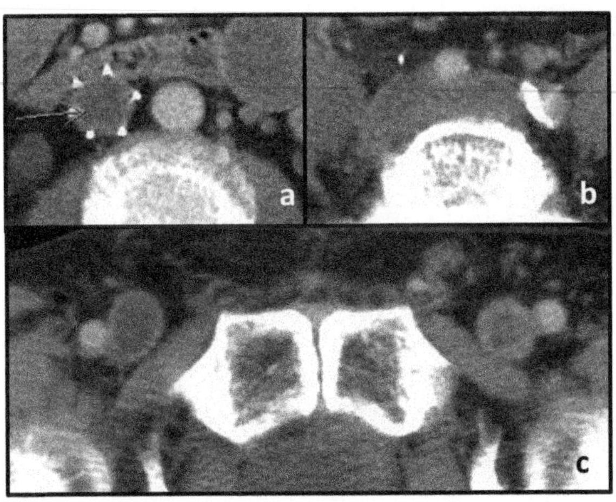

Figure 43-2. IVC thrombosis within filter (**a**), extending into bilateral iliac (**b**) and common femoral veins (**c**).

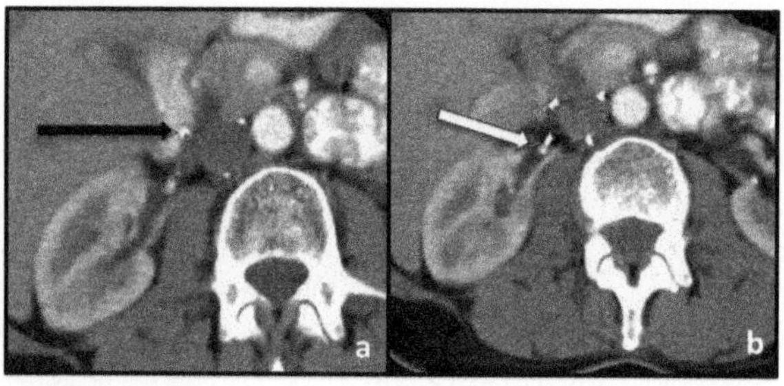

Figure 43-3. Perforation of retrievable filter prongs into duodenum (**a**) and ureter (**b**).

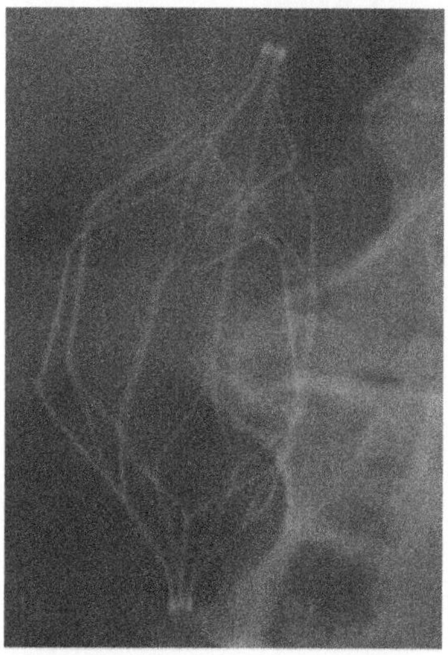

Figure 43-4. Fracture of Optease filter.

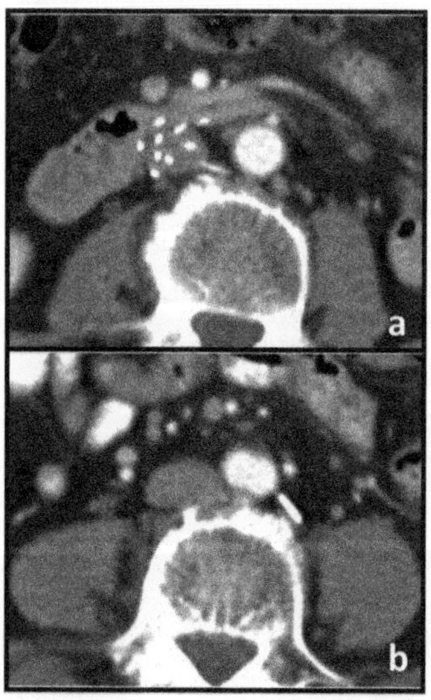

Figure 43-5. Perforation of filter prongs through IVC with fractured strut. (Reproduced with permission from *The Journal of Vascular Surgery*.[25])

associated with retrievable filters in the current era and has been reported to occur rates of 6–10%[20] depending on filter type. It has also been noted to occur at rates of 1%–2.9% with some early permanent IVC filters.[21–23] Embolization of filters or filter fragments is an unusual event, but one with potentially severe consequences.[24] Embolization has been reported to the right heart and pulmonary arteries (Figure 43-6).

There is a relative paucity of studies in the literature directly comparing retrievable and permanent filters. Van Ha et al addressed this topic in a study representing a relatively early experience with retrievable IVC filters.[8] They placed retrievable filters only 16% of the time, with the vast majority of their filters being permanent. They noted an overall 9% complication rate, similar to our results. The majority of their complications were thrombotic (mostly DVT or filter thrombosis). They noted two device-related filter complications in the retrievable group including one strut fracture and one filter that migrated to the right side of the heart. Both complications were noted months after filter implantation. These results are consistent with our experience, which noted that overall symptomatic complications and device complications were significantly more common with indwelling retrievable filters.

Kim and colleagues also compared retrievable and permanent filters, but with the specific focus of examining post filter thrombotic complications, particularly pulmonary emboli.[13] They noted a significantly higher complication rate with both retrievable and permanent filters but did not find any device-related complications. Their study also represented an early experience with retrievable filters, with the primary endpoint clearly being thrombotic complications. More subtle device-related problems may have been more difficult to find at this early stage in the experience with retrievable filters.

A retrospective review from our institution[25] is the largest study to date comparing retrievable and indwelling permanent filters. This review of over 1200

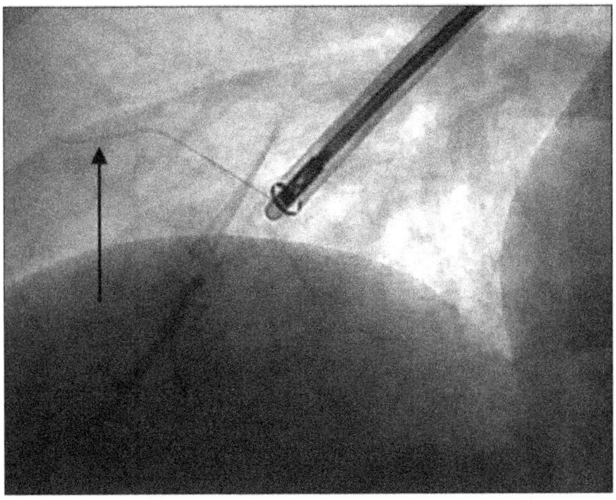

Figure 43-6. Embolized filter strut within right pulmonary artery. (Reproduced with permission from The Journal of Vascular and Interventional Radiology[20]).

patients demonstrated a significantly increased rate of symptomatic and asymptomatic device-related complications with indwelling retrievable filters compared to permanent filters (Table 43-1).

Thrombotic complications were the most common complication type in both groups and more common with retrievable filters compared to permanent, although this difference did not achieve statistical significance. In considering different types of thrombotic complications, IVC thrombosis was more common with retrievable filters than permanent. This may reflect the low thrombotic risk of the Venatech filter that comprised the majority of our permanent filters. Our study could not determine whether the IVC thrombosis was a result of the filter fulfilling its function and capturing an embolus or a result of thrombus forming *de novo* within the filter because of its thrombogenicity. Pulmonary embolism rates remained low with both filter types, supporting their effectiveness over the follow-up period reported. The remainder of the thrombotic complications consisted of recurrent lower extremity deep vein thrombosis and did not differ between the two filter types. Although we were not able to show reduction of thrombotic complications by anticoagulation (likely due to limitations in our data collection with respect to anticoagulation), the predominance of thrombotic complications with both filter types may support the use of anticoagulation when feasible in conjunction with any filters that are left in permanently.

The overall rate of thrombotic complications noted with both permanent and retrievable filters in our study suggests that anticoagulation of patients with indwelling filters may be important. The inability to demonstrate any influence of anticoagulation on thrombotic complications in our study may have represented a limitation of our retrospective study design. Specific information about types, timing, and adequacy of anticoagulation was not known for these patients. One large study of patients who underwent filter placement along with anticoagulation showed increased rates of thrombotic complications with filter placement compared to anticoagulation alone, suggesting a limited value of anticoagulation in minimizing thrombotic complications of filters. Further study is needed to clarify this issue and to determine what type and level of anticoagulation may be of benefit.

Our study noted a relatively low rate of symptomatic device-related problems with both permanent and retrievable filters (0.5% vs. 2.5%) but numerous additional

TABLE 43-1. REVIEW COMPARING RETRIEVABLE AND PERMANENT, INDWELLING FILTERS

	Retrievable Filters			Permanent Filters		
Complication	Kim et al.[13] (N = 427)	Van Ha et al.[8] (N = 97)	Desai et al.[25] (N = 382)	Kim et al. (N = 275)	Van ha et al. (N = 507)	Desai et al. (N = 785)
Overall	17.8%	7.0%	8.9%	16.4%	7.0%	2.9%
Pulmonary Embolism	4.7%	2.1%	0.8%	4.0%	1.4%	0.6%
DVT	12.6%	3.1%	1.9%	11.3%	2.4%	1.2%
IVC Thrombosis	0.5%	2.1%	1.8	1.1%	1.4%	0.4%
Device-Related Complication[a]	0.0%	2.1%	2.6%	0.0%	0.2%	0.5%

[a]Migration, perforation, fracture.

incidental findings of device perforation or strut fracture noted on imaging studies. These findings were significantly more common with retrievable filters compared to permanent filters (6.3% vs. 0.4%). While the full significance of such filter-related events is still not completely clear (only some of these events are associated with symptoms), the overall safety of indwelling retrievable filters has come into question, with the FDA issuing a warning in 2010 about potential device-related complications of retrievable filters that are left in place.[26]

MANAGEMENT OF COMPLICATIONS

Prevention

The most effective means to decrease the complication rate associated with IVC filters is to prevent the complication from occurring. Current recommendations include avoiding prophylactic filter placement unless absolutely necessary, and adhering to accepted indications for filter placement in patients with diagnosed thromboembolic disease. Given that most retrievable filters (with complications rates which are higher than permanent filters), whether placed therapeutically or prophylactically, are not currently retrieved, with retrieval rates ranging from 4 to 50%,[2,3,5–9,11,27] we also recommend limiting placement of retrievable filters to those patients who will reliably be able to follow-up to undergo planned retrieval. Systematic follow-up of patients in whom retrievable filters are placed is critical, with definitive plans for early retrieval. Significant improvement in retrieval rates (70% retrieval rate compared to a baseline of 18%) has been reported with implementation of such programs.[28]

Local Complications of Insertion

Hematoma and insertion site DVT are reported in approximately 1%–3% of IVC filter insertions.[29] Jugular access can facilitate post-insertion monitoring and may facilitate identification of post-insertion hematoma. These are controlled with direct manual pressure, bedrest, and serial examination. One event of arterial compression leading to ischemia has been reported.[30] Anticoagulation should be resumed as soon as feasible due to the risk of further thrombotic events, including suprafilter thrombus, filter thrombosis, as well as insertion site DVT. In our review we noted one case of femoral artery pseudoaneurysm in over 1000 reviewed cases; this was treated conservatively. Finally jugular access may be associated with the complication of pneumothorax which may require thoracic vent or chest tube drainage.

Filter tilt

Filter retrieval depends on the operator's ability to capture a hook centered in the lumen of the vena cava. If the tip is adjacent to the caval endothelium it will often become incorporated into scar tissue, making retrieval more difficult. In a review of 523 patients, 1% had filter tilt > 15 degrees, and 50% had filter tilt > 5%.[31] If significant filter tilt occurs on implantation, the filter should be retrieved and replaced with a new filter. Certain filter designs are said to facilitate centering on deployment. For example, the Denali filter reported 0% tilt at placement (of 175 filters placed), and 0% tilt at retrieval (of 88 attempted retrievals).[32] In our experience, some tilt has been noted with all of the conical design IVC filters we have utilized. Attention to this complication during insertion with prompt repositioning when identified is recommended.

Filter malposition

Malposition occurs when a filter is unknowingly deployed somewhere other than the inferior vena cava. This is rare as fluoroscopic guidance permits accurate identification of the intended deployment position. Malposition can occur when the jugular approach is used and the tip of the deployment sheath is inadvertently moved from the inferior vena cava into a paraspinal vein[33] or gonadal vein (Figure 43-1). Malposition has also occurred when intravascular ultrasound has been used and the filter deployed in the common iliac vein instead of the inferior vena cava.[34,35] These malpositions are treated by retrieval and placement of a new filter, or placement of a second filter cephalad to the first.

Intraarterial placement has rarely been reported. Naidu et al described retrieval of a Trapease filter inadvertently placed in the aorta.[36]

Filter Fracture

Fracture is believed to occur with repeated mechanical deformation, possibly in part due to the adjacent pulsatile aorta and is most commonly noted with retrievable IVC filters. In one review, fracture occurred in less than 1% of 465 filters placed.[37] Another review of 148 IVC filter retrievals described 15 fractured filters; this rate may be falsely high as the authors were referred a number of outside cases for retrieval attempt. The authors successfully retrieved all 15 filters. Most of the fractured struts were retrieved using bronchial forceps, and no complications occurred due to retrieval attempts.[20] Serious cardiac complications have occurred, including tamponade and death.[24,38] Retrieval of fractured IVC filters is recommended, with retrieval of all accessible fragments, which may require adjunctive techniques as described above.

Strut Perforation

Contrast-enhanced CT scanning is the first step in evaluating the extent of IVC perforation. CT images can demonstrate strut protrusion into and through the aortic wall, and can demonstrate intrusion into the lumbar vertebral body. Perforation into the duodenum is more difficult to confirm with CT scan and if struts are seen adjacent to the duodenum EGD is recommended.

It is our experience that most of these filters (long implantation time, and or IVC perforation without perforation of the aorta or duodenum) can and should be removed in symptomatic patients.[39–42]

Principles for removal of retrievable filters which have been in place for an extended period of time include:

1. Ability to access both the internal jugular vein and the femoral vein;
2. Use of large outer sheath, 14–16 Fr;
3. Use of stiff guidewire, e.g., Amplatz wire;
4. Ability to dislodge the filter from the wall of the IVC. This may be accomplished multiple ways, including loop snare technique or dissection with bronchial forceps.[43]

Not infrequently the retrieved filter has significant adherent vascular endothelium (Figure 43-7). To our knowledge, however, there are no reports of clinically significant caval injury following IVC filter retrieval.

Thrombosis

Any degree of thrombosis may be seen following retrievable IVC filter placement, ranging from a small amount of clot in the filter to complete IVC thrombosis. The filter can likely be safely removed if it carries less than 25% thrombus burden within its cone and the vena cava is otherwise patent.

If there is more significant clot burden and the patient is asymptomatic, the filter should be left in place and anticoagulation continued. Some degree of thrombus was found at initial cavogram in 6.5% of retrieval attempts in one series; slightly less than 50% were retrieved during the same procedure.[44] About half of the remaining patients had successful filter retrieval after additional anticoagulation.

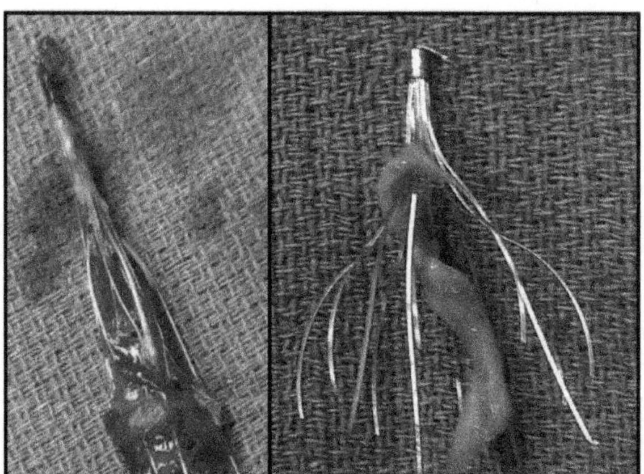

Figure 43-7. Retrieved filters with adherent IVC wall remove.

It is difficult to know the rate of complete IVC filter thrombosis. Ahmad et al reported 2% total filter occlusion in a retrospective imaging review, most of which were asymptomatic.[45] Another review reported 4.75% rate of IVC thrombosis.[29] If the patient presents with symptomatic lower extremity swelling and thrombosis of the vena cava, lytic therapy should be considered in the context of the patient's overall bleeding risk.

At our institution, a suitable risk patient is treated in the interventional radiology suite. Access is usually through the popliteal vein. AngioJet is first used in pulse-spray mode to deliver tPA into the clot. AngioJet may then be used in thrombectomy mode to re-establish venous flow and help resolve symptoms; the goal in this phase is not complete clearance of clot. An infusion catheter is left in the clot and set to deliver 1 mg/hr of tPA. In most cases we also infuse 500 units/hr of heparin to maintain subtherapeutic PTT. If re-thrombosis occurs, the heparin rate can be increased and the PTT kept therapeutic. Patients are monitored in the ICU with careful attention to hemodynamic and coagulation parameters, bedrest, and no new intravenous line starts or blood draws. Lysis and rethrombosis of such a large clot burden may be reflected in falling fibrinogen levels, and may necessitate increased heparin dosing. After clot clearance is maximized, balloon angioplasty and iliac stents may be necessary to maintain patency.

Complications requiring open repair

In the vast majority of cases, complications can be managed with endovascular techniques. Occasionally, the perforation causes significant damage to adjacent structures and endovascular retrieval is not feasible. Becher reported filter erosion into the aorta, right renal artery, and duodenum. After multiple failed endovascular retrieval attempts, the filter was retrieved by cavotomy. The aorta was repaired by femoral vein interposition, and nephrectomy was required to treat a renal artery pseudoaneurysm.[46] Open surgical removal of a filter has not yet been necessary at our institution.

CONCLUSIONS

Retrievable and permanent filters are associated with thrombotic and device-related complications long term, but indwelling retrievable filters are associated with a higher overall complication rate compared to permanent filters. Thrombotic complications are the most common complications with both types of filters. Device-related complications are more common with retrievable filters. In a majority of cases, these may not cause symptoms, but are still cause for significant concern. Retrievable filter use should be limited to patients with appropriate indication for filter placement in whom retrieval is highly likely. Furthermore, systematic follow-up of patients with retrievable filters is necessary to improve current retrieval rates. Retrievable filters with significant perforation or fracture can undergo safe retrieval but may require adjunctive maneuvers if they have been indwelling for long periods of time. Thrombosed filters should undergo attempted thrombolytic therapy but may be difficult to treat if IVC occlusion has become chronic prior to presentation.

REFERENCES

1. Trousseau A. Phlegmasia alba dolens. In: Trousseau, editor. *Clinique Medicale de l'Hotel-Dieu de paris.* Paris: Balliere; 1865. p. 654–712.
2. Greenfield LJ, McCurdy JR, Brown PP, Elkins RC. A new intracaval filter permitting continued flow and resolution of emboli. *Surgery.* 1973;73(4):599–606.
3. Cimochowski GE, DeMeester TR, Evans RH, et al. Greenfield filter vs Mobin-Uddin umbrella. *JAMA.* 1980;244(19):2160.
4. Stein PD, Kayali F, Olson RE. Twenty-one-year trends in the use of inferior vena cava filters. *Arch Intern Med.* 2004;164(14):1541–5.
5. Angel LF, Tapson V, Galgon RE, et al. Systematic review of the use of retrievable inferior vena cava filters. *JVIR.* 2011;22(11):1522–30 e3.
6. Imberti D, Bianchi M, Farina A, et al. Clinical experience with retrievable vena cava filters: results of a prospective observational multicenter study. *JTH.* 2005;3(7):1370–5.
7. Ray CE, Jr., Mitchell E, Zipser S, et al. Outcomes with retrievable inferior vena cava filters: a multicenter study. *JVIR.* 2006;17(10):1595–604.
8. Van Ha TG, Chien AS, Funaki BS, et al. Use of retrievable compared to permanent inferior vena cava filters: a single-institution experience. *Cardiovasc Intervent Radiol.* 2008;31(2):308–15.
9. Kaufman JA, Kinney TB, Streiff MB, et al. Guidelines for the use of retrievable and convertible vena cava filters: report from the Society of Interventional Radiology multidisciplinary consensus conference. *JVIR.* 2006;17(3):449–59.
10. Doody O, Given MF, Kavnoudias H, et al. Initial experience in 115 patients with the retrievable Cook Celect vena cava filter. *JMIRO.* 2009;53(1):64–8.
11. Gaspard SF, Gaspard DJ. Retrievable inferior vena cava filters are rarely removed. *Am Surg.* 2009;75(5):426–8.
12. Janjua M, Younas F, Moinuddin I, et al. Outcomes with retrievable inferior vena cava filters. *JIC.* 2010;22(5):235–9.
13. Kim HS, Young MJ, Narayan AK, et al. A comparison of clinical outcomes with retrievable and permanent inferior vena cava filters. *JVIR.* 2008;19(3):393–9.
14. Sarosiek S, Crowther M, Sloan JM. Indications, complications, and management of inferior vena cava filters: the experience in 952 patients at an academic hospital with a level I trauma center. *JAMA Intern Med.* 2013;173(7):513–7.
15. Zhou D, Spain J, Moon E, et al. Retrospective review of 120 celect inferior vena cava filter retrievals: experience at a single institution. *JVIR.* 2012;23(12):1557–63.
16. Decousus H, Leizorovicz A, Parent F, et al. A clinical trial of vena caval filters in the prevention of pulmonary embolism in patients with proximal deep-vein thrombosis. Prevention du Risque d'Embolie Pulmonaire par Interruption Cave Study Group. *N Engl J Med.* 1998;338(7):409–15.
17. Durack JC, Westphalen AC, Kekulawela S, et al. Perforation of the IVC: rule rather than exception after longer indwelling times for the Gunther Tulip and Celect retrievable filters. *Cardiovasc Intervent Radiol.* 2012;35(2):299–308.
18. Olorunsola OG, Kohi MP, Fidelman N, et al. Caval penetration by retrievable inferior vena cava filters: a retrospective comparison of Option and Gunther Tulip filters. *JVIR.* 2013;24(4):566–71.
19. Ota S, Yamada N, Tsuji A, et al. The Gunther-Tulip retrievable IVC filter: clinical experience in 118 consecutive patients. *Jpn Circ J.* 2008;72(2):287–92.
20. Dinglasan LA, Trerotola SO, Shlansky-Goldberg RD, et al. Removal of fractured inferior vena cava filters: feasibility and outcomes. *JVIR.* 2012;23(2):181–7.
21. Babuty D, Quilliet L, Charbonnier B, et al. Partial interruption of the inferior vena cava using a percutaneous endovenous filter. *Arch Mal Coeur Vaiss.* 1990;83(9):1389–96.
22. Ferris EJ, McCowan TC, Carver DK, McFarland DR. Percutaneous inferior vena caval filters: follow-up of seven designs in 320 patients. *Radiology.* 1993;188(3):851–6.

23. Wolf F, Thurnher S, Lammer J. Simon nitinol vena cava filters: effectiveness and complications. *Fortschr Geb Rontgenstr Nuklearmed.* 2001;173(10):924–30.
24. Nicholson W, Nicholson WJ, Tolerico P, et al. Prevalence of fracture and fragment embolization of Bard retrievable vena cava filters and clinical implications including cardiac perforation and tamponade. *Arch intern med.* 2010;170(20):1827–31.
25. Desai TR, Morcos OC, Lind BB, et al. Complications of indwelling retrievable vs permanent inferior vena cava filters. *J Vasc Surg: Venous and Lym Dis.* 2014;2(2):166–73.
26. US Food and Drug Administration. Removing Retrievable Inferior Vena Cava Filters: Initial Communication. http://www.fda.gov/MedicalDevices/Safety/AlertsandNotices/ucm221676.htm. August 9, 2010.
27. Mohan CR, Hoballah JJ, Sharp WJ, et al. Comparative efficacy and complications of vena caval filters. *J Vasc Surg.* 1995;21(2):235–45; discussion 45–6.
28. Gasparis AP, Spentzouris G, Meisner RJ, et al. Improving retrieval rates of temporary inferior vena cava filters. *J Vasc Surg.* 2011;54(6 Suppl):34S–8S e1.
29. Nazzal M, Chan E, Nazzal M, et al. Complications related to inferior vena cava filters: a single-center experience. *Ann Vasc Surg.* 2010;24(4):480–6.
30. Athanasoulis CA, Kaufman JA, Halpern EF, et al. Inferior vena caval filters: review of a 26-year single-center clinical experience. *Radiology.* 2000;216(1):54–66.
31. Semaan D, Raythatha M, Burgin A, Harb A. Inferior vena cava filter tilt and its future clinical implications: a community based practices experience. *JVIR.* 2013;24(4):S166.
32. Inc BPV. DENALI Filter System 510(k) Summary. USA: Food and Drug Administration; 2013.
33. Funaki B. Inferior vena cava filter malposition in a paraspinal vein. *Semin Intervent Radiol.* 2006;23(3):298–302.
34. Jacobs DL, Motaganahalli RL, Peterson BG. Bedside vena cava filter placement with intravascular ultrasound: a simple, accurate, single venous access method. *J Vasc Surg.* 2007;46(6):1284–6.
35. Wellons ED, Matsuura JH, Shuler FW, et al. Bedside intravascular ultrasound-guided vena cava filter placement. *J Vasc Surg.* 2003;38(3):455–7; discussion 7–8.
36. Naidu SG, Stone WM, Sweeney JP, Money SR. Endovascular retrieval of permanent IVC filter placed within the aorta. *J Vasc Surg.* 2010;52(6):1736.
37. McLoney ED, Krishnasamy VP, Castle JC, Yang X, Guy G. Complications of Celect, Gunther tulip, and Greenfield inferior vena cava filters on CT follow-up: a single-institution experience. *JVIR.* 2013;24(11):1723–9.
38. Chandra PA, Nwokolo C, Chuprun D, Chandra AB. Cardiac tamponade caused by fracture and migration of inferior vena cava filter. *South Med J.* 2008;101(11):1163–4.
39. Kuo WT, Cupp JS, Louie JD, Kothary N, Hofmann LV, Sze DY, et al. Complex retrieval of embedded IVC filters: alternative techniques and histologic tissue analysis. *Cardiovasc Intervent Radiol.* 2012;35(3):588–97.
40. Kuo WT, Robertson SW, Odegaard JI, Hofmann LV. Complex retrieval of fractured, embedded, and penetrating inferior vena cava filters: a prospective study with histologic and electron microscopic analysis. *JVIR.* 2013;24(5):622–30 e1; quiz 31.
41. Lind BB, Ferral H. Gunther-Tulip inferior vena cava filter removal 3334 days after placement. *J Vasc Surg Cases.* 2015;1(1):39–41.
42. Van Ha TG, Kang L, Lorenz J, et al. Difficult OptEase filter retrievals after prolonged indwelling times. *Cardiovasc Intervent Radiol.* 2013;36(4):1139–43.
43. Stavropoulos SW, Dixon RG, Burke CT, et al. Embedded inferior vena cava filter removal: use of endobronchial forceps. *JVIR.* 2008;19(9):1297–301.
44. Teo TK, Angle JF, Shipp JI, et al. Incidence and management of inferior vena cava filter thrombus detected at time of filter retrieval. *JVIR.* 2011;22(11):1514–20.
45. Ahmad I, Yeddula K, Wicky S, Kalva SP. Clinical sequelae of thrombus in an inferior vena cava filter. *Cardiovasc Intervent Radiol.* 2010;33(2):285–9.
46. Becher RD, Corriere MA, Edwards MS, Godshall CJ. Late erosion of a prophylactic Celect IVC filter into the aorta, right renal artery, and duodenal wall. *J Vasc Surg.* 2010;52(4):1041–4.

44

Endovascular Techniques and Outcomes for Acute Pulmonary Embolism

Christopher J. Kwolek, MD

Pulmonary embolism (PE) is a common problem in the United States (US) leading to over 100,000 deaths/year with nearly 25% of patients presenting with sudden death.[1,2] The overall mortality rate in massive PE approaches 60% with most deaths occurring within the first one to two hours.[3] For those patients who do survive, there is a 15%–18% predicted mortality over the next 3 months despite therapy.[4,5] As the US population continues to age, the severity of this problem may increase further. A recent study at our institution demonstrated that patients ≥65 years old were more likely to present with severe PE and had a (3.7×) higher 30-day mortality.[6] Recent guidelines have tried to standardize the algorithms for the evaluation and treatment of this diverse group of patients; however, there is relatively little prospective, randomized data to drive these recommendations in the highest risk group of patients.[7,8] Thus many of the interventional treatments are given a 2C level of support. Furthermore, the decision about which treatments to utilize may vary depending on institutional ability, individual operator experience, and even which specialists are called to consult upon an individual patient.

In order to standardize the quality of care that patients with PE were receiving, individuals from various disciplines at the Massachusetts General Hospital (MGH) chose to establish a multidisciplinary team to manage these complex patients. The MGH Pulmonary Embolism Response Team (MGH PERT) was modeled on other successful rapid-response teams such as those for managing Acute Stroke and ST-segment elevation myocardial infarction (STEMI).[5,9] Representatives from emergency medicine, pulmonary critical care, cardiothoracic surgery, vascular medicine, and cardiology were among the founding members; however, additional participants from vascular surgery, interventional radiology, and echocardiography have been added.

The core mission of the MGH PERT was to advance the care of patients with PE through rapid multidisciplinary consultation, quality improvement programs, research and education. The founding participants felt that the complex group of "high risk" patients with massive and submassive PE would potentially benefit the most from using a multidisciplinary team approach to identify the treatment strategy for each patient. The MGH PERT program includes a 24-hour emergency activation line that allows the electronic notification of an on-call fellow who gathers the appropriate information and a multidisciplinary team which conducts a virtual meeting within 90 minutes or less depending on the urgency of the situation (Figure 44-1). Mechanisms to activate the operating room (OR), the cardiac catheterization lab (Cath), the extracorporeal membrane oxygenation (ECMO) team, the emergency department (ED), the intensive care unit (ICU), and initial transfer are included.

CURRENT THERAPY OF LOW-RISK PATIENTS

The standard of care for the management of acute pulmonary embolism in approximately 70% of patients is systemic anticoagulation. The majority of patients are "low risk" with no evidence of hemodynamic instability, right ventricular dysfunction or myocardial necrosis. Since these patients have excellent short term outcomes once therapeutic anticoagulation has been established, there is no role for more aggressive intervention with either thrombolytics, surgery or endovascular therapy. Attempts should be made to identify the underlying etiology of the PE, while preventing further venous thromboembolism and providing supportive care.[7]

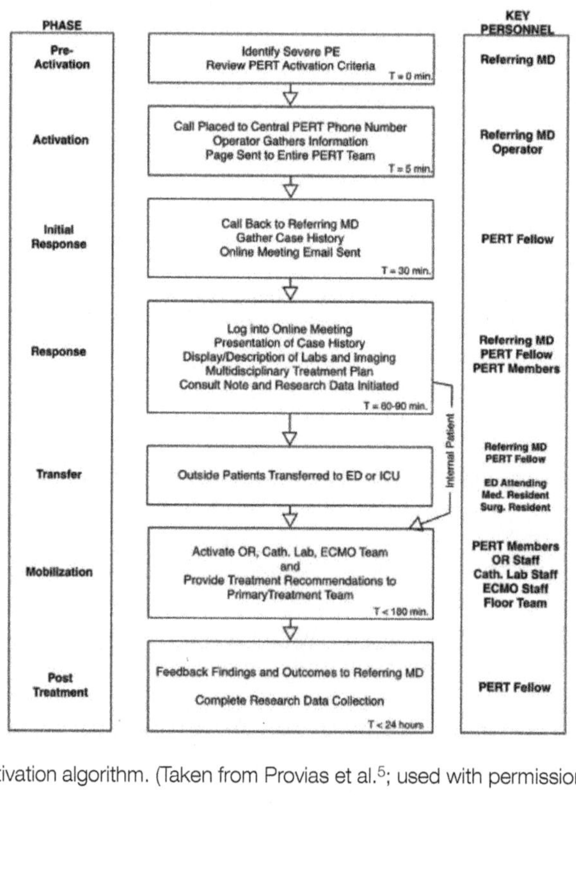

Figure 44-1. PERT activation algorithm. (Taken from Provias et al.[5]; used with permission.)

CURRENT THERAPY OF HIGH RISK PATIENTS

The other 25%–30% of patients fall into the high risk group.[10] This can be further divided into patients with massive PE who comprise (5%) of all patients. These individuals present with major hemodynamic or respiratory instability. The diagnosis is made when patients present in shock or with a sustained blood pressure of <90 mmHG. The American College of Chest Physician (ACCP) guidelines have recommended systemic thrombolytics as the first line therapy for treating eligible patients with massive PE.[7,8,11,12] The US Food and Drug Administration (FDA) has approved a dose of 100 mg of tissue plasminogen activator usually infused over 2 hours. While this approach can be effective, it also carries with it a 20% risk of significant hemorrhage and a 3%–5% risk of intracranial hemorrhage.[1,12]

Surgical thromboembolectomy has been previously described and remains a treatment for patients with acute massive PE who are not candidates for systemic thrombolysis. Historically, this approach has been associated with a very high morbidity and mortality, however more recently published series have demonstrated close to 90% survival,[7,13] This may be due to a combination of factors including better patient selection, more rapid diagnosis and treatment and improved surgical technique. In our institution, the use of ECMO has been used as a successful method of cardiopulmonary support in combination with other pharmacomechanical adjuncts.[5]

Catheter based techniques have long been described in the treatment of patients with acute PE. Early on, simple rotation of a pigtail catheter was described to try and fragment massive PE. Balloon maceration was also used to try and break up large pulmonary emboli. Local intraclot delivery of thrombolytics was eventually added to these techniques. Kuo published a meta-analysis of these techniques to treat massive PE with over 85% of patients having stabilization of their hemodynamics, with improved oxygenation and patient survival.[10] The overall rate of hemorrhagic complication was only 2.4% with a less than 1% incidence of intracranial hemorrhage.[11]

More recently the results of the Pulmonary Embolism Response to Fragmentation, Embolectomy, and Catheter Thrombolysis (PERFECT) registry were reported. One-hundred and one consecutive patients receiving catheter directed therapy for acute PE were prospectively enrolled in a multicenter registry. Twenty-eight patients with massive PE and 73 with submassive PE were treated with immediate catheter-directed mechanical or pharmacomechanical thrombectomy and/or catheter-directed thrombolysis with low dose infusion of tissue plasminogen activator (TPA) or urokinase.[14]

Clinical success was achieved in 24/28 patients with massive PE (85.7%; 95% CI 67.3%–96%) and 71 of 73 patients with submassive PE (97.3%; 95% CI, 90.5%-99.7%). The mean pulmonary artery pressures decreased from 51 mmHG to 37 mmHG (P <.0001) and 89% of patients followed by echocardiography showed improved right sided heart strain. Most importantly, there were no major procedure-related complications, major hemorrhages, or hemorrhagic strokes.

The use of the angiojet device to perform rheolytic thrombectomy has been shown to be very effective in the removal of acute thrombus in both the peripheral arterial and venous circulation. However its use in the pulmonary vasculature may lead to bradycardia, pulmonary vasospasm and hypoxia.[4] Thus, the FDA has issued a "black box" warning for Angiojet (Boston Scientific, Marlborough, MA) thrombectomy for the treatment of PE.[15]

We and others have also described the use of the Vortex Angiovac catheter (Angiodynamics, Marlborough, MA) for the removal of acute pulmonary emboli, right atrial thrombus and IVC thrombus. This catheter can be used either percutaneously through a 27 Fr Gore Dry seal sheath or through direct venous cutdown. The 22 Fr cannula system is connected to a veno-venous perfusion circuit to allow for continuous reinfusion of shed bled to allow for hemodynamic stability while trapping any emboli or thrombus within a separate filter. Current limitations include catheter steerability and the need for adjunct tools to assist with thrombus removal. However renewed interest has developed in this device with the start of a multi-center registry, the RAPID (Registry of AngioVac Procedures in Detail) study, sponsored by Angiodynamics, Marlborough, MA (Figure 44-2).

The last technology to be described for the acute endovascular management of PE is the EkoSonic ultrasound-assisted thrombolysis (EKOS, Bothell, Washington) for catheter directed treatment of PE. This has recently received FDA approval and uses ultrasound energy to thin the thrombus and allow better penetration of the locally delivered thrombolytic into the clot. This in turn has allowed interventionalists to decrease both the total dose and time of thrombolytic used, potentially decreasing the overall risk of bleeding complications associated with the use of TPA.[4] The results of two recent trials involving EKOS will be discussed in the next section.

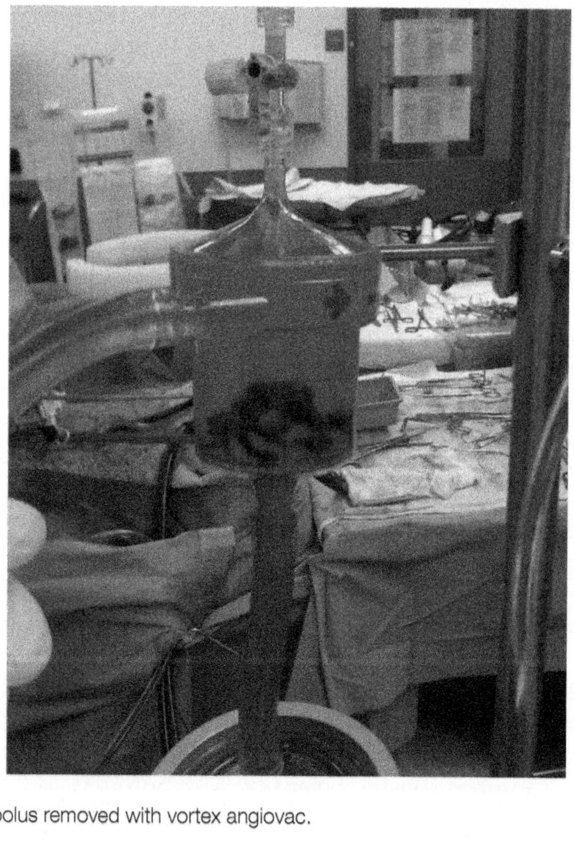

Figure 44-2. Pulmonary embolus removed with vortex angiovac.

MANAGEMENT OF SUBMASSIVE PULMONARY EMBOLISM

Submassive PE is diagnosed when patients are hemodynamically stable, but have evidence of right ventricular (RV) dysfunction or myocardial necrosis. These patients have a significantly higher mortality, up to 21% at 90 days, than patients with normal RV function.[7,10] There is also concern about the long-term sequelae of PE including chronic pulmonary artery hypertension which can occur in up to 44% of patients with submassive PE with RV dysfunction noted at the time of discharge.[4] While the use of systemic anticoagulation is the standard of care for treating these patients, the use of systemic thrombolytics has remained controversial due to concerns about bleeding complications.

The largest randomized trial to date evaluating the use of systemic thrombolytics in patients with acute submassive PE is the Pulmonary Embolism International Thrombolysis (PEITHO) trial.[16] This study randomized 1006 patients with acute submassive PE with evidence of RV dysfunction by echocardiography or myocardial injury with a positive troponin. Patients received systemic anticoagulation with heparin and either weight based thrombolytic with tenecteplase or placebo. The primary endpoint of death or hemodynamic collapse at 7 days was significantly lower in the tenecteplase group (2.6% vs. 5.6%; $P = 0.015$). This was due to an improvement in the hemodynamics since there was no difference in mortality between the tenecteplase vs. control groups (2.4% vs. 3.2%; $P = 0.42$). However, the hemodynamic benefit of the thrombolytic therapy was countered by a higher incidence of bleeding related complications including stroke (2.4% vs. 0.2%; $P = 0.003$) and major hemorrhage (6.3% vs. 1.2%; $P < 0.001$).

Recently, the use of ultrasound-assisted catheter-directed thrombolysis (USAT) in patients with submassive PE was evaluated in a prospective fashion. The Randomized, Controlled Trial of Ultrasound-Assisted, Catheter-Directed Thrombolysis for Acute Intermediate–Risk Pulmonary Embolism (ULTIMA) treated 59 patients with acute main or lower lobe PE and echocardiographic evidence of RV dysfucntion (RV/LV ratio ≥ 1).[17] The primary endpoint was difference in LV/RV ratio at 24 hours for patients randomized between unfractionated heparin alone vs. heparin with USAT. The mean decrease in RV/LV ratio was 0.30 ± 0.20 in the treatment group vs. 0.03 ± 0.16 in the control group ($P < 0.001$) with no difference in mortality or major bleeding complications, between the groups. However several limitations exist including the lack of a non-ultrasound lytic group to demonstrate the additional benefit of ultrasound in addition to the local lytic effect and insufficient data to demonstrate whether the improvement in RV function at 24 hours is sustained at 90 days.

The results of a study—A Prospective, Single-Arm, Multicenter Trial of Ultrasound-Facilitated, Catheter-Directed, Low-Dose Fibrinolysis for Acute Massive and Submassive Pulmonary Embolism (SEATTLE II)—was also recently published.[18] In this study, 31 patients with acute massive PE and 119 patients with submassive PE were treated with USAT. All patients had proximal PE with an LV/RV ratio of ≥ 0.9 by chest CT scan. Patients received 24 mg of TPA either at 1 mg/hr for 24 hours via a unilateral catheter or 1 mg/hour for 12 hours with bilateral catheters. The primary safety endpoint was major bleeding at 72 hours. The primary efficacy outcome was RV/LV ratio measured on repeat chest CT scan within 48 hours of the procedure. Mean RV/LV ratio decreased from baseline to 48 hours (1.55 vs. 1.13; $P < 0.0001$) with a decrease in mean pulmonary artery systolic pressure (51.4 mmHG vs. 36.9 mmHG;

$P < 0.0001$). There was only one severe bleed with transient hypotension and no intracranial bleeds. Further follow-up is already being planned to determine whether improvements in pulmonary artery pressures are sustained at 90 days and what effect there is on quality of life.

CONCLUSION

Pulmonary embolism remains a significant health problem within the United States. While most patients with low-risk PE have a good prognosis with standard anticoagulation, the treatment of patients with massive and submassive PE remains controversial and highly variable. While systemic fibrinolysis for acute PE reduces cardiovascular collapse, hemorrhagic complications such as stroke and bleeding are still a significant concern. New catheter-based techniques using USAT show promise with short-term improvement in RV/LV ratio, decreased pulmonary pressures, and fewer bleeding complications; however, little data exists about long-term benefits or improved patient quality of life. Subsequent studies will be necessary to determine the optimal treatment strategies for the management of acute massive and submassive PE. Our institution believes that developing a consortium of centers with dedicated PERT teams will provide the best method to improve patient care and allow for collaborative programs to further education and research in this area.

REFERENCES

1. Goldhaber SZ, Visani L, DeRosa M. Acute pulmonary embolism: Clinical outcomes in the International Cooperative Pulmonary Embolism Registry (ICOPER). *Lancet* 1999;353:1386–89.
2. US Department of Health and Human Services. The Surgeon General's call to action to prevent deep vein thrombosis and pulmonary embolism. 2008. http://www.surgeongeneral.gov/library/calls/deepvein/call-to-action-on-dvt-2008.pdf.Accessed July 1, 2015.
3. Tapson VF, Acute pulmonary embolism. *N Engl J Med.* 2008;358(10):1037–52.
4. Safadi AH. The next era of pulmonary embolism treatment. *Cardiac Intv Today.* 2014;33–6.
5. Provias T, Dudzinski DM, Jaff MR, et al. The Massachusetts General Hospital Pulmonary Embolism Response Team (MGH PERT): Creation of a multidisciplinary program to improve care of patients with massive and submassive pulmonary embolism. *Hospital Practice.* 2014;42(1):31–7.
6. Cefalo P, Weinberg I, Hawkins BM, et al. A comparison of patients diagnosed with pulmonary embolism who are > 65 years with patients < 65 years. *Am J Cardiol.* 2015;115:681–6.
7. Jaff MR, McMurty S, Archer SL, et al. American Heart Association Council on Cardiopulmonary, Critical Care, Perioperative and Resuscitation; American Heart Association Council on Peripheral Vascular Disease; American Heart Association Council on Arteriosclerosis, Thrombosis and Vascular Biology. Management of massive and submassive pulmonary embolism, iliofemoral deep venous thrombosis, and chronic thromboembolic pulmonary hypertension. A scientific statement from the American Heart Association. *Circulation.* 2011;123(16):1788–830.
8. Kearon C, Akl EA, Comerota AJ, et al. American College of Chest Physicians. Antithrombotic therapy for VTE disease: Antithrombotic Therapy and Prevention of Thrombosis, 9th ed. American College of Chest Physicians Evidence-Based Clinical Practice Guidelines. *Chest.* 2012;141(2Suppl):e419S–e494s.

9. Kabrhel C, Jaff MJ, Channick RN, et al. A multidisciplinary pulmonary embolism response team. *Chest.* 2013;144(5):1738–9.
10. Piazza G. Submassive pulmonary embolism. *JAMA.* 2013;309(2):171–80.
11. Kuo WT. Endovascular therapy for acute pulmonary embolism. *J Vasc Interv Radiol.* 2012;23:167–79.
12. Kim P. Current studies in endovascular therapy for pulmonary embolism. *Endovasc Today.* 2013;56–9.
13. Aklog L, Williams CS, Byrne JG, et al. Acute pulmonary embolectomy: A contemporary approach. *Circulation.* 2002;105:1416–9.
14. Kuo WT, Banerjee A, Kim PS, et al. Pulmonary Embolism Response to Fragmentation, Embolectomy, and Catheter Thrombolysis (PERFECT): Initial results from a prospective multicenter registry. *Chest.* 2015;148(3)667–73.
15. Sobieszczyk P. Catheter-assisted pulmonary embolectomy. *Circulation.* 2012;126:1917–22.
16. Meyer G, Vicaut E, Danays T, et al. Fibrinolysis for patients with intermediate-risk pulmonary embolism. *N Engl J Med.* 2014;370(15):1402–11.
17. Kucher N, Boekstegers P, Muller OJ, et al. Randomized, controlled trial of ultrasound-assisted catheter-directed thrombolysis for acute intermediate-risk pulmonary embolism. *Circulation.* 2014;129:479–86.
18. Piazza G, Hohlfelder B, Jaff M. A prospective, single-arm, multicenter trial of ultrasound-facilitated, catheter-directed, low-dose fibrinolysis for acute massive and sub-massive pulmonary embolism: The SEATTLE II study. *J Am Coll Cardiol Intv.* 2015;8(10):1382–92.

45

Status of Robotic-Assisted Endovascular Procedures

Frederic Baumann, MD, Ripal T. Gandhi, MD, and Constantino Peña, MD

Endovascular therapy was introduced in 1964 by Dr. Charles Dotter when performing the world's first percutaneous transluminal angioplasty procedure in Portland, Oregon, while dilating a high grade stenosis of the superficial femoral artery in an elderly woman with ischemic rest pain and gangrene. Ever since, the aim of endovascular procedures has been to provide a less invasive approach to reduce morbidity and mortality compared to open surgical alternatives. Today, there are almost no limitations to endovascular therapy secondary to the advancements in technology and the development of new techniques. However, there remains ongoing ambition to refine the concept of "minimal-invasiveness."

Along that line, robotic technology has recently been introduced for endovascular procedures. Currently, the main goals of robotic technology in endovascular therapy include facilitating complex cannulation/catheterization, improving catheter stability and control, providing more predictable procedure times with potential for increased case throughput, and reducing physician radiation exposure and fatigue by allowing for remote catheter manipulation.

There are several robotic systems on the market developed specifically for endovascular intervention. The Magellan Robotic system (Hansen Medical, Mountain View, CA) and the Corindus Robotic system (Corindus Vascular Robotics, Waltham, MA) are the two latest robotic systems used for endovascular therapy. The Corindus system is designed for the treatment of coronary arteries, whereas the spectrum of the Magellan system is broader including the treatment of cerebrovascular, visceral and peripheral vascular as well as aortic diseases.

The following chapter is intended to provide an overview on robotic technology and its current applicability for the treatment of vascular diseases as well as some future perspectives.

HISTORY OF ROBOTIC-ASSISTED VASCULAR THERAPY

Robotics in the cardiovascular arena were initially devised for endovascular treatment of cardiac arrhythmias. In 2007, the Sensei robotic catheterization system (Hansen Medical, Mountain View, CA) was introduced for electrophysiological ablation in patients with arrhythmias.[1] The use of the robotic system was intended to provide more stability and guidance during complex arrythmia procedures. In addition, the robotic system enables the operator to reach difficult-to-access areas of the heart with significant control. Thereafter, the CorPath robotic system (Corindus Vascular Robotics, Waltham, MA) was introduced and obtained FDA approval in 2012 for coronary interventions. The CorPath robotic system allows for careful navigation of the coronary arteries and precise placement of angioplasty balloons and coronary stents from a remote position. The recent PRECISE study reported a 95.2% reduction of radiation dose for the operators at the remote workstation when compared to the bedside position.[2] Furthermore, one study has shown that robotic technology reduced contrast volume and fluoroscopy time when compared to conventional percutaneous coronary intervention.[3]

The 9 French (F) Magellan Robotic system (Hansen Medical, Mountain View, CA) received initial 510K clearance from the FDA in May 2012 for the treatment of various vascular diseases and vascular beds. In February of 2014, the smaller 6 F Magellan robotic catheter was FDA approved. The newest generation 10 F robotic catheter received European Conformity (CE) marking for use in the peripheral vasculature in April 2015; however, it is not FDA approved at the time of this writing.

CURRENT CLINICAL APPLICABILITY OF ROBOTIC TECHNOLOGY FOR VASCULAR THERAPY

Primary Objectives of Robotic Technology

Intravascular robotics have been designed to facilitate complex catheterization by improving catheter maneuverability while providing increased catheter stability. This can be advantageous for a multitude of diverse procedures including navigation of tortuous anatomy and catheterizing challenging angulated vessels, which may be difficult or impossible to engage with a manual catheter. In addition, the ability to manipulate the angle and shape of the robotic catheter minimizes the number of catheters and catheter exchanges. These attributes of the robotic system have the potential to decrease fluoroscopy time and contrast use. Finally, the ability to operate the robot from a remote position may result in reduction of radiation exposure to the physician and staff. The latter may also decrease operator fatigue and occupational stress as the physician can be comfortably seated at an ergonomic robotic workstation away from radiation source, which may be even outside of the interventional suite as illustrated in Figure 45-1. This eliminates the need for wearing a heavy lead apron while performing the procedure, and thus increased ergonomics. Operator performance may also be improved during long, complex cases if the physician is less vulnerable to fatigue.

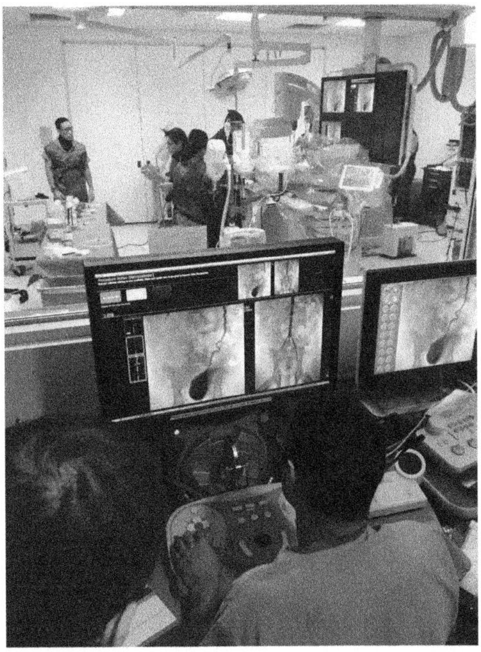

Figure 45-1. Depiction of an operator performing an endovascular intervention using the Magellan robotic system from the remote workstation, which can be located outside of the intervention suite.

The Magellan Robotic System

The Magellan system is extremely versatile and is designed for the treatment of various vascular diseases and for performing a multitude of diverse procedures, which will be discussed later. The Magellan robot consists of a robotic arm, which is fixed to the table (Figure 45-2a and b). As mentioned, it can be navigated from the bedside or from a remote workstation. Therefore, it consists of two control panels: one control panel located at the bedside as with manual catheterization and one remotely. Figures 45-2a,b and 45-3 provide illustrations of the robotic setup at the table (Figures 45-2a,b) and the remote workstation (Figure 45-3).

The initial system which was released and cleared by the FDA was the 9F robotic catheter which featured a telescoping system composed of an outer 9 F guide catheter and an inner 6 F inner "leader" catheter. Commercially available guidewires ranging in size from 0.014" to 0.035" are used to navigate the catheter. This system enables the operator to have independent control of both the outer and inner catheters with 180 degree bending and 360 degree rotational movements as depicted in Figure 45-4, allowing for the creation of virtually any catheter shape. In addition, the robotic catheter can be "stiffened" or "relaxed" during a procedure which allows for enhanced stability and flexibility, respectively, which can be adjusted within the same procedure as needed. Additionally, the 9F system can be used to coaxially deliver and deploy 6F compatible therapies such as stents, balloons and embolization coils and plugs.

Recently, an additional single catheter system was introduced with continued functionality but with a smaller caliber (6F) designed to catheterize and intervene in

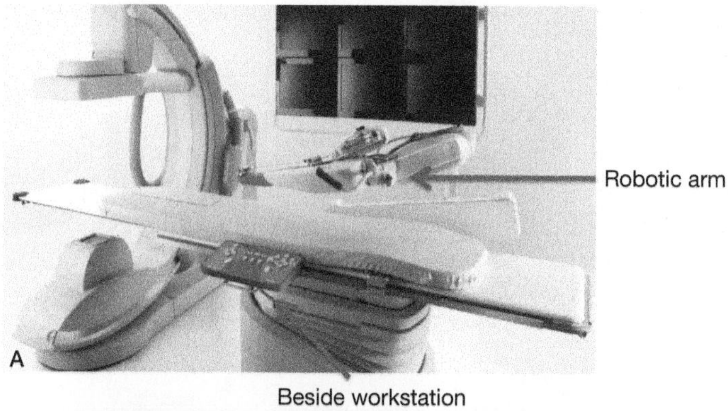

Figure 45-2. (**A**) Illustration of the Magellan robotic system and its setup at the intervention table consisting of the bedside workstation and the robotic arm. (**B**) Depiction of the robotic arm in action.

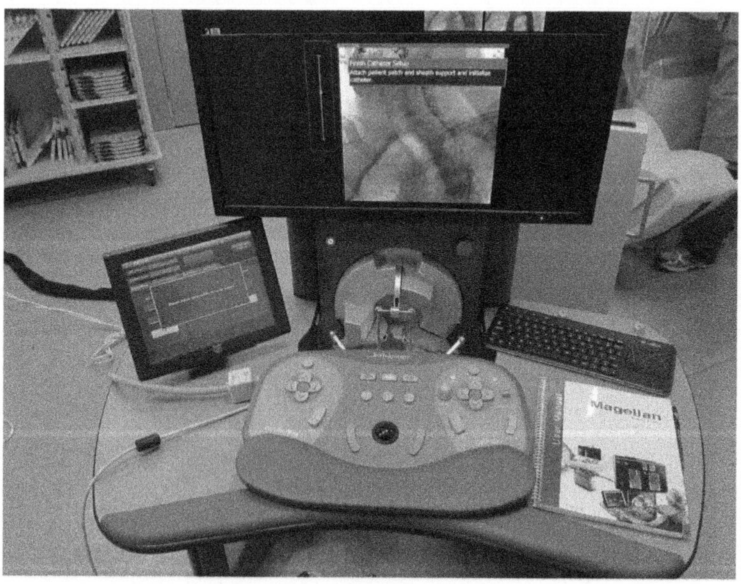

Figure 45-3. Remote workstation of the Magellan robotic system.

smaller vessels. This new 6F robotic catheter is designed to deliver a control guide wire and is equipped with two bends (proximal and distal) of which each can be controlled independently. The proximal joint is utilized solely for bending while the distal end is capable of rotational movements (Figure 45-5). This further improves the maneuverability of the robotic system while allowing for a simpler setup and workflow. The ability to have a smaller diameter vessel access while using a 6F platform is helpful when accessing smaller vessels for procedures such as embolization, mesenteric/renal artery angioplasty and stenting, and interventions for peripheral vascular disease of the lower extremity (including below the knee applications). Additionally, the 6F catheter can create a stable base catheter for a coaxial microcatheter that can be used for more remote diagnostic or intervention work.

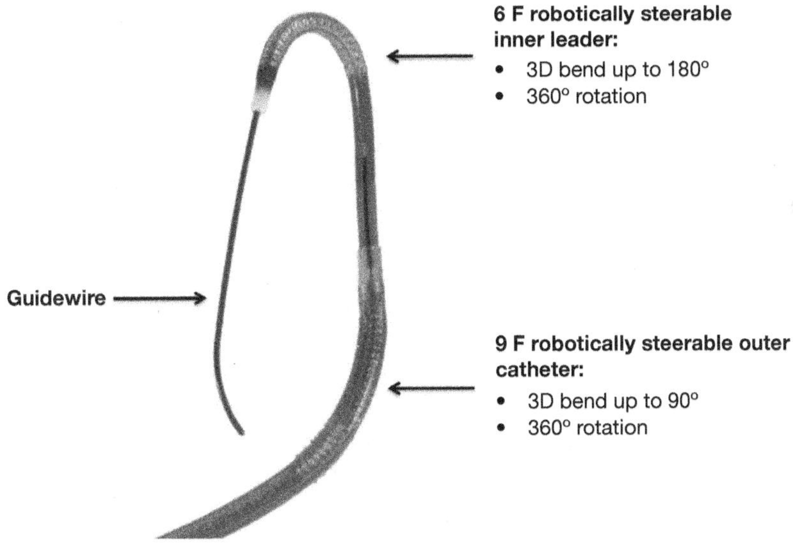

Figure 45-4. Illustration and description of the 9 F Magellan robotic catheter.

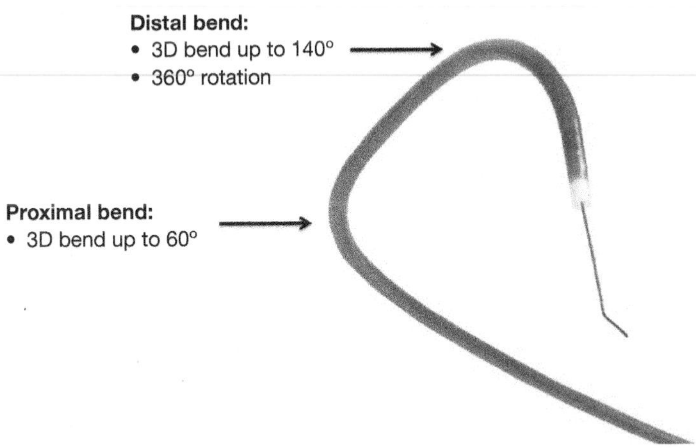

Figure 45-5. Illustration and description of the 6 F Magellan robotic catheter.

The newest generation 10F robotic catheter which received the European CE mark in April 2015 is very similar to the 9F system in terms of allowing independent control of both the outer guide and inner leader catheter. Its primary benefit is the fact that the 10F guide catheter has a 7F inner lumen (largest of all the robotic catheters) and allows delivery of a broader range of larger endovascular devices including stents, balloons, IVC filters, and others. This expands the range of procedures that can be performed; this system is particularly well suited for treatment of peripheral artery disease and complex endovascular aneurysm repair including fenestrated grafts, which not infrequently require a 7F inner lumen.

Carotid Arteries

In patients presenting with complex aortic arch anatomy, catheterization of the innominate artery, carotid arteries, and subclavian arteries can be challenging and may be associated with an increased risk for thromboembolic complications. Robotic assistance may facilitate a more accurate and centerline maneuverability and, thereby, reduce the risk for embolization and catheter dislodgment. Interestingly, the Magellan robotic system was evaluated for complex aortic arch catheterization in two reconstructed pulsatile phantoms.[4] The robotic system was compared to conventional (manual) catheterization by a total of 17 physicians. It was shown that the use of Magellan significantly reduced cannulation times and the number of catheter tip movements. Preclinical laboratory investigations have also demonstrated differences in histology between manual and robotic catheterization, with significantly less vessel injury from the latter.

In clinical practice, we have found that the robotic catheter enables catheterization in extremely challenging type 3 aortic arches, which we could not engage with manual catheterization. Robotic stability paired with the ability to create a wide variety of shapes and angles allows for the operator to steer the catheter through tortuous and difficult anatomy. Figures 45-6a–e provide an example of the advantages of complex aortic arch catheterization.

Visceral Arteries

Commonly the outgoing branches of visceral arteries have a very severe angle challenging its cannulation. Frequently, this necessitates a secondary arterial access from the upper extremities (i.e., axillary, brachial, or radial artery) to gain access which is not only associated with the need for an additional procedure, but also the potential for increased complications. Hereby, the robot system may facilitate the cannulation and preclude the need for a secondary access. In addition, the excellent stability and control of the robotic catheter allows for additional device and catheter exchanges for further interventions. According to one study, the cannulation times of the renal, celiac and superior mesenteric arteries were reduced from 15–20 minutes to less than 5 minutes resulting in a reduction of cannulation time of 83% when using Magellan.[5] However, this benefit in cannulation time was not confirmed for simple cannulation tasks in the hands of experienced interventionists.

The robotic catheter has been shown to be at least as safe as manual catheterization of the bilateral renal arteries, superior mesenteric artery (SMA), and contralateral iliac artery in an in-vivo porcine model.[6] In this study, the animals were sacrificed after robotic and manual catheterization of these arteries. Upon pathologic review, more extensive vascular injury was actually observed with the manual technique.

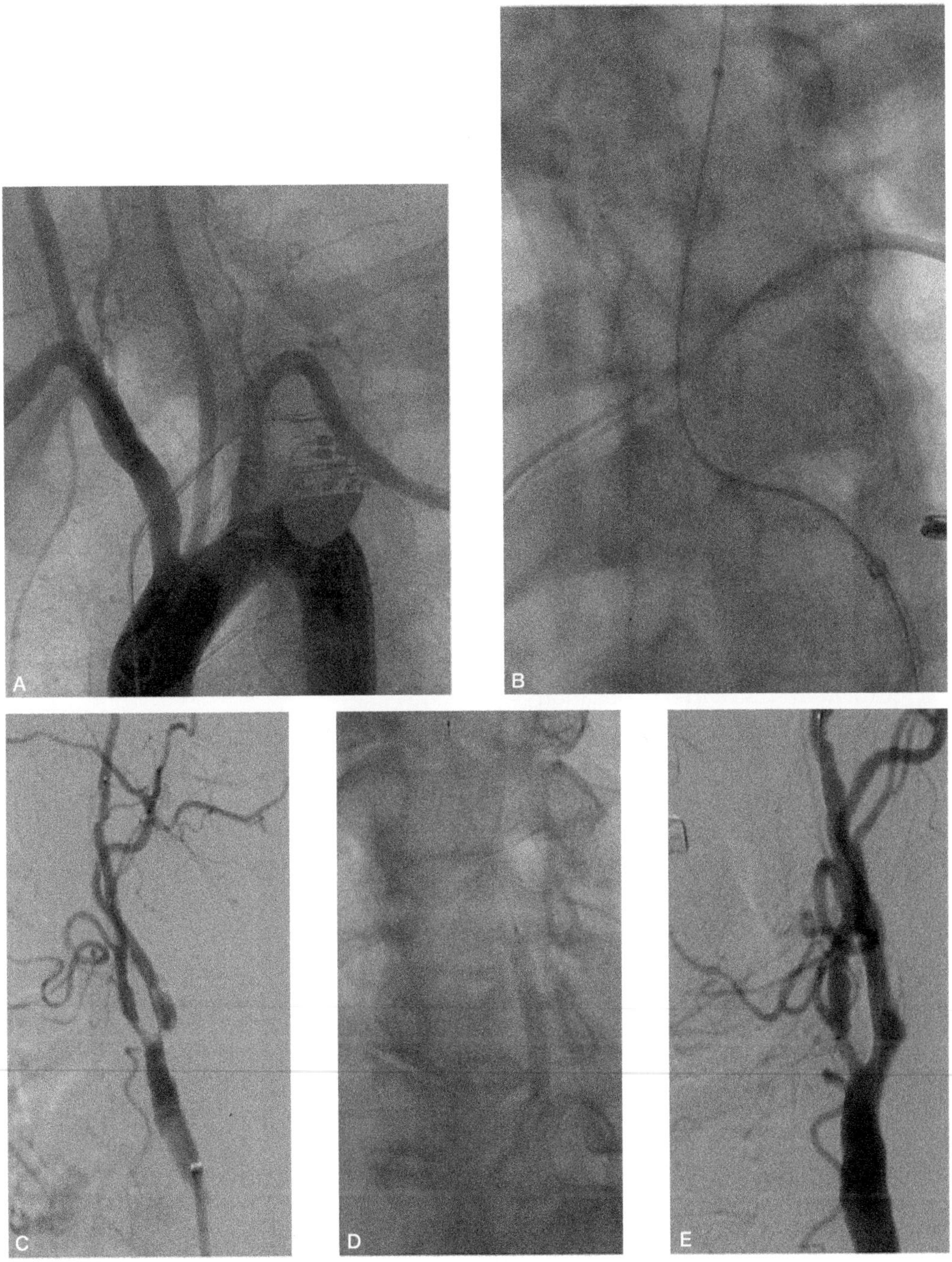

Figure 45-6. (**A**) Angiogram of a complex aortic arch anatomy (type 3) in a patient with left carotid artery stenosis. (**B**) Angiogram showing the catheterization of the left common carotid artery using the Magellan robotic system. Please note the guidewire supported by the 6 F inner leader advancing, whereas the 9 F outer catheter of the robot is still at the level of the aortic arch. (**C**) Illustration of the left carotid bifurcation with proximal stenoses of both the internal and external carotid arteries. Please note the robotic guidewire advanced into the internal carotid artery (target artery). (**D**) Stenting of the stenosis of the proximal internal carotid artery. (**E**) Final angiogram showing the treated internal carotid artery with flow improvement when compared to baseline, whereas the external carotid artery was not treated.

Aorta

In complex endovascular aortic aneurysm repair (EVAR) the benefit of using the Magellan robot may constitute improved stability as well as facilitated cannulation of visceral branches (i.e., fenestrated graft). A phantom study, using silicon models of reconstructed thoraco-abdominal aneurysms, was performed evaluating the cannulation time of visceral and renal arteries comparing robot-assisted versus manual catheterization.[5] Using the robot resulted in a reduction of cannulation time from 17.2 to 2.9 minutes (P< 0.001) and the number of wire/catheter movements was significantly reduced (454 to 38 movements, P< 0.001). Subsequent to this publication, several case reports have been published reporting information and details on the benefit of using the Magellan robot for fenestrated EVAR.[7–9] In addition, it has been shown that robot assistance may facilitate the cannulation of the contralateral limb in EVAR procedures.

The robot may also be of benefit during secondary interventions after EVAR. In the case of endoleak complications, robotic-assistance may assist in cannulating visceral arterial branches or hypogastric arterial branches feeding an enlarging aneurysm sac, for coiling or embolization purposes. In our own experience, we had a patient with a type II endoleak originating from the SMA, which could not be catheterized from a femoral approach due to significant aortic angulation and tortuosity and also could not be successfully treated via a brachial approach because the microcatheter was not of sufficient length. In this case, the robotic catheter provided excellent stability from a femoral approach, allowing stable cannulation of the SMA followed by microcatheterization and embolization of the endoleak.

Lower Extremities

The benefit and applicability of the Magellan robot for peripheral artery disease warrants further scrutiny. To date, there is only one first-in-man study evaluating the Magellan robotic system for iliofemoral revascularization.[10] Thereby, the robot was investigated for catheterization of iliofemoral *de novo* lesions. In a total of 20 patients, the procedure was performed by one of three experienced operators. Overall technical success was 100% with no complications at the access site. The navigation time and radiation exposure per case differed significantly comparing the more and the less experienced interventionists.

Nevertheless, the following may represent potential benefits for the Magellan robot and its use for treating PAD lesions: (1) enhanced pushability and maneuverability in procedures with crossover access may allow treatment of difficult lesions[11]; (2) centerline guidance may allow for improved true lumen revascularization, decreased risk of dissection, and fewer thromboembolic complications when treating occlusive lesions.

In certain clinical scenarios such as prior endovascular aneurysm repair, aortobifemoral surgical bypass, kissing iliac stents, and tight/steep aortic bifurcations it can be difficult or impossible to utilize a crossover approach with manual catheterization. In such situations, the stability and unique ability to adjust the catheter angulation and stiffness may allow an operator to treat contralateral peripheral arterial disease without having to utilize an antegrade femoral approach. We have utilized the robotic system to treat contralateral SFA disease in an obese patient with a prior bifurcated aortic endograft with minimal difficulty using a crossover femoral approach.

Embolization Procedures

The stability and navigability of the robotic catheter of the Magellan robotic system are critical features which allow for the precision and delicate touch necessary when performing embolization procedures. Non-target delivery of embolic agents can lead to severe adverse complications; the stability provided by the robotic catheter is unparalleled and may be superior to manual catheterization in the setting of precarious anatomy. The robot has been used in a diversity of embolization procedures including chemoembolization, Yttrium-90 radioembolization, uterine artery embolization, prostatic artery embolization, and hypogastric artery embolization. Robotic catheterization is currently limited for smaller vessels for which the smaller 6F system is often still too large and often requires delivery of a microcatheter through the robotic system. Hansen Medical is currently investigating smaller catheters which would be valuable in selecting and tracking into smaller vessels in this setting.

Rolls et al. published the first report on robot-assisted bilateral uterine artery embolization in 5 women with symptomatic uterine fibroids or adenomyosis.[11] Technical success was achieved in all patients, no complications were encountered, and the authors noted additional navigational capability and maneuverability with the robotic catheter. The ability to deflect the leader catheter and create a 180 degree bend enabled successful ipsilateral hypogastric catheterization without catheter exchange. Although this was a very small safety and feasibility study, median fluoroscopy time was 11 minutes which compares favorably with 13.4–27 minutes reported in the literature for conventional manual technique.

CORINDUS ROBOTIC SYSTEM

The CorPath 200 robotic system, the only FDA-cleared vascular robotic system for percutaneous coronary intervention,[12] consists of a remote interventional cockpit and a bedside disposable cassette that enables the operator to advance, retract, and rotate guidewires and catheters potentially enhancing the visibility and level of intravascular accuracy during interventional cardiology procedures. Based on the remote control panel, radiation exposure to the physician-operator can be decreased by up to 95% thus minimizing the occupational hazards associated with traditional PCI.[2,13] However, robotic assisted PCI has been shown to not only benefit physicians, but also patients in whom there is a reduction in fluoroscopy time, radiation dose, and contrast volume when compared to the traditional manual approach.[3] Suboptimal positioning of coronary stents with geographical miss of lesion has been shown to increase the rate of target vessel revascularization. Because this robotic system allows for precise sub-millimeter measurements and 1 mm advancement accuracy, it is hypothesized that robotic assisted PCI may provide a solution for more precise stent deployment and reduction in total number of stents needed.[14] If the latter is indeed true, there is potential for cost savings. Unlike the Magellan robot, the CorPath robot has been shown to enhance the visibility,[14] which may provide further benefit.

Of note, the previous investigations focused on simple coronary lesions (type A and B1) and moreover there are no prior randomized clinical trials to our knowledge.

CONCLUSION

Robotic technology was introduced to further improve the concept of minimally invasive endovascular therapy. Early clinical experience has shown robotic assistance may facilitate the catheterization of complex lesions and of angulated branches. At the same time, the ability to guide the robot from a remote workstation has been shown to reduce radiation dose to the operators while decreasing fatigue by providing a more ergonomic seated working position.

Although robotic catheters have been associated with excellent technical success rates and safety profile, one must be aware that we are only at the infancy of understanding the true clinical value of this novel technology. A meaningful comparison of the clinical outcomes and cost of robotic assisted endovascular therapy versus the conventional standard of care (manual catheterization) in a randomized clinical trial is necessary.

REFERENCES

1. Malcolme-Lawes LC, Lim PB, Koa-Wing M, et al. Robotic assistance and general anaesthesia improve catheter stability and increase signal attenuation during atrial fibrillation ablation. *EP Europace*. 2013;15:41–7.
2. Weisz G, Metzger DC, Caputo RP, et al. Safety and feasibility of robotic percutaneous coronary intervention: PRECISE (Percutaneous Robotically-Enhanced Coronary Intervention) Study. *J Am Coll Cardiol*. 2013;61:1596–600.
3. Smilowitz NR, Moses JW, Sosa FA, et al. Robotic-Enhanced PCI Compared to the Traditional Manual Approach. *JIC*. 2014;26:318–21.
4. Riga CV, Bicknell CD, Hamady MS and Cheshire NJ. Evaluation of robotic endovascular catheters for arch vessel cannulation. *J Vasc Surg*. 2011;54: 799–809.
5. Riga CV, Cheshire NJ, Hamady MS, Bicknell CD. The role of robotic endovascular catheters in fenestrated stent grafting. *J Vasc Surg*. 2010;51:810–9; discussion 9–20.
6. Bismuth J, Kashef E, Cheshire N, Lumsden AB. Feasibility and safety of remote endovascular catheter navigation in a porcine model. *JEVT*. 2011;18:243–9.
7. Riga C, Bicknell C, Cheshire N, Hamady M. Initial clinical application of a robotically steerable catheter system in endovascular aneurysm repair. *JEVT*. 2009;16:149–53.
8. Riga CV, Bicknell CD, Rolls A, Cheshire NJ and Hamady MS. Robot-assisted fenestrated endovascular aneurysm repair (FEVAR) using the Magellan system. *JVIR*. 2013;24:191–6.
9. Carrell T, Dastur N, Salter R, Taylor P. Use of a remotely steerable "robotic" catheter in a branched endovascular aortic graft. *J Vasc Surg*. 2012;55:223–5.
10. Bismuth J, Duran C, Stankovic M, et al. A first-in-man study of the role of flexible robotics in overcoming navigation challenges in the iliofemoral arteries. *J Vasc Surg*. 2013;57:14S–9S.
11. Rolls AE, Riga CV, Bicknell CD, et al. Robot-assisted uterine artery embolization: a first-in-woman safety evaluation of the Magellan System. *JVIR*. 2014;25:1841–8.
12. Tada T, Natsuaki M, Morimoto T, et al. Duration of dual antiplatelet therapy and long-term clinical outcome after coronary drug-eluting stent implantation: landmark analyses from the CREDO-Kyoto PCI/CABG Registry Cohort-2. *Circ Cardiovasc Interv*. 2012;5:381–91.
13. Granada JF, Delgado JA, Uribe MP, et al. First-in-human evaluation of a novel robotic-assisted coronary angioplasty system. *JACC Cardiovasc Interv*. 2011;4:460–5.
14. Kapur V, Smilowitz NR and Weisz G. Complex robotic-enhanced percutaneous coronary intervention. *Catheter Cardiovasc Interv*. 2014; 83:915–21.

46

Abdominal Aortic Aneurysms in Women

Ulka Sachdev, MD and Jean Starr, MD

Abdominal aortic aneurysm (AAA) has traditionally been considered a degenerative arterial disease that affects males. As a result, the vast majority of current treatment paradigms, screening regimens, and devices have been geared and produced to manage aneurysms in men. While the incidence of AAA is certainly higher in men, the presence of aneurysmal aortic degeneration in women can be a formidable clinical challenge, with significant consequences if not suspected or treated in a timely manner. Over the last three decades, a number of studies have documented a sobering trend: women with AAA have a higher tendency to present with deadly rupture, indicating a failure to identify the pathologic condition at a time when options for elective repair can be optimized. A definitive reason as to why women present with more advanced disease remains elusive. A number of research studies have tested the hypothesis that hormonal factors play a critical role in the gender differential that is apparent in the natural history and response to treatment of AAA. Paralleling the experience in many other disease processes, what appears clear in animal models is muddled in clinical studies. In fact, as they relate to the study of AAA in men and women, the clinical and basic science studies manifest opposite results.[1,2] Fortunately, the new decade is likely to see the advent of endovascular devices that favor the anatomy so commonly encountered in women with aneurysmal disease such as small, tortuous iliacs and short aortic necks.[3-5] Furthermore, screening recommendations offered by the Society of Vascular Surgery (SVS) have continued to push for more aggressive attempts to detect aneurysmal disease in women at an earlier stage.[6] The following sections will describe what is known about gender differences in aneurysmal disease, including clinical factors, emphasizing difference in presentation and response to intervention, the contribution of hormones and wall stress, aneurysm size indexed to body surface area, response to open surgical and endovascular treatments, and changes in the recommendations for screening. A critical assessment of our current treatment models is paramount to address the significant risk of morbidity and mortality associated with AAA in women.

WHAT IS KNOWN

Outcomes are different

Repeated observations in large randomized controlled trials in which the number of women enrolled was appreciable demonstrate that females have a higher risk of rupture than males, and that rupture can occur at a smaller size. For example, in follow-up studies to the United Kingdom Small Aneurysm Trial (UKSAT), rupture risk for women was shown to be three to four times higher than for men at smaller sizes.[7,8] In UKSAT, women comprised approximately 17% of the study population. In the follow-up study including an additional 1167 patients with slightly more female participation, female gender was a strong predictor of rupture. Additionally, rupture occurred at a smaller diameter in women than in men (5.0 cm in women vs. 6.0 cm in men, $p = 0.001$).[8] These types of findings would call into question whether the clinical practice of observing aneurysms 4.5–5.5 cm is applicable to women, although large randomized trials still do not appear to support the contention.[9]

It has also consistently, although not uniformly, been shown that women are more likely to die and have complications after repair of both intact and ruptured aneurysms, regardless of the approach to repair[10] (see Tables 46-1 and 46-2). In 2006, Dillavou et al. demonstrated that a decade's worth of aneurysm repairs demonstrated a higher decrease in mortality for men following aneurysm surgery than for women. In that study, while mortality for open repair in men decreased significantly from 1994 to 2004,

TABLE 46-1. OUTCOME AFTER ELECTIVE REPAIR FOR AAA, EVAR, AND OAR

Elective repair	Women postoperative mortality, %	Men postoperative mortality, %	*P*
Mehta et al.[59] EVAR *N* = 2,631	3.2	0.96	< 0.005
Dillavou et al.[48] All elective *N* = 322,000	6.6	4.7	< 0.01
Dillavou et al. EVAR	2.6	1.3	< 0.013
Larsson et al.[8] *N* = 14,000	5.7	4.9	< 0.01[a]
Johnston[57] *N* = 679	5.2	4.4	NS
McPhee et al.[58] *N* = 146,000 EVAR	6.1	4	< 0.001
McPhee et al.[58] OAR	2.1	0.8	< 0.001
Norman et al.[58] OAR	3.6	4.4	NR[b]

[a] After age adjustment in a multivariate model, mortality rates were similar for women and men.
[b] *P* values were not reported.
Source: Adapted from: Hultgren R.[10]; used with permission from Georg Thieme Verlag KG.
Note: References within table are from Hultgren review.

TABLE 46-2. MORTALITY AFTER REPAIR FOR RUPTURED AAA, IN HOSPITAL OR 30 DAYS POSTOPERATIVELY

Ruptured AAA	Women postoperative mortality %	Men postoperative mortality %	*P*
Murebee et al.[60] *N* = 75,000	52.3	43.5	< 0.001
Larsson et al.[8]	41.9	36.8	< 0.001[a]
McPhee et al.[58]	43	35.6	< 0.001
Dillavou et al.[48]	52.8	44.2	< 0.001
Norman et al.[61] OAR	43.9	34.7	NR[b]

[a] After age adjustment in a multivariate model, mortality rates were similar for women and men.
[b] *P* values were not reported.
Source: Adapted from: Hultgren R.[10]; used with permission from Georg Thieme Verlag KG.
Note: References within table are from Hultgren review.

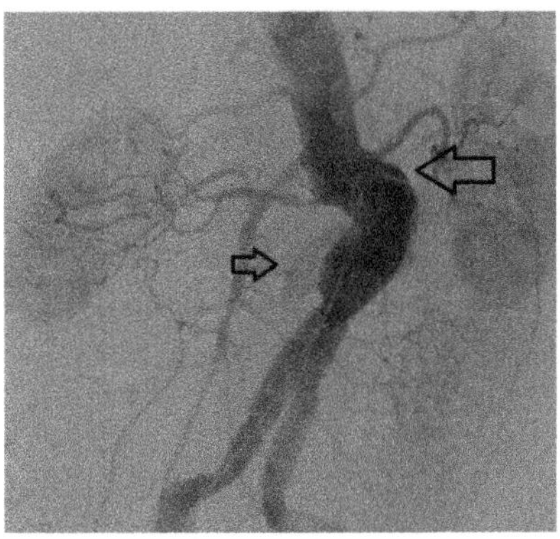

Figure 46-1. Abdominal aortogram during EVAR: arrows demonstrate short and angulated aortic neck and distal aorta.

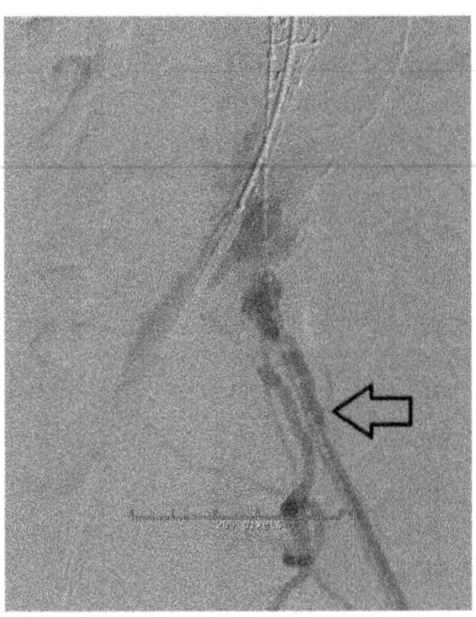

Figure 46-2. Angiogram during EVAR: arrow demonstrates small size of left external iliac artery.

the decrease in mortality following open aneurysm repair (OAR) for women was marginal.[11]

Anatomical considerations of the aorto-iliac segment in women have been shown to contribute to the ineligibility of endovascular aneurysm repair (EVAR) for female patients. Women have been shown to present with shorter, smaller, more angulated aortic necks (see Figure 46-1), as well as small, tortuous iliac arteries (see Figure 46-2).[4,12] Thus, EVAR has often been associated with a higher complication rate, higher re-intervention rate, and higher mortality.[4,5] In one study by Mehta et al. in which women represented 24% of the study population, iliac artery rupture and leg ischemia complicated EVAR performed in women more commonly than similar procedures performed in men.[5] In this particular study, the same disadvantage was not demonstrated after OAR. These types of complications result in longer hospital stays for women, which is another trend in AAA surgery that has been noted across studies.[4,11]

In a more recent study evaluating the results from Eurostar, a voluntary registry of EVARs initiated in 1996, similar results were demonstrated. Specifically, women had more device related complications, failure to complete the procedure and arterial complications. Additionally, women had worse survival and an unfavorable composite endpoint of event-free survival and re-intervention.[13]

Biological factors have an influence

The literature supports the finding that women present with AAA at an older age than men.[4,13] However, this difference alone does not appear to be the sole factor contributing to higher postoperative complications rates for women. These observations would suggest that the hormonal milieu between men and women offer some protection against aneurysmal dilation than men, at least at younger ages. Due to space limitations, the following findings are reported from comprehensive review articles focusing on gender differences in AAA, rather than the original research articles. The original reports are referenced in these sources. Studies in animals have focused on identifying the roles of estrogen and androgen on the development of AAA, but their findings have not been consistently applicable to patients.[2] In a review of sex hormones and abdominal aortic aneurysm, Bloomer et al. report that in animal models, androgens have been shown to promote aneurysmal degeneration. In contrast, human studies demonstrate that low testosterone is clinically correlated with the development of AAA, and that androgens may be protective.[1] While estrogen appears to be protective in animal models, clinical studies evaluating the role of exogenous estrogens on aneurysmal formation have been inconclusive. While some studies suggest a protective effect, others demonstrate a deleterious or no effect.[2] The evidence available to evaluate the roles of endogenous androgen and estrogen in human aneurysmal disease is too sparse to make any meaningful conclusion.[1]

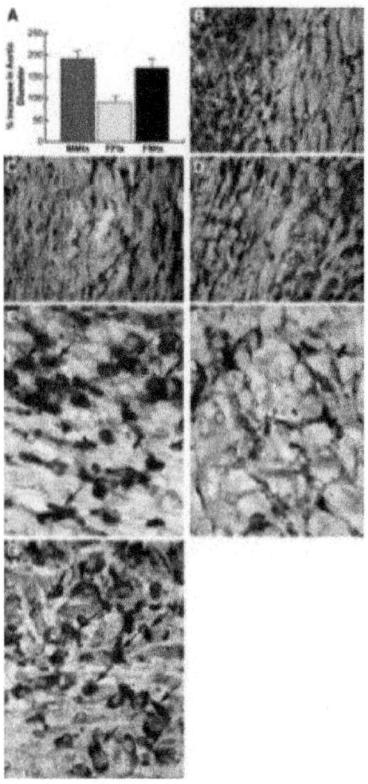

Figure 46-3. Transplanted aortas subjected to elastase perfusion. (**A**) Percent increase in aortic diameter in transplanted animals after elastase perfusion compared with baseline aortic diameter before aneurysm induction. All male-to-male transplanted aortas after elastase perfusion (MMtx) developed AAAs, whereas female-to-female transplanted aortas (FFtx) remained AAA-resistant. Female-to-male transplanted aortas (FMtx) uniformly developed AAAs ($P = 0.0118$). Immunohistochemistry for MMP-9 (red) demonstrates more staining in MMtx (**B**) and FMtx (**C**) than in FFtx (**D**) (100×). Colocalization of ED-1 (blue) and MMP-9 (red) demonstrates prominent costaining in MMtx (**E**), less staining in FFtx (**F**), and more prominent costaining in FMtx (**G**) (100×). From Ailawadi et al, ATVB.[22] Used with Permission.

In animal studies, however, the roles of androgens and estrogens in contrived models of aneurysmal disease have shown them to be critical mediators of aortic wall degeneration after injury. Evidence points to gender-mediated alterations in leukocyte recruitment, extracellular matrix, matrix metalloproteinase activity and NFκB translocation. Of note, animal models often utilize the infusion of elastase directly into the aorta, or the administration of angiotensin-II in supra-physiologic levels.[1,2] This results in rapid aortic degeneration involving large amounts of inflammatory cells and mediators (see Figure 46-3). It is unclear how well these studies truly mirror human disease. In one study by Ailawadi et al., elastase perfusion into rats resulted in more aneurysmal formation in males than in females (82% vs. 29%). Aortas transplanted from females to males demonstrated similar rates of aneurysmal degeneration as males, while treatment with estradiol appeared to protect against large aneurysm formation.[14] This same paper demonstrated increased MMP9 activity in male compared with female rodents, as well as increases in macrophage infiltration into the aortic wall. Daugherty et al. demonstrated the feasibility of angiogensin-II infusions to promote aneurysms in ApoE -/- mice. Studies from his group demonstrated that castration reduced angiotensin-II-induced aneurysms in male rodents, and that androgens promoted the expression of angiotensin 2 receptors in vulnerable aortas.[1,2]

The tensile strength of the aortic wall has been implicated in the etiology of aneurysmal disease as well as in rupture. Studies from the University of Pittsburgh demonstrated that diminished tensile strength was associated with rupture. These studies were performed by evaluating the mechanical properties of aortic wall strips harvested during open operations for both intact and ruptured aneurysms. Using similar techniques to study gender differences, strips of aorta were harvested during open aneurysmal repair from male and female human subjects. Although not statistically significant likely due to small numbers, women were shown to have a trend towards decreased aortic tensile strength than men.[3] These data suggest that decreased tensile strength contributes to rupture risk in women.

Aortic Size Index may be more predictive

A great deal of interest has been applied to the concept that the recommendation to repair aneurysms at 5.5 cm and above does not take into account the fact that women, on average, have a smaller body surface area than men. As a result, a number of studies have evaluated the benefit of using an aortic size index (ASI) rather than absolute diameter in determining which patients are more at risk for rupture.[15] In a retrospective review of the Vascular Study Group of New England (VSGNE) database, Lo et al. demonstrated that the variable most predictive of rupture in women was the ASI, determined by dividing the absolute diameter of the aneurysm by the individual's body surface area. The same did not hold true for men, in whom absolute diameter was more predictive of rupture. An ASI less than or equal to $3.5/m^2$ was found to correlate with an aneurysm size of 5.3 cm for women and 6.0 cm for men.[15] These data corroborate other findings that women may rupture at absolute diameters that are smaller than men, and may benefit from AAA repair at smaller sizes than what guidelines suggest currently.[16]

Similar findings were reported by Matyal et al. in a recent study published in 2015. Again using the database provided by the VSGNE, they evaluated results of both open and endovascular repair for aneurysms indexed by size and by ASI. Notably, while women underwent repair at absolute sizes that were less than men (5.8 cm vs. 6.2 cm), their ASI values were significantly higher than those of men (3.38 vs. $3.10/m^2$). Women had higher transfusion rates, as well as longer intensive care unit and hospital stays.[17] The authors suggest that using the current threshold for AAA repair may ignore the fact that women have a smaller body surface area, and thus may be undergoing repairs at a physiologically more advanced state than men.[17] Taken together, these results may suggest that an ASI may be a more useful tool for screening and determining the indication for aneurysm repair, although further studies are warranted to change the current recommendations.

SCREENING

U.S. Preventive Services Task Force (USPSTF) Recommendations for Screening

Given what is known about the differences between clinical presentation of aneurysms between men and women, it might be reasonable to consider expanding current screening recommendations to include more women who are at risk. Currently, the USPSTF Recommendation supports screening for men aged 65–75 years of age who have ever smoked. However, they also found the data to be insufficient to recommend routine screening for AAA in women of the same age group who have ever smoked.[18] In some studies, smoking has been shown to be more of a risk factor for aneurysmal degeneration in women than in men. A Swedish cohort of 35,550 women, in which 199 developed aneurysms, demonstrated a hazards ratio (HR) of over 10 for aneurysmal disease in women with more than a 20 pack-year smoking history. In the same study, men with similar histories had a HR closer to 7. Interestingly, cessation of smoking reduced the risk of aneurysmal formation in women more than men, suggesting a possible gender difference in the sensitivity to toxins in cigarette smoke. Finally, women smokers had an appreciably higher risk of aneurysmal degeneration than men who had never smoked.[19] Despite these findings, the report issued by the USPSTF cites a paucity of randomized controlled trials that include screening for AAA in women, as well as a low incidence of aneurysms in women against making a strong recommendation supporting the practice. Currently, Medicare supports screening for both women and men who have a family history of aneurysmal disease as part of the "Welcome to Medicare" exam. Women with a history of smoking are not routinely recommended for screening.[18]

Despite new USPSTF recommendations and efforts to include women in future screening efforts, the SAAVE act (Screening Abdominal Aortic Aneurysms Very Efficiently) of 2007 has only brought about a modest increase in AAA screening with abdominal ultrasound use in 65-year-old men joining Medicare. After 2007, although 2/3 of men entering Medicare were appropriate for screening, only 10% actually received an abdominal ultrasound. Additionally, this new screening program has had no effect on rate of AAA repair, rate of rupture, or all-cause mortality.[20] It is also unclear how often patients receive appropriate follow up after initial AAA diagnosis. Thus, it appears that screening in its current state has not had the intended effect to improve the care of AAA patients overall. A new screening scoring system proposed by Kent et al. may help identify more patients with AAA, inclusive of women, younger patients, and non-smokers, who are currently excluded from screening.[21]

SVS Recommendations for Screening and Follow-up

Based on a number of high-quality studies, the SVS and the Society for Vascular Medicine and Biology have supported screening for aneurysmal disease.[6] Importantly, they include more aggressive recommendations regarding screening for AAAs in women. In particular, official practice guidelines include screening for aneurysms in 65-year-old women who have a history of smoking or a family history of aneurysmal disease. For patients in which an aneurysm has been detected, follow-up imaging should occur yearly for those with aneurysm diameters of 3.5 to 4.4 cm, and every 6 months for aneurysm diameters of 4.5 to 5.4 cm.[6]

The data to support the recommendations of the SVS is not overwhelming regarding its contention that screening should be offered more broadly to women. A study from the *British Journal of Surgery* in 2002 reported the results of a randomized controlled trial in which approximately 9000 women were screened as part of a larger study including both men and women. The prevalence of AAA was six times lower in women than in men. Importantly, rupture rates were similar between women who were screened and those who were not. The authors report no benefit either clinically or economically in offering screening for AAA to women.[22]

However, more recent studies have suggested that the higher risk of rupture may offset the lower incidence of disease in women, promoting a potential benefit of expanding screening more broadly to include women. Using a Markov simulation model, Wanhainen et al. sought to evaluate the cost effectiveness of screening for AAA in women.[23] The model incorporated evidence-based assumptions, including prevalence of the disease between the genders and rupture risk. This study demonstrated an incremental cost-effectiveness ratio in women that was similar to that of men, and the authors concluded that screening for AAA in women may be economically beneficial.[23]

The true prevalence of associated aneurysms in patients with AAA is unknown. Diwan et al. examined 313 patients with AAA (20% women) who had prospective peripheral arterial ultrasound and discovered 14% of men had femoral or popliteal aneurysm, whereas no women were diagnosed with lower extremity aneurysm. Although the incidence in men was higher than previously thought, there was a stronger affiliation with a positive family history of AAA in women than in men with AAA.[24] The etiology of these sex differences is unknown. In contrast, there may be higher association of AAA in women with concurrent descending thoracic aortic aneurysm, compared to men (39% vs. 16%). Consideration should be given to thoracic aortic screening in patients, especially women, who are reasonable operative candidates.[10]

EVOLUTION OF AAA REPAIR

As with many surgical interventions, results of AAA repair continue to improve as we adapt new procedures and devices to the appropriate patient populations. A National Inpatient Sample study found the use of EVAR has significantly increased over the course of 11 years, while the volume of OAR has equally decreased.[11] There has been an improvement in mortality for ruptured and intact AAA, realized more for those undergoing EVAR. Women tend to undergo EVAR less frequently, and thus may not similarly benefit from recent advances in AAA repair. They are more prone to significant complications, particularly involving access vessels, and are less likely to be discharged to home.[5] These issues are starting to be addressed by medical device companies, and recent generations of stent graft devices may now accommodate access vessels with smaller lumens, as well as angulated necks. With further advances, differences in sex-specific outcomes have more potential to become equalized in endovascular repair.

As technology evolves to allow vascular specialists to treat more complicated AAA anatomy, more patients will receive branched and fenestrated grafts for treatment of paravisceral aneurysms. Currently, however, there is little to no data reported on how women will fare after branched or fenestrated EVAR. A recent National Surgical Quality Improvement Program study found 27.5% of open paravisceral AAA repairs were women and female sex was one predictor of post-operative mortality.[25] It is too early to determine if branched and fenestrated technology will have a positive impact on survival in this group or if anatomic considerations will overshadow the ability to offer this advancement to women.

SHOULD THE THRESHOLD FOR REPAIR BE LOWER FOR WOMEN?

Current SVS guidelines recommend considering AAA repair when the absolute aortic diameter reaches 5.5 cm, when there is rapid growth, or when symptoms occur. These guidelines also suggest that operating on women with aneurysms less than 5.5 cm (5–5.4 cm) can be considered.[16] As with most surgical interventions, the decision to proceed is based on the potential risks incurred by the operation, weighed against the risks of no intervention; in this case, rupture. Certainly, this formula should take into account the life expectancy and general health of the patient, as well as the surgeon's/hospital's experience and surgical quality outcomes. No definitive evidence exists to lower the threshold of aneurysm repair to less than 5.5 cm for women. However, a growing body of literature continues to identify disparities in outcomes in both endovascular and open repair between men and women. Furthermore, clear anatomical differences between men and women with aneurysms consistently appear in the literature. Anatomically, women have smaller native aortic sizes, rupture at smaller diameters, and present with worse access anatomy, often precluding them from the safer endovascular approach. Because of this, EVAR is offered less frequently to women, excluding many from the benefits that endovascular management offers patients. Smaller AAAs are often more suited for EVAR, but women have larger AAAs at presentation, predisposing them to more complications. While randomized controlled trials may not demonstrate a benefit in either screening more women for aneurysms, or operating on them at smaller aneurysm sizes, the circumstantial evidence favoring such practices continues to build.[16] Perhaps incorporating a new paradigm of diagnosis and surveillance that takes into account body mass index or surface area will evolve into a new treatment strategy for managing aneurysms in women. Coupled with advances in endovascular technology favoring lower profile, and flexible devices, outcomes in both men and women will continue to improve.

REFERENCES

1. Bloomer LD, Bown MJ, Tomaszewski M. Sexual dimorphism of abdominal aortic aneurysms: A striking example of "male disadvantage" in cardiovascular disease. *Atherosclerosis.* 2012;225:22–8.
2. Makrygiannis G, Courtois A, Drion P, et al. Sex differences in abdominal aortic aneurysm: The role of sex hormones. *Ann Vasc Surg.* 2014;28:1946–58.
3. Starr JE, Halpern V. Abdominal aortic aneurysms in women. *J Vasc Surg.* 2013;57:3S–10S.
4. Chung C, Tadros R, Torres M, et al. Evolution of gender-related differences in outcomes from two decades of endovascular aneurysm repair. *J Vasc Surg.* 2015;61:843–52.
5. Mehta M, Byrne WJ, Robinson H, et al. Women derive less benefit from elective endovascular aneurysm repair than men. *J Vasc Surg.* 2012;55:906–13.
6. Chaikof EL, Brewster DC, Dalman RL, et al. Svs practice guidelines for the care of patients with an abdominal aortic aneurysm: Executive summary. *J Vasc Surg.* 2009;50:880–96.

7. McPhee JT, Hill JS, Eslami MH. The impact of gender on presentation, therapy, and mortality of abdominal aortic aneurysm in the united states, 2001-2004. *J Vasc Surg.* 2007;45:891–9.
8. Brown LC, Powell JT. Risk factors for aneurysm rupture in patients kept under ultrasound surveillance. UK small aneurysm trial participants. *Ann Surg.* 1999;230:289–96; discussion 296–7.
9. Bown MJ, Powell JT. Part two: Against the motion. Evidence does not support reducing the threshold diameter to 5 cm for elective interventions in women with abdominal aortic aneurysms. *Eur J Vasc Endovasc Surg.* 2014;48:614–8.
10. Hultgren R. Abdominal aortic aneurysms-gender aspects on prevalence, treatment, and concurrent aneurysms. *Thorac Cardiovasc Surg.* 2013;61:15–21.
11. Dillavou ED, Muluk SC, Makaroun MS. A decade of change in abdominal aortic aneurysm repair in the united states: Have we improved outcomes equally between men and women? *J Vasc Surg.* 2006;43:230–8; discussion 238.
12. Hultgren R, Vishnevskaya L, Wahlgren CM. Women with abdominal aortic aneurysms have more extensive aortic neck pathology. *Ann Vasc Surg.* 2013;27:547–52.
13. Grootenboer N, Hunink MG, Hendriks JM, et al. Sex differences in 30-day and 5-year outcomes after endovascular repair of abdominal aortic aneurysms in the eurostar study. *J Vasc Surg.* 2013;58:42–9 e41.
14. Ailawadi G, Eliason JL, Roelofs KJ, et al. Gender differences in experimental aortic aneurysm formation. *Arterioscler Thromb Vasc Biol.* 2004;24:2116–22.
15. Lo RC, Lu B, Fokkema MT, et al. Relative importance of aneurysm diameter and body size for predicting abdominal aortic aneurysm rupture in men and women. *J Vasc Surg.* 2014;59:1209–16.
16. Vavra AK, Kibbe MR. Part one: For the motion. Evidence supports reducing the threshold diameter to 5 cm for elective interventions in women with abdominal aortic aneurysms. *Eur J Vasc Endovasc Surg.* 2014;48:611–4.
17. Matyal R, Shakil O, Hess PE, et al. Impact of gender and body surface area on outcome after abdominal aortic aneurysm repair. *Am J Surg.* 2015;209:315–23.
18. LeFevre ML, Force USPST. Screening for abdominal aortic aneurysm: U.S. Preventive services task force recommendation statement. *Ann Intern Med.* 2014;161:281–90.
19. Stackelberg O, Bjorck M, Larsson SC, et al. Sex differences in the association between smoking and abdominal aortic aneurysm. *Br J Surg.* 2014;101:1230–7.
20. Shreibati JB, Baker LC, Hlatky MA, Mell MW. Impact of the screening abdominal aortic aneurysms very efficiently (SAAVE) act on abdominal ultrasonography use among medicare beneficiaries. *Arch Intern Med.* 2012;172:1456–62.
21. Kent KC, Zwolak RM, Egorova NN, et al. Analysis of risk factors for abdominal aortic aneurysm in a cohort of more than 3 million individuals. *J Vasc Surg.* 2010;52:539–48.
22. Scott RAP, Bridgewater SG, Ashton HA. Randomized clinical trial of screening for abdominal aortic aneurysm in women. *Br J Surg.* 2002;89:283–5.
23. Wanhainen A, Lundkvist J, Bergqvist D, Björck M. Cost-effectiveness of screening women for abdominal aortic aneurysm. *J Vasc Surg.* 2006;43:908–14
24. Diwan A, Sarkar R, Stanley JC, et al. Incidence of femoral and popliteal artery aneurysms in patients with abdominal aortic aneurysms. *J Vasc Surg.* 2000;31:863–9.
25. Gupta PK, Mactaggart JN, Natarajan B, et al. Predictive factors for mortality after open repair of paravisceral abdominal aortic aneurysm. *J Vasc Surg.* 2012;55:666–73.

47

Inflammatory Abdominal Aortic Aneurysms

Robert Jason T. Perry, MD and Kenneth J. Cherry, MD

Inflammatory abdominal aortic aneurysm (IAAA) is one of the most challenging conditions confronting the modern vascular surgeon. In this chapter we will review the presentation, epidemiology, pathophysiology, treatment options, technical considerations and expected outcomes in the treatment of patients with this diagnosis.

PRESENTATION

In contrast to patients with non-inflammatory abdominal aortic aneurysms (AAA), those with IAAA typically are symptomatic with the classic triad consisting of a pulsatile abdominal mass, weight loss and elevated erythrocyte sedimentation rate (ESR).[1] The most common symptoms include abdominal, back or flank pain, tender pulsatile mass and weight loss.[2] At presentation, imaging with CT scan is usually obtained with a sensitivity of detecting retroperitoneal inflammation and the classically described Mantle sign approaching 80%[3] (Figure 47-1A and 47-1B). Secondary signs of retroperitoneal inflammation such as irregularity of the contour of the inferior vena cava (IVC), deep venous thrombosis, development of aortocaval fistula (ACF), medialization of the ureters and hydronephrosis may also be present.[1,3–5]

IAAA patients are at elevated risk for development of ACF with reported incidence as high as 17% compared to 1% in non-inflammatory AAA patients.[6] Hydronephrosis with obstructive uropathy complicates approximately 20% of cases of IAAA.[2–3] Compared to non-inflammatory AAA, IAAA are less likely to rupture, with rupture rates of 17%–20% for the former and 3%–8%, for the latter.[6] Whether this is secondary to a protective effect of the thickened aneurysm wall or whether patients with IAAA are generally brought to medical attention when their aneurysms are smaller is unclear.

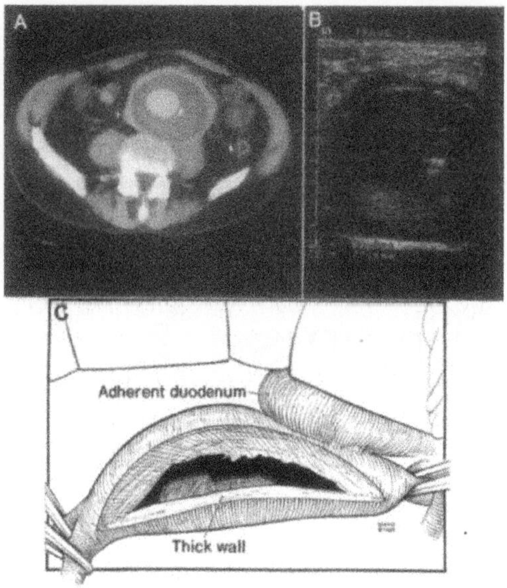

Figure 47-1. (**A**) Representative CT scan of the abdomen demonstrating thickened aortic wall characteristic of IAAA. (**B**) Representative duplex ultrasound of the same patient demonstrating the characteristic inflammatory 'halo' of IAAA. (**C**) Diagrammatic representation of the thickened aortic wall with adherent duodenum at operation. (From Nitecki SS, Hallett JW, Stanson AW, et al.[10]; used with permission from Elsevier.)

EPIDEMIOLOGY

While some degree of inflammation is expected with any AAA, true IAAA with extensive periaortic and retroperitoneal inflammation and fibrosis is encountered in 2.5%–14% of patients undergoing aneurysm repair and in 2.5%–10% of patients with AAA at autopsy.[1,6–9] While IAAA can be secondary to syphilis, tuberculosis or giant cell arteritis, most are idiopathic.

Family history of aneurysm is more strongly associated with IAAA than non-inflammatory AAA, as is ongoing tobacco abuse at time of diagnosis.[10] There does appear to be an association between IAAA and autoimmune disease. Haug, et al., described associated autoimmune disease including rheumatoid arthritis, systemic lupus erythematosus and giant cell arteritis in 19% of patients with IAAA compared to none of their control AAA subjects.[11]

PATHOPHYSIOLOGY

The pathophysiology of IAAA remains unclear. Current hypotheses include an exaggerated inflammatory response to the presence of AAA or, alternatively, a poorly understood primary inflammatory process driving the development of AAA.[11–13] Most authors now agree that IAAA manifest the extreme spectrum of the normal inflammatory response associated with AAA development. Grossly, at operation, the retroperitoneum overlying the aorta is glistening white and fibrotic.[2–3] While symptoms, elevated ESR and characteristic imaging findings are suggestive, the intraoperative findings of thickened aneurysm wall, extensive perianeurysmal and retroperitoneal fibrosis and dense adhesions of adjacent abdominal organs confirm the diagnosis of IAAA (Figure 47-1C).[1,13] Histologic analysis of the aorta and surrounding tissues demonstrates adventitial and medial fibrosis with lymphoplasmacytic infiltrate extending into the retroperitoneum.[12] More recently, IAAA has been potentially identified as IgG4-related disease in which IgG4-restricted plasma cells are found within the inflamed tissues.[14]

TREATMENT OPTIONS AND TECHNICAL CONSIDERATIONS

Like non-inflammatory AAA, IAAA have been repaired via open, endovascular and hybrid approaches. All patients that are stable enough for CT scan should undergo axial imaging for treatment planning, assessment for suitability for endovascular repair and to assess the presence of hydronephrosis, renal anomalies and aortocaval fistula (ACF).[6] Placement of prophylactic ureteral stents should be considered in all patients suspected of having IAAA, although efficacy data in this patient population is limited.[1] Certainly those patients with hydronephrosis or obstructive uropathy should have ureteral stents placed to aid with decompression. Prolonged operative time and increased intraoperative blood loss should be anticipated.[2,11]

For open repair, IAAA are most often approached transperitoneally, although some authors have advocated a retroperitoneal approach to avoid injury to the structures adherent to the anterior wall of the aorta including the duodenum, left renal vein and IVC.[3,9] In addition, the descending colon or its mesentery may be densely adhered to the IAAA.

For transperitoneal repair, a generous midline laparotomy incision is made from the xyphoid process to the symphysis pubis. Proximally, the incision should extend along the full length of the xypoid—to the level of the dome of the diaphragm—to facilitate subsequent pararenal exposure. The small bowel may be eviscerated into a bowel bag or, if the patient's anatomy permits it, simply packed in the right upper quadrant to minimize intraoperative desiccation and potential injury. A self-retaining retracting system, such as the Omni-Tract retractor©, facilitates exposure. With these dense adhesions and the resulting rigidity of the tissues, additional focused manual retraction is often necessary. Crawford, et al. emphasize minimal dissection of the structures adherent to the anterior aortic wall and repair via inclusion technique to avoid iatrogenic injury.[2] The duodenum is invariably densely adhered to the aneurysm surface, the IVC in roughly two-thirds and the left renal vein in approximately half of patients with IAAA (Figure 47-2).[1,9–10] In the past, partial excision prior to aortic clamping of that part of the thickened aortic wall adhesed to the duodenum in a tangential shaving or paring technique to allow mobilization of the duodenum has been recommended. If the aortic wall is not of uniform thickness, however, this may prove to be a dangerous maneuver and is not to be advocated.

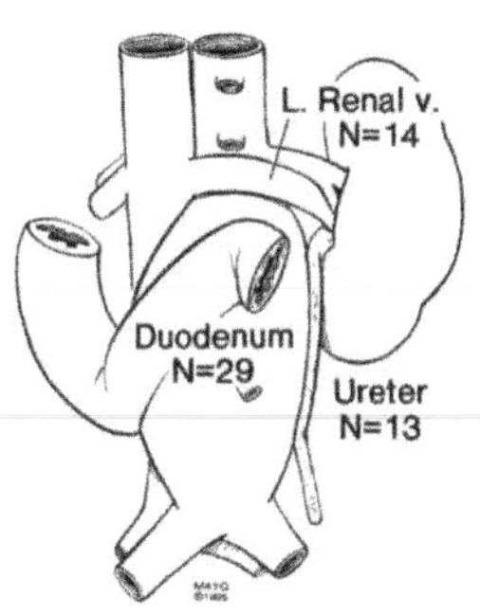

Figure 47-2. Structures adherent to the aorta among 29 patients with inflammatory abdominal aortic aneurysms: Duodenum (100%), left renal vein (48%), ureter (45%). (From Nitecki SS, Hallett JW, Stanson AW, et al.[10]; used with permission from Elsevier.)

We have found that dealing with the left renal vein may represent the greatest technical challenge in both exposure and repair. It may be difficult to dissect free, and sometimes even visualize, in the thickened tissue, often being effaced. It may be necessary to divide it adjacent to the IVC, and well towards the left kidney. The surgeon has to be cognizant of its presence even if not well seen or exposed. Piercing the vein with the usual vertically placed aortic clamps may lead to extensive blood loss. Despite the frequency of duodenal involvement, primary aortoduodenal fistula and injury of the duodenum during the operation are uncommon.[1] In the event that either of these is present, *in situ* omental-wrapped rifampin-soaked Dacron graft, autogenous homograft or cryopreserved allograft, or extraanatomic bypass, should be considered for reconstruction to decrease the risk of graft infection.[15,16]

The extent of the inflammatory process dictates in large part the extent of aortic dissection required to obtain proximal and distal control. Fortunately, the inflammatory component is often confined proximally to the aorta distal to the left renal vein and distally to the iliac arteries.[3,13] Despite this, 17%–37% of patients will require suprarenal clamping.[2,3] Uncommonly, ACF complicates IAAA repair. The ACF may be approached via the standard technique of repairing the IVC from within the aneurysm sac but this may be associated with significant blood loss in a patient already at elevated risk of the same. Madani and colleagues describe a novel technique for dealing with this challenging situation by obtaining standard proximal control of the IVC outside of the zone of inflammation and endovascular balloon occlusion of the more distal IVC involved in the inflammatory process.[4]

In the event that the aneurysm extent dictates use of a bifurcated graft, great care should be taken to avoid injury to the ureters as they are often encased in the inflammatory process. Prophylactic ureteral stents may aid in identification of the ureters and avoidance of injury.[1] Once sufficient proximal aorta and distal aorta or iliac arteries are exposed, the patient is systemically heparinized and proximal and distal control are obtained. The aneurysm is opened longitudinally slightly to the right of midline. The aortotomy must often be made carefully in the thin strip of uninvolved aorta between the adherent duodenum and the left colon or its mesentery. The aortotomy needs to stop short of the anticipated level of the left renal vein if that has not been seen. Adherent thrombus is extracted and back bleeding from the lumbar arteries and inferior mesenteric artery is controlled. The proximal and distal extents of the sac are then opened partially in transverse orientation. An appropriately sized graft is brought into the field and the proximal anastomosis is performed with running 3-0 Prolene suture via the inclusion technique.

Suturing the greatly thickened and fibrotic aortic wall is difficult, and can be facilitated by dividing the aorta circumferentially. Inclusion of two aortic surfaces, as is commonly done with undivided posterior aorta in non-inflammatory aneurysms, is not possible. Large needles such as an MH aid greatly in traversing these tough thick walls. A vascular clamp is applied to the graft and the proximal clamp is removed to ensure proximal suture line hemostasis. Once hemostasis is ensured, the distal anastomosis or anastomoses are performed in similar fashion. The retroperitoneum is reapproximated over the graft with absorbable suture to ensure exclusion of the graft from the peritoneal contents.

A retroperitoneal approach affords at least two distinct theoretical advantages over a transperitoneal one.[9] First, the intense inflammation which is typically encountered on the anterior surface of the aneurysm may be partially or entirely avoided by entering the retroperitoneal space laterally. However, the inflammatory process may be circumferential with extensive retroperitoneal involvement, negating this advantage in some patients. Second, should control of the abdominal aorta in the pararenal area be technically not possible, proximal supraceliac or thoracoabdominal control can be obtained in the chest where inflammation is unlikely.[1] It is important to ascertain the distal extent of the aneurysm as exposure of the right iliac artery is difficult via this approach. The proximal extent of the aneurysm dictates the level of thoracotomy necessary. Two incisional options are available, depending on the proximal extent of the aneurysm: a left flank incision for infrarenal and a true thoracoabdominal incision for juxtarenal or visceral segment aneurysms. If a thoracoabdominal approach is planned, an eighth interspace thoracotomy is typically suitable for most AAA, including those involving the visceral segment. One-lung ventilation can help prevent iatrogenic lung injury during entry into the chest but is not mandatory.

The patient should be positioned on the operating room table in a modified left thoracotomy position with the shoulders at 70 to 80 degrees to the table and the hips rotated posteriorly as far as possible. The break in the operating room table should be located between the iliac crest and the inferior border of the costal margin to increase exposure.[17] For the flank approach, an oblique incision is made midway between the anterior iliac spine and the umbilicus, extended medially to the lateral edge of the left rectus abdominis muscle. The external oblique aponeurosis is opened in the direction of its fibers up to the rectus muscle. The internal oblique and transversus abdominus muscles and the transversalis fascia are then opened and the peritoneum identified. It is easier to enter the correct plane of dissection laterally that it is medially. The remainder of the dissection is carried out as described below with the thoracoabdominal approach.

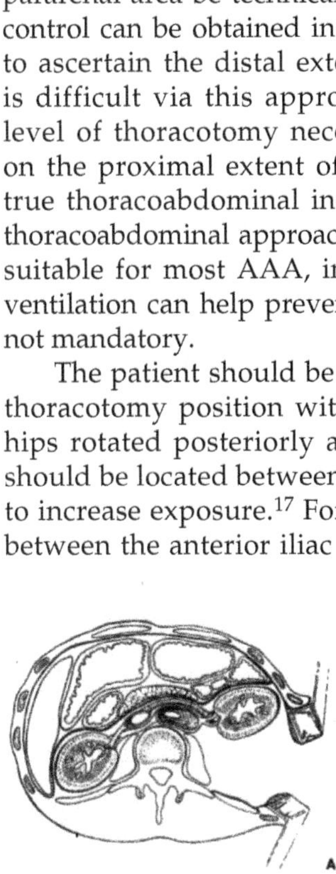

A

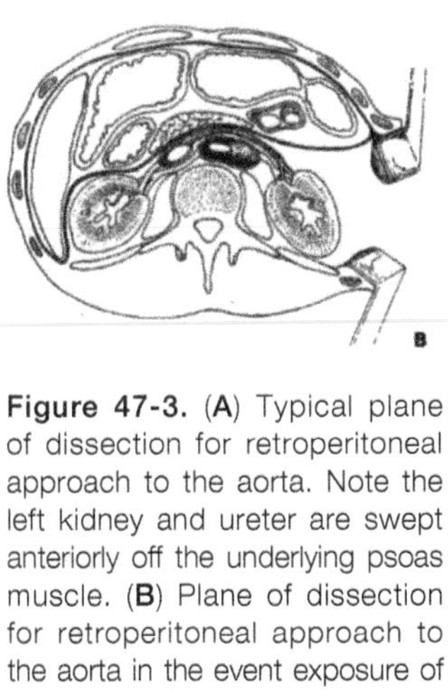

B

Figure 47-3. (A) Typical plane of dissection for retroperitoneal approach to the aorta. Note the left kidney and ureter are swept anteriorly off the underlying psoas muscle. (B) Plane of dissection for retroperitoneal approach to the aorta in the event exposure of the proximal superior mesenteric artery is required. (From Shepard AD, Tollefson DFJ, Reddy DJ, et al.[17]; used with permission from Elsevier.)

For more proximal aneurysms, a hockey stick thoracoabdominal incision is made incorporating the appropriate thoracotomy level with the paramedian abdominal component made lateral to the rectus abdominis musculature. The chest wall musculature is divided along the superior surface of the appropriate rib, the chest entered and the rib divided in the course of the incision. Resection of a portion of the rib can prevent a painful posterior rib fracture. For the abdominal component, the external oblique aponeurosis is opened longitudinally lateral to the rectus sheath as is the underlying internal oblique and transversus abdominus musculature and transversalis fascia. Taking care to avoid injury to the peritoneum, the peritoneal contents and left kidney are then swept medially off the underlying retroperitoneal structures and psoas muscle (Figure 47-3A and 47-3B). The diaphragm may be divided, ensuring an adequate lateral cuff for subsequent repair, down to and including the median arcuate ligament. Applying surgical clips to both sides of the diaphragm division line facilitates proper

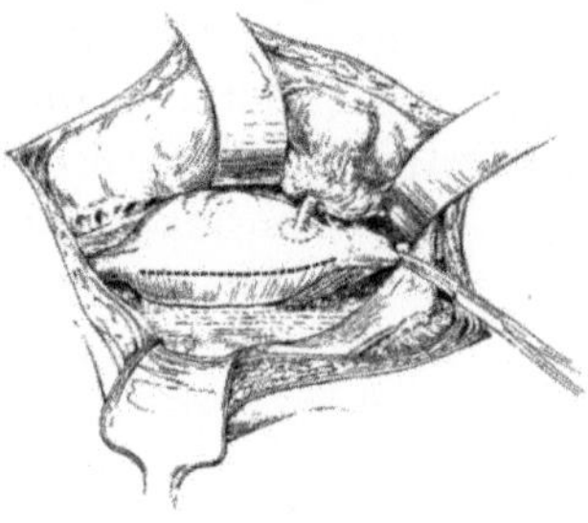

Figure 47-4. Exposure of the anterolateral aorta with peritoneal contents reflected anteriorly. The path of the aortotomy is indicated by the dashed line. (From Shepard AD, Tollefson DFJ, Reddy DJ, et al.[17]; used with permission from Elsevier.)

alignment for subsequent repair. With further dissection, control of the visceral arteries can be obtained. Once adequate exposure is obtained proximally and distally, repair can be carried out as previously described. This stage of the dissection is illustrated in Figure 47-4.

Endovascular (EVAR) and hybrid repair of IAAA have been described, although it is unclear if EVAR leads to resolution of the periaortic and retroperitoneal inflammation, as is often seen following open repair.[18] A recent Cochrane review comparing open IAAA repair to EVAR identified no high-quality studies comparing the two methods of repair.[19] EVAR is carried out in standard fashion with no particular modifications necessary for IAAA as compared to non-inflammatory AAA. Tadros et al. describe a hybrid approach for a patient with a rapidly expanding infrarenal IAAA in the presence of crossed renal ectopia with fusion. The aorta was first debranched with renal revascularization followed, 3 days later, by EVAR deployed just distal to the superior mesenteric artery origin.[20] It is important to note that, rarely, EVAR may be complicated by post-operative retroperitoneal fibrosis that mimics IAAA with compression of the IVC or hydronephrosis. Mansour and colleagues describe the early onset of IVC compression secondary to post-EVAR retroperitoneal fibrosis. The patient was successfully treated with a course of corticosteroids.[21]

OUTCOMES

Crawford, et al. describe excellent short-term outcomes following IAAA with a 96.7% 30-day survival rate.[2] Older data would suggest a higher operative mortality rate among those patients with IAAA than non-inflammatory AAA, although this has not been borne out in more recent reports.[1] There is conflicting data regarding long-term survival differences between patients with IAAA and non-inflammatory AAA.[1,3,10] Nuellari, et al. documented 1, 3, 5 and 7 year actuarial survival rates of 94%, 85%, 72% and 65%.[3] Nitecki and colleagues established 5 year survival rates of 79% among IAAA patients compared to 83% in those patients with non-inflammatory AAA.[10] Yusuf, et al. examined outcomes in IAAA compared to non-inflammatory AAA patients with a case-matched outcomes study. Similar to Crawford and colleagues, they found no difference in early outcomes but, at 8 years post-operatively, outcomes were worse in the IAAA group than in the non-inflammatory group with 60% and 74% survival rates.[22] Post-operative inflammation persists radiographically in roughly half of patients with treated IAAA, with ongoing ureteral entrapment in a third and signs of renal atrophy in half.[10] Persistence of post-operative inflammation characterized by persistent ESR elevation, presence of renal failure and fibrosis with ureteral entrapment all increase the risk of IAAA repair mortality.[3,22] In a small case-matched study, Bonati, et al. compared long-term outcomes between patients with IAAA and non-inflammatory AAA. While overall survival rates were similar, IAAA patients were more likely to develop graft related pseudoaneurysms or true aneurysms proximal to the graft.[23] In a smaller study of IAAA treated with EVAR, 5-year survival was 67% with no aneurysm-related deaths.[18] Tambyraja and colleagues examined outcomes in patients with IAAA presenting with rupture. They found that IAAA patients were at similar risk of immediate perioperative mortality and median survival in the ruptured IAAA group was 42 months, similar to survival among non-inflammatory ruptured AAA.[6]

CONCLUSIONS

Inflammatory abdominal aortic aneurysms remain a challenging condition for the treating vascular surgeon. The gold standard for repair, in the absence of high quality data to the contrary, remains open repair. With meticulous operative technique, acceptable survival rates approaching those of patients undergoing repair of non-inflammatory abdominal aortic aneurysms can be achieved.

REFERENCES

1. Pennell RC, Hollier LH, Lie JT, et al. Inflammatory abdominal aortic aneurysms: a thirty-year review. *J Vasc Surg.* 1985;2:859–69.
2. Crawford JL, Stowe CL, Safi HJ, Hallman CH, Crawford ES. Inflammatory aneurysms of the aorta. *J Vasc Surg.* 1985;2:113–24.
3. Nuellari E, Prifti E, Giampiero E, Saimir K, Kapedani E. Surgical treatment of inflammatory abdominal aortic aneurysms: Outcome and predictors analysis. *Interv Med Appl Sci.* 2014;6:104–110.
4. Madani A, Leung S, Obrand D. Open repair of inflammatory abdominal aortic aneurysm and aortocaval fistula using retrograde balloon occlusion. *Vasc Endovasc Surg.* 2014;48:80–2.
5. Kashyap VS, Fang R, Fitzpatrick CM, Hagino RT. Caval and ureteral obstruction secondary to an inflammatory abdominal aortic aneurysm. *J Vasc Surg.* 2003;38:1416–21.
6. Tambyraja AL, Murie JA, Chalmers RT. Ruptured inflammatory abdominal aortic aneurysm: Insights in clinical management and outcome. *J Vasc Surg.* 2004;39:400–3.
7. Railo M, Isoluoma M, Keto P, Salo JA. Surgical treatment of inflammatory abdominal aortic aneurysms: a long-term follow up of 19 patients. *Ann Vasc Surg.* 2005;19:361–6.
8. von Fritschen U, Malzfeld E, Clasen A, Kortmann H. Inflammatory abdominal aortic aneurysm: A postoperative course of retroperitoneal fibrosis. *J Vasc Surg.* 1999;30:1090–8.
9. Todd GJ, DeRose JJ. Retroperitoneal approach for repair of inflammatory aortic aneurysms. *Ann Vasc Surg.* 1995;9:525–34.
10. Nitecki SS, Hallett JW, Stanson AW, et al. Inflammatory abdominal aortic aneurysms: a case-control study. *J Vasc Surg.* 1996;23:860–9.
11. Haug ES, Skomsvoll JF, Jacobsen G, et al. Inflammatory aortic aneurysm is associated with increased incidence of autoimmune disease. *J Vasc Surg.* 2003;38:492–7.
12. Ketha SS, Warrington KJ, McPhail IR. Inflammatory abdominal aortic aneurysm: A case report and review of the literature. *Vasc Endovasc Surg.* 2014;48:65–69.
13. Rasmussen TE, Hallett JW. New insights into inflammatorhy abdominal aortic aneurysms. *Eur J Vasc Endovasc Surg.* 1997;14:329–32.
14. Stone JH, Khosroshahi A, Hilgenberg A, et al. IgG4-related systemic disease and lymphoplasmacytic aortitis. *Arthritis Rheum.* 2009;60:3139–45.
15. Oderich GS, Bower TC, Cherry KJ, et al. Evolution from axillofemoral to *in situ* prosthetic reconstruction for the treatment of aortic graft infections at a single center. *J Vasc Surg.* 2006;43:1166–74.

16. Harlander-Locke MP, Harmon LK, Lawrence PF, et al. The use of cryopreserved aortoiliac allograft for aortic reconstruction in the United States. *J Vasc Surg.* 2014;669–74.
17. Shepard AD, Tollefson DFJ, Reddy DJ, et al. Left flank retroperitoneal exposure: a technical aid to complex aortic reconstruction. *J Vasc Surg.* 1991;14:283–91.
18. Coppi G, Rametta F, Aiello S, et al. Inflammatory abdominal aortic aneurysm endovascular repair into the long-term follow-up. *Ann Vasc Surg.* 2010;24:1053–59.
19. Capoccia L, Riambau V. Endovascular repair versus open repair for inflammatory abdominal aortic aneurysms. *Cochrane Database Syst Rev.* 2015.
20. Tadros R, Malik R, Ellozy S, et al. A novel approach to management of an inflammatory abdominal aortic aneurysm associated with crossed-fused renal ectopia. *Ann Vasc Surg.* 2011;25:984e9–14.
21. Mansour W, Capoccia L, Garofano R, Pranteda C, Speziale F. Early onset of periaortic inflammation after EVAR with inferior vena cava involvement: A case report. *Ann Vasc Surg.* 2015;29:127e1–127.
22. Yusuf K, Murat B, Unal A, et al. Inflammatory abdominal aortic aneurysm: predictors of long-term outcome in a case-control study. *Surgery.* 2007;141:83–9.
23. Bonati L, Rubini P, Japichino G, et al. Long-term outcome after inflammatory abdominal aortic aneurysm repair: case-matched study. *World J Surg.* 2003;27:539–44.

48

Utility of IVUS for EVAR and TEVAR

Charles C. Leithead, MD and William D. Jordan Jr, MD

Intravascular ultrasound (IVUS) has become an integral component of many endovascular procedures. The catheter-based technology of an ultrasound probe within the vessel lumen in close proximity to the arterial or venous wall allows more thorough internal visualization of vessel characteristics (lesion morphology and wall structure) as well as the anatomic relation to surrounding vasculature. IVUS provides accurate measurement of lumen diameter, which is of great importance during intraoperative assessment and planning. Vessel characteristics able to be assessed by IVUS include extent of atherosclerosis, blood flow, intraluminal thrombus, plaque, intimal defects and stent apposition. Obtaining accurate measurements of luminal diameter and visualizing origins of branch vessels is of utmost importance when evaluating the true lumen of an aortic dissection and landing zones for endovascular stent placement during aneurysm repair. As the complexity of Vascular Surgery procedures increases along with patient age and comorbidities, IVUS allows more complete imaging of vasculature, compared to catheter angiography which defines vessel lumen. The benefits of IVUS are seen without exposing patients to radiation, Gadolinium or contrast which can be detrimental to comorbid conditions. Radiation exposure to the operator is limited with the use of intravascular ultrasound due to decreasing digital subtracted angiography and fluoroscopic acquisition. IVUS allows real time intraoperative imaging of all layers of the aorta simultaneously, providing the opportunity to adjust treatment plans for the betterment of the patient.[1] These imaging qualities of IVUS are extremely useful and beneficial for endovascular abdominal aortic aneurysm repair (EVAR) and endovascular thoracic aortic aneurysm repair (TEVAR).

BASICS OF IVUS

IVUS is a catheter based tool using small piezoelectric transducers located at the tip of the catheter that provide ultrasound-based imaging of vasculature. There are two commercially available IVUS systems through Boston Scientific Corporation (Natick, Mass) and Volcano Corporation (Rancho Cordova, Calif) which transmit sound waves encompassing 360 degrees of the vessel creating high resolution axial images of the vessel lumen and wall. The image resolution is dependent on beam frequency. Penetration distance is decreased when the frequency is increased. A frequency of 8 to 12 MHz is ideal for aortic imaging due to its larger vessel diameter.[1] Iliac artery and infrainguinal imaging can be investigated with a higher frequency (20 to 30 MHz). Lower frequency catheters require larger sheaths. The Pioneer catheter (Medtronic, Minneapolis, MN) is a specialized two-lumen catheter used to gain reentry from a sub-intimal plane when crossing chronic occlusions and treating aortic dissection.

Our institution primarily employs the Volcano catheter for aortic procedures. Catheter designs without a monorail delivery wire eliminate wire artifact and provide 360-degree visualization of the arterial anatomy. Optimal visualization is obtained with the IVUS catheter positioned parallel to the vessel wall with the ultrasound directed 90 degrees to the luminal surface. In tortuous vessels, higher quality imaging is best obtained by withdrawing the IVUS catheter, opposed to advancement, due to difficulty in catheter centering.[11]

IVUS produces a two-dimensional, gray-scale image with visualization of the vessel lumen and wall structure. IVUS image interpretation and familiarity with artifacts produced by wires and catheters within the lumen is critical to IVUS use.[10] IVUS creates an image by the amplitude or intensity of the returning signal. Intima is echogenic, in contrast to the media which is echolucent, with the adventitia brighter than intima. Vessel lumen appears dark when blood flow is present, and bright lesions can represent atherosclerotic lesions with a characteristic posterior shadowing when encountering heavy calcification. Soft plaque is often darker and echolucent. Attenuation of the ultrasound signal by calcification in the arterial lumen, enhancement by graft material, and careful visualization of the high fibrous tissue content of intimal flaps and tears optimizes appropriate device selection and expedites accurate graft placement.[10] IVUS is an important adjunct to computed tomography (CT), as discrepancies have been detected between preoperative CT imaging and intraoperative IVUS measurements requiring adjustment in graft selection. Nolthenius et al.[14] compared preoperative CT scan measurements with intraoperative IVUS measurements and found CT to underestimate aortic length and overestimation of aortic diameter resulting in a 65% change in stent graft selection. Comparison with CT, angiography and IVUS has shown measurements utilizing IVUS to be the most accurate method in determining luminal dimension and fixation sites.[8,12] We agree that final intraoperative measurements with IVUS prior to graft deployment are of utmost importance and can lead to adjustment in graft selection; an invaluable feature of IVUS. In conjunction with fluoroscopy, IVUS can be used to assess accuracy of endograft deployment. In experimental models, incomplete proximal balloon-expandable stent expansion was determined by IVUS in cases which were not apparent by cinefluoroscopy.[13] Reinsertion of the IVUS catheter to inspect the deployed device can detect unsuspected vessel injury in patients with difficult access, as well as component separation during procedures when several device deliveries are required, and assist in planning subsequent intervention.[10]

Extensive preoperative planning is frequently required for endovascular aortic treatment, and IVUS has the potential to make EVAR and TEVAR safer procedures. Successful endovascular treatment of aortic disease depends on accurate assessment of aortic lesion morphology, luminal disease, vessel diameter and important anatomic characteristics of landing zones.[10] Real time measurement of aortic diameter, length of proximal and distal landing zones with visualization of branch vessels and assessment of aortic thrombus or calcification renders IVUS a critical component for aortic repair and a very useful adjunct to preoperative imaging (computed tomography [CT], computed tomography angiography [CTA], magnetic resonance angiography [MRA], ultrasound [U/S]), especially during technically challenging cases. IVUS supplements non-contrast CT scans and previous imaging in patients with a contrast allergy or kidney disease, and allows the vascular surgeon to accurately size endografts by obtaining additional intraoperative information without limitation of contrast. Confirming proximal stent placement distal to great vessels and lowest renal artery, apposition of landing zones, entry into true lumen for dissections involving the iliac system or abdominal aorta, and cannulation of the contralateral gate prior to limb deployment avoids adverse events and directs further intervention when necessary. Assessment of access vessels to ensure adequate size prior to sheath placement versus need for conduit are other useful features of this technology. These advantages of IVUS are of great utility for EVAR and TEVAR as endovascular technology continues to advance and less invasive procedures for patients of advanced age with comorbid conditions have become more prevalent. Complex aortic aneurysm pathology in patients with multisystem disease is a challenge faced by vascular surgeons, and endovascular repair has been shown to have lower morbidity and mortality rates.

Use of IVUS has shown a real benefit within our institution for treatment of abdominal and thoracic aortic disease. Thoracic aortic disease encompasses aneurysms, penetrating ulcers, dissections and intramural hematoma. IVUS has assisted our intraoperative management of several blunt thoracic aortic injuries by visualizing the entry tear and distance from left subclavian artery, while assuring endograft deployment within the true lumen. IVUS can also be used for anatomic certainty when subclavian or celiac coverage is necessary to extend landing zones. Additionally, it confirms apposition of aortic stent grafts revealing any proximal graft infolding or endoleak as well as patency of great and visceral vessels. The abilities of IVUS during aortic dissection repair can detect flap movement and possible dynamic obstruction of great or visceral vessels which guides further therapy after entry tear has been repaired. We use IVUS on a routine basis due to the many advantages that it offers during endovascular aortic repair, with a decreased incidence of renal injury and reduction in radiation exposure.

Accurate graft sizing, analysis of the aortic wall and graft post-deployment rely upon proficient use and interpretation of intravascular ultrasound. IVUS is an adjunct imaging modality for nearly all of our EVAR and TEVAR cases. We routinely use the Visions PV 8.2 Fr (Volcano, San Diego, CA) catheter at 8.3 MHz due to large vessel imaging.[2] We use it frequently to confirm vessel length and diameter prior to choosing an endograft. IVUS enables us to visualize branch vessels and reduce contrast load.

ENDOVASCULAR AORTIC ANEURYSM REPAIR

We typically approach EVAR for abdominal aortic aneurysm by bilateral common femoral artery exposure, ipsilateral femoral cut-down with contralateral percutaneous access or bilateral percutaneous access (PEVAR). Determining which access to utilize depends upon the expected endograft, its delivery sheath size and the patient's anatomic characteristics. Preoperative measurements are obtained from CT with plans to use IVUS for confirmation, which can be accessed through either groin. The IVUS is advanced over a guidewire suprarenal and imaging is obtained by a pull-back method. We perform a manual pull-back technique, opposed to an automated system, which produces images of high quality. Orientation is determined by lowest renal artery and location of the left renal vein, with appropriate adjustment of the left renal vein positioned at the top of the IVUS screen (Figure 48-1).

The lowest renal artery marks the proximal aspect of the neck fixation and the image is frozen during systole in order to perform a diameter measurement. Proximal and distal aspects of the aneurysm neck are then measured using pull-back technique followed by infrarenal aortic length. Common iliac artery diameter is then measured as well as distance to hypogastric artery (Figure 48-2). Length is often underestimated by CT scan, even with centerline measurement techniques with tortuous iliac arteries.[2] Using a floppy wire with pullback techniques allows the natural tortuosity of the aortic iliac segment to be evaluated for more realistic length measurements.

An initial subtraction angiography is performed, unless renal function does not allow, once the main body of the graft is deployed and findings are compared with IVUS. Wire access of the contralateral gate is then obtained. The IVUS is advanced up the contralateral wire to confirm entry into the gate and measurements of the contralateral iliac system are recorded. IVUS allows us to perform contralateral gate cannulation and limb deployment without further contrast use if necessary. We then perform completion aortography to evaluate for endoleak and patency of major branch vessels along with the use of the color-flow feature of the IVUS.[2] Assessment for endoleak can be performed solely with fluoroscopy, although we use IVUS for additional information on a selective basis.

IVUS is an invaluable tool to assess apposition of the graft, and its color flow feature can be used to assess for endoleak. It also demonstrates a need for balloon dilation

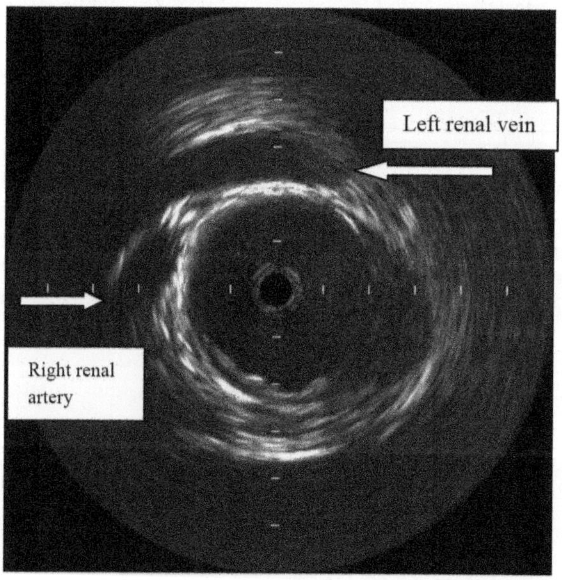

Figure 48-1. IVUS image of lowest renal artery with left renal vein positioned at the top of the IVUS screen.

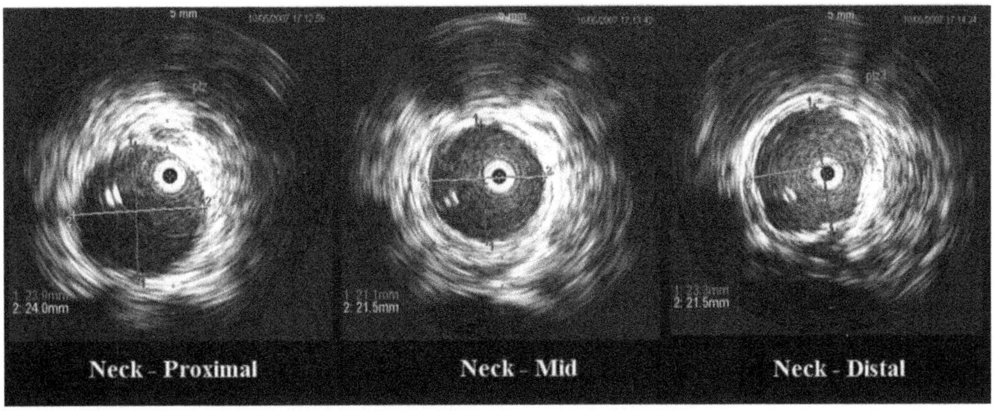

Figure 48-2. IVUS imaging of proximal and distal aspect of the aneurysm neck.

of the proximal and distal landing zones as well as areas of overlap that may have a type III endoleak present. We have been able to eliminate subtraction runs during EVAR with the use of IVUS, reducing the volume of contrast to the patient and radiation exposure to persons in the operating room. In patients with reduced glomerular filtration rates, we perform a single 10- to 15-mL subtraction angiography to confirm renal artery anatomy in order to reduce contrast exposure. Our fluoroscopy time ranges from 10 to 15 minutes. There is potential for unrecognized endoleak when solely using IVUS after graft deployment, although dialysis-dependent renal failure or anaphylaxis to contrast exposure may outweigh the risk.[2] Our regular use and interpretation of IVUS imaging during endovascular aortic repair aids in determining if further imaging with angiography is warranted in patients with renal disease.

ENDOVASCULAR REPAIR OF THORACIC AORTIC ANEURYSMS

We determine whether femoral access or iliac conduit is warranted to approach TEVAR by preoperative CT scan and real-time imaging with IVUS. IVUS is also used to determine the size of iliac vessels and evaluate for pathology that could preclude safe sheath placement. We often obtain contralateral percutaneous femoral access to utilize a diagnostic catheter instead of "piggy-backing" the catheter through the delivery sheath or obtaining left subclavian versus brachial access.[2] We place a flexible guide wire into the ascending aorta and advance the IVUS proximal to the innominate artery. Great vessel origins are visualized with the pull-back technique. The length and diameter of the proximal landing zone is measured at this time. The distal landing zone is then determined and measured with confirmation of the celiac and superior mesenteric artery origins. The infrarenal aorta and iliac vessel diameters are then assessed with IVUS. Once our thoracic stent graft is deployed, IVUS can be used to ensure appropriate graft placement, apposition of the graft to the aortic wall and patency of great/visceral vessels. A completion digital subtraction angiogram is performed in appropriate patients. Experience with IVUS has allowed us to eliminate many angiographic steps, limiting contrast and radiation exposure.[2]

The routine intraoperative use of IVUS for endovascular aneurysm repair without the use of angiography was investigated by Segesser et al. These patients underwent

CT-scan and angiography at the beginning of their work-up. It was found that patients whose aortic or thoracic aortic aneurysm was repaired with IVUS use intraoperatively, as opposed to angiography, had lower hospital mortality rates, less fluoroscopy exposure (8 min vs. 24 min), and fewer early endoleaks.[7] Lower contrast volumes reduce renal insult which may have an impact on other morbidity parameters. We do not perform zero contrast endovascular aneurysm repairs with only intraoperative IVUS at our institution, although this analysis confirms that successful aneurysm exclusion can occur without exposing patients to further contrast and potential renal impairment.

CASE 1

An 81-year-old white male status post two prior aortic repairs including a thoracoabdominal repair in 2003 who had degeneration of the proximal aortic segment to 5.9 × 7.2 cm on CT angiogram. He denied chest or back pain.

A right femoral incision was made and the common femoral artery was identified and encircled. The left femoral artery was then accessed under ultrasound guidance. On the right side a 9 French sheath was placed. A J-wire was passed under fluoroscopic control and intravascular ultrasound was obtained. The proximal landing zone was just beyond the left subclavian artery origin. The intravascular ultrasound showed the proximal landing zone to be 35 × 32. Five centimeters distally it was 35 × 33. Additional landing zone was 29 mm proximally, but 33.6 × 34.2 mm distally. Then a pigtail catheter was placed and aortogram obtained that confirmed the length of the aorta and planned landing zones. We elected to do a two piece case. Initially a Medtronic Valiant 40 × 40 × 200 graft was deployed distally without difficulty. Then we selected a proximal area with a Captivia Securement System at the proximal aspect. A 40 × 40 × 200 stent graft was deployed just beyond the left subclavian artery origin, with careful manipulation to not involve the aortic arch. Our grafts were deployed with approximately 7 cm of overlap. An intravascular ultrasound was performed to assess graft apposition which showed that the graft was not fully expanded in the midsection (Figure 48-3). We angioplastied the overlap segments and the distal landing zone. Completion angiography was without endoleak, and there was good filling through the visceral vessels. The wires, catheter, and sheath were removed from the groin, and the arteriotomy on the right side was closed primarily. On the left side, a 6 French ProGlide was used. Good Doppler signals of the feet were noted.

USE OF IVUS IN AORTIC DISSECTION AND BLUNT TRAUMATIC AORTIC INJURY

We find IVUS to be extremely useful during endovascular therapy of type B aortic dissection, penetrating aortic ulcer, blunt aortic injury including traumatic aortic transection. At our institution IVUS is used to identify and characterize these unique aortic processes as well as accurately size endografts prior to implantation. We have successfully used IVUS to confirm entry into true lumen and graft cannulation for type B dissection and traumatic aortic transection. Thoracic stent grafting has become

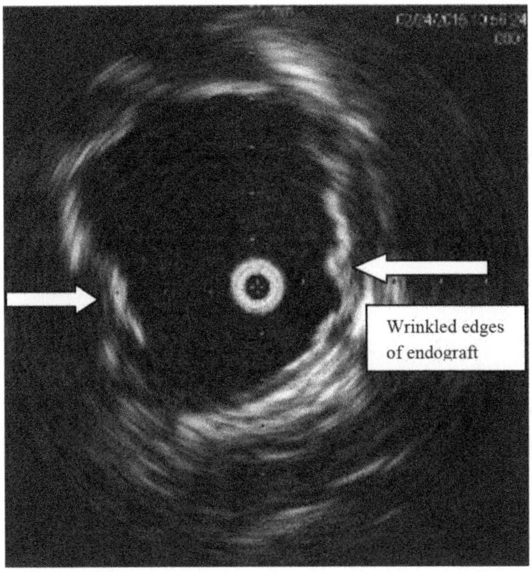

Figure 48-3. IVUS demonstrating inadequate thoracic aortic endograft apposition post-deployment.

the treatment of choice for most complicated type B dissections within our institution. There has been a transition to endovascular repair due to the improved early mortality rate compared to traditional open surgical replacement of the descending thoracic aorta. The major advantages we have noted with stent-graft placement are stabilization of the intimal flap, preservation of the true lumen, positive remodeling of the aorta with thrombosis of the false lumen and prevention of dissection-related complications in the future. We have published early results in 2008 of our first fifteen patients treated with endovascular stent-graft repair for acute, complicated type B dissection. All patients had an entry flap at or distal to the left subclavian artery confirmed by computed tomography angiogram (CTA) and/or IVUS. IVUS was used to confirm entry into the true lumen, localize the entry flap, and for sizing measurements in all patients. Particularly for dissection pathology, IVUS provides precise visualization of the outer aortic wall. We use these measurements as a reference point for sizing which tends to be 10% or less for acute dissection. Our overall mortality was significantly lower than historic controls of open repair which has also been demonstrated by other institutions.[3–5,9] IVUS allows visualization of the proximal entry site as well as determining the size of the normal proximal and distal aorta.

Exclusion of the proximal entry tear promotes thrombosis of the false lumen and restores flow within the true lumen, improving distal perfusion. IVUS is used to confirm graft deployment and apposition within the true lumen. We had 93% success in excluding the proximal entry tear with a perioperative 30-day mortality rate of 13% in our early study which is similar to other published reports.[9] The use of IVUS in stent-graft sizing prevents over or undersizing which can result in worsening malperfusion if an intimal flap is fractured. Such overexpansion can result in distal aortic occlusion, and graft collapse with underexpansion leading to obstruction of the true lumen.[2] We utilize IVUS to assist in characterizing the intimal flap after stent-graft placement and balloon dilation of the distal graft. IVUS is also used to precisely measure iliac vessel size when kissing iliac stent placement is warranted to restore lower extremity perfusion due to acute aortic dissection.

Considering that our institution is a regional referral center and the only hospital currently designated as a Level 1 Adult Trauma Center by the American College of Surgeons in the state, we frequently treat traumatic aortic injury. This involves penetrating and blunt traumatic aortic injury including intimal tears, intramural hematomas, pseudoaneurysms, and traumatic aortic transections. When treating these pathologic aortic conditions, IVUS is a helpful imaging modality to visualize and guide treatment for these defects in the aortic layers. IVUS allows us to measure the length of aortic injury limiting the extent of aortic coverage to exclude the defect in order to prevent spinal cord ischemia and coverage of branch vessels.

TEVAR has also become a common treatment option for traumatic aortic transection. IVUS precisely identifies great vessel origins and accurately measures aortic diameter during systole leading to optimal graft deployment. Due to these patients often having multiple other injuries, prompt use of IVUS with visualization of the aortic injury and confirming graft placement can lead to improved outcomes with less renal injury from contrast use. IVUS does not have the ability to visualize the complete external vessel wall pathology and is limited by larger field of views, which can have an impact on an intervention involving a larger thoracic aorta.

CTA has been the primary early diagnostic modality for these injuries, although equivocal scans require additional imaging. Prior to the advent of IVUS, angiography had been the most common modality to confirm the aortic injury with equivocal CTA. The utility of IVUS compared to angiography in the diagnosis of blunt traumatic aortic injury was analyzed by Azizzadeh et al. and showed that in cases with equivocal CTA imaging, IVUS changed the diagnosis in 13% of cases compared to angiography, identifying injuries in 11% of cases and ruling out injuries in 2%.[6] Angiography demonstrated equivocal results twice as often as IVUS. Based on these findings, IVUS is a better adjunct than angiography in defining traumatic aortic injury in patients who have equivocal CTA or angiography.[6] We have detected new findings with IVUS use during operations and agree that IVUS enables clarification of subtle aortic abnormalities diagnosed on preoperative CT-scans.

CASE 2

A 65-year-old while male with a past medical history of rectal cancer s/p low anterior resection, chemotherapy and radiation therapy, hypertension, coronary artery disease, history of myocardial infaraction status post coronary angioplasty and prior tobacco use presented as a transfer from an outside hospital with a Type B aortic dissection and recurrent chest pain despite medical management. He was taking daily antiplatelet therapy, and his lower extremity perfusion was noted to be intact upon presentation. A CTA of the chest, abdomen, and pelvis was obtained that demonstrated an aortic dissection originating between the left carotid artery and the left subclavian artery, extending to the left renal artery. Malperfusion to the right kidney was also evident, and the patient had renal insufficiency.

The patient was taken to the operating room for intravascular ultrasound of the aorta, left subclavian artery and left axillary artery as well as a limited aortogram. The intravascular ultrasound showed that the dissection originated in the ascending aorta proximal to the innominate artery (Figure 48-4), extending into the left subclavian artery, with a very dynamic flap in the thoracic aorta. In the perivisceral aorta, there was thrombus evident, flow in the left renal artery although limited flow into the right renal artery.

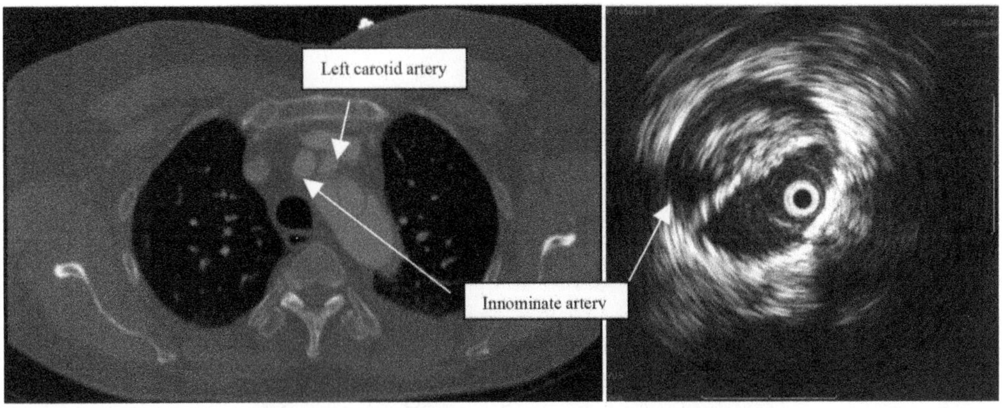

Figure 48-4. Discrepency between CT and IVUS. CT showing aortic dissection originating between the left carotid artery and left subclavian artery with IVUS demonstrating aortic dissection originating in the ascending aorta proximal to the innominate artery.

Right renal angioplasty and stent placement was performed with improved perfusion of the right kidney. These findings were reviewed with Cardiac Surgery and it was determined that his ascending aorta would require repair first. The patient ultimately underwent coronary artery bypass grafting, replacement of ascending aorta and transverse aortic arch with aortic valve resuspension. With the use of IVUS, we were able to visualize a more proximal entry tear in the aortic arch not detected on CTA, which changed the patient's treatment plan, and used 45 mL of contrast, preventing further renal injury.

CASE 3

A 48-year-old black male diagnosed with an uncomplicated acute type B dissection 6 weeks prior treated medically presented to the Emergency Department with recurrent chest pain. CT chest showed the development of a false aneurysm proximal to his initial fenestration site in the mid-descending thoracic aorta. We considered this a failure of medical therapy, and he was taken to the operating room for exclusion of the involved area to relieve his pain and prevent aneurysm rupture.

The procedure was initiated by creating a standard left groin incision through which the common femoral artery was skeletonized. A 5-French diagnostic sheath followed by a 0.35 J-wire was inserted retrograde. A marking pigtail catheter was positioned in the ascending thoracic aortic arch, and an angiogram was obtained. This revealed no abnormality of the proximal ascending and transverse thoracic arch, normal anatomy with no stenosis or abnormalities in the supra aortic trunks. While the origin of the dissection originally was at the level of the left subclavian artery, this had thrombosed, and there was a fenestration approximately 10 cm distal to the left subclavian artery origin. Intravascular ultrasound was then performed. The immediate diameter just at the level of the left subclavian artery was 32 mm; 2 cm distally it was 26 mm. We were able to evaluate the fenestrations, as well as the true lumen, and we were certain that we were in the true lumen based upon our IVUS images (Figure 48-5).

We elected to exclude approximately 20 to 23 cm of the descending thoracic aorta since the lower aorta diameter was smaller. A 31×31×10 device was positioned 22 cm distal to the left subclavian artery origin and deployed without difficulty. Next, a 37×37×15 device was

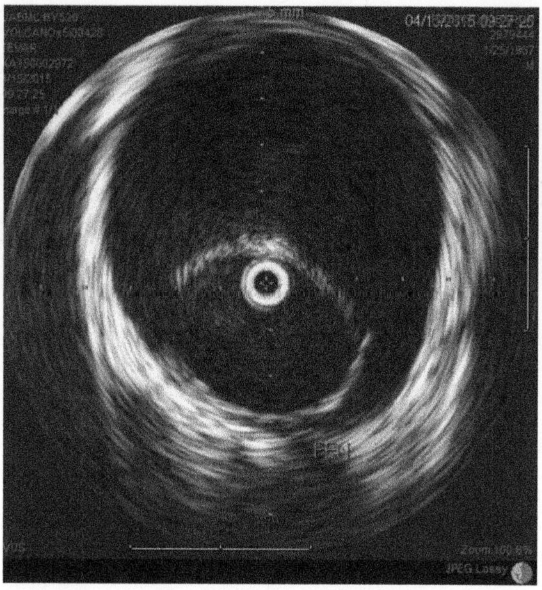

Figure 48-5. IVUS confirming catheter within true lumen of aortic dissection.

situated with the leading edge of the graft just at the orifice of the left subclavian artery. It was positioned and deployed without difficulty. Completion angiogram revealed satisfactory exclusion of the proximal fenestration, satisfactory patency of all the visceral vessels with the terminal portion of the aorta normal in caliber. The sheath was removed, and the cannulation site was closed primarily. Appropriate perfusion of the feet was confirmed.

CASE 4

A 54-year-old black female presented to UAB trauma status post motor vehicle crash versus tree with grade 4 blunt aortic injury, grade 5 liver laceration, grade 5 splenic laceration and hemodynamic instability. She was taken to the operating room emergently for endovascular thoracic aortic repair secondary to ongoing hemorrhage and grade 4 thoracic aortic injury. A right common femoral exposure was performed. Percutaneous access of the left common femoral was then performed. The procedure was performed without heparin secondary to concern of ongoing bleeding. Intravascular ultrasound of the ascending aorta, aortic arch, descending thoracic aorta, abdominal aorta, and the right iliac system was performed. The intravascular ultrasound images showed that the right common iliac artery was appropriate size for acceptance of a 20-French sheath (Figure 48-6).

The IVUS images were used to assist in selecting our thoracic stent graft device. A thoracic aortogram was then performed. A 26 × 26 × 10 Gore CTAG device was deployed up to the innominate artery which had a common origin of the left common carotid artery. This deployed without difficulty. We then extended with a 26 × 21 × 10 Gore CTAG device. We performed a completion angiogram and had complete exclusion of the area of injury with immediate improvement in the patient's hemodynamics. The left subclavian artery was intentionally covered and did reconstitute through the left vertebral artery. We then removed our sheath from the right common femoral artery and closed the arteriotomy primarily.

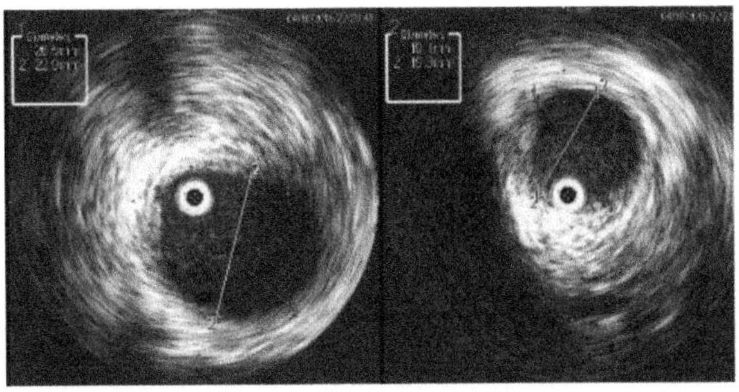

Figure 48-6. Intravascular ultrasound of bilateral common iliac arteries ensuring appropriate size prior to sheath placement.

CONCLUSION

IVUS is an invaluable tool to the endovascular surgeon and offers unique imaging advantages during endovascular treatment of aortic pathology. We routinely use IVUS during endovascular repair of thoracic and abdominal aortic aneurysms, type B dissections, penetrating aortic ulcers and traumatic aortic injury. IVUS is safe, accessible and a useful adjunct to other imaging modalities for the diagnosis of aortic disease. IVUS assists during therapeutic interventions and provides additional data with real time, accurate measurements as well as precise evaluation of lesion morphology. The many benefits of IVUS are seen intraoperatively as well as post-procedure with the reduction of radiation exposure and limitation of contrast use in patients with renal disease or contrast allergy.

We have appreciated a substantial benefit in the endovascular treatment of aortic disease with IVUS, especially in patients with renal impairment. The use of IVUS is dependent upon proficiency in device utilization and its advantages may result in an expanding role in the treatment of EVAR and TEVAR. As we have become more facile with the use of IVUS in endovascular aortic repairs and as more endovascular surgeons become familiar with interpretation of IVUS imaging, more procedures will be performed with IVUS and limited contrast.

REFERENCES

1. Reid DB, Arko FR: Intravascular ultrasound. In: Cronenwett JL, Johnston KW, eds. *Rutherford's Vascular Surgery*, 8th ed. Philadelphia: Saunders/Elsevier, 2014;377–85.
2. Pearce BJ, Jordan WD Jr. Using IVUS during EVAR and TEVAR: improving patient outcomes. *Semin Vasc Surg*. 2009;22(3):172–80.
3. Eggebrecht H, Nienaber CA, Neuhauser M, Baumgart D, Kische S, Schmermund A, et al. Endovascular stent-graft placement in aortic dissection: a meta-analysis. *Eur Heart J*. 2006;27(4):489–98.
4. Nathanson DR, Rodriquez-Lopez JA, Ramaiah VG, et al. Endoluminal stent-graft stabilization for thoracic aortic dissection. *J Endovasc Ther*. 2005;12(3):354–9.
5. Feezor RJ, Martin TD, Hess PJ Jr, et al. Early outcomes after endovascular management of acute, complicated type B aortic dissection. *J Vasc Surg*. 2009;49(3):561–6.

6. Azizzadeh A, Valdes J, Miller CC III, Nguyen LL, et al. The utility of intravascular ultrasound compared to angiography in the diagnosis of blunt traumatic aortic injury. *J Vasc Surg*. 2011;53(3):608–14.
7. von Segesser LK, Marty B, Ruchat P, Bogen M, Gallino A. Routine use of intravascular ultrasound for endovascular aneurysm repair: angiography is not necessary. *Eur J Vasc Endovasc Surg*. 2002;23(6):537–42.
8. White RA, Donayre CE, Walot I, et al. Preliminary clinical outcome and imaging criterion for endovascular prosthesis deployment in high risk patients with aortoiliac and traumatic arterial lesions. *J Vasc Surg*. 1996;24(4):556–9.
9. Pearce BJ, Passman MA, Patterson MA, et al. Early outcomes of thoracic endovascular stent-graft repair for acute complicated type B dissection using the Gore TAG endoprosthesis. *Ann Vasc Surg*. 2008;22(6):742–9.
10. Song TK, Donayre CE, Kopchok GE, White RA. Intravascular ultrasound use in the treatment of thoracoabdominal dissections, aneurysms, and transections. *Semin Vasc Surg*. 2006; 19(3):145–9.
11. Lee JT, White RA. Basics of intravascular ultrasound: an essential tool for the endovascular surgeon. *Semin Vasc Surg*. 2004;17(2):110–8.
12. White RA, Scoccianti M, Back M, et al. Innovations in vascular imaging: Arteriography, three-dimensional CT scans, and two- and three-dimensional intravascular ultrasound evaluation of an abdominal aortic aneurysm. *Ann Vasc Surg*. 1994;8(3):285–9.
13. White RA, Verbin C, Kopchok G, et al. The role of cinefluoroscopy and intravascular ultrasound in evaluating the deployment of experimental endovascular prostheses. *J Vasc Surg*. 1995;21(3):365–74.
14. Tutein Nolthenius RP, van den Berg JC, Moll FL. The value of intraoperative intravascular ultrasound for determining stent graft size (excluding abdominal aortic aneurysm) with a modular system. *Ann Vasc Surg*. 2000;14(4):311–7.

49

Streamlining EVAR for Ruptured Aneurysms

Claire Matsumura and Jon Matsumura, MD

Since the pioneering work published by Juan Parodi in 1991, innovation has marked the development of abdominal aortic aneurysm (AAA) repair using a remotely-delivered intraluminal stent combined with a prosthetic graft.[1] Endovascular aortic aneurysm repair (EVR) has become a standard of care for elective repair of patients with large abdominal aortic aneurysms, based on collective results from four randomized trials. In the three larger trials, EVR has significantly reduced perioperative morbidity and mortality and improved recovery. EVR was associated with a greater number of secondary aortic reinterventions, but there is similar late survival.[2–4] Recent analysis has shown EVR is cost-effective and delivers greater quality-adjusted life years in the United States.[5] Several FDA-approved endografts are on the market for the treatment of infrarenal abdominal aortic aneurysms, although none are approved for use in ruptured aneurysms.

AAA rupture is responsible for approximately 15,000 deaths each year, which is the thirteenth leading cause of death in the United States.[6] Use of EVR for treatment of ruptured aneurysms has been studied in three European randomized trials—the Dutch AJAX trial, the French ECAR trial and the UK IMPROVE trial.[7–9] There was no difference in 30-day mortality between open repair and EVR; however, EVR was associated with faster discharge, improved quality of life, and was more cost-effective. Outcomes of EVR for ruptured AAA have been favorable in institutions where a systematic algorithm ensures that the appropriate endovascular team is alerted when a ruptured aneurysm presents in the emergency room or from external transport. Meta-analyses and administrative datasets have produced discordant conclusions, which may be related to whether there is advanced programs for EVR care for ruptured aneurysms.[10–17] Surgeons active in the care of ruptured aneurysms are intimately familiar with the potential system factors which challenge the expeditious care of these dire patients. This chapter describes programmatic efforts to improve aortic emergency care at the University of Wisconsin (UW) Hospitals and Clinics. Components of an aortic emergency program may be divided into Facilities, Personnel, and Integration.

FACILITIES

A hybrid operating room (OR) affords the most flexibility and safety for aortic emergencies. Imaging is critical. High fidelity flat detector imaging facilitates precision and speed with endovascular procedures. Fusion with preprocedure imaging may minimize contrast nephrotoxicity. Fluoro CT capability allows immediate assessment of an endovascular exclusion and objective quantification of retroperitoneal hematoma. Surface ultrasound is routinely used for arterial puncture, and intravascular ultrasound conserves contrast dosing for patients with severe chronic kidney disease. The ability to convert from an endovascular to an open approach when indicated is an important consideration. The aseptic operating room permits EVR to be performed beginning with local or general anesthesia, with immediate access to an iliofemoral cutdown, open vascular repair, and decompressive laparotomy if abdominal compartment syndrome develops. This location has the full spectrum of OR support, including LED lighting, suction, electrocautery, cell saver, retractors, and specialty instrumentation (see Figure 49-1).

The hybrid OR is also stocked with a complete endovascular toolbox and wide range of device implants. The on-site inventory must be large enough to accommodate the broad range of patients who present with appropriate anatomy for EVR. This is not synonymous with having every component of each available system, but only requires a prudent selection of larger diameter components, mixed with low profile options, and extenders. Many of these components can be used between systems if there is familiarity with compatibility. Some specialty equipment is particularly useful for emergency cases, such as expandable sheaths for challenging access, occlusion balloons for unstable patients, and a range of embolization supplies to accommodate whatever may be encountered. Of course, the usual array of supplies for elective EVR may already include these items, depending on the degree of advanced intervention that is routinely performed.

PERSONNEL

Of paramount importance to the success of every aortic program is a dedicated Anesthesiology team. In many cases, a highly specialized anesthetist—familiar with vascular patients and pathology—contributes more to the positive outcome than

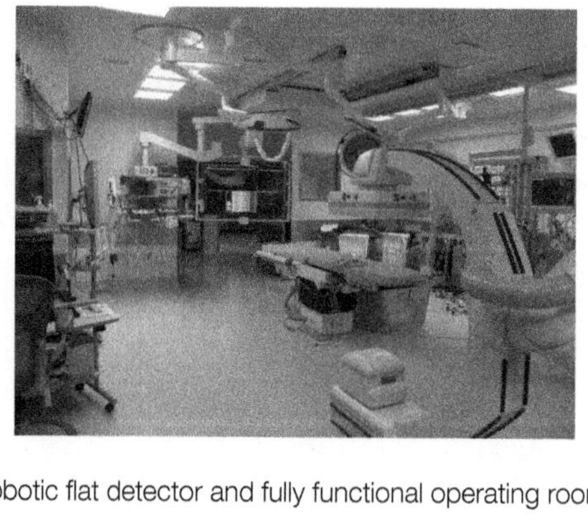

Figure 49-1. Hybrid OR with robotic flat detector and fully functional operating room capabilities.

the experienced vascular surgeon. Attending to permissive hypotension, rapidly obtaining vascular access and securing the airway, adjusting to balloon occlusion and declamping, and assessing and treating the multi-organ dysfunction sequalae of aortic catastrophes requires commitment and skill, practiced in programs with a high volume of aortic intervention. Institutions privileged to have this quality of staff will find that the smaller "details" have been enveloped in the local culture, such as month long rotations of the same senior resident, dedicated anesthesiology attending aortic emergency call, and seamless transitions to intensive care. This culture nourishes candid inter-specialty communication, a longitudinal interest of all providers in the patient outcome throughout the postoperative period, and further investment in programmatic development of a true aortic center.

Equally important is identifying and training a dedicated endovascular team of nurses, operating room "scrub" technicians, and radiology technologists. For some institutions, this will require a major shift in operating room boundaries, budgets, and reporting lines. Having personnel whom routinely work together facilitates the efficiency and professionalism necessary for the middle-of-the-night emergency. One can sense when an integrated team is working with non-verbal communication, anticipating downstream patient needs, and bringing "A" game attentiveness and confidence to the dire situation.

The vascular team extends beyond the walls of the hybrid operating room. Referring physicians are greeted by an Access Center, staffed by trained registered nurses, who can rapidly take essential information, confirm transfer of imaging studies (see later), and coordinate helicopter transport. UW helicopters include a flight surgeon, usually a veteran emergency room physician, who can take over medical control at the referring institution, and assess and treat patients during transport. The vascular surgeon has two way communication with the flight surgeon which provides invaluable updates and smooths transfer from the helipad directly to the OR, usually bypassing the emergency room.

A fully staffed blood bank must muster the Massive Transfusion Protocol (MTP), 24 hours a day. Activation of the UW MTP results in automatic call in of an additional technician, and alerts the attending pathologist. MTP produces coolers of blood components every twenty minutes, with an appropriate ratio of PRBC, FFP and platelets. In order for the OR team to maintain all focus on the patient, the MTP flows without hindrance or additional communication until the attending surgeon or anesthesiologist calls to discontinue the MTP.

For postoperative care, the critical care team, including nurses, surgeons and anesthesiologists familiar with thoracoabdominal aortic intervention, attends to the most critically ill. However, patients treated with EVR may often be transferred early to intermediate care on a dedicated vascular surgery floor staffed by an experienced cadre of disciplines, and supervised by vascular surgery advanced practice practitioners seven days a week.

INTEGRATION

Facilities and personnel, as described above, are essential, but the "streamlining" gains are exponentially larger, when the care is integrated into a routine workflow. This begins with vision, diligent planning, operational execution, and cyclical

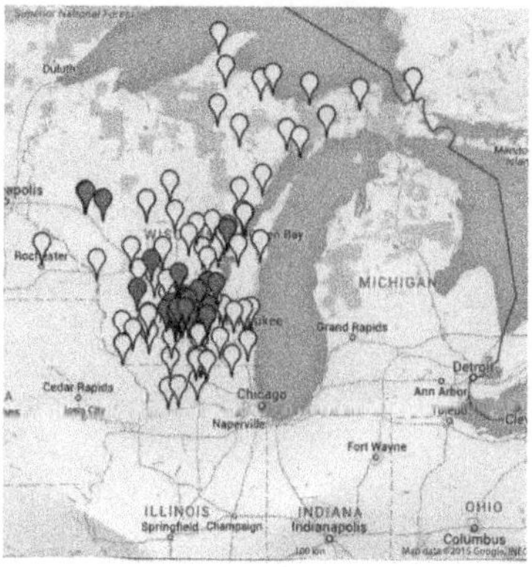

Figure 49-2. Map of virtual private network (VPN) medical imaging links.

program improvement. Establishment of virtual private network (VPN) connections with over 150 regional hospitals, allows near immediate transmission of medical imaging, with appropriate regulatory compliance. This is superior to commercial "cloud" services which require an exchange of ftp codes. See Figure 49-2. We have expectations of attending vascular surgeon response to the Access Center within minutes, and the surgeon may review the medical imaging remotely. This review includes using our own PACS system, familiar measurement tools, and post-processing thin client support. This remote review permits the surgeon to confirm the diagnosis, determine if EVR or open repair (or both) are indicated, and call in the appropriate team to fit the planned procedure. For example, the surgeon can perform device sizing, do procedure planning for percutaneous access, and may call in the radiology technologist early for an EVR case under local anesthesia. Other specialists in cardiac surgery, emergency general surgery, urology, perfusionists, or others can be given advanced notice. Often, remote imaging review facilitates a multispecialty consultation with cardiac surgery about a complex arch dissection. The Access Center also opens an electronic medical record and documents initial communication and updates from the referring facility and flight surgeon. The institution has prioritized certain quarternary care capabilities, and unless OR capacity for specific vascular emergencies is currently overcommitted, we do not decline emergency aortic cases due to bed availability. Stable patients have been staged into the ICU for line placement, when both the angio OR and backup rooms are occupied but anticipated to open shortly.

The benefits of remote imaging review and the electronic record are substantial. The surgeon has an additional quarter hour to two hours to study the images, contemplate different options, such as a Brazilian internal iliac artery snorkel or renal chimney graft, and notify the OR team to the plan for brachial access. Any member of the team may review the imaging and records from any location, facilitating education and coordination. This is particularly useful for broadcasting the estimated time of arrival of the patient, and continuing preparations while the surgeon and others are commuting to the hospital. Occasionally, further imaging is needed, particularly for complex thoracoabdominal and acute dissection patients, and a decision is made to divert the patient to the ER from the helipad. Prior to one local hospital enlisting the VPN, a patient had been transferred with the classic CD-ROM of the medical imaging. The CD could not be opened because the patient label had been applied in hurried fashion, off center, and it jammed the reader. What ensued was an unpredictable delay and an anxious decision choice on repeat imaging, empiric open repair, or waiting for IT support. Fortunately, it was brief and, later, the VPN was installed at this facility for future transmission. Although not common, but of striking value, the remote imaging review and discussion may lead to a decision to cancel the transfer, and initiate hospice consultation and comfort care of a moribund, unsalvageable patient. This avoids the patient, team, and family rushing through bad weather in futility.

Periodic review and modification are an important process for "streamlining." Risk-adjusted outcomes are discussed in a regular multidisciplinary meeting entitled the Vascular Collaborative. Morbidity and mortality peer review, aortic bundle programs, supply chain management, and other administrative meetings provide additional opportunities to refine the care pathways with a goal for continual improvement.

CASE EXAMPLE: PUTTING IT ALL TOGETHER

Table 49-1 outlines a typical workflow and timing for a patient with ruptured aneurysm who was transferred to UW. This patient is a middle-aged man with acute back pain, who was hemodynamically stable, and flown to UW. The time from initial Access Center call to arrival in OR was 93 minutes. The flight surgeon managed the patient with permissive hypotension. Figure 49-3 shows the OR team, having arrived in advance of the patient and pre-briefed on the specific therapeutic plan, calmly greeting the patient and flight surgeon in the hybrid room. The patient underwent EVR under local anesthetic and was discharged on the first

TABLE 49-1. WORKFLOW AND TIMELINE FOR A PATIENT WITH A RUPTURED ANEURYSM TRANSFERRED TO THE UNIVERSITY OF WISCONSIN[a]

Time	Event
3:29 AM	First contact with Access Center
3:40 AM	Attending surgeon discusses case with referring physician, accepts patient based on ER MD assessment, and helicopter dispatched.
3.42 AM	OR notified of a transfer in progress of probable aortic emergency. Preliminary setup of OR begins with call in of vascular specialty nurse and scrub tech.
4:09 AM	CT scan reviewed by vascular surgeon and decision for EVR made
4:10 AM	Access Center calls surgeon to alert that films are in VPN—surgeon has already reviewed films as they became available, and notifies Access Center to coordinate direct admit to OR, and update flight surgeon who is arriving at outside facility, and assuming care of patient.
4:12 AM	Attending anesthesiologist and vascular surgeon coordinate EVR plan and then begin commute to hospital.
4:14 AM	OR staff notified of confirmed AAA rupture and definitive plan for EVR under local anesthetic. OR calls in radiology technologist, and sets up of specific endovascular trays and supplies.
4:15 AM	Access Center updates entire team on estimated time of arrival and initial stable vital signs relayed from flight surgeon
4:25 AM	Chief vascular resident arrives in OR and confirms EVR plan and specific devices.
4:31 AM	Updates on unstable vital signs and permissive hypotension discussed between vascular and flight surgeon
4:39 AM	Vascular surgeon and attending anesthesiologist arrive in OR.
4:41 AM	Flight surgeon updates on improved vital signs and estimated time of arrival
5:02 AM	Patient enters OR

[a]Image review is conducted early in transfer workflow, allowing specific staff and setup to proceed expeditiously. Note frequent communication with UW flight surgeon who assumes care upon arrival at outside facility and decision to implement permissive hypotension.

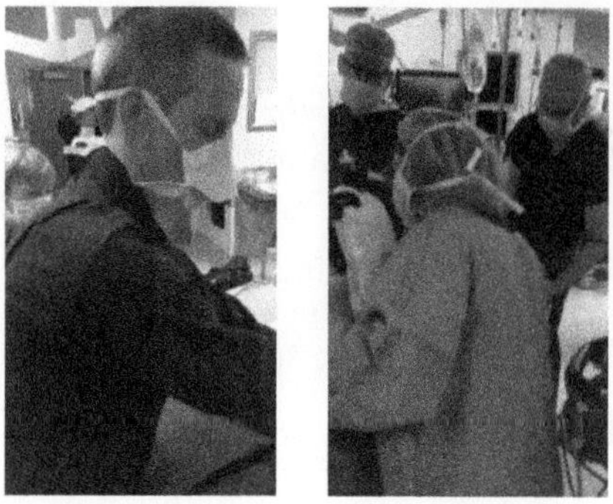

Figure 49-3. Patient with ruptured aneurysm entering prepared hybrid OR with a prepared team waiting to assume care from UW flight surgeon.

postoperative day. He was able to attend and dance with the bride at his daughter's wedding a month later.

The "Wisconsin Idea" is a philosophy embraced by the University of Wisconsin that holds that university research should be applied to solve problems and improve health. As explained by Adlai Stevenson, "It also meant a faith in the application of intelligence and reason to the problems of society. It meant a deep conviction that the role of government was not to stumble along like a drunkard in the dark, but to light its way by the best torches of knowledge and understanding it could find."[18] This aortic emergency program is an excellent example of the practice of the Wisconsin Idea.

SUMMARY

In summary, contemporary vascular surgery clinical practice requires more than a well-trained surgeon. Facility investment, specialized personnel, and integration of these resources will provide streamlined care and optimize the outcomes of patients who suffer an aortic catastrophe.

REFERENCES

1. Parodi JC, Palmaz JC, Barone HD. Transfemoral intraluminal graft implantation for abdominal aortic aneurysms. *Ann Vasc Surg.* 1991;5(6):491–9.
2. United Kingdom EVAR Trial Investigators, Greenhalgh RM, Brown LC, et al. Endovascular versus open repair of abdominal aortic aneurysm. *N Engl J Med.* 2010;362:1863–71.
3. De Bruin JL, Baas AF, Buth J, et al. Long-term outcome of open or endovascular repair of abdominal aortic aneurysm. *N Engl J Med.* 2010;362:1881–9.
4. Lederle F, Freischlag J, Kyriakides TC, et al. Long-term comparison of endovascular and open repair of abdominal aortic aneurysm. *N Engl J Med.* 2012;367(21):1988–97.
5. Stroupe KT, Lederle FA, Matsumura JS, et al. Cost-effectiveness of open versus endovascular repair of abdominal aortic aneurysm: Results of a multicenter randomized trial. *J Vasc Surg.* 2012;56(4):901–909.
6. Ernst CB. Abdominal aortic aneurysm. *N Engl J Med.* 1993;328:1167–72.
7. Reimerink J, Hoornweg L, Vahl A, et al. Endovascular repair versus open repair of ruptured abdominal aortic aneurysms: A multicenter randomized controlled trial. *Ann Surg.* 2013;258(2):248–56.
8. Desgranges P, Kobeiter H, Katsahian S, et al. ECAR (Endovascular ou Chirugie dans les Anevrysmes aorto-iliaques Rompus): A French randomized controlled trial of endovascular versus open surgical repair of ruptured aorto-iliac aneurysms. *Eur J Vasc Endovasc Surg.* http://dx.doi.org/10.1016/j.ejev.2015.03.028

9. Grieve R, Gomes M, Sweeting M, et al. Endovascular strategy or open repair for ruptured abdominal aortic aneurysm: one year outcomes from the IMPROVE randomized trial. *Eur Heart J*. 8 April 2015 ehv 125. DOI:http/dx.doi.org/10.1093/eurheartj/ehv125
10. Mehta M, Taggert J, Darling RC, 3rd, et al. Establishing a protocol for endovascular treatment of ruptured abdominal aortic aneurysms: outcomes of a prospective analysis. *J Vasc Surg*. 2006;44(1):1–8; discussion
11. Mehta M. Technical tips for EVAR for ruptured AAA. *Semin Vasc Surg*. 2009;22(3):181-6.
12. Oyague KS, Mubarak OA, Nowak LR, et al. Endovascular repair of ruptured and symptomatic abdominal aortic aneurysms using a structured protocol in a community teaching hospital. *Ann Vasc Surg*. 2015;29:76–83.
13. Antoniou GA, Ahmed N, Georgiadis GS, Torella F. Is endovascular repair of ruptured abdominal aortic aneurysms associated with improved in-hospital mortality compared with surgical repair? *ICVTS*. 2015;20:135–9.
14. Thomas D, Hulten E, Ellis S, et al. Open versus endovascular repair of abdominal aortic aneurysm in the elective and emergent setting in a pooled population of 37,781 patients: A systematic review and meta-analysis. *Cardiol* 2014 April 2; 2014:149243. doi: 10.1155/2014/149243.
15. Luebke T, Brunkwall J. Risk-adjusted meta-analysis of 30-Day mortality of endovascular versus open repair for ruptured abdominal aortic aneurysms. *Ann Vasc Surg*. 2015;29(4):845–63.
16. Gupta PK, Ramanan B, Engelbert TL, et al. A comparison of open surgery versus endovascular repair of unstable ruptured abdominal aortic aneurysms. *J Vasc Surg*. 2014; 60(6): 1439–45.
17. Pini R, Faggioli G, Longhi M, et al. The influence of study design on the evaluation of ruptured abdominal aortic aneurysm treatment. *Ann Vasc Surg*. 2014;28:1568–80.
18. Stark, Jack 1995. The Wisconsin Idea: the University's service to the state. Wisconsin Blue book 1995-1996, Madison: Wisconsin Legislative Reference Bureau. pp 1–80.

50

Benefits and Pitfalls of Upper Extremity Access for Fenestrated EVAR

Joseph Karam, MD and Luis A. Sanchez, MD

Fenestrated EndoVascular Aneurysm Repair (FEVAR) is increasingly used for the treatment of juxtarenal and paravisceral aneurysms not amenable to standard endovascular aneurysm repair (EVAR) in patients who cannot tolerate open repair and are anatomically suitable. First described in 1996 by Park et al.,[1] the FEVAR experience has grown exponentially with an extensive international experience with well over 10,000 devices implanted to date.[2–4] In the United States, the landmark trial started by Greenberg et al.[5] and ultimately completed after several modifications in 2010, led to the FDA approval of the Cook Zenith Fenestrated Endograft in April 2012.[6]

The FEVAR technique involves meticulous pre-operative planning and is often technically challenging with the need for multiple vessel cannulation done from inside of a partially deployed custom-made endograft. Cannulation of vessels in the currently available devices is performed in a retrograde fashion from the contralateral femoral access but specific anatomical or technical situations require alternate branch vessel access. Upper extremity access has been traditionally used in cardiac and mesenteric interventions but can be a valuable option for complex fenestrated cases. Over the past few years, upper extremity access has been more frequently used for snorkel and chimney techniques before fenestrated devices were readily available for treatment of juxtarenal abdominal aortic aneurysms. Its indications, advantages and pitfalls in FEVAR will be discussed in this chapter.

UPPER EXTREMITY ACCESS: GENERAL CONSIDERATIONS

Considerable experience has been amassed from the cardiology literature describing radial, ulnar and brachial interventions for coronary diagnostic imaging and therapeutic interventions. Multiple studies have showed comparable outcomes between femoral and upper extremity access in coronary interventions.[7] Upper extremity access in vascular surgery had been traditionally reserved for patients in whom femoral puncture was contraindicated or technically not feasible, however it has become increasingly relied on with the advent of mesenteric and complex aortic interventions.[8,9] Access from "Above" is a useful adjunct in endovascular aortic aneurysm repair (EVAR) helping overcome tortuous iliac anatomy,[8] cannulation of contralateral gates and assisting with device deployment.

The left brachial artery is the preferred site for access. Most authors describe access to the brachial artery just proximal to the antecubital fossa, a location where the pulse is more readily felt, the course of artery is more predictable, and where it can be easily compressed over the distal humerus. The artery at that location is relatively far from adjacent nerves as opposed to more proximally where access complications can lead to neuropraxia and other compressive neuropathies. The choice of a percutaneous access versus open exposure is dependent on surgeon preference and level of comfort with the technique. Ultrasound evaluation of the brachial artery can be very helpful to assess the size and any anatomical anomalies that may preclude access at that level including an early brachial bifurcation, severe calcification or other abnormalities. Female patients frequently have small upper extremity vessels leading to proximal access at the axillary or proximal brachial level when such access is needed. Most authors proceed with open exposure when anticipating the use of a 7 Fr sheath or larger.[10]

Several series have documented complication rates of upper extremity access to be as high as 11%[11–13]; however, recent vascular surgery literature has shown that open and percutaneous brachial access to be a safe and effective adjunct to aortic endovascular interventions[8–10] with a high technical success rate (up to 99%) and a low incidence of access related complications (4%–6%). A recent publication by Knowles et al.[10] suggests that upper extremity access for FEVAR is not associated with increased morbidity compared to femoral access alone. Only 1 out of 98 patients in the upper extremity access group suffered from a hemorrhagic stroke 5 days after the procedure, most likely due to uncontrolled hypertension rather than arch manipulation. There were four access-related complications, two of which required operative intervention for hematoma evacuation. The right upper extremity was accesses in six patients with no periprocedural complications.

Upper extremity access adds the risk of stroke to procedures that do not necessarily require arch manipulation. Wire manipulation across the arch, especially from the right side is theoretically associated with possible athero-embolism into the cerebral circulation. Some retrospective series have suggested a stroke rate as high as 10% when snorkel and chimney techniques are performed.[14–16] Iatrogenic dissections or perforations have also been described but this seems to be quite rare. Access through the right upper extremity, although much less performed than on the left has not been shown to be associated with a higher incidence of cerebrovascular adverse events.[9]

UPPER EXTREMITY ACCESS IN FEVAR

Early EVAR experience with short aortic necks and juxtarenal aneurysms included the use of snorkels and chimneys to preserve flow to branch vessels. Appropriate and sometimes multiple upper extremity access is critical for these procedures. There has been however a high rate of complications related to such access including a stroke rate as high as 10% in some series.[14–16] An additional high incidence of Type Ia

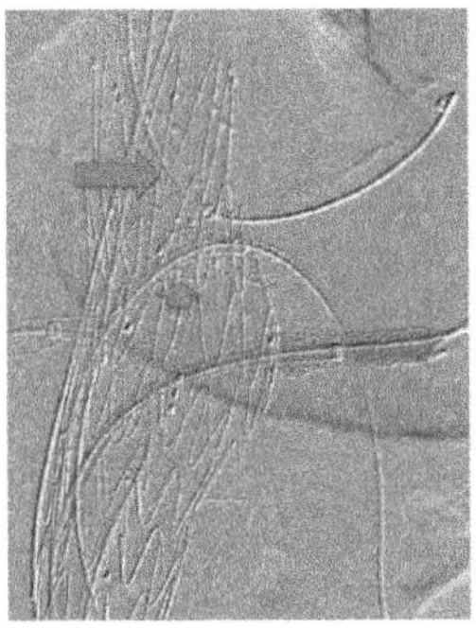

Figure 50-1. Celiac artery access at the upper edge of a fenestrated device. Red arrow points to the sheath accessing the celiac artery. Short arrow points to SMA fenestration.

endoleaks due to challenging anatomy and poor sealing in the proximal neck has shifted the attention towards fenestrated devices after their approval in 2012 and their associated excellent results.[15–20]

FEVAR requires maintaining sheath access from the groin with the main fenestrated device on one side and contralateral sheath access for multiple vessel cannulation. Preoperative planning is critical in deciding if upper extremity access is necessary. Some situations that benefit from upper extremity access include: diseased vessels that need to be cannulated and protected, anticipation of difficult cannulation of down-sloping vessels, notably the SMA and celiac, as well as some renal arteries, and possible branch salvage for misaligned fenestrations.

Upper extremity access can be also used as an adjunct to maintain patency of branch vessels in cases where landing in a healthy neck entails partial or total coverage of the celiac or SMA. Patency of these vessels can be maintained using snorkel and chimney techniques (Figure 50-1).

Upper extremity access can also be useful during fenestrated procedures for diagnostic purposes or planned cannulation when iliac and femoral occlusive disease limits the size of the contralateral femoral access. Additionally, it can be used to obtain "through and through" aortic access in patients with aortoiliac disease and severe tortuosity that benefit from the use of the "body-floss technique" to advance the endovascular device to its planned location. Wire snaring and secondary sheath advancement is also performed with the assistance of upper extremity access for the alignment and branch stent deployment in patients treated with pre-cannulated FEVAR and branch devices that are currently under investigation.[10]

TECHNICAL CONSIDERATIONS

Preoperative CT imaging of the chest is important in identifying the type of aortic arch with type I and II arches offering easier access to the descending aorta. It also allows us to identify occlusive disease, tortuosity or heavy atheromatous load that may lead to perioperative complications. Additionally, we routinely use ultrasound to image the brachial artery. Assessing the size of the artery is important as we feel that at least a 4 mm lumen is needed to safely proceed. Ultrasound also allows us to select a disease-free segment of the artery and detect high brachial bifurcations that may require more proximal access. We consider using the right arm if the artery on the left is heavily calcified or occluded at the subclavian level. If more than a single vessel cannulation is needed from above, bilateral upper extremity access can be used or a more proximal artery is chosen (Axillary or Subclavian artery). A sheath up to 12 Fr in size can be used for multiple vessel cannulation through the same sheath. Alternatively, the vessel can be accessed multiple times with smaller sheaths to avoid the potential leak from the large sheath at its valve.

The most common configuration of approved fenestrated devices is one scallop and two fenestrations. This configuration accounted for 70% of the devices used in the US-fenestrated trial.[6] In situations where difficult cannulation of a renal artery is anticipated, upper extremity access can be used, and cannulation of that renal artery can be obtained through the scallop of the partially deployed graft (Figures 50-2 and 50-3).

Using grafts without a scallop makes cannulating vessels from above more challenging. This situation can be addressed by partially deploying the suprarenal fixation system, allowing for passage of wire, catheter and sheath into the target vessel (Figure 50-4).

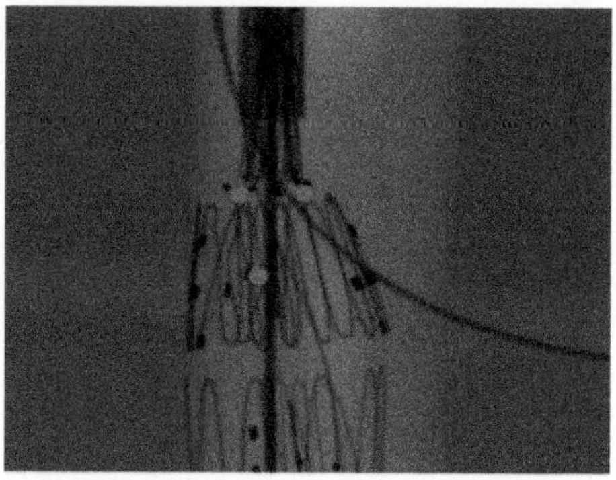

Figure 50-2. Cannulation of a renal artery through a scallop. The red dots correspond to the gold markers delineating the scallop.

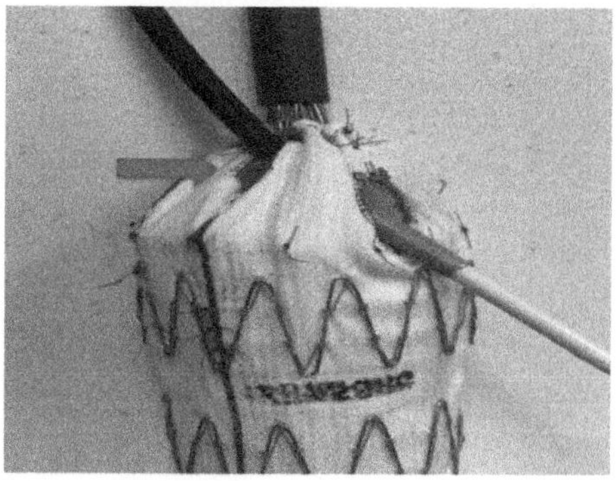

Figure 50-3. Model showing cannulation of a fenestration through the scallop. The red arrow marks the scallop aperture in a partially deployed graft.

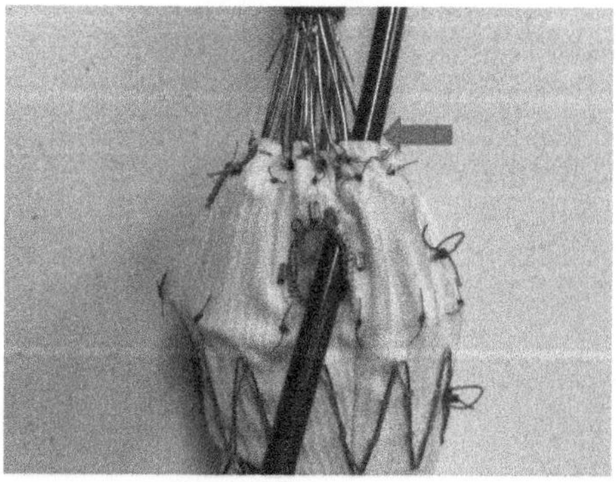

Figure 50-4. Model showing cannulation of a partially deployed cap allowing passage of wire and sheath in between struts of the suprarenal fixation system, accessing a fenestration. The red arrow points to the sheath going through the struts.

SUMMARY

Upper extremity access in FEVAR is very valuable in carefully selected situations where difficult cannulation is anticipated or coverage of a branch vessel is needed for a good seal. A complete arterial evaluation, appropriate patient selection, and meticulous technique are necessary to obtain excellent outcomes as noted by Knowles et al.[10] As endovascular repair for complex aortic aneurysm evolves, alternative access to the aorta, including upper extremity access will be a valuable adjunct to the endovascular reconstructions.

REFERENCES

1. Park JH, Chung JW, Choo IW, Kim SJ, Lee JY, Han MC. Fenestrated stent-grafts for preserving visceral arterial branches in the treatment of abdominal aortic aneurysms: preliminary experience. *J Vasc Interv Radiol.* 7(6):819–23.
2. Amiot S, Haulon S, Becquemin JP, et al. Fenestrated Endovascular Grafting: The French Multicentre Experience. *Eur J Vasc Endovasc Surg.* 2010;39(5):537–44. doi:10.1016/j.ejvs.2009.12.008.
3. Verhoeven ELG, Vourliotakis G, Bos WTGJ, et al. Fenestrated Stent Grafting for Short-necked and Juxtarenal Abdominal Aortic Aneurysm: An 8-Year Single-centre Experience. *Eur J Vasc Endovasc Surg.* 2010;39(5):529–36. doi:10.1016/j.ejvs.2010.01.004.
4. Vallabhaneni SR. Early results of fenestrated endovascular repair of juxtarenal aortic aneurysms in the United Kingdom. *Circulation.* 2012;125(22):2707–15. doi:10.1161/CIRCULATIONAHA.111.070334.
5. Greenberg RK, Sternbergh WC, Makaroun M, et al. Intermediate results of a United States multicenter trial of fenestrated endograft repair for juxtarenal abdominal aortic aneurysms. *J Vasc Surg.* 2009;50(4):730–7.e1. doi:10.1016/j.jvs.2009.05.051.
6. Oderich GS, Greenberg RK, Farber M, et al. Results of the United States multicenter prospective study evaluating the Zenith fenestrated endovascular graft for treatment of juxtarenal abdominal aortic aneurysms. *J Vasc Surg.* 2014;60(6):1420–8.e5. doi:10.1016/j.jvs.2014.08.061.
7. Kiemeneij F, Laarman GJ, Odekerken D, et al. A randomized comparison of percutaneous transluminal coronary angioplasty by the radial, brachial and femoral approaches: The access study. *J Am Coll Cardiol.* 1997;29(6):1269–75. doi:10.1016/S0735-1097(97)00064-8.
8. Criado FJ, Wilson EP, Abul-Khoudoud O, et al. Brachial artery catheterization to facilitate endovascular grafting of abdominal aortic aneurysm: Safety and rationale. *J Vasc Surg.* 2000;32(6):1137–1141. doi:10.1067/mva.2000.109335.
9. Alvarez-Tostado JA, Moise MA, Bena JF, et al. The brachial artery: A critical access for endovascular procedures. *J Vasc Surg.* 2009;49(2):378–85. doi:10.1016/j.jvs.2008.09.017.
10. Knowles M, Nation DA, Timaran DE, et al. Upper extremity access for fenestrated endovascular aortic aneurysm repair is not associated with increased morbidity. *J Vasc Surg.* 2015;61(1):80–7. doi:10.1016/j.jvs.2014.06.113.
11. Grollman JH, Marcus R. Transbrachial arteriography: techniques and complications. *Cardiovasc Intervent Radiol.* 1988;11(1):32–5.
12. Watkinson AF, Hartnell GG. Complications of direct brachial artery puncture for arteriography: a comparison of techniques. *Clin Radiol.* 1991;44(3):189–91. doi:10.1016/S0009-9260(05)80868-2.
13. Heenan SD, Grubnic S, Buckenham TM, Belli AM. Transbrachial arteriography: Indications and complications. *Clin Radiol.* 1996;51(3):205–9. doi:10.1016/S0009-9260(96)80324-2.

14. Bruen KJ, Feezor RJ, Nelson PR, et al. Endovascular chimney (Snorkel) technique vs open surgery for repair of juxtarenal and suprarenal aneurysms. *J Vasc Surg*. 2010;51(6):18S–19S. doi:10.1016/j.jvs.2010.02.073.
15. Coscas R, Kobeiter H, Desgranges P, Becquemin JP. Technical aspects, current indications, and results of chimney grafts for juxtarenal aortic aneurysms. *J Vasc Surg*. 2011;53(6):1520–7. doi:10.1016/j.jvs.2011.01.067.
16. Lee JT, Greenberg JI, Dalman RL. Early experience with the snorkel technique for juxtarenal aneurysms. *J Vasc Surg*. 2012;55(4):935–46. doi:10.1016/j.jvs.2011.11.041.
17. Moulakakis KG, Mylonas SN, Avgerinos E, et al. The chimney graft technique for preserving visceral vessels during endovascular treatment of aortic pathologies. *J Vasc Surg*. 2012;55(5):1497–503. doi:10.1016/j.jvs.2011.10.009.
18. Hogendoorn W, Schlösser FJ, Moll FL, et al. Thoracic endovascular aortic repair with the chimney graft technique. *J Vasc Surg*. 2013;58(2):502–11. doi:10.1016/j.jvs.2013.03.043.
19. Oderich GS, Correa MP, Mendes BC. Technical aspects of repair of juxtarenal abdominal aortic aneurysms using the Zenith fenestrated endovascular stent graft. *J Vasc Surg*. 2014;59(5):1456–61. doi:10.1016/j.jvs.2013.10.060.
20. Vemuri C, Oderich GS, Lee JT, et al. Postapproval outcomes of juxtarenal aortic aneurysms treated with the Zenith fenestrated endovascular graft. *J Vasc Surg*. 2014;60(2):295–300. doi:10.1016/j.jvs.2014.01.071.

51

Categorizing Acute Thoracic Aortic Dissections: DISSECT

Michael D. Dake, MD

Establishing the best method of treatment for individual patients with Type B aortic dissections has always presented a vexing challenge for physicians. Physicians are often faced with balancing the conservative approach of medical management with the more aggressive approaches of surgical or endovascular treatments. With the high surgical mortality for patients presenting with acute complicated Type B dissections, physicians have readily adopted thoracic endovascular aortic repair (TEVAR) as the accepted therapy for this condition.

With newer TEVAR devices achieving a broad indication from the FDA approval for the treatment of all Type B dissections and new insights regarding physiological predictors of future complications, physicians have expanded their consideration of TEVAR to treat the multiple challenges of this etiology. In this regard, based on their performance in the study of acute complicated Type B dissection, both W.L. Gore and Medtronic were awarded an FDA indication to treat all Type B dissections with their devices. The broad treatment indication was given to balance pre-market and post-market studies in order to more quickly provide on-label alternatives to physicians and their patients. This allows physicians to treat all Type B dissection while continued data is being collected by Vascular Quality Initiative (VQI), using a collaborative multiple company sponsored Post Approval Study.[1]

When considering a complex variety of relevant factors, such as the patient's condition and various physiological predictors, an algorithmic approach may prove useful in deciding among treatment options. In essence, an algorithm is meant to provide a simplified, streamlined guide to decision making when numerous input considerations exist and often complicate therapeutic considerations. A useful algorithm should help discriminate between choices on a high-level and prioritize the relevance of various concerns while also providing the necessary detail for justifying every decision step. The algorithm with this paper attempts just that, by providing a simple linear structure, which has depth to support each step. Additionally, the algorithm is stratified left–to-right and top-to-bottom to reflect the clinical urgency of treatment (Figure 51-1).

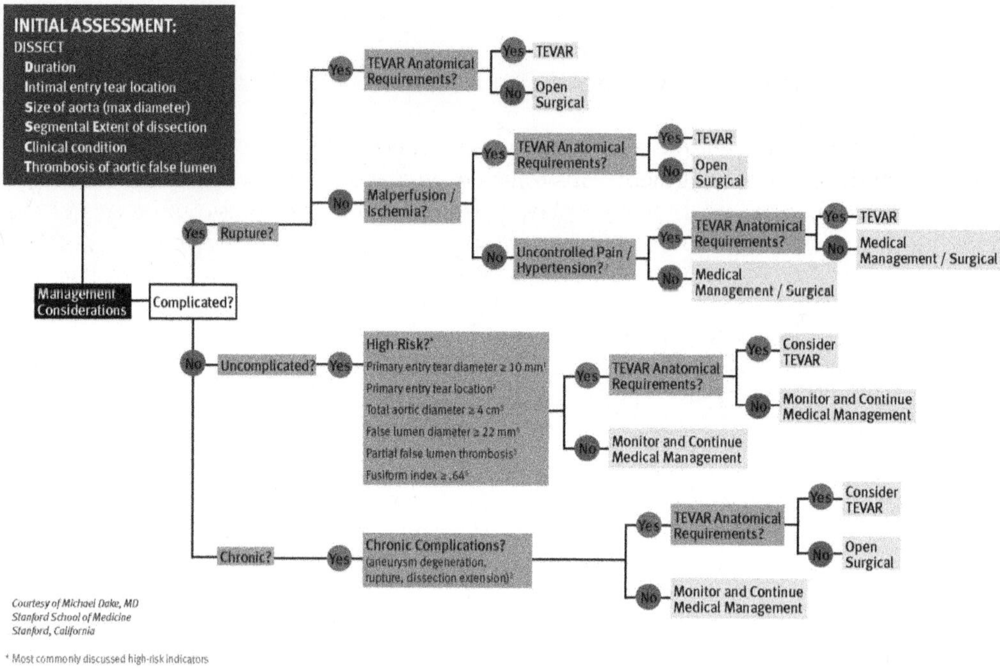

Figure 51-1. An algorithm to guide evaluation and management of type B aortic dissection.

Starting in the top left corner, the evaluation begins with a patient assessment using a simple mnemonic of *DISSECT*. The mnemonic provides an easy to follow stepwise assessment of six clinical and anatomic characteristics of dissection deemed most relevant to treatment planning in the era of endovascular options. It was originally designed to facilitate communication amongst care-givers and colleagues of different backgrounds and at different points of care, including outside hospital personnel, transfer team members, EMT service providers, emergency department physicians, medical trainees, nursing staff as well as attending and consulting physicians.

Beyond traditional considerations of medical therapy and open surgical care, this mnemonic approach insures that the key features of disease that determine the suitability and appropriateness of endovascular therapies are included in the initial evaluation and discussions of treatment alternatives. Late night phone discussions amongst colleagues regarding a patient in transfer or presenting to the emergency department are facilitated by the routine presentation of the DISSECT sequence's individual dissection features that allow for confident analysis and triage.

The publication, "DISSECT: A New Mnemonic-based Approach to the Categorization of Aortic Dissection" describes the meaning of each letter in detail, but here is quick summary.[2] The "D" stands for the Duration the patient has had the dissection. Traditionally, "acute" is used to classify the disease process in patients whose initial symptoms are 14 days or less in duration, whereas the term "chronic" dissection is applied to those with a dissection older than 14 days. These time designations were established in a 1958 paper by Albert Hirst called "Dissecting Aneurysm of the Aorta: A review of 505 cases," in which Hirst notes gross anatomic morphological changes in the septum at approximately 14 days.[3] However, instead of classifying duration into these general categories, the field is moving towards a more precise definition of the duration of a dissection to help better understand the patient's true morphological disease state and the potential responses to the newer range of therapeutic options.

The "I" in DISSECT describes the Intimal Tear or Primary Entry Tear (PET). Crucial information includes not only the exact location of the tear, but also the location of the tear relative to the greater curve ("convexity") or inner curve ("concavity") of the aorta.

The first "S" is related to the Size of the aorta, specifically the maximum diameter at any level in the dissected segment. This trans-aortic diameter is measured in an orthogonal plane to the aorta center line display. This dimension may prove to be one of the simplest, yet most important feature of the initial assessment. The application of this variable within the algorithmic sequence is especially relevant upon initial presentation of patients with uncomplicated dissection when evaluating the risk of disease progression, as we will discuss later.

The "SE" portion of DISSECT stands for the Segment of Extension. As we know, aortic dissections occur in the medial layer of the vessel and can propagate distally well into the abdominal aorta and even down into the femoral arteries. They can also extend proximally from the primary entry tear to involve the aortic arch and ascending segment. Capturing information on the extent of dissection and affected visceral vessels is important in determining if an endovascular approach is feasible.

The "C" letter is used to capture the clinical Complications of the dissection. It directs the physician to identify any of the clinically important complications of the disease that may mandate immediate intervention. Aortic rupture (Figure 51-2) and clinically relevant branch vessel involvement are two classic examples of complications that dramatically influence early mortality.

In terms of physiologically important aortic branch vessel involvement, there are two general mechanisms of branch compromise—static and dynamic. Static branch vessel involvement is caused by direct extension of the aortic dissection flap into a branch. If the resultant branch false lumen re-enters distally with a tear, there is double barrel flow to the branch. This is called static with re-entry involvement and it is not typically associated with critical malperfusion and vessel bed acute ischemia (Figure 51-3).

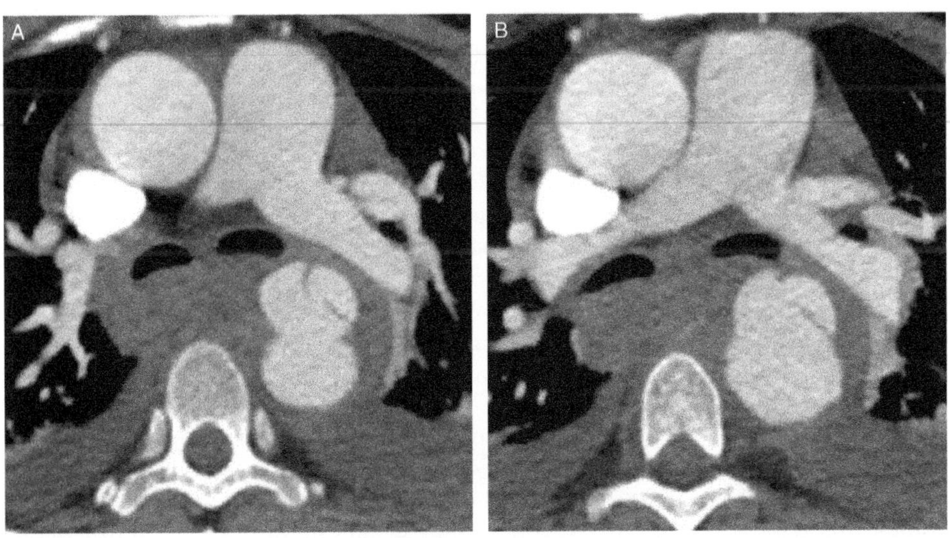

Figure 51-2. Aortic rupture associated with acute type B aortic dissection in a 34-year-old post-partum woman. (A,B) Axial CT scans identify primary tear in the mid-descending aorta associated with posterior aortic rupture.

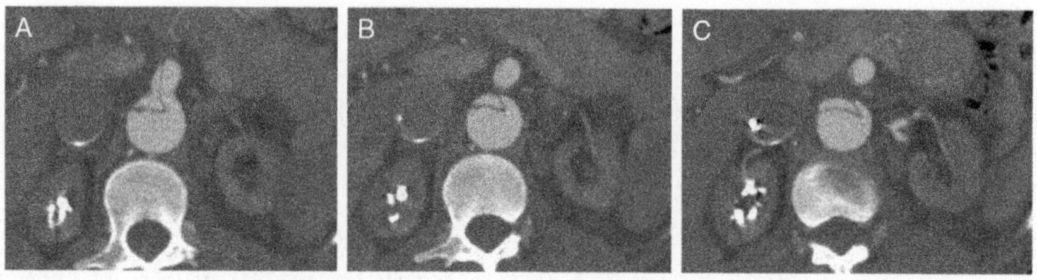

Figure 51-3. Static branch vessel involvement with re-entry. (A-C) CT images at the level of the superior mesenteric artery (SMA) show direct extension of the aortic septum into the branch. The flap within the SMA extends down the main trunk however contrast is noted within both the true and false lumen channels. Although the false lumen within the branch is larger, the presence of contrast distally within both true and false lumens suggests double barrel branch flow and a distal tear or re-entry of the false lumen.

Alternatively, if the false lumen within the branch does not terminate with a tear distally, a blind-ending false lumen segment is created. This is state is called static with no re-entry involvement. Because the false lumen expands without a re-entry, the true lumen in the branch is compressed and often critically narrowed. Without adequate true lumen flow and no false lumen perfusion, the organ or vascular bed supplied by the involved branch is commonly ischemic and at risk of necrosis. In such cases, immediate intervention is often warranted to relieve critical ischemia (Figure 51-4).

Dynamic branch vessel involvement occurs when the aortic flap prolapses over the ostia of abdominal branch vessels originating from the aortic true lumen (Figure 51-5). This phenomenon is synonymous with the term true lumen collapse or true lumen obliteration. It is often associated with large or circumferential primary entry tears. As the name implies, the degree of obstruction is variable and may be altered by changes in blood pressure, heart rate, and so forth. When severe, the level of branch vessel obstruction can result in profound ischemia that may affect multiple branches originating from the aortic true lumen and the vessel beds they supply.

These high-risk features of disease, rupture and branch vessel compromise, warrant careful evaluation and prompt management to avoid potentially irreversible sequelae, including death. Extension of the dissection and rapid enlargement of the aortic false lumen are also findings that may merit expeditious intervention, but both of these possibilities require re-imaging subsequent to the initial diagnosis to establish a change in appearance.

Lastly, the "T" captures the extent of Thrombus formation within the false lumen (Figure 51-6). In this regard, the status of any clot within the false lumen is an important predictor of disease progression. Partial thrombosis in conjunction with mural clot and a patent false lumen channel at any aortic level is associated with a higher risk of disease progression than with a patent false lumen which has a worse prognosis than a completely thrombosed false channel.

Once the initial patient assessment is complete by following the "DISSECT" mnemonic approach, we move onto the *management considerations* portion of the algorithm. For simplicity, decision junctions in the algorithm are presented as binary yes-or-no questions.

The answer to the first and primary question, "Is the patient presenting with a complication?" is captured in the "C" portion of the mnemonic analysis. While the definition of "complicated" varies in the literature, we focus on whether the patient is presenting with a rupture or visceral malperfusion, including spinal cord ischemia,

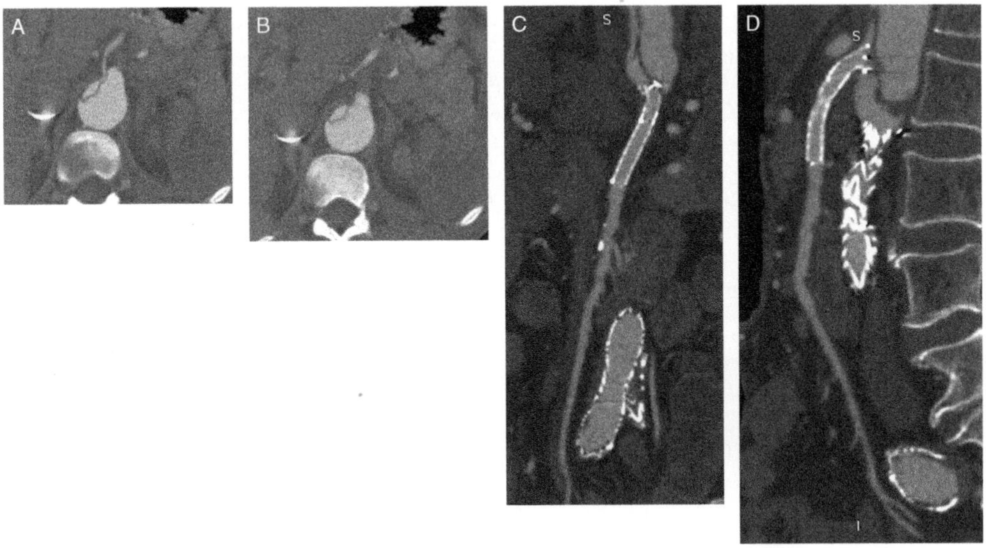

Figure 51-4. Static branch involvement with no re-entry. (A,B) CT scan at level of superior mesenteric artery (SMA) in a 68-year-old man with acute type B aortic dissection and prior EVAR placement who presented with chest, back, and abdominal pain associate with blood per rectum. The axial images show the aortic true lumen on the right with extension of the aortic flap into the SMA. The true lumen in the branch is string-like and narrowed by a nonopacified false lumen. The lack of contrast within the proximal false lumen segment indicates the presence of clot or static blood and suggests that there is no distal communication or tear in the false lumen. Without flow from the false lumen and compromised perfusion via the true lumen, the mesenteric bed is ischemic and at risk of irreversible necrosis. (C,D) Coronal and sagittal CT images after emergent placement of self-expanding metallic stents in the true lumen of the SMA show return of normal true lumen caliber. The stented segment is extended into the aortic true lumen by 2 mm to 3 mm to insure adequate flow at the ostia.

which are consensually agreed upon complications. Since rupture is the most severe of all the complications in aortic dissection and requires immediate treatment, it is appropriately located at the top of the algorithm. If the patient is experiencing rupture, the next piece of information needed in considering treatment options is whether or not the aortic anatomy meets *TEVAR anatomical requirements*, which vary according to endovascular device indication and may be discerned from respective Instructions for Use (IFU).

The goal for TEVAR treatment of a rupture that complicates aortic dissection is to completely cover the primary entry tear and depressurize the false lumen (FL). This should initiate progressive thrombosis over the length of the aortic segment covered by the endograft. Rupture sites in the false lumen wall are often difficult to identify, but are typically found directly opposite to the initial entry tear site.

When treating ruptures, multiple devices are typically needed to ensure a long length of coverage, usually to the level of the diaphragm or immediately supraceliac, to prevent potential retrograde flow in the false lumen through distal tears. If using multiple devices the order of placement is critical. The most proximal device should be placed first over the initial tear site with subsequent delivery of same-size devices placed distally. Paraparesis or paraplegia is always a relevant risk to consider when covering a long segment of thoracic aorta (≥20 cm), but literature detailing this approach reports low percentages of debilitating long-term effects.[4] If patients do experience motor or sensory neurological symptoms

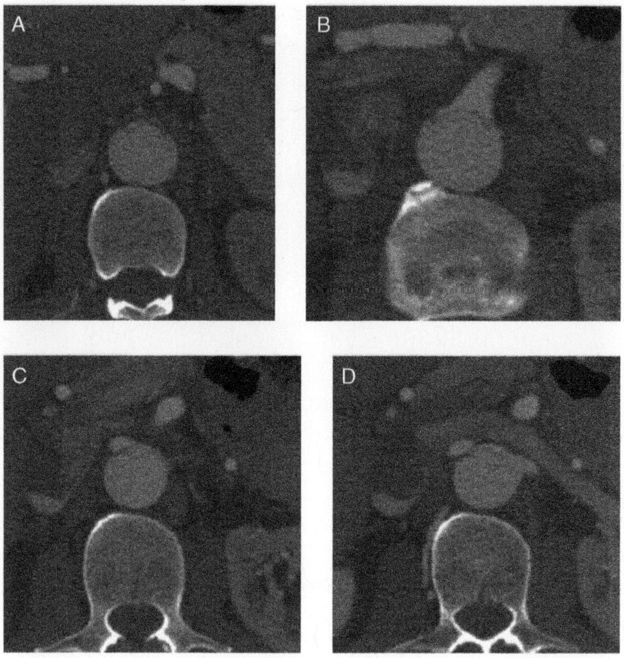

Figure 51-5. Dynamic branch vessel involvement in 62-year-old man with acute type B aortic dissection. (A-D) Four axial CT images through the mid-abdominal aorta show a crescent-like narrowed true lumen bordering the anterior aortic wall at the level of the mesenteric and renal branches. A dominant aortic false lumen is noted posteriorly. All branches supplied exclusively by the aortic true lumen are disadvantaged by the compromised channel. This includes the celiac trunk (A), superior mesenteric artery (B), right renal artery (C), and left renal artery (D). The extent of branch malperfusion is changeable and may be improved by the patient's lowering blood pressure until more definitive therapy is possible.

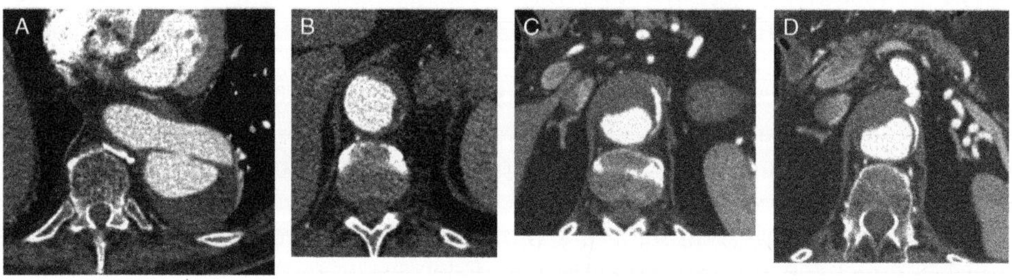

Figure 51-6. (A-D) Axial CT images through the descending and abdominal aorta demonstrate thrombus within the aortic false lumen. This is termed partial false lumen thrombosis and its presence has been shown to be associated with a higher risk of progression of disease than either a completely patent or completely thrombosed aortic false lumen.

post-TEVAR, rapid initiation of a protocol to treat spinal cord ischemia (including, placement of a lumbar catheter for CSF drainage, insuring a mean blood pressure of ≥ 80 to 90 mmHg and a normal hematocrit, etc.) frequently results in successful symptom reversal.

Clinically relevant branch vessel malperfusion is a similarly dangerous complication and is the next consideration after rupture in the algorithm. Up to 30% of patients with dissection exhibit some level of malperfusion or ischemia.[5,6] Malperfusion may be evidenced by the patient exhibiting symptoms, blood chemistry abnormalities and/or hemodynamic or physiological deficits. In addition, appropriate corresponding imaging findings, typically identified on CTA, are a necessary association that must be appreciated to diagnose clinically relevant branch compromise.

Like rupture, the patient meeting *anatomical requirements* is a prerequisite to determining if TEVAR is appropriate. While the procedural goals for treating malperfusion or ischemic events are similar to the treatment of rupture, a step-by-step treatment approach is typically preferred. In this regard, an aortic endograft is first placed over the primary entry tear site. The malperfusion may not adequately be corrected in the affected branch artery(ies) with a single device. In this case, careful evaluation of the flow within the aortic lumens, as well as, the involved branch(es) post-endograft placement, is required before undertaking further intervention. Remember, just because an endograft is placed remotely in the proximal descending aorta to cover the site of the primary intimal tear, occlusive lesions within involved branch vessels may remain critically compromised and may require an interventional procedure within the affected artery. No literature references for rupture or malperfusion are provided in the algorithm as their treatment with TEVAR has been widely studied and agreed upon.

In continuing to follow the algorithm along the next possible path, we address patients that have recurrent pain or difficulty managing their hypertension as possible candidates for intervention beyond medical management. Trimarchi et al. retrospectively looked at patients from the International Registry of Aortic Dissection (IRAD) that exhibit recurrent and/or refractory pain or uncontrollable hypertension.[7] They found that even with patients receiving medical management, patients experiencing recurrent and/or refractory pain or hypertension had a significantly higher in-hospital mortality rate of 35.6% ($P = 0.0003$) when compared with patients who presented without clinical complications with a rate of 1.5%. Most of the deaths were attributed to aortic rupture. They concluded that patients with refractory pain and/or refractory hypertension were at increased risk of disease progression and may be suitable for "aortic intervention, such as via an endovascular approach."

If the patient is not experiencing any of the previously mentioned complications, attention is directed to the bottom portion of the algorithm. Here, the first question asks "Is there Disease Progression?" *Disease Progression* is a generic term in this algorithm that denotes false lumen degeneration that becomes "aneurysmal" or extension of the false lumen which could cause malperfusion or ischemic events. While this consideration may span the classic boundaries between acute (≥14 days from symptom onset) and chronic dissection (>14 days), it also includes a rapidly growing false lumen in the acute phase. Practically, however, the majority of the disease progression events are late dilation or continued expansion of the false lumen. Occasionally, new septal tears or poor hypertension management can propagate the dissection proximally or distally, causing new symptoms for the patient.

Up to 25%–30% of patients require late aortic interventions for aneurysm expansion, extension of the progressive dissection or other related complications.[8] One literature reference is proposing a rapid growth metric is included in the algorithm, as there is no real consensus on what rapid growth entails. Akin, et al. describe abnormal false lumen enlargement in the chronic phase as expansion of any portion of the false lumen by 1 cm from diagnosis to the one year follow-up or enlargement that contributes to an overall aortic diameter (TL plus FL) of 5.5 cm.[9]

In the acute setting, most authorities agree that false lumen enlargement of ≥5 mm at 30 days from the initial diagnosis represents rapid growth. Consequently, if these patients do not warrant immediate intervention, they require close follow-up, imaging surveillance at frequent intervals to diagnose any progressive expansion.

As centers continue to have success, more chronic Type B dissections with aneurysm degeneration are being treated with TEVAR as an alternative to open surgery. In these cases, TEVAR should be considered if the patient meets the anatomical requirements of a good landing zone and adequate access. While the method of building from the proximal landing zone and extending aorta coverage with a same size device distally is performed with acute dissections, different techniques have been used when treating chronic dissections. The goal of covering the primary entry tear and depressurizing the false lumen remains the same; however, typically there is a thick aortic septum in chronic dissections and remodeling of the true lumen may become a challenge. While the anatomical TEVAR requirements are the same as for the other dissection categories, case planning differs widely depending on center experience and even by country.

One arguable advantage of treatment at a later time period is that the septum and aorta have had time to "heal" in the chronic phase. With the aorta less vulnerable to intraoperative mishaps, other approaches have been established. Many centers report building coverage with multiple devices, distal to proximal. The advantage of this approach is a smaller device diameter may be placed distally in a relatively noncompliant, smaller diameter true lumen. The smaller diameter device is placed first with the larger, more proximal endograft extending to the proximal landing zone to close the intimal tear site in the setting of classic dissection anatomy. In an acute dissection, this is not a viable strategy due to the risk of influencing flow through the entry tear which may risk propagating the dissection proximally and into the transverse arch or ascending aorta. With this in mind, it should be noted that, in the absence of significant diameter mismatches between the proximal and more distal true lumen, the preferred sequence for device implantation when treating chronic aortic dissection with false lumen aneurysm is the more routine top-to-bottom placement when more than one device is required.

If no *disease progression* is noted, the bottom-most and last path to *High Risk* should be navigated. At present, one of the most interesting debates among cardiovascular specialists concerns the endovascular treatment of patients presenting with uncomplicated Type B dissections. Published data from the INSTEAD, INSTEAD-XL, and ADSORB trials have fueled the current opinionated discussions and led all interested parties to ponder the real meaning of uncomplicated dissection.[10–12] Specifically, debate revolves around the emerging concept that the prognosis of an initially uncomplicated dissections at the time of diagnosis is highly variable, with many cases progressing in the first 2 to 5 years.

Traditionally, patients who are asymptomatic and have "stable aortic dissections" are managed with a medical therapy regimen and are monitored regularly with imaging. As previously noted, 25% 30% of these patients will experience some level of disease progression. Identifying these *High-Risk* patients has proven to be a challenge. With the new broad approvals of TEVAR devices, physicians have become increasing open to the idea of using these devices to proactively treat the future "bad actors" or high-risk patients.

Many attempts to simply identify these bad actors by applying a single prognostic metric have been less than successful and, consequently, none of these predictors are widely adopted. A profile based on a multi-factorial composite analysis, however, may provide a more powerful predictor based on its potential to develop a preponderance of evidence that allows identification of high-risk patients with multiple positive features that correlate with progression. Most of these predictors have come from published experiences in Japan. The algorithm provides a framework to analyze high risk factors and proposes treatment in this group of "high-risk" uncomplicated patients at an optimal time to increase the odds of full aortic remodeling, while minimizing intraprocedural risks and future potential problems.

Timing for treating high-risk uncomplicated Type B dissection patients is being actively investigated in many centers.[13] Some patients may benefit from delaying TEVAR treatment to establish control of hypertension and to allow the septum to go through an initial "seasoning" process. The rationale is that this delay will enable a safer procedure, with lower risk of dissection progression events, including retrograde Type A extension, and allow collateral development to perhaps lower the risk of spinal ischemic events.

The algorithm identifies six of the most prominent ideas around identifying these high-risk patients. The first two characterize the primary entry tear, focusing on whether its initial size is greater than 10 mm and its location in the aorta. If a large entry tear (≥ 10 mm) exists at initial presentation, further false lumen growth is likely.[11–14] Along with the size of the tear, Loewe et al. and Weiss et al. found the location of the tear effects the risk of future events; namely, tear location on the inner curve ("concavity") may characterize dissections that are more susceptible to retrograde dissection into the transverse and/or ascending aorta.[15,16]

The next predictor recognizes the importance of the initial total aortic diameter or trans-aortic diameter, which has been described in multiple peer-reviewed articles. Most publications detail initial total diameters of 40 mm or greater as prognostic of aneurysmal degeneration of the false lumen.[17–20]

Potentially, one of the most useful predictors for identifying patients at risk for aneurysmal degeneration was developed by Song et al. from Korea.[21] Their technique is to measure the aortic false lumen at initial presentation. This simple metric is obtained by measuring from the outer wall of the false lumen perpendicular to the septum. They found that a perpendicular measurement of 22 mm or greater predicted late phase growth of the false lumen.

A more common predictor of long-term progression is the characterization of thrombus within the false lumen, which was briefly discussed earlier. While one would assume a fully patent false lumen would lead to false lumen dilatation, partial false lumen thrombosis was shown to lead to higher patient mortality.[22,23] The plausible theory is that partial thrombosis in the distal false lumen blocks potential exit or runoff flow creating back pressure on the proximal false lumen. Fully patent false lumens or thrombosed false lumens are associated with lower rates of aortic false lumen dilation.

The last indicator for late aortic events is based on a recurrent idea to compare the true lumen diameter to the total aortic lumen diameter in the form of a ratio. One such ratio is called the Marui Fusiform Index.[24] Developed by Marui et al., it measures the maximum total diameter, including the false lumen, of the descending aorta and divides this term by the summation of diameter of the aortic arch and the trans-aortic diameter of the descending aorta at the level of the pulmonary artery. A ratio greater than 0.64 is associated with higher patient risk.

By identifying and proactively using TEVAR to treat high-risk uncomplicated patients, we may be able to promote more comprehensive positive aortic remodeling and minimize or eliminate the need for late aortic interventions. However, in the absence of complications or reliable predictors, traditional approaches of medical management and close clinical and imaging surveillance should be continued.

As new information becomes available through multi-center experience and post-approval studies a more definitive decision tree will emerge. As technology continues to evolve with better devices and better techniques less invasive approaches will continue to open up new treatment opportunities and better outcomes for physicians and their patients.

REFERENCES

1. Abel DB. Innovation in regulation applied to descending thoracic aortic endografts. *Endovasc Today*. 2013 12:68–9, 81.
2. Dake MD, Thompson M, van Sambeek M, et al. DISSECT: a new mnemonic-based approach to the categorization of aortic dissection. *Eur J Vasc Endovasc Surg*. 2013 46:175–190.
3. Hirst AE Jr, Johns VJ Jr, Kime SW Jr. Dissecting aneurysm of the aorta: a review of 505 cases. *Medicine*. 1958 37:217–79.
4. Hanna JM, et al. Five-year results for endovascular repair of acute complicated type B aortic dissection. *J Vasc Surg*. 2014 59:96–106.
5. Cambria RP, Brewster DC, Gertler J, et al. Vascular complications associated with spontaneous aortic dissection. *J Vasc Surg*. 1988 7:199–209.
6. Lauterbach SR, Cambria RP, Brewster DC, et al. Contemporary management of aortic branch compromise resulting from acute aortic dissection. *J Vasc Surg*. 2001 33:1185–92.
7. Trimarchi S, Eagle KA, Nienaber CA, et al. International Registry of Acute Aortic Dissection (IRAD) Investigators. Importance of refractory pain and hypertension in acute type B aortic dissection: insights from the International Registry of Acute Aortic Dissection (IRAD). *Circulation*. 2010 122:1283–9.
8. Fattori R, Montgomery D, Lovato L, et al. Survival after endovascular therapy in patients with type B aortic dissection: a report from the International Registry of Acute Aortic Dissection (IRAD). *JACC Cardiovasc Interv*. 2013 6:876–82.
9. Akin I, Kische S, Ince H, Nienaber CA. Indication, timing and results of endovascular treatment of type B dissection. *Eur J Vasc Endovasc Surg*. 2009;37(3):289–96.
10. Nienaber CA, Rousseau H, Eggebrecht H, et al. INSTEAD Trial. Randomized comparison of strategies for type B aortic dissection: the INvestigation of STEnt Grafts in Aortic Dissection (INSTEAD) trial. *Circulation*. 2009 120:2519–28.
11. Nienaber CA, Kische S, Rousseau H, et al. INSTEAD-XL trial. Endovascular repair of type B aortic dissection: long-term results of the randomized investigation of stent grafts in aortic dissection trial. *Circ Cardiovasc Interv*. 2013 6:407–16.
12. Brunkwall J, Kasprzak P, Verhoeven E, et al. Endovascular repair of acute uncomplicated aortic type B dissection promotes aortic remodeling: 1 year results of the ADSORB trial. *Eur J Vasc Endovasc Surg*. 2014 48:285–91.
13. Desai N, Menon R, Szeto W, et al. Retrograde aortic dissection after thoracic endovascular aortic repair: operative management techniques and pitfalls. Presented at the 27th European Association for Cardio-Thoracic Surgery (EACTS) Annual Meeting; October 5–9, 2013; Vienna, Austria. *Interact Cardiovasc Thorac Surg*. 2013;17(Suppl2):S118.
14. Evangelista A, Salas A, Ribera A, et al. Long-term outcome of aortic dissection with patent false lumen: predictive role of entry tear size and location. *Circulation*. 2012 125:3133–41.
15. Loewe C, Czerny M, Sodeck GH, et al. A new mechanism by which an acute type B aortic dissection is primarily complicated, becomes complicated, or remains uncomplicated. *Ann Thorac Surg*. 2012;93(4):1215–22.
16. Weiss G, Wolner I, Folkmann S, et al. The location of the primary entry tear in acute type B aortic dissection affects early outcome. *Eur J Cardio-Thorac*. 2012;42(3): 571–6.
17. Kato M, Bai H, Sato K, et al. Determining surgical indications for acute type B dissection based on enlargement of aortic diameter during the chronic phase. *Circulation*. 1995;92(9 Suppl):II107–II112.

18. Kudo T, Mikamo A, Kurazumi H, et al. Predictors of late aortic events after Stanford type B acute aortic dissection. *J Thorac Cardiovasc Surg.* 2014;148(1):98–104.
19. Onitsuka S, Akashi H, Tayama K, et al. Long-term outcome and prognostic predictors of medically treated acute type B aortic dissections. *Ann Thorac Surg.* 2004 78:1268–73.
20. Takahashi J, Wakamatsu Y, Okude J, et al. Maximum aortic diameter as a simple predictor of acute type B aortic dissection. *Ann Thorac Cardiovasc Surg.* 2008 14:303–10.
21. Song JM, Kim SD, Kim JH, et al. Long-term predictors of descending aorta aneurysmal change in patients with aortic dissection. *J Am Coll Cardiol.* 2007 50:799–804.
22. Tanaka A, Sakakibara M, Ishii H, et al. Influence of the false lumen status on clinical outcomes in patients with acute type B aortic dissection. *J Vasc Surg.* 2014 59:321–6.
23. Tsai TT, Evangelista A, Nienaber CA, et al. International Registry of Acute Aortic Dissection. Partial thrombosis of the false lumen in patients with acute type B aortic dissection. *N Engl J Med.* 2007 357:349–59.
24. Marui A, Mochizuki T, Koyama T, Mitsui N. Degree of fusiform dilatation of the proximal descending aorta in type B acute aortic dissection can predict late aortic events. *J Thorac Cardiovasc Surg.* 2007 134:1163–70.

52

Treatment Strategies for Thoracic Aortic Dissections

Mark A. Farber, MD and Raghuveer Vallabhaneni, MD

For the last several decades, initial management of Stanford Type B aortic dissections (DeBakey IIIa or IIIb) has involved medical therapy aimed at reduction of blood pressure and impulse stress ((Dp/dT). This concept has been indoctrinated into the medical field but is now being challenged with advancements in endovascular therapies and devices. Although there have been advances in the medical management and ICU care, medical modalities alone may still pose a 25%–50% complication rate to the patients resulting in some physicians seeking alternative approaches to reduce this risk in certain subsets of these patients.[1]

CLASSIFICATION

Aortic dissections have traditionally been divided into different categories based by their anatomy, acuity, and whether they are complicated or uncomplicated (see later). The reasoning behind this approach allows for stratification based upon medical and surgical risks and outcomes. As our understanding of dissections has evolved, management approaches have changed and more detailed classification schemes are being developed to help differentiate patients that may benefit from therapy beyond medical management to improve outcomes. One that is becoming increasingly popular is the DISSECT mnemonic by Dake on behalf of the DEFINE investigators: Duration, Intimal tear, Size of aorta, Segmental extent of involvement, Clinical complications, and Thrombosis of the false lumen. (Table 52-1)[2]

Type B Dissections (DeBakey 3a and 3b) typically have an entry tear that begins distal to the left subclavian artery. Several studies have identified anatomic features that may predict development of complications from Type B dissections.[3–5] These include size of entry tear > 10 mm, size of aortic enlargement > 40 mm, extent of dissection into the abdomen, as well as amount of false lumen thrombosis.

TABLE 52-1. DISSECT MNEMONIC FOR AORTIC DISSECTION CLASSIFICATION

D	Duration	• Ac = acute: < 2 weeks from initial onset of symptoms • Sa = subacute: 2 weeks to 3 months after symptom onset • Ch = chronic: > 3 months from initial symptoms
I	Intimal tear	• A = ascending Aorta • Ar = aortic arch • D = descending aorta • Ab – abdominal aorta • Un = unknown
S	Size of aorta	• Maximum center line diameter in millimeters
SE	Segmental Extent of involvement	• A = ascending aorta exclusively • Ar = aortic arch exclusively • D = descending exclusively • Ab = abdomen exclusively • AAr = ascending to arch • AD = ascending to descending • AAb = ascending to abdomen • AI = ascending to iliac • ArD = arch to descending • ArAb = arch to abdomen • ArI = arch to iliac • DAb = descending to abdomen • DI = descending to iliac

C	Clinical complications	• C = complicated:
		  • aortic valve involvement
		  • cardiac tamponade
		  • rupture
		• UC = uncomplicated

T	Thrombosis of false lumen	• P = patent aortic false lumen
		• CT = complete thrombosis of false lumen
		  • A = ascending aorta
		  • Ar = aortic arch
		  • D = descending
		  • Ab = abdomen
		• PT = partial thrombosis of false lumen
		  • A = ascending aorta
		  • Ar = aortic arch
		  • D = descending
		  • Ab = abdomen

Chronicity

Dissections are also organized based on their chronicity. Dissections are generally considered acute if they are less than 14 days old. Some groups have recently considered a category of subacute dissections (between 15 and 90 days) in an attempt to define a more stable phase of the disease process where treatment may be associated with a lower incidence of acute complications.[6,7] Chronic dissections are dissections that have been present for greater than 90 days from presentation. The most devastating complication from early intervention is retrograde aortic dissections, which decreases in incidence as the patient enters into a more stable condition; the subacute and chronic phases. Treatment during the subacute phase compared to more chronic interventions may have more potential for aortic remodeling secondary to increased plasticity of aortic wall and flap. As mentioned above these categories are important because the risk profile of the operations needed to treat these patients improves as the time progresses but the potential of aortic remodeling may be decreased.[7]

Complicated or Uncomplicated

The majority of Type B dissections are uncomplicated dissections that traditionally have not required repair on the basis of risk/benefit analysis. These patients have typically been managed with blood pressure control and close surveillance for complications. However, up to 25% of aortic dissections are considered complicated.[8] Complicated Type B dissections include those that cause malperfusion (to either visceral vessels, lower extremities or spinal cord), aortic rupture, rapid aneurysmal enlargement, refractory pain, or refractory hypertension. Complicated dissections require repair secondary to the high failure rate of medical management in patients with these symptoms. As one would suspect, due to the acuity of the patients requiring repair of a type B aortic dissection, mortality rates can be high, reaching 32% in certain studies.[8,9]

MEDICAL MANAGEMENT

Patients that present with acute type B aortic dissections, but are medically stable are initially treated with medical therapy. Medical management of uncomplicated aortic dissections is based principally on blood pressure management. This often requires multidrug therapy, but is primarily done with the use of beta blockade. This is typically initiated in the form of a short acting agent to titrate for impulse control such as esmolol. If further medication is needed to improve the patient's blood pressure, nitroprusside can be used to decrease the blood pressure acutely, however this should not be used without first using rate controlling medications as the reflex catecholamine release associated with vasodilators can cause an increase is left ventricular contraction. Calcium channel blockers are also a powerful adjunct in the management of these patients, especially for patients that are difficult to treat with beta blockade. Patients should have their systolic blood pressure maintained between 100 and 140. In conjunction with blood pressure control, heart rate control has also been believed to have protective benefits in these patients, although no studies to date have shown a clear benefit.[10]

The long-term mortality of patients with acute TBAD is 20%–40% percent at 5 years.[10–12] However, this number may be misleading, as patients that are likely sicker and have worse dissections, are more likely to undergo operative management. Further, the presence of an aortic dissection is often associated with other underlying disorders, which can often lead to a patient's demise.

In addition, long term surveillance and strict blood pressure control is paramount to assist in appropriate management of these patients, especially if they are being managed non-operatively. These patients usually have a repeat axial imaging performed within 2 weeks after the initial imaging to evaluate for changes to the dissection and progression that may warrant intervention. This scan should also be repeated in 3 months. Data suggests that if there is aneurysmal degeneration > 4.5 cm, the likelihood of needing future repair is substantial.[13,14] Our approach is to manage patients with anatomic features indicative of disease progression (see above) with TEVAR exclusion of their proximal entry tear covering the majority of the descending thoracic aorta to aid in aortic remodeling. This is typically targeted at the 3 month time point to minimize the risks of TEVAR related complications such as retrograde dissection and to maximize aortic remodeling.

OPERATIVE MANAGEMENT FOR COMPLICATED PRESENTATIONS

In the past, patients that have developed a complication from a Type B aortic dissection or enlargement of the dissection sac to aneurysmal extent (> 6 cm) have been treated with an open repair, +/− reperfusion of the ischemic vessel. Over the past decade endovascular treatment for Type B dissections has become more common. Although originally the primary endovascular technique involved septal fenestrations to improve perfusion to the false lumen, now the most common endovascular repair is placement of a thoracic stent graft in the proximal descending thoracic aorta to repressurize the true lumen and exclude the primary entry tear.

Open operative treatment is generally focused upon treating the sequelae of the dissections. Unfortunately, it is associated with a significant postoperative mortality reaching 33% within 1 year and has a reported adverse event rate of 42%. Open surgical repair is performed via a left thoracotomy and resection of the aortic tear with a segmental replacement of the aorta with a prosthetic graft. The resection of the septum or surgical bypass from a reliable inflow source is necessary to resolve visceral vessel ischemic complications. Patients that present with acute lower extremity ischemia can also be managed with an extra-anatomic bypass to restore flow into the affected limb(s), be it an axillo-bifemoral bypass or a femoral to femoral artery bypass.

The septal fenestration approach is aimed at resolving malperfusion by equalization of pressure between the two lumens. Since this is performed in symptomatic patients it is not surprising that the mortality was high 32% and not dissimilar for open surgical results published at the same period.[15] While correcting the pressure in both lumens, septal fenestration maintains patency of the false lumen which may be counterproductive for the disease process in the long term.

TEVAR FOR COMPLICATED DISSECTIONS

In the vast majority of cases, quoted in some studies as up to 90%, the primary entry tear for type B aortic dissections is in the proximal descending thoracic aorta.[16] While exclusion of this tear resolves the malperfusion in many cases, the open surgical mortality was prohibitively high. With the development of TEVAR however, the paradigm has shifted, and covering over the initial fenestration has taken on popularity as a result of the reduced procedural morbidity and mortality. This is supported heavily by several recent studies including the ADSORB and INSTEAD trials.[17–19] Furthermore, these studies have also shown a significant improvement in aortic remodeling after thoracic endovascular aortic repair (TEVAR).[20–23] Whereas in patients managed with medical therapy there has been a less than 5% rate of aortic remodeling, and false lumen thrombosis, patients managed with endovascular stenting have a rate of endovascular remodeling and false lumen thrombosis reaching above 50% in these studies ranging 2 to 5 years.

Adjunct studies during TEVAR are paramount in the appropriate management of patients treated by this method. Presumably, placing a stent graft in the aorta and occluding the primary fenestration redirects flow into the true lumen reduces, thus depressurizing the false lumen. The use of intravascular ultrasound (IVUS) during the procedure confirms appropriate positioning of the thoracic stent-graft in the true lumen prior to its deployment. Incorrect positioning of the thoracic endoprosthesis in the false lumen can result in devastating consequences. In order to achieve primary entry tear exclusion, it is recommended that the left SCA be overstented in most cases due to both the proximity of the tear to the LSCA as well as the extension of dissected aorta and the need to have the proximal extent of the device implanted in undissected aorta. In complicated TBAD, coverage of the subclavian artery may be performed with expectant management of rare ischemic, vertebrobasilar or paraplegic symptoms. In the uncomplicated chronic or sub-acute setting, subclavian artery revascularization should be performed when the patient has a previous LIMA bypass to a coronary, large segment coverage of the aorta will be performed, dominant vertebral artery on the left, extensive throacoabdominal repair is anticipated in future to help decrease risk of paraplegia. Management strategies for the left SCA are still controversial with some data suggesting that coverage carries an increased stroke and ischemic risk while others use a selective approach to management.[3,22,24,25] Controversy remains in the placement of stent grafts in uncomplicated dissections. Although there has been no demonstrable short-term survival benefit in TEVAR in uncomplicated dissections, long-term data may be promising compared to medical management alone (see later).

Management of dissections that involve the visceral vessels is more complex. In most situation endovascular exclusion of the primary entry tear results in false lumen depressurization and allows the true lumen to re-expand resolving the most common presentation of dynamic obstruction of the visceral segment as well as the lower extremities. Performing balloon fenestrations to equalize the pressure in the acute setting is also a viable option in patients with distal entry tears in the visceral region. For patients with static obstructions involving branched vessel, additional strategies often become necessary. This most commonly involves stenting of the branched vessel after traversing the obstruction and reestablishing true lumen perfusion. Fenestrated repair is seldom used currently because of device availability but has been employed in chronic dissection cases.

The efficacy of endovascular management for patients with visceral vessel ischemia has been studied in a limited setting with mixed results. A series of 40 patients who developed ischemia to the visceral segment of the aorta after previous type A dissection repair or TEVAR in a chronic type b dissection underwent percutaneous decompressive fenestration of the false lumen, had a 93% success rate, but a 25% postoperative mortality, likely related pre-existing comorbidities.[16]

TEVAR IN UNCOMPLICATED DISSECTIONS

There are several recent trials that have compared the efficacy of current management options for uncomplicated type B aortic dissections. Initial publications of the short and mid-term outcomes suggest the efficacy of stent graft placement (TEVAR) in these patients, by improve aortic remodeling, and providing a survival benefit since optimal medical therapy is associated with a 10%–50% mortality for patients with a chronic type B dissection over 5 years.

The INSTEAD trial by Nienaber et al., using the Talent device was the first of such trials and looked at patients in the subacute and chronic period (greater than 14 days).[19] Conducted at seven high volume European centers, 140 patients were enrolled over a three-year period. Patients were randomized to either optimal medical therapy (OMT) with appropriate antihypertensive medications, or TEVAR + OMT. Endpoints included all-cause mortality, related mortality, aortic remodeling, and progression of disease. Patients undergoing TEVAR would have < 20 cm of their aorta covered, with the primary focus on occluding the primary entry tear. Further, management of the left subclavian artery was at the discretion of the surgeon.

The TEVAR data revealed a 2.8% mortality at 30 days with no conversion to open surgery. Furthermore, 4.4% of patents would develop a major neurologic event including stroke or paraplegia. Eleven patients in the OMT group would crossover to the TEVAR group after sequelae of the dissection (aneurysmal expansion > 6 cm), and none of these patients would undergo any significant events. Further, at the 24-month mark, the trial would go on to show a higher mortality in the TEVAR group than OMT (16% vs. 4%) and place patients at elevated operative risks.

The INSTEAD XL trial followed this same set of patients for a 5-year period.[18] Although there was a higher mortality in the TEVAR and OMT group in the first two years, late follow-up showed a trend towards improved overall mortality and a reduction in aortic related mortality after two years. OMT failed to prevent late aortic mortality.

This study also shows that patients that underwent TEVAR and OMT, had a stable aortic diameter compared to OMT alone. A total of 20.8% of patients had an increase in aortic diameter by greater than 1 cm on TEVAR and OMT as compared to 66%. Only 22% of patients developed complete thrombosis of the false lumen in the OMT group, whereas in the TEVAR group over 90% of patients had complete thrombosis of their dissection sac with a significantly larger true lumen diameter. Almost 80% of patients had positive remodeling in the TEVAR group versus 10% in OMT group.

This trial concludes that although there may be an earlier risk of mortality with TEVAR, long term results demonstrate improved aortic related mortality and more favorable remodeling than OMT alone.

The ADSORB trial by Brunkwall et al. evaluated uncomplicated type B dissection patients treated in the acute setting (less than 14 days).[17] This study involved 17 high-volume European centers and compared OMT and OMT + TEVAR in patients that had symptoms for less than 14 days as opposed to the INSTEAD trial which compared patients with subacute type B dissections. A total of 250 patients were randomized with a 1:1 ratio with a 3-year follow up. Patients with connective tissue disorders or the need for another open operation were excluded, as well as patients with aneurysmal dilation above 5.5 cm. The end points evaluated included incomplete false lumen thrombosis, aortic dilation at 1 year, and aortic rupture at 1 year. The Gore TAG device was used.

The trial is still in progress, however 1-year data has been reported. The 30-day mortality for both OMT and TEVAR + OMT was 0%, however there were three cross-overs from the OMT group to the TEVAR group secondary to disease progression in 1 week. One-year follow-up data revealed two failures in the BMT group (aneurysmal dilation, and malperfusion) and one death in the TEVAR group. The only statistically significant difference of note was the rate of incomplete false lumen thrombosis, which was 97% in the OMT group and 43% in the TEVAR group. Further the false lumen was noted to increase in size in the OMT group, whereas in the TEVAR group was noted to become smaller. Similarly, the true lumen became larger in the TEVAR group, and remained unchanged in the OMT group. Although the study is still in progress and several factors need to evaluated at longer follow up including mortality, some conclusions that can be drawn from this data is that TEVAR with the Gore device is safe at 1 year, with improved aortic remodeling compared to OMT and the implantation of a stent-graft appears to promote aortic remodeling with false lumen thrombosis with reduction of its diameter.

Several studies have identified characteristics of patients with uncomplicated Type B dissections that would benefit from TEVAR.[26–29] The size of the entry tear has been shown to be associated with development of complications with the size of the entry tear in the proximal descending thoracic aorta > 10 mm associated with increased aneurysmal degeneration and increased mortality in untreated patients. Initial aortic diameter > 40 mm has also been associated with increasing size of aneurysm. Recently there has been an interest in FDG-PET CT technology to evaluate aortic dissections to detect inflammation in the wall of the aorta. Increased FDG-avid aortas were associated with enlarging aortas and possible rupture in patients that were medically managed for uncomplicated Type B dissections.[30]

There are, however, associated risks that make one pause prior to placing a stent graft in all patients. In one study, major complications occurred in 11.1% of patients, including neurologic deficits, stroke, paraplegia, and failure to abolish the false lumen. Failure to exclude the false lumen can be a particularly challenging complication as partial thrombosis of the false lumen has been associated with poor outcomes.[31] Also, patients that underwent repair in the acute setting were more likely to develop in-hospital and postoperative complications compared to those patients that were treated 30 or more days after the aortic dissection was detected, with an operative mortality nearly double for those stented acutely compared to patients being stented after initially being managed with medical therapy. This may be in part due to retrograde type A dissection, which although uncommon can be a devastating complication with a mortality of 33.6%. The development of a retrograde type A dissection has been associated with oversizing the aortic stent graft greater than 9%.[32]

It has been our approach to initially medically manage patients with uncomplicated dissections. Close follow-up with excellent blood pressure control is crucial. These patients are imaged during their sub-acute stable phase (3 months after presentation) to determine if they possess any characteristics suggestive of poor outcome or progression of disease as mentioned previously. In these circumstances TEVAR is often conducted in associated with subclavian revascularization with coverage to within 5–8 cm of the celiac artery. Subsequent treatment with fenestrated or branched devices is determined by the progression of disease in the aorta. By extending the initial repair to within 5–8 cm of the celiac artery there is reduction in the number of stent-grade induced new entry tears and the need for secondary thoracic interventions because the implant is sitting in a straighter portion of the aorta and the position of the false lumen is on the inner curvature where the stent graft forces are probably reduced. Approaching patients in this fashion has also stabilized many patients and in those with continued progression of disease, we find that the true lumen has enlarged somewhat in the visceral region allowing easier implantation of a fenestrated component facilitating complete exclusion of the dissection. It should be noted that particular attention should be focused on the internal iliac arteries. Often the dissection extends beyond the iliac bifurcation with the internal iliac origin opposite of a re-entry tear. In these situations, a fenestrated iliac limb is often essential in excluding the dissection while preserving the internal iliac patency to reduce the risk of paraplegia.

CONCLUSION

Overall, the optimal management of type B aortic dissections has changed over time and is in a state of evolution. Acute complicated type B dissections with signs of malperfusion, refractory pain and hypertension, or rupture, benefit from early interventions, most commonly TEVAR as well as optimal medical therapy. At present, the placement of a thoracic stent graft with or without occlusion of the subclavian artery is likely to improve aortic remodeling in these patients, and may provide a survival benefit. Patients with uncomplicated Type B dissections who have > 40 mm initial aortic diameter, >10 mm proximal aortic entry tear, or rapid aneurysmal growth in follow-up may benefit from TEVAR. In our opinion, these patients are better treated in the sub-acute phase secondary to the decreased mortality and complication risk compared to the acute phase as well as the increased plasticity of the aorta to remodel during the first 90 days. Patients that have symptoms of continued inflammation on follow-up with FDG-positive uptake in the aorta may benefit from TEVAR but larger studies are needed. All patients should be managed on optimal medical therapy and should be closely monitored for development of complications of malperfusion or aneurysmal growth.

It may be too early to say that all patients with uncomplicated Type B dissections should be treated with TEVAR, as further follow up from ongoing clinical trials are needed. Stent graft placement is not without its own risks including paraplegia, TIA, stroke, renal failure, and vascular injury. These risks must be weighed with the benefits provided by aortic remodeling and freedom from aortic related complications. Future studies on high-risk characteristics of progression of dissection and aneurysmal degeneration as well as long-term outcomes of TEVAR for asymptomatic Type B dissections will help further select patients that would benefit from this therapy.

REFERENCES

1. Elefteriades JA, Hartleroad J, Gusberg RJ, et al. Long-term experience with descending aortic dissection: the complication-specific approach. *Ann Thorac Surg.* 1992;53(1):11–20–discussion20–1.
2. Dake MD, Thompson M, van Sambeek M, et al. DISSECT: a new mnemonic-based approach to the categorization of aortic dissection. *Eur J Vasc Endovasc Surg.* 2013;46(2):175–90.
3. Xu SD, Huang FJ, Yang JF, et al. Endovascular repair of acute type B aortic dissection: early and mid-term results. *J Vasc Surg.* 2006;43(6):1090–5.
4. Kunishige H, Myojin K, Ishibashi Y, et al. Predictors of surgical indications for acute type B aortic dissection based on enlargement of aortic diameter during the chronic phase. *Jpn J Thorac Cardiovasc Surg.* 2006;54(11):477–82.
5. Marui A, Mochizuki T, Mitsui N, et al. Toward the best treatment for uncomplicated patients with type B acute aortic dissection: A consideration for sound surgical indication. *Circulation.* 1999;100(19 Suppl):II275–80.
6. Umaña JP, Miller DC, Mitchell RS. What is the best treatment for patients with acute type B aortic dissections—medical, surgical, or endovascular stent-grafting? *Ann Thorac Surg.* 2002;74(5):S1840–3–discussion S1857–63.

7. Eggebrecht H, Nienaber CA, Neuhäuser M, et al. Endovascular stent-graft placement in aortic dissection: a meta-analysis. *Eur Heart J*. 2006;27(4):489–98.
8. Greenberg R. Treatment of aortic dissections with endovascular stent grafts. *Semin Vasc Surg*. 2002;15(2):122–7.
9. Wheat MW. Acute dissection of the aorta. *Cardiovasc Clin*. 1987;17(3):241–62.
10. Winnerkvist A, Lockowandt U, Rasmussen E, Rådegran K. A prospective study of medically treated acute type B aortic dissection. *Eur J Vasc Endovasc Surg*. 2006;32(4):349–55.
11. Elefteriades JA, Hartleroad J, Gusberg RJ, et al. Long-term experience with descending aortic dissection: the complication-specific approach. *Ann Thorac Surg*. 1992;53(1):11–20–discussion20–1.
12. Dake MD. Endovascular stent-graft management of thoracic aortic diseases. *Eur J Radiol*. 2001;39(1):42–9.
13. Wheat MW. Acute dissection of the aorta. *Cardiovasc Clin*. 1987;17(3):241–62.
14. Winnerkvist A, Lockowandt U, Rasmussen E, Rådegran K. A prospective study of medically treated acute type B aortic dissection. *Eur J Vasc Endovasc Surg*. 2006;32(4):349–55.
15. Patel HJ, Williams DM, Meerkov M, et al. Long-term results of percutaneous management of malperfusion in acute type B aortic dissection: implications for thoracic aortic endovascular repair. *J Thorac Cardiovasc Surg*. 2009;138(2):300–8.
16. Deeb GM, Patel HJ, Williams DM. Treatment for malperfusion syndrome in acute type A and B aortic dissection: A long-term analysis. *J Thorac Cardiovasc Surg*. 2010;140(6 Suppl):S98–S100–discussion S142–S146.
17. Brunkwall J, Lammer J, Verhoeven E, Taylor P. ADSORB: a study on the efficacy of endovascular grafting in uncomplicated acute dissection of the descending aorta. *Eur J Vasc Endovasc Surg*. 2012;44(1):31–6.
18. Nienaber CA, Kische S, Rousseau H, et al. Endovascular repair of type B aortic dissection: long-term results of the randomized investigation of stent grafts in aortic dissection trial. *Circ Cardiovasc Interv*. 2013;6(4):407–16.
19. Nienaber CA, Rousseau H, Eggebrecht H, et al. Randomized comparison of strategies for type B aortic dissection: the INvestigation of STEnt grafts in Aortic Dissection (INSTEAD) trial. *Circulation*. 2009;120(25):2519–28.
20. Conrad MF, Crawford RS, Kwolek CJ, et al. Aortic remodeling after endovascular repair of acute complicated type B aortic dissection. *J Vasc Surg*. 2009;50(3):510–7.
21. Huptas S, Mehta RH, Kühl H, et al. Aortic remodeling in type B aortic dissection: effects of endovascular stent-graft repair and medical treatment on true and false lumen volumes. *J Endovasc Ther*. 2009;16(1):28–38.
22. Lopera J, Patiño JH, Urbina C, et al. Endovascular treatment of complicated type-B aortic dissection with stent-grafts: midterm results. *J Vasc Intervent Radiol*. 2003;14(2 Pt 1):195–203.
23. VIRTUE Registry Investigators. Mid-term outcomes and aortic remodelling after thoracic endovascular repair for acute, subacute, and chronic aortic dissection: the VIRTUE Registry. *Eur J Vasc Endovasc Surg*. 2014;48(4):363–71.
24. Gawenda M, Brunkwall J. Device-specific outcomes with endografts for thoracic aortic aneurysms. *J Cardiovasc Surg*. 2005;46(2):113–20.
25. Shigemura N, Kato M, Kuratani T, et al. New operative method for acute type B dissection: left carotid artery-left subclavian artery bypass combined with endovascular stent-graft implantation. *J Thorac Cardiovasc Surg*. 2000;120(2):406–8.
26. Kunishige H, Myojin K, Ishibashi Y, et al. Predictors of surgical indications for acute type B aortic dissection based on enlargement of aortic diameter during the chronic phase. *Jpn J Thorac Cardiovasc Surg*. 2006;54(11):477–82.
27. Marui A, Mochizuki T, Mitsui N, et al. Toward the best treatment for uncomplicated patients with type B acute aortic dissection: A consideration for sound surgical indication. *Circulation*. 1999;100(19 Suppl):II275–80.

28. Conrad MF, Ergul EA, Patel VI, et al. Management of diseases of the descending thoracic aorta in the endovascular era: a Medicare population study. *Ann Surg.* 2010;252(4):603–10.
29. Bernard Y, Zimmermann H, Chocron S, et al. False lumen patency as a predictor of late outcome in aortic dissection. *Am J Cardiol.* 2001;87(12):1378–82.
30. Kato K, Nishio A, Kato N, et al. Uptake of 18F-FDG in acute aortic dissection: a determinant of unfavorable outcome. *J Nucl Med.* 2010;51(5):674–81.
31. Tsai TT, Trimarchi S, Nienaber CA. Acute aortic dissection: perspectives from the International Registry of Acute Aortic Dissection (IRAD). *Eur J Vasc Endovasc Surg.* 2009;37(2):149–59.
32. Canaud L, Ozdemir BA, Patterson BO. Retrograde aortic dissection after thoracic endovascular aortic repair. *J Vasc Surg.* 2014;60(6):1710.

53

Left Subclavian Revascularization in the Setting of Thoracic Aortic Endograft Placement

Kimberly C. Zamor, MD, MS and Andrew W. Hoel, MD

The early reports of thoracic endovascular aortic repair (TEVAR) in 1994 heralded an important shift toward minimally invasive treatment of aortic disease. These endovascular strategies have over time reduced morbidity and mortality compared to open repair.[1–4] Over the last 20 years TEVAR has continued to advance in surgical precision and improved patient outcomes as a growing number of FDA approved grafts have become available.[5] Although TEVAR is now considered an acceptable treatment option for descending aortic aneurysmal disease, dissection and traumatic aortic injury, TEVAR is limited when there is disease involving the proximal descending thoracic aorta and aortic arch. Limitating factors include maintaining patency of major arch vessels and variations in arch anatomy.[6]

Treatment of proximal aortic pathology is a constant challenge because of limited ability to acheive an adequate proximal landing zone. Lack of an optimal endograft seal places patients at risk for endoleak and the need for subsequent complex reintervention. Coverage of zone 2 of the aortic arch, defined as the segment of the arch from the distal side of the left carotid origin to the distal side of the left subclavian origin, with a thoracic endograft is required in 26%–40% of patients with thoracic aortic diease.[1–11] There has been debate over the associated risks of coverage of the left subclavian artery (LSA) during TEVAR and whether revascularization is necessary. The Society for Vascular Surgery (SVS) practice guidelines provided three recommendations to address key concerns with zone 2 aortic coverage. First, when LSA coverage is required for elective TEVAR, routine revascularization of the LSA is recommended.[7,8] This recommendation is unfortunately based largely on low quality evidence. Second, there are a specific set of anatomic situations where LSA revascularization is strongly recommended. Lastly, in emergent cases the SVS guidelines recommend considering left subclavian revascularization on a case-by-case basis. Specific guidelines regarding LSA management for traumatic injury are addressed in separate SVS guidelines.[12]

The goals for this chapter are to review subclavian artery revascularization techniques during TEVAR, carotid–subclavian bypass (CSB) and subclavian–carotid transposition (SCT), provide a review of our experience, and lastly to discuss future directions of TEVAR management of arch vessels.

INDICATIONS FOR LSA REVASCULARIZATION

Prior to TEVAR, the primary indication for LSA revascularization was for atherosclerotic occlusive disease. The inceased use of TEVAR with proximal seal in zone 2 with coverage of the LSA has broadened the context for LSA revascularization.[13,14] In cases of arterial occlusive disease and TEVAR, the goals of LSA revascularization are to preserve antegrade vertebral artery perfusion and optimal left upper extremity blood flow.

Absolute indications for LSA revascularization during TEVAR include: patent LIMA coronary artery bypass graft, left arm arteriovenous fistula, non-revascularized aberrant right subclavian artery, hypoplastic or absent right vertebral, termination of left vertebral into posterior inferior cerebellar artery, and anomalous origin of the left vertebral at the aortic arch. Additionally, relative indications for LSA revascularization are left dominant vertebral artery, occluded internal iliac arteries, and extensive coverage of the aorta due to increased risk for spinal cord ischemia. Risk of spinal cord ischemia is further increased with prior or concurrent treatment of abdominal or thoracoabdominal aortic disease (Table 53-1). Revascualrization may not always be feasible in the setting of an urgent procedure or with the need to treat injuries of highest acuity first. In such cases if the LSA is covered without revascularization, assessment of right vertebral artery and the Circle of Willis is warranted.[6]

Carotid subclavian bypass (CSB) and subclavian carotid transposition (SCT) are the approaches of choice for LSA revascularization. The selection of CSB versus SCT can often times be based on surgeon preference. However, a key exception where CSB is specifically indicated is for patients with a patent left internal mammary artery coronary bypass graft.[15,16]

TABLE 53-1. INDICATIONS FOR SUBCLAVIAN REVASCULARIZATION AFTER TEVAR

Absolute indications
Patent LIMA coronary artery bypass graft
Left arm arteriovenous fistula
Nonrevascularized aberrant right subclavian artery
Hypoplastic or absent right vertebral
Termination of left vertebral into posterior inferior cerebellar artery
Anomalous origin of the left vertebral at the aortic arch
Relative indications
Left dominant vertebral artery
Occluded internal iliac arteries
Extensive (concurrent or prior) aortic reconstruction

LIMA: Left internal mammary artery.

TECHNICAL APPROACH

Subclavian Carotid Transposition

Performing SCT requires a transverse incision at the level of the clavicle. Exposure of the common carotid and left subclavian arteries is achieved by splitting the sternal and calvicular heads of the sternocliedomastoid muscle.[15] Adequate exposure requires division of the omohyoid and the thoracic duct and vertebral vein are also ligated to aid exposure and mobilization of the subclavian artery. The subclavian artery is divided well proximal to the vertebral artery and the proximal end is oversewn. The transected distal end of the subclavian is mobilized to the common carotid artery. Clamping the carotid artery with a Satinski or pair of profunda clamps allows elevation of the common carotid artery facilitating easier anastomosis. Care must be taken to avoid traction or compression of the vagus nerve. We then an oval arteriotomy is created in the common carotid artery using an aortic punch. The single anastomosis is then created between the subclavian and carotid arteries (Figure 53-1). Since completion of this anastomosis revascularizes the left subclavian artery, SCT avoids the need for a prosthetic bypass and eliminates the need for embolization of the proximal LSA.

Carotid-Subclavian Bypass

The technical approach for CSB requires an oblique incision lateral to the sternal head of the sternoclidomastoid muscle approximately 1-finger breath above the clavicle. Careful mobilization of the supraclavicular fat pad provides access to the deeper structures.

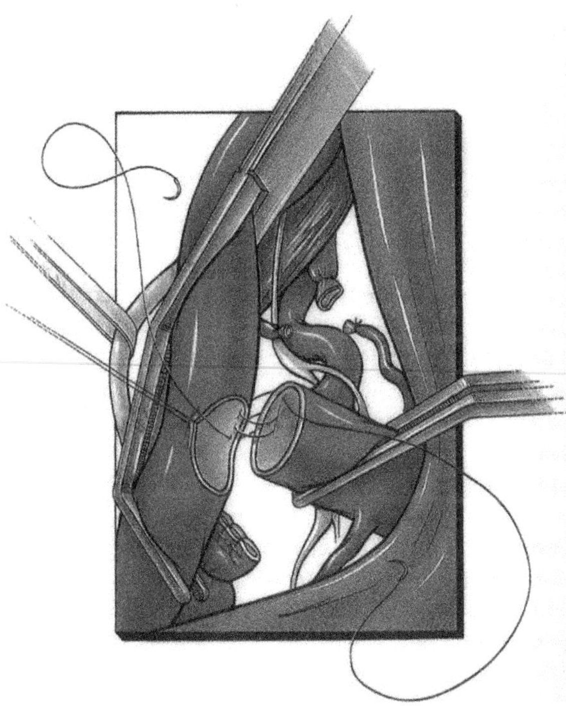

Figure 53-1. Primary anastomosis of the subclavian to carotid transposition demonstraing the relative anatomy. The vagus nerve in close proximity to the carotid artery and the sympathetic chain in close proximity to the vertebral artery. (From Morasch MD[15]; used with permission from Elsevier.)

The subclavian artery is isolated lateral to the vertebral artery (and usually lateral to the internal mammary artery, particularly if there is a LIMA bypass). This commonly requires division of the lateral portion of the anterior scalene muscle and care must be taken to avoid manipulation of or electrocautery adjacent to the phrenic nerve. (We typically will identify the nerve, but leave it in situ as it is quite sensitive to any manipulation.) We also minimize dissection of the brachial plexus and subclavian vein.

The common carotid artery is isolated by anterior and medial reflection of the jugular vein after entering the carotid sheath taking care to avoid the vagus nerve. The thoacic duct is often identified and ligated in the course of this dissection.

The subclavian anastomosis is performed first followed by the carotid anastomosis. The carotid anastomosis is facilitated by use of a Satinski clamp or two profunda clamps to elevate the carotid into the field. An oval arteriotomy in the common carotid artery is created using an aortic punch. The carotid anastomosis is created from posterior wall to anterior wall (Figure 53-2).

Following carotid subclavian bypass, we will either puncture the hood of the subclavian anastomosis or the more distal brachial artery and place a 4-french sheath. Through this sheath, we advance a flush catheter to aid in TEVAR placement. It is through this sheath that we also perform coil embolization of the proximal subclavian artery after TEVAR.

At the time of subclavian artery embolization, we carefully pack coils directly on the thoracic endograft. While we do not consider the subclavian origin to be effective for proximal seal of the endograft, we do believe that a solid coil pack at the subclavian origin does aid in stability of the endograft.

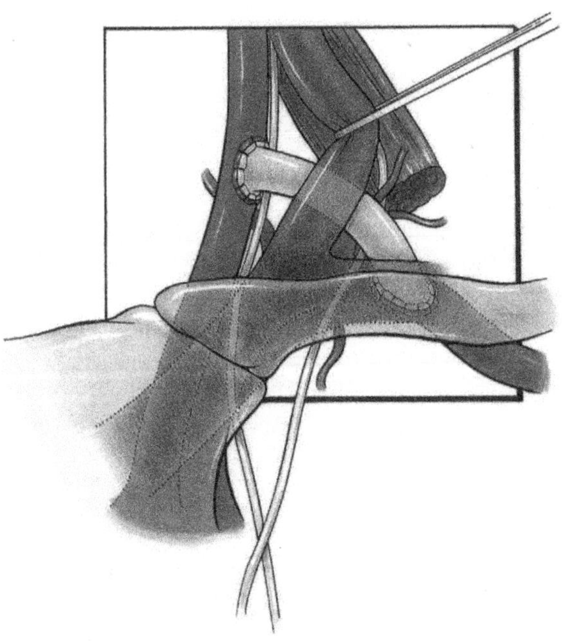

Figure 53-2. Completed left carotid subclavian bypass demonstrating relative anatomy and course of the bypass. Note the divided anterior scalene muscle and the phrenic nerve in close proximity to the subclavian anastomosis. (From Morasch MD[15]; used with permission from Elsevier.)

COMPLICATIONS

Associated Complications of Unrevascularized Subclavian Artery

LSA Coverage without reavscularization has been associated with increased risk for spinal cord ischemia, stroke and upper extremity ischemia. The EUROSTAR registry, a multicenter registry for patients underoging TEVAR, has demonstrated an increased risk for stroke and spinal cord ischemia in patients requiring left subclavian artery coverage that do not undergo revascularization. Multivariable analysis demonstrates a persistent correlation between spinal cord ischemia and left subclavian artery coverage without revascularization.[10] The protective effect of left subclavian artery revascularization is also supported by a report from the University of Florida demonstrating that selective LSA revascularization with TEVAR involving Zone 2 reduced neurologic events from 6% to 2%.[11] This is in contrast with the multicenter retrospective review by Maldonado and colleagues which was unable to demonstrate a benefit for LSA revascularization in TEVAR with Zone 2 coverage. Patient selection may have been a factor in this result however, with non-revascularization potentially occuring more commonly in patients at low risk for neurologic complications related to left subclavian artery coverage.

Complications of Revascularization Techniques

The differences in technical approach for LSA revascularization expose the patient to some variation in the spectrum of complications associated with LSA revascularization. It has been a longstanding question, which is better, bypass (CSB) or transposition (SCT)? CSB has the advantage of straightforward anatomy and low rates of complications. We additionally like CSB because it allows placing a solid coil pack directly onto the endograft to aid stability. Compared to SCT, the anatomy suggests an increased risk of phrenic nerve injury due to the proximity of dissection. In contrast, SCT has the advantage of a single anastomosis without the use of prosthetic material for bypass. We like it for these reasons; and, though it is difficult to clearly demonstrate, we suspect a lower risk of infection and lower procedure cost. It is somewhat more technically demanding, requiring work in a somewhat smaller space in anatomic territory that is less commonly encountered in the broader practice of vascular surgery. Ligation of the subclavian artery in the chest has potential to be a harrowing experience. Compared to CSB, the anatomy favors increased risk of vagus nerve injury and vocal cord paralysis as well as increased risk of Horner syndrome.

OUR EXPERIENCE

We recently published a retrospective cohort study to evaluate 30-day and mid-term outcomes of TEVAR involving LSA coverage within our institution.[17] The study compared TEVAR and LSA coverage +/− revascularization and LSA revascularization techniques, CSB versus SCT. The outcomes evaluated were stroke, upper extremity ischemia, spinal cord ischemia, primary graft patency, vocal cord paralysis and mortality.

From 2001 to 2013, 80 patients underwent TEVAR with LSA coverage, of which 20 were unrevascularized: 22 had CSB, and 38 had SCT. The key study findings demonstrated that unreavascularization of the LSA during TEVAR was associated with a 25% stroke rate at 30 days, compared to revasculized 2% ($P = 0.003$). Stroke events included anterior, posterior and multi-territory infarcts. Additionally, unrevascularized LSA was associated with a 30-day upper extremity ischemia rate of 15% compared to 0% in revascularized patients ($P = 0.014$). There was no statistically significant difference for revascularization technique for any of the outcomes of interest (Table 53-2).

Multivariate logistic regression was performed to evaluate factors associated with adverse perioperative events, such as stroke, spinal cord ischemia, upper extremity ischemia and mortality. The presence of LSA revascularization was associated with a lower risk of adverse perioperative events (odds ratio 0.23, $P = 0.034$) after adjustement for urgent or emergent procedures, advance age (over 65 years old), and coronary artery disease.

Our experience demonstrated the importance of LSA revascularization during TEVAR whenever feasable. It appears that the technique of revascularization is less important with equivalent 30-day and midterm outcomes. While there are strong advocates for CSB and for SCT, each has distinct advangates and disadvantages to be considered. Ultimately, we suspect that the best results are achieved when the surgeon is performing the procedure with which they are most comfortable.

TABLE 53-2. OUTCOMES FOR TEVAR AND LSA REVASCULARIZATION TECHNIQUES, CSB AND SCT

Outcome	CSB (N = 22)	SCT (N = 38)	P^a
30 Day			
Stroke	0	1(2.63%)	1.000
SCI	0	2(5.26%)	0.528
UE Ischemia	0	0	–
Vocal Cord Paralysis	1(4.55%)	4(10.53%)	0.643
Primary patency	22(100%)	38(100%)	–
Death	0	0	–
Midterm	**CSB (N = 15)**	**SCT (N = 32)**	**P^a**
Stroke	0	1(3.12%)	1.000
SCI	0	0	–
UE Ischemia	0	0	–
Vocal Cord Paralysis	0	1 (3.12%)	1.000
Primary patency	15 (100%)	32 (100%)	–

TEVAR, Thoracic Endovascular Aortic Repair; LSA, Left Subclavian Artery; CSB, Carotid-Subclavian Bypass; SCT, Subclavian-Carotid Transposition; SCI, spinal cord ischemia; UE, upper extremity.

[a]x^2 or Fisher exact tests, when appropriate.

ON THE HORIZON

The use of branched and fenestrated grafts has become increasingly common in the visceral segment aorta largely because of the availability of an FDA approved device. The use of branched and fenestrated devices in the aortic arch is developing as devices are proceeding toward pivotal clinical evaluation. Two devices are currently on this path: the Medtronic Valiant Mona LSA device and the Gore TAG Thoracic Branch Endoprosthesis. Both devices are intended for revascularization of the left subclavian artery with Zone 2 coverage during TEVAR. Each device employs left brachial or axillary artery cannulation for branch device delivery. Approval of these devices will advance the minimally invasive and, potentially, the totally endovascular treatment of proximal descending thoracic aortic technology. With advancing technology it is important to be mindful of the possilility that at some point in the future, CSB and SCT will be legacy perocedures without clinical utility.

CONCLUSIONS AND SUMMARY

TEVAR has improved the ability to treat a number of life-threatening aortic pathologies with reduction in morbidity and mortality compared to open thoracic aortic repair. With increasing comfort with TEVAR, it is being more commonly utilized for the treatment of proximal aortic pathology including disease in the aortic arch. In this setting it is increasing clear that the majority of patients undergoing Zone 2 aortic coverage deserve left subclavian revascularization for perioperative risk reduction, particularly for neurologic events. The technique of revascularization is less critical and in the majoriry of circumstances should be based on surgeon preference.

ACKNOWLEDGMENT OF SUPPORT

This work is supported by funding from a National Institutes of Health Grant (T32-2T32HL094293-06A1).

REFERENCES

1. Dake MD, Miller DC, Semba CP, et al. Transluminal placement of endovascular stent-grafts for the treatment of descending thoracic aortic aneurysms. *N Engl J Med.* 1994;331(26):1729–34.
2. Hoel AW. Aneurysmal Disease: Thoracic Aorta. Surg Clin North Am. 2013;93(4):893–910.
3. Upchurch G. Thoracic and Thoracoabdominal Aortic Aneurysms: Evaluation and Decision Making. In: Rutherford's Vascular Surgery. *Vol 2.* 8th ed. New York: Saunders; 2014. pp. 2084–101.
4. Acher C, Wynn M. Outcomes in open repair of the thoracic and thoracoabdominal aorta. *J Vasc Surg.* 2010; 52(4, Suppl): 3S–9S.

5. Liao JM, et al. Nationwide trends and regional/hospital variations in open versus endovascular repair of thoracoabdominal aortic aneurysms. *J Thorac Cardiovasc Surg.* 2012;144(3):612–6.
6. Cronenwett, JL ed. *Rutherford's Vascular Surgery.* 8th ed. 2014: Elsevier.
7. Matsumura JS, Rizvi AZ, Society for Vascular Surgery. Left subclavian artery revascularization: Society for Vascular Surgery® Practice Guidelines. *J Vasc Surg.* 2010;52(4):65S–70S.
8. Matsumura, JS, Lee WA, Mitchell RS, et al. The Society for Vascular Surgery Practice Guidelines: management of the left subclavian artery with thoracic endovascular aortic repair. *J Vasc Surg.* 2009;50(5): 1155–8.
9. Kotelis D, Geisbusch P, Hinz U, et al. Short and midterm results after left subclavian artery coverage during endovascular repair of the thoracic aorta. *J Vasc Surg.* 2009;50(6):1285–92.
10. Buth J, Harris PL, Hobo R, et al. Neurologic complications associated with endovascular repair of thoracic aortic pathology: Incidence and risk factors. A study from the European Collaborators on Stent/Graft Techniques for Aortic Aneurysm Repair (EUROSTAR) Registry. *J Vasc Surg.* 2007;46(6):1103–11.e2.
11. Feezor RJ, Martin TD, Hess PJ, et al. Risk factors for perioperative stroke during thoracic endovascular aortic repairs (TEVAR). *J Endovasc Ther.* 2007;14(4): 568–73.
12. Lee WA, Matsumura JS, Mitchell RS, et al. Endovascular repair of traumatic thoracic aortic injury: Clinical practice guidelines of the Society for Vascular Surgery. *J Vasc Surg.* 2011;53(1): 187–92.
13. Madenci AL, Ozaki CK, Belkin M, McPhee JT. Carotid-subclavian bypass and subclavian-carotid transposition in the thoracic endovascular aortic repair era. *J Vasc Surg.* 2013; 57(5):1275–82.
14. Scali ST, Chang CK, Pape SG, et al. Subclavian revascularization in the age of thoracic endovascular aortic repair and comparison of outcomes in patients with occlusive disease. *J Vasc Surg.* 2013;58(4):901–9.
15. Morasch MD. Technique for subclavian to carotid transposition, tips, and tricks. *J Vasc Surg.* 2009;49(1): 251–4.
16. Morasch MD, Peterson B. Subclavian artery transposition and bypass techniques for use with endoluminal repair of acute and chronic thoracic aortic pathology. *J Vasc Surg.* 2006;43(2, Suppl): A73–A77.
17. Zamor KC, et al. Outcomes of thoracic endovascular aortic repair and subclavian revascularization techniques. *J Am Coll Surg.* 2015;221(1):93–100.

54

Patient Selection and Repair Timing for Blunt Thoracic Aortic Injuries

Donald G. Harris, MD and Robert S. Crawford, MD

Blunt thoracic aortic injury (BTAI) is a leading cause of traumatic death, with most mortality occurring at the scene.[1,2] Based on seminal autopsy studies in the mid-twentieth century, Parmley described the natural history of blunt aortic injuries as progression to rupture.[3] As such, traditional management consisted of screening based on characteristic chest x-ray findings to select high-risk patients for diagnostic contrast aortography.[4] With few exceptions, recommended treatment was early open aortic repair,[4] but at the expense of significant procedural morbidity and mortality.[1,5,6] However, application of thoracic endovascular aortic repair (TEVAR) and computed tomography (CT) has revolutionized the management of patients with BTAI.

The use of TEVAR has dramatically lowered the morbidity and mortality of aortic injury repair,[7,8] and is now the standard treatment for patients requiring aortic intervention.[9–11] Perhaps as importantly, the development of highly accurate CT techniques has had two transformative effects on BTAI management. First, the routine use of CT for screening and diagnosis has defined a complete spectrum of traumatic aortic lesions. Second, subsequent better understanding of the specific natural histories of these lesions has led directly to new treatment paradigms: definitive non-operative management and delayed aortic repair. As such, for many patients, early aortic repair is no longer the standard of care.[9,12] The current challenge, and focus of this review, is lesion grading and risk assessment to select the appropriate management strategy for each patient.

COMPUTED TOMOGRAPHY SCREENING AND DIAGNOSIS

Contrast CT aortography is the optimal test for detection and characterization of BTAI.[1,9] Importantly for screening, it has 100% sensitivity for aortic injuries,[13,14] and can be incorporated into a single-pass, single-contrast bolus, whole body CT protocol for evaluation of other injuries in patients at risk for polytrauma.[1,15] Its specificity matches or exceeds that of conventional invasive aortography, while offering further characterization of extra-luminal signs of injury.[13,14] While alternative techniques, such as transesophageal echocardiography or intravascular ultrasound,[16] are available, their test characteristics and practical limitations hinder their utility.[1] As such, between the first and second American Association for the Surgery of Trauma BTAI studies (AAST-1 1994–1996, and AAST-2 2005–2007), the primary diagnostic modality shifted from conventional aortography (87% in AAST-1) to CT (93% in AAST-2),[5,7] a trend that persists in modern data.[11] As a result, current guidelines endorse CT as the screening and diagnostic test of choice for BTAI.[9]

Implementation of routine CT screening for at-risk patients has resulted in the characterization of a full spectrum of aortic lesions, ranging from intimal tears to complete transection. Intimal lesions constitute the most limited form of BTAI, and are characterized by a limited intimal defect and no external aortic contour abnormality.[17] These lesions were clinically occult in the era of chest x-ray screening and selective diagnostic aortography, but are diagnosed with increasing frequency by modern techniques.[18] Together with intramural lesions without external contour abnormality, these lesions comprise a recently defined category of minimal aortic injuries.[1,17] Follow-up imaging of these lesions indicate a high rate of resolution and low rate of progression, and several studies have demonstrated the safety of definitive non-operative management for these lesions.[11,17,19–23]

More extensive aortic disruption results in pseudoaneurysm formation,[3,24] which is characterized by focal, contained dilation of the aorta with an external contour abnormality.[19,25] These are clinically significant lesions that are associated with aortic-specific morbidity and mortality,[11,19] including the risk for progression to rupture.[3] While there are high-risk features that define a subgroup of patients with unstable pseudoaneurysms,[19,26,27] most deaths occur at the scene such that those surviving to admission have been automatically selected for a degree of aortic stability.[19,28,29] Indeed, studies of patients with high-grade BTAI and concurrent injuries who are selected for delayed repair or non-operative management indicate early repair is not required in all cases.[30–34] Complete aortic disruption, either from progression of an unstable pseudoaneurysm or primary transection, represents the most severe BTAI. While such patients frequently present in extremis, some ruptures are contained and will be diagnosed by CT. Emergency repair is indicated in this situation.[27]

This spectrum of BTAI is summarized by several CT-based systems that grade the anatomic severity of the aortic lesion (Table 54-1).[19,23,25,27,35,36] For example, the scale described by Azizzadeh et al. and adopted by the Society for Vascular Surgery has four injury types: I, intimal tear; II, intramural hematoma; III, pseudoaneurysm; and IV, rupture.[12,36] Other systems, including those described by the Vanouver, Stanford, and Presley trauma centers, and ours at the Maryland Shock Trauma Center, build on this gradation by stratifying pseudoaneurysms based on size.[25,27,35] In contrast, the group at Harborview trauma center proposed a simplified scheme that categorizes lesions as minimal or significant based on the absence or presence of an external aortic contour abnormality.[19] However, classification of the lesion type or grade does not accurately inform stability, particularly for pseudoaneurysms, which may be stable despite being a high grade injury. While CT assessment of the primary lesion is sufficient to direct therapy for lesions that are clearly low or high grade (i.e., observation of minimal lesions, or emergent repair of for ruptured injuries), further characterization is required to optimize treatment of intermediate BTAI.[10]

TABLE 54-1. SUMMARY OF BTAI INJURY GRADING SCALES

	Classification System					
Lesion	SVS	Stanford	Presley	Vancouver	Shock Trauma	Harborview
Isolated MH			I			
Intraluminal defect		I				
Intimal injury	I	II	IIa IIb with MH	I: <1 cm II: > 1cm	I	I
Intramural hematoma or defect	II	III			I	
Pseudoaneurysm	III	IV: <50% circumference V: >50% circumference	IIa: <1 cm IIb: < 1 cm + mediastinal hematoma IIIa: >1cm IIIb: >1cm & proximal to LSCA	III	II: <50% circumference III: >50% circumference	II
Rupture/ transection	IV		IV	IV	IV	

Note: Roman numerals specify grade or categorization within respective scheme, while blank cells indicate a lesion not included in the scale. Presley grade I (isolated mediastinal hematoma) and Stanford grade I (intraluminal defect) are not included in the table. SVS: Society for Vascular Surgery, MH: mediastinal hematoma, LSCA: left subclavian artery.

AORTIC INJURY MANAGEMENT PARADIGMS

Recent studies indicate a growing trend of nonoperative management for BTAI.[10, 11, 19, 20, 23] For example, a review by de Mestral et al. of the Canadian National Trauma Registry demonstrated a significant decrease in the rate of aortic repair, from 55% in 2002 to 36% in 2010 despite stable injury incidence.[10] A recent multicenter study by DuBose et al. reported an overall nonoperative management rate of 32% for 2008–2013.[11] Most patients (60%–90%) selected for non-operative management have intimal or intramural lesions, and among this group there have been no reported aortic-specific deaths in modern series.[11,19,20,22] As such, current guidelines endorse non-operative management for minimal aortic injuries.[12] However, while most of these lesions heal, there is a 1%–5% risk for progression and need for salvage TEVAR,[11,22] such that follow-up imaging to document resolution or stability is recommended.[12]

Although traumatic pseudoaneurysms are frequently stable over the near term and have been managed nonoperatively,[11,19,27,30] they warrant definitive repair because of a higher risk of rupturing.[3,9,12,19] For these patients, intervention timing has an important effect on outcome.[33] Between the AAST-1 and -2 studies, delayed repair became normative, with the mean time to aortic repair increasing from less than 24 to more than 48 hours. Further, in AAST-2, delayed repair was associated with 65% lower mortality.[5,7] Single institution series support the general safety and benefit of delayed repair.[8,32] As such, delayed repair is currently recommended for patients who have favorable anatomy and are candidates for preoperative medical management.[9,19,27]

A study by our group indicates that delayed aortic repair may have a specific benefit among patients with concurrent traumatic brain injury (TBI).[31] In an analysis of patients with BTAI and moderate to severe TBI, 29% were managed nonoperatively, 39% underwent early aortic repair (17 open and 12 endovascular repairs), and 32% had delayed repairs (3 open and 21 endovascular repairs). Despite similar TBI profiles, patients undergoing early aortic repair had a higher rate of postoperative TBI progression, regardless of anticoagulation or repair modality. In contrast, none of the patients having delayed repairs had worsening TBI, despite universal procedural anticoagulation. Overall, early aortic repair was an independent risk factor for progressive TBI, and was associated with increased aortic specific morbidity and mortality.[31]

For patients selected for delayed repair, standard practices include antiplatelet therapy and β-blockade targeting a systolic blood pressure of 100–120 mmHg and heart rate of 60–90 beats per minute as tolerated by concurrent injuries.[19,31,34] The timing of delayed repair is largely dependent on stabilization of concurrent injuries and stability of the aortic lesion on follow-up imaging,[12,19,32,34] but definitive intervention is recommended during the index hospitalization.[12] While TEVAR has become the primary method of BTAI repair and is recommended by current management guidelines,[7,9–11] open repair has a continuing role for patients with specific injury patterns, aortic anatomy, or as salvage after TEVAR.[9,11] Finally, although procedural anticoagulation is a potential concern for patients with an associated hemorrhagic brain injury, TEVAR after 48–72 hours with systemic heparinization appears safe without risk for new or progressive intracranial hemorrhage.[31]

Three categories of patients require emergency or early aortic repair. First, patients who have complete aortic disruption, either from ruptured pseudoaneurysm or primary transection, will die without intervention. Although many of these patients present in extremis and may not be salvageable,[11,19] in the absence of concurrent non-survivable injuries they may benefit from emergency repair.[25–27] Those who can undergo repair have an in-hospital survival rate of up to 50%.[11] Second, patients with TBI with elevated intracranial pressures who require pharmacologic blood pressure support should be considered for early aortic repair.[19] However, this was an infrequent scenario in our series of patients with concurrent BTAI and TBI.[31] Finally, pseudoaneurysms with high-risk features represent a more severe and unstable lesion than bland pseudoaneurysms, and should be evaluated for urgent repair.[19,26,27] Determining which features characterize aortic instability has been the subject of recent studies to optimize selection of these patients.

ASSESSMENT OF AORTIC INJURY STABILITY

Evaluation of patients with traumatic aortic pseudoaneurysms must weigh the potential benefit of lower procedural morbidity and mortality associated with delayed repair against the risk of interval aortic rupture. BTAI grading schemes alone, however, are insufficient to assess pseudoaneurysms, which are high-grade by operational definition, yet may be stable or unstable. As such, further assessment of aortic stability and appropriate patient selection depends on the presence of defined high-risk features.

Two studies, one each from the groups at Harborview and Maryland Shock Trauma Center, have studied primary and secondary injury features that are associated with aortic mortality. In an analysis of BTAI clinical and CT characteristics associated with aortic mortality, Starnes et al. found that mediastinal hematoma size (>15 mm at the aortic arch) and hypotension (systolic blood pressure < 90 mmHg) were independently associated with death from BTAI.[19] Using similar methodology, Rabin et al. described a large left hemothorax, or mediastinal hematoma with mass effect or aortic pseudocoarctation as high-risk features that should prompt urgent repair among patients with large pseudoaneurysms.[27]

An additional study by our group analyzed specific risk factors for aortic instability.[26] Harris et al. evaluated patients presenting in stable condition with pseudoaneurysms who either a) remained stable without intervention for at least 48 hours, or b) progressed to rupture. This enabled comparison of a subgroup of high-grade lesions that had inherent short-term stability versus a subgroup of similarly graded but unstable lesions. Admission physiology, primary lesion characteristics, and secondary injury signs were compared to determine variables that were associated subsequent aortic rupture. Admission lactate (> 4 mM), lesion size (> 1.4 times normal aortic diameter), and mediastinal hematoma (>10 mm at the descending aorta) were independent predictors of rupture. The presence of at least two of these factors identified patients who progressed to rupture with 100% sensitivity and 84% specificity, and was significantly more accurate than blinded clinical assessment.[26]

Integrating these analyses indicates that the presence of shock, pseudoaneurysm size, and extent of mediastinal hematoma are critical risk factors that can be used to assess aortic stability (Table 54-2). Importantly, these factors are clinically relevant, readily available early in the assessment of patients with BTAI, and intuitively valid. While it is unclear if one factor in isolation is enough to classify a pseudoaneurysm as high or low-risk, our risk model indicates most, if not all, patients with unstable lesions have multiple high-risk features.[26]

On the basis of these studies, patients with traumatic pseudoaneurysms with high-risk characteristics should be evaluated for urgent aortic repair. Conversely, patients without such features can be reliably selected for delayed repair provided they are candidates for preoperative medical therapy. Indeed, while the primary goal of assessing lesion stability is to identify patients at risk for rupture who should undergo early repair to prevent fatal rupture, these studies suggest that the more common scenario is the identification of patients with high-grade but otherwise stable pseudoaneurysms.[19,26,27] As such, an important secondary outcome of lesion risk assessment is optimizing the identification of patients who can be safely selected for, and benefit from delayed aortic repair.[26]

TABLE 54-2. RISK FACTORS ASSOCIATED WITH TRAUMATIC AORTIC PSEUDOANEURYSM INSTABILITY

Physiology	PSA Size	Mediastinal Hematoma	Reference
SBP < 90 mmHg	n/a	> 15 mm at the aortic arch	Starnes *et al.*[19]
n/a	≥ 50% aortic circumference	mass effect, hemothorax, or pseudocoarctation	Rabin *et al.*[31]
Lactate > 4 mM	> 1.4 × normal aortic diameter	> 10 mm at descending aorta	Harris *et al.*[26]

Abbreviations: SBP: systolic blood pressure; PSA: pseudoaneurysm.

These studies have important limitations. All are retrospective, single-institution analyses, with our studies from the Maryland Shock Trauma Center derived from the same BTAI cohort. While the results are consistent with each other and the broader current BTAI literature, these findings lack external or prospective validation. Given recent advances in injury diagnosis, medical management, and endovascular repair, the current challenge in the field is optimizing patient selection. Future studies, including prospective, multi-institutional studies, should validate and further define specific factors associated with lesion stability.

SUMMARY AND CONCLUSION

The standard of care for BTAI has evolved from near universal early repair to tailored management individualized to patient physiology, injury severity, and lesion stability (Figure 54-1). Recent studies have helped optimize patient selection by assessing lesion grade and stability. After initial resuscitative maneuvers and the

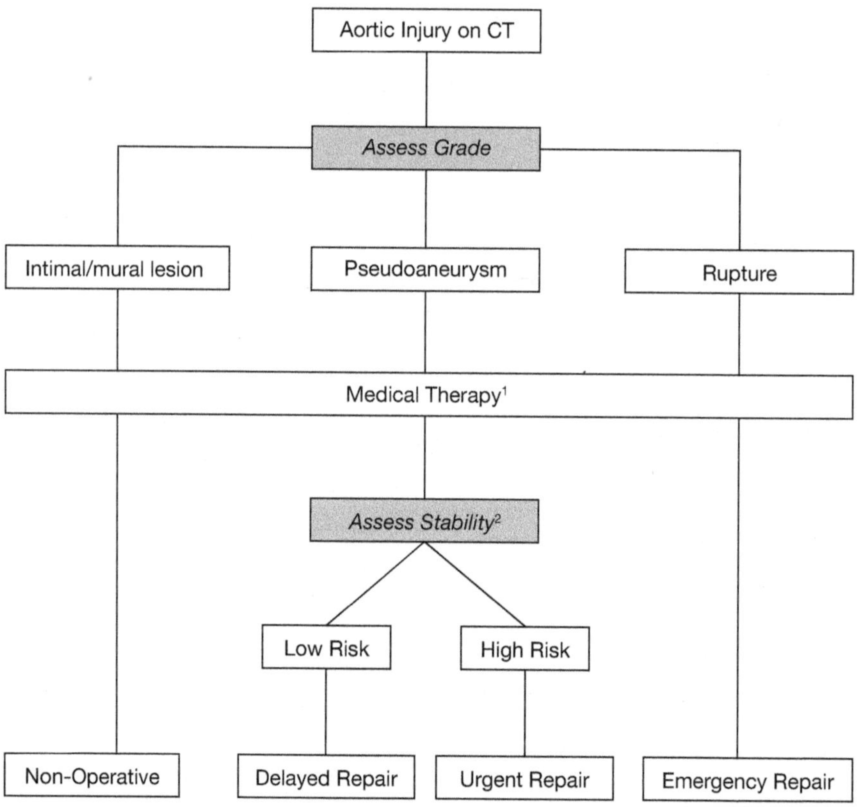

Figure 54-1. Recommended BTAI management based on lesion grade and stability. Antiplatelet therapy and β-blockade targeting a systolic blood pressure of 100–120 mmHg and heart rate of 60–90 beats per minute with additional antihypertensive agents as required for blood pressure control. Repeat CT within at 48–72 hours for patients managed nonoperatively or by delayed repair access stability. High risk factors include signs of hypotension, large pseudoaneurysm, and extensive mediastinal hematoma (refer to Table 54-2).

primary and secondary surveys, patients suspected of having BTAI should undergo chest CT, typically as part of a whole-body screening study. All patients with BTAI should receive β-blockade and antiplatelet therapy as tolerated as soon as possible after diagnosis. Assessment of lesion grade enables identification of patients with minimal lesions appropriate for nonoperative management, and those with aortic rupture requiring emergency repair. Traumatic pseudoaneurysms represent an intermediate lesion that require further evaluation to determine stability. For these, relatively smaller lesions and the absence of shock and large mediastinal hematoma are associated with a low risk for progression to rupture and can help select patients for delayed aortic intervention. In the presence of these features, urgent repair should be pursued. Future studies should validate this approach and continue to refine optimal patient selection and management.

REFERENCES

1. Neschis DG, Scalea TM, Flinn WR, Griffith BP. Blunt aortic injury. *N Engl J Med.* 2008;359:1708–16.
2. Smith RS, Chang FC. Traumatic rupture of the aorta: still a lethal injury. *Am J Surg.* 1986;152:660–3.
3. Parmley LF, Mattingly TW, Manion WC, Jahnke EJ. Nonpenetrating traumatic injury of the aorta. *Circulation.* 1958;17:1086–101.
4. Nagy K, Fabian T, Rodman G, et al. Guidelines for the diagnosis and management of blunt aortic injury: an EAST Practice Management Guidelines Work Group. *J Trauma.* 2000;48:1128–43.
5. Fabian TC, Richardson JD, Croce MA, et al. Prospective study of blunt aortic injury: multicenter trial of the American Association for the Surgery of Trauma. *J Trauma.* 1997;42:374–83.
6. Cardarelli MG, McLaughlin JS, Downing SW, et al. Management of traumatic aortic rupture: a 30–year experience. *Ann Surg.* 2002;236:465.
7. Demetriades D, Velmahos GC, Scalea TM, et al. Operative repair or endovascular stent graft in blunt traumatic thoracic aortic injuries: results of an American Association for the Surgery of Trauma Multicenter Study. *J Trauma.* 2008;64:561.
8. Estrera AL, Gochnour DC, Azizzadeh A, et al. Progress in the treatment of blunt thoracic aortic injury: 12–year single–institution experience. *Ann Thorac Surg.* 2010;90:64–71.
9. Fox N, Schwartz D, Salazar JH, et al. Evaluation and management of blunt traumatic aortic injury: A practice management guideline from the Eastern Association for the Surgery of Trauma. *J Trauma Acute Care Surg.* 2015;78:136–46.
10. de Mestral C, Dueck A, Sharma SS, et al. Evolution of the incidence, management, and mortality of blunt thoracic aortic injury: a population–based analysis. *J Am Coll Surg.* 2013; 212: 1110–5.
11. DuBose JJ, Leake SS, Brenner M, et al. Contemporary management and outcomes of blunt thoracic aortic injury: A multicenter retrospective study. *J Trauma Acute Care Surg.* 2015;78:360–9.
12. Lee WA, Matsumura JS, Mitchell RS, et al. Endovascular repair of traumatic thoracic aortic injury: Clinical practice guidelines of the Society for Vascular Surgery. *J Vasc Surg.* 2011;53:187–92.
13. Mirvis SE, Shanmuganathan K, Buell J, Rodriguez A. Use of spiral computed tomography for the assessment of blunt trauma patients with potential aortic injury. *J Trauma.* 1998;45:922–30.
14. Fabian TC, Davis KA, Gavant ML, et al. Prospective study of blunt aortic injury: helical CT is diagnostic and antihypertensive therapy reduces rupture. *Ann Surg.* 1998;227:666.

15. Nguyen D, Platon A, Shanmuganathan K, et al. Evaluation of a single–pass continuous whole–body 16–MDCT protocol for patients with polytrauma. *Am J Roentgenol.* 2009;192:3–10.
16. Smith MD, Cassidy JM, Souther S, et al. Transesophageal echocardiography in the diagnosis of traumatic rupture of the aorta. *N Engl J Med.* 1995;332:356–62.
17. Gunn ML, Lehnert BE, Lungren RS, et al. Minimal aortic injury of the thoracic aorta: imaging appearances and outcome. *Emerg Radiol.* 2014:1–7.
18. Malhotra AK, Fabian TC, Croce MA, et al. Minimal aortic injury: a lesion associated with advancing diagnostic techniques. *J Trauma.* 2001;51:1042–8.
19. Starnes BW, Lundgren RS, Gunn M, et al. A new classification scheme for treating blunt aortic injury. *J Vasc Surg.* 2012;55:47–54.
20. Paul JS, Neideen T, Tutton S, et al. Minimal aortic injury after blunt trauma: selective nonoperative management is safe. *J Trauma.* 2011;71:1519.
21. Kepros J, Angood P, Jaffe CC, Rabinovici R. Aortic intimal injuries from blunt trauma: resolution profile in nonoperative management. *J Trauma.* 2002;52:475–8.
22. Osgood MJ, Heck JM, Rellinger EJ, et al. Natural history of grade I–II blunt traumatic aortic injury presenting over 10 years at a single institution. *J Vasc Surg.* 2014;59:334–42.
23. Lamarche Y, Berger FH, Nicolaou S, et al. Vancouver simplified grading system with computed tomographic angiography for blunt aortic injury. *J Thorac Cardiovasc Surg.* 2012;144:347–54.
24. Richens D, Field M, Neale M, Oakley C. The mechanism of injury in blunt traumatic rupture of the aorta. *Eur J Cardiothorac Surg.* 2002;21:288–93.
25. Gavant ML. Helical CT grading of traumatic aortic injuries: impact on clinical guidelines for medical and surgical management. *Radiol Clin North Am.* 1999;37:553–74.
26. Harris DG, Rabin J, Kufera JA, et al. A new aortic injury score predicts early rupture more accurately than clinical assessment. *J Vasc Surg.* 2015; 61: 332–8.
27. Rabin J, DuBose J, Sliker CW, et al. Parameters for successful nonoperative management of traumatic aortic injury. *J Thorac Cardiovasc Surg.* 2014;147:143–50.
28. Dosios TJ, Salemis N, Angouras D, Nonas E. Blunt and penetrating trauma of the thoracic aorta and aortic arch branches: an autopsy study. *J Trauma.* 2000;49:696–703.
29. McGwin G, Jr, Reiff DA, Moran SG, Rue LW, III LW. Incidence and characteristics of motor vehicle collision–related blunt thoracic aortic injury according to age. *J Trauma.* 2002;52:859–66.
30. Holmes JH, Bloch RD, Hall RA, et al. Natural history of traumatic rupture of the thoracic aorta managed nonoperatively: a longitudinal analysis. *Ann Thorac Surg.* 2002;73:1149–54.
31. Rabin J, Harris DG, Crews GA, et al. Early aortic repair worsens concurrent traumatic brain injury. *Ann Thorac Surg.* 2014; 98: 46–51.
32. Marco Di Eusanio M, Folesani G, Berretta P, et al. Delayed management of blunt traumatic aortic injury: open surgical versus endovascular repair. *Ann Thorac Surg.* 2013; 95:1591–7.
33. Demetriades D, Velmahos GC, Scalea TM, et al. Blunt traumatic thoracic aortic injuries: early or delayed repair–results of an American Association for the Surgery of Trauma prospective study. *J Trauma.* 2009;66:967–73.
34. Pate JW, Gavant ML, Weiman DS, Fabian TC. Traumatic Rupture of the Aortic Isthmus: Program of Selective Management. *World J Surg.* 1999;23:59–63.
35. Caffarelli AD, Mallidi HR, Maggio PM, et al. Early outcomes of deliberate nonoperative management for blunt thoracic aortic injury in trauma. *J Thorac Cardiovasc Surg.* 2010;140:598–605.
36. Azizzadeh A, Keyhani K, Miller CC, et al. Blunt traumatic aortic injury: initial experience with endovascular repair. *J Vasc Surg.* 2009;49:1403–8.

55

Open Repair of Adult Aortic Coarctation

Harleen K. Sandhu, MD, MPH,
Kristofer M. Charlton-Ouw, MD and
Hazim J. Safi, MD

DESCRIPTION AND NATURAL HISTORY

Coarctation of the aorta (CoA) is defined as a circumscript narrowing of any region of the aorta, from the distal arch to the abdominal aortic bifurcation. The morphological spectrum of CoA has been described to vary from a discrete segment of stenosis, a long segment, or diffuse hypoplasia involving the aortic arch or isthmus, with or without collateral vessels.[1] The classification of CoA into discrete, tubular or diffuse stenosis (the narrowing is >10 mm), and isthmic hypoplasia (the narrowing is <75% of the transverse aortic diameter) is important for endovascular intervention.[2]

CoA is the fifth most common congenital anomaly that accounts for approximately 5%–8% of all congenital heart defects with an estimated incidence of 3–4/10,000 live births and a 2:1 male predominamnce.[3–5] Typically congenital, however, CoA may have an acquired aetiology (e.g., Takayasu arteritis, or atherosclerosis) and has sporadic evidence of familial occurrence, especially in syndromic forms.[6] Based on its association with other congenital anomalies, including bicuspid aortic valve (50%–60%), ventricular septal defect (13%), patent ductus arteriosus (7%), and intracranial aneurysms (up to 10%). CoA is called *simple* in the absence and *complex* in the presence of other accompanying intracardiac or aortic lesions.[7] CoA is known to be highly associated with Turner syndrome.[8] It is also known to be associated with "cystic medial necrosis" and early elastic fibre fragmentation or fibrosis, especially among cases presenting in the ascending and descending aorta, resulting in an increased aortic wall stiffness.[9] Complex CoA is usually diagnosed in infancy and the prognosis, in most cases, depends on the outcome of the simultaneous management of the associated lesion. Simple coarctation is the most commonly diagnosed form of CoA among adults. In rare cases, about 10%, adult CoA narrowing occurs ectopically in the distal ascending, descending, or abdominal aorta.[10]

The natural history of untreated CoA leads to early death, with nearly 25% mortality before age 20, 50% by age 31, 75% by age 45, and 90% by 60 years.[11–13] The causes of mortality were chiefly due to complications of the coarctation, including bacterial endarteritis (18%), aortic rupture (21%), cardiac failure (26%), and intracranial haemorrhage (12%).[14,15] The advent of surgical repair for CoA and the evolution of management techniques highlight considerably improved survival and reduction in morbidity.[16,17] Early series on long-term outcomes following surgical repair of CoA, from nearly 3 decades ago, report 91%–95% survival 10 years after initial repair, 84%–89% after 20 years, and 72%–82% after 30 years.[18,19] Contemporary results demonstrate long-term actuarial survival of 98% at 40 years, 98% at 50 years, and 89% at 60 years with reintervention-free survival of up to 50 years in 63%, following surgical repair in adults with CoA.[17]

Clinical Presentation

The crude and obsolete anatomical classification into post-ductal (adult, narrowing occurs at or just distal to the ductus arteriosus) and pre-ductal (infantile, narrowing proximal to the ductus arteriosus) types fails to accurately reflect the clinical presentations because most cases of CoA among adults are "infantile-type." Although classically considered a disease of infancy that is usually repaired prior to school age, CoA in the adult population might occur either because of a delay in diagnosis or restenosis of previously treated CoA. The reasons could be restenosis due to failure of growth at the anastomosis, or delayed manifestation secondary to development of collaterals that maintain distal perfusion resulting in patients being asymptomatic well into their fifth decade.

With most cases of adult CoA being asymptomatic, signs typically manifest in adults or adolescents secondary to development of cardiac or aortic complications. These may present as upper limb hypertension, lower extremity hypotension/pulse-deficits (radio-femoral delay) and claudication, exercise intolerance, left ventricular dysfunction or cardiac failure, systolic or continuous murmur radiating to back (palpable collaterals or suprasternal thrill), hypertensive retinopathy, intracranial bleed or cerebrovascular accidents, aortic dissection or rupture with or without associated post-stenotic aneurysm, and infective endocarditis.[4] These complications are usually the presenting features of unrepaired adult CoAs with increased risk for early mortality, recurrence of CoA or late aneurysm formation following childhood repair might also occur in adulthood.[20–22]

Diagnosis and Work-up

Besides the clinical signs, almost all patients require multiple investigations to be performed for a complete assessment of CoA and planning the treatment. Chest X-ray evaluation may show pathognomonic features, such as rib notching of the third to the eighth ribs (due to well-developed collateral circulation) and the classic "figure 3" sign (double contouring) of the proximal descending aorta demonstrating the pre- and post-stenotic dilatation. Other abnormal x-ray findings might include ascending aortic ectasia, widening of the left subclavian artery, or cardiomegaly with enlarged cardiac silhouettes that could raise the suspicion for the presence of associated cardiac anomalies.

Echocardiography is essential for diagnostic confirmation as well as quantification and assessment of aortic, mitral, and left ventricular structure and function, as well as exclusion of other intracardiac anomalies that might require correction. Magnetic resonance imaging angiography (MRA) or multi-detector computed tomography angiography (MDCTA) can depict the site, extent, and degree of the aortic narrowing, the aortic arch, the pre- and post-stenotic aorta, along with the assessment of neck vessels and major arterial collaterals.[23,24] Both MRA and MDCTA are the preferred non-invasive techniques for the initial evaluation and follow-up (post-intervention) assessment to detect complications, such as aneurysms, restenosis, or residual stenosis.

Cardiac catheterization with manometry and aortography is the gold standard imaging technique for a complete anatomical and functional evaluation of the aortic arch as well as exclusion of associated aortic wall complications.[3] In addition, aortography allows measurement of the pressure gradient across the lesion. A hemodynamically significant CoA is >20 mmHg peak-to-peak gradient in the absence of collaterals. Pressure gradients can be useful to diagnose and track restenosis after interventions.

MANAGEMENT

Even though CoA was first described pathologically in the 1700s and received clinical recognition in the early 1900s,[11,13] it was not until the mid-to-late twentieth century that an interventional repair of CoA was established. Since surgery for CoA was first described in 1945,[25,26] techniques for repair have progressively evolved over the past few decades. Several techniques for open repair of adult CoA have been described, including patch aortoplasty, resection with end-to-end anastomosis (REE), extra-anatomic bypass, and resection and interposition graft (RIPG).[16,17,27,28] Beginning with balloon angioplasty in the 1980s and the use of endovascular stents in the 1990s, the advancement of these minimally invasive percutaneous techniques over the past two decades has become an alternative to opensurgery.[2,29] Advances in surgical experiences and endovascular stent technology have influenced the success rate and safety of transcatheter approaches. Data on long-term endovascular outcomes remain scarce, thereby, limiting a direct comparison of available techniques (open vs. percutaneous) with regard to aneurysm formation, recoarctation, aortic dissection, and post-intervention morbidity and mortality. As such, the optimal approach for adult CoA management, whether open surgery or by stent placement, remains unclear.

Indications for Interventional Treatment

Adults with CoA require repair in cases of aneurysm, recurrent stenosis, and when the diagnosis was missed in childhood. In our recently published experience with open repair of CoA in adults, the common indications for repair included native CoA,[16] restenosis or pseudoaneurysm with or without aneurysm (150% of reference artery diameter) after previous endovascular or open repair in childhood. However, the final decision to offer endovascular vs. open repair for adult CoA should be based on anatomy, patient preference, age, and presence of aneurysm. Based on published guidelines,[3,30] intervention for CoA is recommended in cases with:

- Pressure gradient >20 mmHg between upper and lower extremities, upper extremity hypertension (>140/90 mmHg in adults), peak-to-peak coarctation gradient ≥20 mmHg, pathological blood pressure response during exercise, significant LVH, or peak-to-peak coarctation gradient <20 mmHg in the presence of anatomic imaging evidence of significant coarctation with radiological evidence of significant collateral flow (class I recommendation, level of evidence C).

- ≥50% aortic narrowing relative to the aortic diameter at the diaphragm with (class IIa recommendation) or without hypertension (class IIb recommendation, level of evidence C).
- Choice of percutaneous intervention vs. surgical repair of native discrete CoA should be determined by consultation with a team of adult congenital heart disease cardiologists, interventionalists, and surgeons (class I recommendation, level of evidence C).

Even though endovascular techniques and extra-anatomic open repairs have the advantage of being minimally invasive and avoiding dissection around the extensive collateral blood supply, there is not enough evidence on the durability of these techniques compared to *in situ* open repair.[31] The common indications for open repair, in our experience, have been young age, when the coarctation is associated with aneurysm, and unsuitable anatomy for endovascular repair or proximity of CoA to major branch arteries, such as the left common carotid artery.[16]

Objectives of Correction of Defect

The objective of surgical correction of CoA is to permit unobstructed passage of proximal blood flow to the distal aorta beyond the coarctation or the aortic narrowing. This requires traversing through and widening the narrowed region of the aortic lumen (*endovascular balloon angioplasty or stent placement*), or bypassing the obstruction or narrowing and creating an alternate path (*RIPG, extra-anatomical bypass, etc.*), or resection of the stenosis in the diseased aortic segment and reconstituting the blood flow by using a prosthetic conduit (REE, aortoplasty). Regardless of the treatment technique (open surgical or endovascular), the goal of the intervention is to improve survival by correction of CoA.

Open Surgical Repair

Surgical repair of CoA involves clamping the aorta above and below the narrowed and diseased segment, such that the lower body is perfused only via collaterals (when they have developed), or through utilization of adjuncts such as distal aortic perfusion.[16] The standard approaches for open surgical repair include subclavian flap aortoplasty (ligation of distal subclavian artery to use the proximal portion to patch the coarctation segment), REE, patch aortoplasty with foreign material (usually a Dacron patch), RIPG, and, less frequently, carotid-to-descending aorta shunting.[16,17,27,28,32]

Incision

Traditionally, open CoA repair (especially in isolated or simple CoA) is performed through a left thoracotomy through the third or fourth intercostal space to provide adequate exposure to the thoracic aorta. This exposure requires careful dissection and isolation of numerous large arteries (collaterals) within the muscles and between the ribs that tend to be friable or thin walled owing to the increased blood pressure. In complicated CoA, whereby combination procedures (valvular repair or replacement, ascending aortic aneurysm) are to be performed, repair via median sternotomy should be considered.

End-to-End Anastomosis

The most common surgical repair method, originally described by the pioneers of surgical repair of CoA (Crafoord and Nylin),[25] employs resection of the narrowed CoA segment and creation of an end-to-end anastomosis, provided there is sufficient amount of normal aortic tissue left in order to complete the repair without undue tension. The advantage is that it creates a wide anastomosis at the inferior aspect of the aortic arch, which provides maximum reduction in systemic afterload and recurrence of stenosis. Furthermore, in cases of hypoplastic aortic arch and isthmus, an extended anastomosis allows for maximum growth potential (when performed in early childhood or infancy) and relieves hypoplasia.[33] Due to the benefits of simultaneous correction of the coexistent arch hypoplasia, preservation of the left subclavian artery, and resection of ductal tissue, extended REE is the preferred technique in pediatric patients and is associated with a low mortality and a low recoarctation rate over long-term followup.[19,34,35] However, the outcome is less favorable in patients with associated cardiac lesions and is less frequently used in adults as it is difficult to perform in this age group.

Resection and Interposition Graft (RIPG)

In situ repair with RIPG is a commonly employed technique in adolescents and adults and is increasingly replacing REE. Briefly, aortic clamps are applied proximal and distal to the coarctation, the narrowed segment is resected, and a prosthetic tube graft is interposed. Despite that, it can be surgically difficult to perform, due to extensive collaterals, and requires careful dissection to expose the relevant anatomical structures. It is, however, the technique of choice in many centers for adult CoA patients. Furthermore, this technique allows for the utilization of adjunctive techniques, such as distal aortic perfusion or deep hypothermic circulatory arrest (DHCA), to protect organs from ischemic consequences during aortic clamping.

Subclavian Flap Aortoplasty

Subclavian flap surgery is the second most frequent surgical technique performed in infants with long-segment coarctation.[36] Although this technique creates a tension-free repair, obviates the need for prosthetic material, and is associated with less extensive aortic resection and mobilization, it is associated with a high (40%) risk of restenosis and aortic aneurysm formation.[37] The efficacy of the subclavian flap procedure has been questioned due to the associated postoperative complication rate and, hence, most centers have abandoned this approach. It is believed that the cause of the increased incidence of recoarctation is due to failure of complete resection of ductal tissue in the majority of the cases.

Patch Angioplasty

Prosthetic patch angioplasty, introduced in the 1960s, is a straightforward approach and is characterized by successful gradient resolution. The initial steps were the same as those described above in REE. A generous aortotomy is then made across the coarctation and the coarctation shelf is excised. A prosthetic (woven Dacron) patch is fashioned to extend 0.5 to 1 cm on either side of the coarctation segment. The technique reduces the potential for complications associated with extensive resection, such as iatrogenic injury to intercostal arteries, and is associated with a low risk for restenosis following resection of the narrowed segment. However, in view of the frequent association with aortic aneurysm and rupture (reported in nearly 51% of the patients),[38] the use of patch aortoplasty is decreasing. The late aneurysm formation after patch angioplasty can be potentially fatal when associated with aortic dissection.[39] The mechanism behind aneurysm formation after patch angioplasty might be related to the difference in the flow dynamics between the aortic wall and the stiff, less compliant graft, which creates turbulence that is transmitted to the adjacent elastic aorta resulting in weakening and progressive dilatation of the aortic wall over time.

Extra-Anatomical Bypass

This technique is similar to RIPG and is usually performed in adults. This is accomplished through a median sternotomy and cardiopulmonary bypass and involves creation of a bypass graft across the area of coarctation without resection of the narrowed or disease aortic segment. The proximal end of the conduit is frequently anastomosed to the ascending aorta, then the heart is lifted and posterior pericardium opened in order to access the descending thoracic aorta distal to the coarctation. In rare cases of mid-aortic syndrome, a similar extra-anatomic bypass is performed involving the thoracic aorta proximally extending to the abdominal aorta distal to the narrowing. This technique is indicated in cases when the coarctation is too complex for a graft conduit interposition,[40] extensive collateralization, or when multiple lesions need simultaneous repair, such as significant intracardiac or aortic abnormalities.

Our Technique

In our experience with open repair of CoA in adults, we observed low perioperative major morbidity and no repair-related mortality with the preferred technique of RIPG.[16] The reason for our general adoption of this technique was the prevalence of aneurysm in our patients (thoracic aortic aneurysms in 76% with a mean maximum diameter 4.8 cm; other aneurysms including intercostal arteries in 14% and left common carotid and subclavian arteries in 10%). Other techniques, such as REE, patch aortoplasty or extra-anatomic bypass, are not appropriate for aneurysm patients. Overall, long-term survival in our experience was excellent (89% ± 0.058 standard error at 16.8 years after surgical repair).[16] No patient in our series had restenosis on follow-up imaging or required reintervention in the repaired aortic segment. Although ours is one of the largest series of RIPG in adults, data is insufficient to adequately compare outcomes of different repair techniques.

Our protocol for adult CoA of the distal arch and descending thoracic aorta involves insertion of cerebrospinal fluid (CSF) drain, distal aortic perfusion, and moderate passive hypothermia. In our experience before 1996, we frequently used the clamp-and-sew technique without distal aortic perfusion or spinal neuro-monitoring. Per our current protocol, we monitor spinal activity with somatosensory- and motor-evoked potentials, when available.

As previously described, our usual surgical technique begins with placing the patient in the right lateral decubitus position and the chest is entered through a left thoracotomy incision made in the fifth intercostal space to expose the proximal descending thoracic aorta. Prominent intercostal collaterals around the coarctation are ligated, beginning at the distal clamp site. Distal aortic perfusion is then established using the left inferior pulmonary vein for inflow, and the left common femoral artery for outflow. Intravenous anticoagulation is with 1 mg/kg of sodium heparin. After applying two distal clamps to the aorta below the diseased segment (level of T6-7), an atriofemoral bypass (using a partial bypass circuit with a heat exchanger connected to the centrifugal pump) is started. A complete transection of aorta is performed between the aortic clamps (Figure 55-1). Ligation of intercostal arteries to include the diseased segment is performed proximally. Reimplantation of intercostal arteries above T8 is not performed routinely. Dissection is then carried out proximally to the distal aortic arch opposite the left subclavian artery. A proximal aortic clamp is then placed just distal to the left common carotid artery and the left subclavian artery is clamped as well (Figure 55-2). The diseased coarctation segment is completely excised. A Dacron tube graft of appropriate size is selected for replacement and is anastomosed proximally using a 3-0 running polypropylene suture and distally with 3-0 or 4-0 polypropylene suture. Following completion of anastomosis, the clamps are released, and distal aortic perfusion is stopped.

In the recent years, we have used a side-arm graft attached to the distal anastomosis for arterial outflow for distal aortic perfusion, which obviates the need for femoral artery cannulation. Using this technique, the distal anastomosis is performed first. In our published CoA experience, we performed distal aortic perfusion using atriofemoral bypass in 78% and used the "distal first" technique in 22%.[16] When using the "distal first" approach, the inflow cannula in the left inferior pulmonary vein is placed as usual, followed by transection of the aorta below the diseased segment. The distal anastomosis is performed using a Dacron tube graft with a side arm graft (Figure 55-3). Distal aortic perfusion is begun with the outflow cannula attached to this side arm of the aortic tube graft (Figure 55-4). After the completion of an *en bloc* resection of the diseased aortic segment, the proximal anastomosis (Figure 55-5) is performed and the clamps are removed.

Following the return of antegrade flow and cessation of distal aortic perfusion, decannulation and anticoagulation reversal is achieved. The chest is closed in the standard fashion after placing 32-French chest tubes. The patient is monitored in the intensive care unit until the CSF drain is removed, usually by the second or third postoperative day.

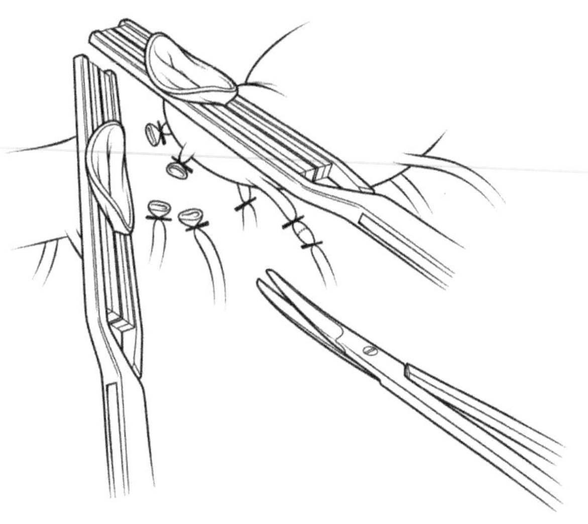

Figure 55-1. Dissection and transection of the aorta below the diseased aortic segment and ligation of intercostal arteries.

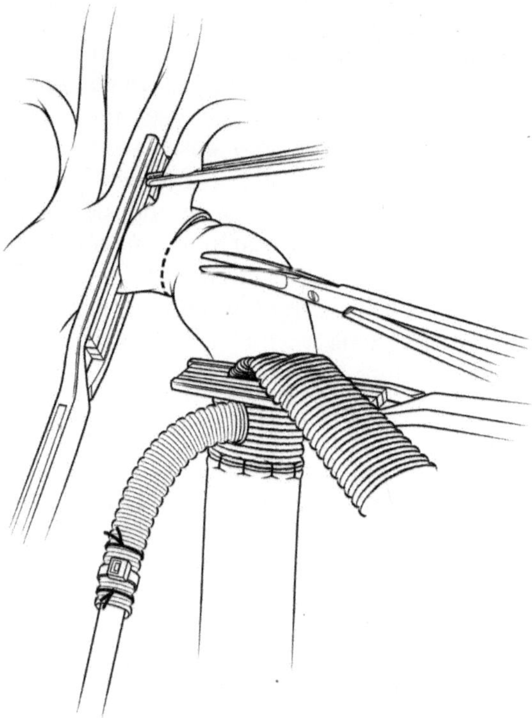

Figure 55-2. Schematic illustration of proximal aortic and the left subclavian artery clamp placement.

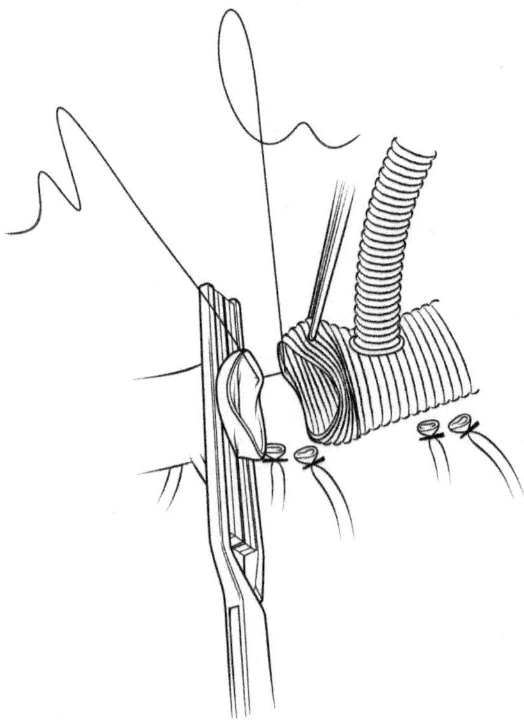

Figure 55-3. Schematic illustration of "distal-first" technique for creation of distal aortic anastomosis.

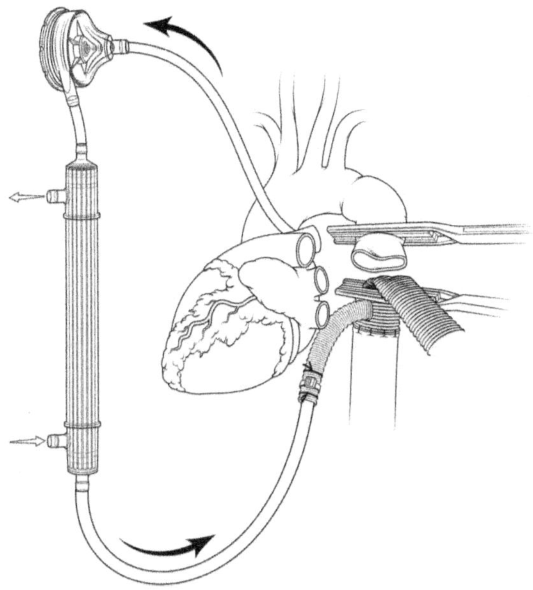

Figure 55-4. Schematic image of distal aortic perfusion through left inferior pulmonary vein and a side-arm graft to the distal aortic anastomosis.

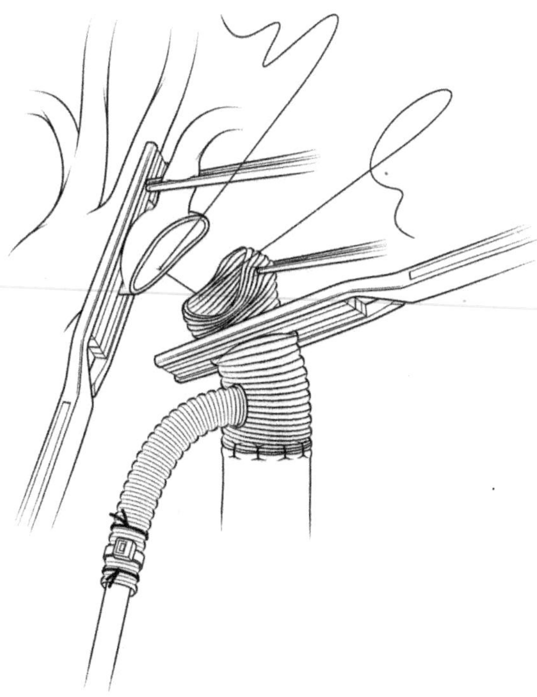

Figure 55-5. An illustration depicting creation of proximal aortic anastomosis.

For patients with associated aortic valve disease and ascending aortic or proximal arch aneurysms, repair via median sternotomy with deep hypothermic circulatory arrest is performed. For patients with coarctation in the distal descending thoracic or proximal abdominal aorta without an associated aneurysm, repair with extra-anatomic bypass from the thoracic aorta to the distal abdominal aorta is considered.

Our standard surveillance protocol after open thoracic or thoracoabdominal aortic repair is annual computed tomography or magnetic resonance imaging for the first 3 years then once every 3 years thereafter.

Endovascular Repair

Although conventional treatment for primary adult CoA, like the neonatal presentation, has been open surgical repair, these patients have well-developed collaterals and are at greater surgical risk secondary to extensive dissection and bleeding related complications. In an effort to minimize the surgical risk and shorten procedural recovery times, the percutaneous catheter-based approaches have gained increasing popularity. Endovascular repair with balloon angioplasty and stenting is a reasonable alternative to open repair in selected patients without aneurysm. Although, balloon angioplasty has high initial success rates (>80%), it is complicated by restenosis in 15% of patients, and aneurysm formation in 5%–35%.[21,41,42] Stenting can reduce the restenosis rate to <10%. However, aneurysm formation continues to pose a risk.[20,21] When compared to open surgery, the mean risk of restenosis after stenting was 11% vs. 2% after surgery (OR 6.0, P = .04).[31] In a single-center series, aortic reintervention for restenosis was 12% with stenting and 5% with open surgery.[17] Other reported procedural complications, such as stent migration, can occur in up to 4%–20%.[43]

In the absence of randomized trials, and long-term results still pending, it is difficult to conclude that stent placement is superior to balloon dilation. However, short-term and intermediate-term outcomes favor stent placement for adult CoA.[43] Concomitant aortic aneurysm is a relative contraindication for balloon angioplasty or bare metal stenting and was observed in nearly 76% of our adult CoA patients.[16] Many patients are poor endovascular candidates due to anatomy or patient preference. In such cases, open repair remains a safe and durable option in aortic centers of excellence.

Hybrid Repair

A hybrid approach involving open and endovascular procedures in a single (or staged) surgical session have been described in adults with CoA and for repair of complications, such as recoarctation and post-repair aneurysm or anastomotic pseudoaneurysm.[44,45] Although the available early results portray the hybrid technique as a safe and less-invasive treatment approach for patients with complicated CoA and concomitant cardiac comorbidities, the current evidence is limited.

PROCEDURAL RISKS AND POTENTIAL COMPLICATIONS

The paucity of adequate data with regard to long-term follow up and complications makes it challenging to directly compare all available treatment strategies for adult CoA. As previously described, a comparison of outcomes after balloon angioplasty to surgery demonstrated a significantly higher reintervention rate due to restenosis as well as an increased risk for aortic rupture and aortic aneurysm formation.[21] Thus far, surgery remains the treatment of choice in neonates as well among those beyond the neonatal period. However, the surgical procedures are associated with early and late complications as well.

Early surgical mortality is usually rare and the reported rate is <1%.[46] Most adults with CoA also suffer from hypertensive cardiac disease. Therefore, they are at increased risk of early surgical morbidity and of developing ischemia and fibrillation following increase in the afterload (aortic clamping). Pre-emptive medical therapy and use of cardiopulmonary bypass can reduce associated cardiac stress.

Postoperative bleeding complications can occur after open surgical repair, especially with enlarged collateral vessels. Careful intraoperative hemostasis during thoracotomy and strict blood pressure control during the intra-and postoperative period is warranted. Furthermore, recurrent laryngeal nerve injury has been reported to occur, especially in reoperations involving re-coarctation repair because the anatomy is difficult to delineate. Additional intervention to correct this complication is only indicated in cases of aspiration or asphyxia.

Paraplegia can occur in nearly 0.3% cases when spinal perfusion is impaired due to interruption of collateral and intercostal vessels during chest wall dissection, or in the absence of collaterals leading to reduction in distal pressure following aortic clamping.[47,48] The risk is further increased to as high as 2.6% in cases of redo-surgery, which involve extensive dissection and prolonged aortic clamp times, or when there is limited collateral flow.[47,49] Use of adjuncts, such as distal aortic perfusion, left heart bypass, femoro-femoral bypass, and moderate hypothermia along with spinal cord monitoring with CSF drainage can reduce the incidence of paraplegia.[50,51]

Postoperative paradoxical hypertension can occur as both an early and late (7%–33%) complication following coarctation repair.[52,53] Medical therapy through preoperative beta blocker and sodium nitroprusside in the early postoperative period, in addition to oral anti-hypertensives before discharge, is recommended. Late postoperative hypertension may also be related to recurrent or residual CoA of patients. Restenosis is an important long-term complication with a reported incidence ranging from 5% to 50%.[53–55] Repair of restenosis in adults can be complex and extra-anatomic (ascending-to-descending) grafts are sometimes used in cases with difficult anatomy.[53] Hybrid approaches for such cases have also been described to be effective alternatives.[45]

Another long-term complication after surgical repair is late aortic aneurysm formation or pseudoaneurysm at the repair site, with an incidence of 5%–50%.[39,56,57] A large study examining the long-term outcomes of 891 patients requiring open CoA repair showed a 5.4% overall rate of pseudoaneurysm development at the site of repair.[56] Of these, 89.6% had patch aortoplasty, 8.3% had REE, and 2.1% had RIPG. Pseudoaneurysm formation is most frequent with patch aortoplasty in several reports (24%–90%), with a spontaneous rupture rate of 31% and rupture-related mortality of 78%–100%.[39,57,58]

CONCLUSIONS

Due to the absence of level-1 evidence, the current literature has conflicting results on outcomes of various treatment options for CoA repair in adults. In our experience,[16] open repair of adult aortic coarctation with aneurysm using resection and interposition graft placement for both native and recurrent disease is associated with acceptable major morbidity, paraplegia, perioperative mortality, and excellent long-term durability with no patient requiring aortic reintervention for restenosis or pseudoaneurysm. The results from a recent Cochrane review, conducted to analyze the effectiveness and safety of endovascular stent placement compared with open surgery in patients with coarctation of the thoracic aorta, were inconclusive, owing to insufficient evidence.[32] However, all available literature demonstrates a tangible risk of pseudoaneurysm formation, restenosis, aneurysmal degeneration, hypertension, and valvular abnormalities associated with all types of interventions in varying degrees.

Thus, the selection of appropriate intervention for CoA repair should be individualized and depend on the underlying morphology, patient age, and the presence or absence of other cardiac abnormalities. In view of the known risk of long-term complications and in accordance with the published guidelines on the management of adults with congenital heart disease, all patients should undergo mandatory regular clinical follow-up and lifelong imaging surveillance following CoA repair, regardless of technique.[3,30]

Acknowledgements

The authors acknowledge Troy Brown for editorial assistance and Chris Akers for the illustrations.

REFERENCES

1. Mullen MJ. Coarctation of the aorta in adults: do we need surgeons? *Heart.* 2003;89(1):3–5.
2. Zabal C. The adult patient with native coarctation of the aorta: balloon angioplasty or primary stenting? *Heart.* 2003;89(1):77–83.
3. Baumgartner H, Bonhoeffer P, De Groot NMS, et al. ESC Guidelines for the management of grown-up congenital heart disease (new version 2010). *Eur Heart J.* 2010;31(23):2915–957.
4. Jenkins NP. Coarctation of the aorta: natural history and outcome after surgical treatment. *QJM.* 1999;92(7):365–71.
5. Rosenthal E. Coarctation of the aorta from fetus to adult: curable condition or life long disease process? *Heart.* 2005;91(11):1495–502.
6. McBride KL, Pignatelli R, Lewin M, et al. Inheritance analysis of congenital left ventricular outflow tract obstruction malformations: Segregation, multiplex relative risk, and heritability. *Am J Med Genet A.* 2005;134A(2):180–6.
7. Teo LLS, Cannell T, Babu-Narayan SV, et al. Prevalence of associated cardiovascular abnormalities in 500 patients with aortic coarctation referred for cardiovascular magnetic resonance imaging to a tertiary center. *Pediatr Cardiol.* 2011;32(8):1120–7.
8. Gravholt CH. Turner syndrome and the heart: cardiovascular complications and treatment strategies. *Am J Cardiovasc Drugs.* 2002;2(6):401–13.
9. Niwa K, Perloff JK, Bhuta SM, et al. Structural Abnormalities of Great Arterial Walls in Congenital Heart Disease: Light and Electron Microscopic Analyses. *Circulation.* 2001;103(3):393–400.
10. Ramnarine I. Role of surgery in the management of the adult patient with coarctation of the aorta. *Postgrad Med J.* 2005;81(954):243–7.

11. Abbott ME. Coarctation of the aorta of the adult type II. A statistical study and historical retrospect of 200 recorded cases, with autopsy, of stenosis or obliteration of the descending arch in subjects above the age of two years. *Am Heart J.* 1928;3(4):381–421.
12. Reifenstein GH, Levine SA, Gross RE. Coarctation of the aorta. *Am Heart J.* 1947;33(2):146–68.
13. Paris M. Rétrècissement considerable de l'aorte pectorale observé à l'Hotel Dieu de Paris. *J Chir Desault.* 1791;2:107.
14. Campbell M. Natural history of coarctation of the aorta. *Heart.* 1970;32(5):633–40.
15. Verheugt CL, Uiterwaal CSPM, Grobbee DE, Mulder BJM. Long-term prognosis of congenital heart defects: a systematic review. *Int J Cardiol.* 2008;131(1):25–32.
16. Charlton-Ouw KM, Codreanu ME, Leake SS, et al. Open repair of adult aortic coarctation mostly by a resection and graft replacement technique. *J Vasc Surg.* 2015;61(1):66–72.
17. Choudhary P, Canniffe C, Jackson DJ, et al. Late outcomes in adults with coarctation of the aorta. *Heart.* 2015;101(15):1190–5.
18. Toro-Salazar OH, Steinberger J, Thomas W, et al. Long-term follow-up of patients after coarctation of the aorta repair. *Am J Cardiol.* 2002;89(5):541–7.
19. Cohen M, Fuster V, Steele PM, et al. Coarctation of the aorta. Long-term follow-up and prediction of outcome after surgical correction. *Circulation.* 1989;80(4):840–5.
20. Holzer R, Qureshi S, Ghasemi A, et al. Stenting of aortic coarctation: acute, intermediate, and long-term results of a prospective multi-institutional registry—Congenital Cardiovascular Interventional Study Consortium (CCISC). *Catheter Cardiovasc Interv.* 2010;76(4):553–63.
21. Hu Z, Wang Z, Dai X, et al. Outcomes of surgical versus balloon angioplasty treatment for native coarctation of the aorta: a meta-analysis. *Ann Vasc Surg.* 2014;28(2):394–403.
22. Rodés-Cabau J, Miró J, Dancea A, et al. Comparison of surgical and transcatheter treatment for native coarctation of the aorta in patients > or = 1 year old. The Quebec Native Coarctation of the Aorta study. *Am Heart J.* 2007;154(1):186–92.
23. Ilica AT, Bilici A, Ilhan A, et al. Thoracoabdominal aorta coarctation with bilateral renal artery involvement: diagnosis with multidetector CT angiography (MDCTA). *Int J Cardiovasc Imaging.* 2007;23(5):645–8.
24. Godart F, Labrot G, Devos P, et al. Coarctation of the aorta: comparison of aortic dimensions between conventional MR imaging, 3D MR angiography, and conventional angiography. *Eur Radiol.* 2002;12(8):2034–9.
25. Crafoord C. Congenital coarctation of the aorta and its surgical treatment. *J Thorac Surg.* 1945;14:347–61.
26. Gross RE. Surgical correction for coarctation of the aorta. *Surgery.* 1945;18:673–8.
27. Chowdhary V, Rose M, Murtagh G, et al. Impact of ascending to descending aortic bypass for aortic coarctation on 3-dimensional hemodynamics. *Circulation.* 2015;131(11):1036–8.
28. Duara R, Theodore S, Sarma PS, et al. Correction of coarctation of aorta in adult patients—impact of corrective procedure on long-term recoarctation and systolic hypertension. *Thorac Cardiovasc Surg.* 2008;56(2):83–6.
29. Singer MI, Rowen M, Dorsey TJ. Transluminal aortic balloon angioplasty for coarctation of the aorta in the newborn. *Am Heart J.* 1982;103(1):131–2.
30. Warnes CA, Williams RG, Bashore TM, et al. ACC/AHA 2008 Guidelines for the Management of Adults with Congenital Heart Disease: a report of the American College of Cardiology/American Heart Association Task Force on Practice Guidelines (writing committee to develop guidelines on the management of a. *Circulation.* 2008;118(23):e714–e833.
31. Carr JA. The results of catheter-based therapy compared with surgical repair of adult aortic coarctation. *J Am Coll Cardiol.* 2006;47(6):1101–7.
32. Pádua LMS, Garcia LC, Rubira CJ, de Oliveira Carvalho PE. Stent placement versus surgery for coarctation of the thoracic aorta. *Cochrane database Syst Rev.* 2012;5(CD008204):CD008204.

33. Lansman S, Shapiro AJ, Schiller MS, et al. Extended aortic arch anastomosis for repair of coarctation in infancy. *Circulation.* 1986;74(3 Pt 2):137–41.
34. Backer CL, Mavroudis C, Zias EA, et al. Repair of coarctation with resection and extended end-to-end anastomosis. *Ann Thorac Surg.* 1998;66(4):1365–70.
35. Hager A, Kanz S, Kaemmerer H, et al. Coarctation Long-term Assessment (COALA): significance of arterial hypertension in a cohort of 404 patients up to 27 years after surgical repair of isolated coarctation of the aorta, even in the absence of restenosis and prosthetic material. *J Thorac Cardiovasc Surg.* 2007;134(3):738–45.
36. Meier MA, Lucchese FA, Jazbik W, et al. A new technique for repair of aortic coarctation. Subclavian flap aortoplasty with preservation of arterial blood flow to the left arm. *J Thorac Cardiovasc Surg.* 1986;92(6):1005–12.
37. Van Heurn LW, Wong CM, Spiegelhalter DJ, et al. Surgical treatment of aortic coarctation in infants younger than three months: 1985 to 1990. Success of extended end-to-end arch aortoplasty. *J Thorac Cardiovasc Surg.* 1994;107(1):74–86.
38. Parks WJ, Ngo TD, Plauth WH, et al. Incidence of aneurysm formation after Dacron patch aortoplasty repair for coarctation of the aorta: long-term results and assessment utilizing magnetic resonance angiography with three-dimensional surface rendering. *J Am Coll Cardiol.* 1995;26(1):266–71.
39. Del Nido PJ, Williams WG, Wilson GJ, et al. Synthetic patch angioplasty for repair of coarctation of the aorta: experience with aneurysm formation. *Circulation.* 1986;74(3 Pt 2):132–6.
40. Robicsek F, Hess PJ, Vajtai P. Ascending-distal abdominal aorta bypass for treatment of hypoplastic aortic arch and atypical coarctation in the adult. *Ann Thorac Surg.* 1984;37(3):261–3.
41. Cowley CG, Orsmond GS, Feola P, et al. Long-term, randomized comparison of balloon angioplasty and surgery for native coarctation of the aorta in childhood. *Circulation.* 2005;111(25):3453–6.
42. Rao PS, Galal O, Wilson AD. Feasibility and effectiveness of repeated balloon dilatation of restenosed congenital obstructions after previous balloon valvuloplasty/angioplasty. *Am Heart J.* 1996;132(2 Pt 1):403–7.
43. Kische S, Schneider H, Akin I, et al. Technique of interventional repair in adult aortic coarctation. *J Vasc Surg.* 2010;51(6):1550–9.
44. Roselli EE, Qureshi A, Idrees J, et al. Open, hybrid, and endovascular treatment for aortic coarctation and postrepair aneurysm in adolescents and adults. *Ann Thorac Surg.* 2012;94(3):751–8.
45. Idrees J, Arafat A, Svensson LG, et al. Hybrid repair of aortic aneurysm in patients with previous coarctation. *J Thorac Cardiovasc Surg.* 2014;148(1):60–4.
46. R J, AM D, A L, et al. Coarctation of the aorta in adults: what is the best treatment? Case report and literature review. *J Med Life.* 2011;4(2):189–95.
47. Keen G. Spinal cord damage and operations for coarctation of the aorta: aetiology, practice, and prospects. *Thorax.* 1987;42(1):11–8.
48. Brewer LA, Fosburg RG, Mulder GA, Verska JJ. Spinal cord complications following surgery for coarctation of the aorta. A study of 66 cases. *J Thorac Cardiovasc Surg.* 1972;64(3):368–81.
49. Wong CH, Watson B, Smith J, et al. The use of left heart bypass in adult and recurrent coarctation repair. *Eur J Cardiothorac Surg.* 2001;20(6):1199–201.
50. Estrera AL, Miller CC, Azizzadeh A, Safi HJ. Adjuncts during surgery of the thoracoabdominal aorta and their impact on neurologic outcome: distal aortic perfusion and cerebrospinal fluid drainage. *Multimed Man Cardiothorac Surg MMCTS / Eur Assoc Cardio-Thoracic Surg.* 2006;2006(1009):mmcts.2006.001933.
51. Coselli JS, LeMaire SA, Köksoy C, et al. Cerebrospinal fluid drainage reduces paraplegia after thoracoabdominal aortic aneurysm repair: results of a randomized clinical trial. *J Vasc Surg.* 2002;35(4):631–9.

52. Hashemzadeh K, Hashemzadeh S, Kakaei F. Repair of aortic coarctation in adults: the fate of hypertension. *Asian Cardiovasc Thorac Ann.* 2008;16(1):11–5.
53. Brown JW, Ruzmetov M, Hoyer MH, et al. Recurrent coarctation: is surgical repair of recurrent coarctation of the aorta safe and effective? *Ann Thorac Surg.* 2009;88(6):1923-30; discussion 1930–1.
54. Kron IL, Flanagan TL, Rheuban KS, et al. Incidence and risk of reintervention after coarctation repair. *Ann Thorac Surg.* 1990;49(6):920-5; discussion 925–6.
55. Brown ML, Burkhart HM, Connolly HM, et al. Coarctation of the aorta: lifelong surveillance is mandatory following surgical repair. *J Am Coll Cardiol.* 2013;62(11):1020–5.
56. Knyshov GV, Sitar LL, Glagola MD, Atamanyuk MY. Aortic aneurysms at the site of the repair of coarctation of the aorta: a review of 48 patients. *Ann Thorac Surg.* 1996;61(3):935–9.
57. Oliver JM, Gallego P, Gonzalez A, et al. Risk factors for aortic complications in adults with coarctation of the aorta. *J Am Coll Cardiol.* 2004;44(8):1641–7.
58. Webb G. Treatment of coarctation and late complications in the adult. *Semin Thorac Cardiovasc Surg.* 2005;17(2):139–42.

Index